Herbs
Demystified

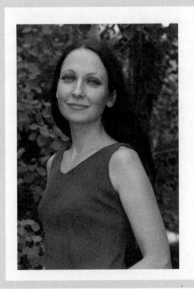

Holly Phaneuf, PhD, a biochemist, drug researcher, and teacher, earned bachelor degrees in both biology and chemistry as well as a doctorate in medicinal chemistry from the University of Utah. Her research included the study of sulfur-containing antioxidant and protective medicines, and the synthesis of novel drugs designed to protect the liver from toxicity. A full-time college chemistry professor, Dr. Phaneuf has contributed to a variety of scientific publications. She has provided countless lectures at national park ranger stations, among other venues, bringing both biochemistry and astronomy to local communities.

Herbs Demystified

A Scientist Explains
How the Most Common
Herbal Remedies Really Work

Holly Phaneuf, PhD

MARLOWE & COMPANY
NEW YORK

HERBS DEMYSTIFIED:
*A Scientist Explains How the Most Common
Herbal Remedies Really Work*
© 2005 by Holly Phaneuf

Published by
Marlowe & Company
An Imprint of Avalon Publishing Group Incorporated
245 West 17th Street, 11th floor
New York, NY 10011–5300

AVALON
publishing group incorporated

The information in this book is intended to help readers make informed decisions about their
health and the health of their loved ones. It is not intended to be a substitute for treatment, or
the advice and care of a professional health care provider. While the author and publisher have
endeavored to ensure that the information presented is accurate and up to date, they are not
responsible for adverse effects or consequences sustained by any persons using this book.

Library of Congress Cataloging-in-Publication Data
Phaneuf, Holly.
Herbs demystified : a scientist explains how the most common herbal
remedies really work / Holly Phaneuf.
p. cm.
Includes bibliographical references and index.
ISBN 1–56924–408–1
1. Herbs—Therapeutic use. 2. Materia medica, Vegetable. I. Title.
RM666.H33P478 2005
615.'321—dc22
2005027782
ISBN 13: 978–1-56924–408–1

9 8 7 6 5 4 3 2 1

DESIGNED BY PAULINE NEUWIRTH, NEUWIRTH AND ASSOCIATES, INC.

Printed in the United States of America

CONTENTS

Introduction

Why Should You Care
about What Herbs *Really* Do?

Knowing What Herbs Do inside Your Body Is Important

Herbs are mysterious. According to herb vendors, you take their product and are promised relief from insomnia, indigestion, low energy, or whatever—and sometimes the stuff actually works. What takes place in between taking the herb and noticing its effect? You trust that the herb is doing *something* good. But you have no information about what happens to the herb during the time between your taking it and your perceiving an effect. Without this information, its actions seem like magic.

Of course, you probably realize that some sort of plant bits must go to particular places in your body, and *do* things there, in order to have an effect. Knowing the details of these processes will do more than just satisfy your curiosity. It will help you decide between useful and useless herbs, safe and unsafe ones.

Why I Care about What Herbs Do to You

My own fascination with herbs began early in life. Over the years I've collected herb books and tried to gather as much information as I could. However, I've discovered most books vaguely state that a given herb is "good" for a particular problem, with no mention of what "good" means, or of what the herb is actually doing. "Milk thistle is good for the liver," they inform you. That's nice, but you can't help wonder, *why is it good,* and *what exactly is it doing in there? Is it good for all liver-*possessing creatures, universally?* For me, reading these books has been like hearing the proverbial doctor's dismissal, "Take two aspirins and call me in the morning."

If you are like me, you need more information. Herbs don't usually come with convenient, informative package inserts the way prescription and over-the-counter drugs do. Most products have vaguely worded phrases like, "Used to support liver function." Your liver has zillions of different functions, so which ones does milk thistle support? If you *really* want to know more, there are wonderful resources out there—if you happen to be a PhD biochemist and can read them without getting dizzy. That's why I've taken the time to read and analyze the latest scientific studies for you—to give you that information clearly, with no science degree required.

Learn Processes, Which Are More Powerful than Names

"You can know the name of a bird in all the languages of the world, but when you're finished, you'll know absolutely nothing whatever about the bird. . . . So let's look at the bird and see what it's doing—that's what counts. I learned very early the difference between knowing the name of something and knowing something."
—Richard Feynman

As the physicist Richard Feynman observed, learning the name of something does not provide you with real knowledge about the thing. You can know the common and Latin names of an herb, and you can even give it more impressive, scientific-sounding names like "*anti-inflammatory*," or "*sedative*," but what is it really *doing* to you? There are dozens of different ways to be sedated, for example. You could slow down the activity of different areas in your brain, or perhaps bonk yourself on the head and give yourself a concussion. Obviously, some processes are better than others.

Now, learning the names of things isn't a bad thing for you to do. It just is not enough. Really understanding the action of an herb on your body requires learning the actual *process* the herb undergoes to affect your body. What molecules do to your body is a topic called *pharmacodynamics*. Results from clinical trials of herbs are available to the public, and this information is very informative and useful, and a great deal of it is included in this book. However, clinical trials provide information like "this herb cleared up acne in 30 percent of the people taking it," for example. They do not tell you *how* an herb's effect was accomplished— they do not describe an herb's pharmacodynamics. My goal is to at last disclose these processes in language that anyone can understand. I hope that you find these molecular journeys as helpful and entertaining as I do.

Learning Herbal Processes Empowers You

This book does not insist that you take certain herbs. Instead, it provides you with mechanisms for their actions, good and bad, and it is up to you to decide whether an herb's mechanism of action is appropriate to initiate in your own, unique body. Understanding an herb's precise behavior in the body allows you to custom fit an herb to your particular concern. What works well for your best friend may be a bad decision for you. For example, licorice root protects the

stomach lining with the very same molecule that can raise blood pressure dangerously, so it should be off-limits for people with hypertension. And peppermint oil, which eases stomach cramps by halting the constriction of muscles surrounding the digestive tract, might not be the right choice for people with acid reflux disease, since its relaxation of the gut muscles also allows stomach acid into the esophagus. As you can see, a little bit of mechanistic information helps you select your herbs wisely, without painful self-experimentation. As you more actively educate yourself about what health products you use, you need to know not only the *names* of the things that you put into your body, but what they are *doing* in there. This book will give you that knowledge.

Learning Herbal Processes Protects You

Most people mistakenly think that herbs are rigorously tested for safety, effectiveness, and truthful labels. This is not so at all! In the United States and many other countries, herbs are for the most part unregulated, which is all the more reason why you should have some idea of exactly what an herb will do inside your body before you consume it.

Before you can enjoy hobbies like rock climbing or scuba diving, you expect to be informed that there are risks involved, and you listen to expert counsel. You should demand no less for yourself when approaching herbal medicine. Since natural remedies can be dangerous and even deadly, you need to protect yourself from misinformation before you can enjoy the thrill of self-treatment. Taking herbs is like bungee jumping: You need to learn what risks you face before you make the leap.

A product can enjoy widespread popularity

before you learn of any warning of its potential danger. Kava, a South Pacific plant, induces a pleasant, relaxed state. Demand for this herb grew feverishly until the FDA alerted consumers in March 2002 that kava could cause liver damage. In the United States, Germany, Switzerland, France, Canada, and the United Kingdom, kava was linked to a growing number of liver injuries, some requiring transplants. In fact, my stepmother's teenage niece became jaundiced after daily cups of kava tea. My family assumed it was a minor gallbladder problem, but it turned out to be far more serious, and this young girl has joined the ranks of those who required a life-saving liver transplant after consuming kava. Nevertheless, kava is still marketed to people of all ages, even children. While most people do not have a problem with kava, the question is, do you want to take the risk? The United States government leaves risk assessment up to its citizens. The 1994 Dietary Supplement Health and Education Act (DSHEA) places the burden of obtaining information on herbs and supplements on you, the consumer.

Use of Herbs during Pregnancy or While Nursing

AS WITH medications, some herbs can injure a developing fetus, induce premature labor, or be transported through breast milk and harm a nursing child. Most herbs have not been tested for safety in pregnant or nursing women. Although this book warns when a particular herb is clearly associated with risk to pregnant or nursing women, do not assume that the herbs in this book that have no warnings associated with them are safe. They are simply unknowns. The typical use of everyday culinary herbs in food, in moderate and customary amounts is probably safe. You should also comply with your doctor's request to take certain vitamins or medicine during pregnancy. On the other hand, if you are pregnant or nursing, you should avoid herbal supplements, extracts, large "medicinal" doses, or daily doses of herbs. As with prescription medications and over-the-counter (OTC) drugs, always consult your personal health care authority prior to taking herbs.

None of this is intended to scare you. You can find good information out there if you know how to separate it from the nonsense. Some scientists seem to feel that providing detailed herbal information is too much of a bother and prefer to throw up their hands and warn, "Just don't take any herbs!" But I don't think you can ever stop people from trying whatever is on hand to heal themselves. The movement among scientists to provide you with honest information about the risks and benefits of current health fads has been growing steadily. Excellent resources now enable you to make your own decisions about safely medicating yourself. If you learn the process the herb undergoes to affect you, you will know *why* scientists judge an herb as "good," "bad," or "questionable."

You Can Learn Herbal Processes Easily

I understand that biochemistry can seem daunting, but just as nontechnical people can learn to fix their computer or fiddle with their stereo, so too can nonscientists understand basic biochemistry. In my mind there are two issues that make biochemistry intimidating. The first is scale—things in biochemistry are too small to be seen with the naked eye. Do not let that bother you. You have an imagination, and if you can picture a person in a story having an adventure and doing all sorts of things, you can certainly picture molecules having tiny molecular adventures as well. The other issue is scientific jargon. When you are unfamiliar with a word, it tends to make your brain freeze up, and you can't think clearly. I will avoid scientific jargon and define terms as clearly as possible when required.

If I do my job properly, then the description of the journey of a plant molecule in your body should be no more perplexing than the description of the journey of someone who gets in his or her car and goes to the store and buys milk. The scale is just smaller, and instead of people getting into cars, we have things called *molecules* getting into things called *cells*. You do not need any science background in order to interpret this book. You only need a good imagination.

WHAT ARE ALL THESE "DOUBLE-BLIND, RANDOMIZED, PLACEBO-CONTROLLED" STUDIES WITH "SIGNIFICANT" EFFECTS?

A "double-blind, randomized, placebo-controlled study" is the gold standard of studies and is especially important when humans are the subjects of the study. Where possible, this book references the most up-to-date studies with the highest standards. However, there simply is a lack of data for certain herbs, like wild yam, so in these cases I've described the results of the few studies that do exist, even though they haven't held to these standards.

The presence or absence of a placebo in an herb study makes or breaks its credibility. A placebo is a material or treatment that is considered ineffective but harmless, like the classic "sugar pill." Other materials, like paraffin or wax, which pass straight through the body without getting absorbed, are also occasionally employed as placebos. The result of taking a placebo, the famous "placebo effect," is nothing to scoff at. We are only now learning how powerfully our minds affect our bodies, such that at times the act of taking something, *anything,* flips some mysterious switch in our minds to banish pain completely, lower blood pressure, improve blood chemistry, and perform other remarkable phenomena.

A placebo-controlled herb study requires a group of people to take an ineffective placebo while a separate "experimental" group takes the herb being tested. If both groups experience the same results, positive or otherwise, the herb probably didn't work. On the other hand, if the group taking the herb did better than the placebo group, you can say that the herb worked. But how much better is considered "better"? This brings up the issue of "significance."

Why are some results "significant"? In this book, you will see that herbs' effects are described as "nonsignificant," "significant," or "highly significant." These terms have special meaning. Statistical methods have evolved to help estimate whether an effect is truly caused by the agent tested, because an effect *could* be due to chance alone. "Significant" means the effect is more likely real and less likely caused by chance. A number called a *probability value,* or *P value,* is calculated, to estimate this. A P value of less than 0.05 is considered significant. If you read scientific papers, you often see something like "P less than 0.05," or "$p < 0.05$," which means the parameter measured was statistically significant, and the smaller the P value is, the less likely the effect is due to chance. Sometimes the number is exactly 0.05, right on the borderline, so you will see terms like "borderline significance," or "barely significant." Effects that are intriguing enough to mention but that are higher than 0.05 are "nonsignificant" effects. The more people in the study, the more you can trust the P value and the significance. So some researchers complain that "the effects of this herb might have become significant had we only used more subjects," leaving you to speculate whether or not that would really be the case. Significance is no guarantee, but it's an agreed-upon standard that helps you estimate which effects you should pay attention to and which you should ignore.

Placebos help determine an herb's side effects, too. The placebo effect can be negative. Some people expect to feel side effects, if they know they are taking something, and their minds either manufacture side effects, or they make careful note of "symptoms" they might otherwise ignore. If the placebo creates the same side effects as an herb, you may expect the herb to be relatively free of genuine side effects.

Double-blind studies are best. The placebo effect probably won't work if you know you are getting a placebo. Thus, ideally, test subjects should be "blind" to what they are taking. When subjects are not told whether they are taking the herb or the placebo, the study is "single-blinded." Single-blind studies are less common, because researchers know that double-blind studies are so much more trustworthy. Double-blinding requires that in addition to subjects not knowing what they are taking, the researchers themselves do not know who is taking what until all the data is compiled. Thus scientists can't inadvertently bias their data with their expectations.

Randomizing subjects is a reasonable precaution. A test group comprised of only men and the placebo group containing only women would throw off the results. A "randomized" study simply means that subjects in both the placebo group and experimental group were chosen randomly. Each group should have roughly equal numbers of people of both sexes with similar ages, weights, and other relevant factors. Thus we would like to see phrases like "randomized to age, sex, and athletic ability" when an herb is tested for increasing physical endurance, for example. That way, you know the researchers didn't cheat by putting athletes in the group receiving the herb and placing couch potatoes in the placebo group.

Variations on a theme exist. It's expensive to perform large, double-blind, randomized, placebo-controlled studies. One quite respectable way to preserve credibility and save money is to perform a "crossover" study. Halfway through your study, the placebo group and the experimental group unknowingly trade treatments, preferably after a "washout" period where no treatment is taken, giving time for any residual herb or medicine to "wash out" of the subject's bodies. This effectively doubles the size of the study. If the herb produces a genuine effect, you will see the effect "cross over" from one group to the other.

Bogus studies abound! This is because the herb business, very much like the pharmaceutical industry, is huge and highly lucrative. And unlike pharmaceuticals, the majority of herbs don't require testing in most countries, including the United States! The number of well-intentioned, rigorous, and credible herb studies easily drown amid the great numbers of shoddy and untrustworthy ones, which are often funded by companies trying to sell you the herb in the first place. Although I've done my best in this book to present the most credible studies, and to warn where I found the study design suspect, you are now better armed to discriminate between good studies and bad ones when you are on your own.

You Don't Need to Worry about "Ruining the Mystery"

I have occasionally met people who express discomfort over the idea of uncovering how herbs work. Perhaps these people are in love with the mystery of it all, and I find that perfectly understandable. Who doesn't love a good mystery? If you love the mysteries of nature, you are in excellent company:

"The most beautiful thing we can experience is the mysterious. It is the fundamental emotion which stands at the cradle of true art and true science."
— Albert Einstein

But I believe that Einstein knew that unraveling mysteries does not make the universe less mysterious. If you think that explaining mysterious natural phenomena automatically makes them more boring, let me reassure you. In my experience, the opposite is true; in science, *more* mysteries always appear in the answers! Thus it is often said that the more you know, the more you realize you have yet to learn. Despite our phenomenal ability to explain how herbs and other things work these days, you do not have to worry about running out of these "beautiful" mysteries. The universe is full of them. We are drawn to them and long to explain them.

Have you ever had a teacher say, "This is the way things are, don't ask why, just memorize it"? Most people can't stand this sort of treatment. So I am puzzled that people are willing to simply accept "Milk thistle is good for the liver," and they just take it without asking questions. If you are as interested in herbs as I am, you ought to be full of questions. Beyond driving human development, I think curiosity is a virtue in itself. I hope your curiosity also fuels your enjoyment of this book.

Index of Symptoms

ALTHOUGH THESE herbs are traditionally used for the following problems, the effectiveness of many remains unproven, and some can even cause harm or make these symptoms worse. Do not use herbs from this list without first considering the more detailed information in each herb's chapter. Do not attempt to treat more serious problems without a trained health professional's guidance, and remember that healthy eating and regular exercise are also essential to maintaining your well-being.

AIDS/HIV
cat's claw

Allergies
astragalus
borage seed oil
evening primrose oil
nettle

Alzheimer's disease
evening primrose oil
ginkgo
lemon balm
sage

Anemia
dandelion
nettle
parsley

Anti-inflammatory, see "inflammation"

Anxiety
catnip
chamomile
gotu kola
kava kava
lavender
lemon balm
St. John's wort
valerian

Aphrodisiac
artichoke
ginseng
guarana
hoodia
kava kava
red pepper

saw palmetto
wild yam
yohimbe

Appetite stimulants
dandelion
eleuthero

Appetite suppressants
flaxseed
guarana
hoodia
tea
yerba maté

Arteries, hardening, see "atherosclerosis"

Arthritis
borage seed oil
cat's claw
cinnamon
eleuthero
evening primrose oil
feverfew
flaxseed oil
ginger
kava kava
nettle
red pepper
tea
turmeric
wintergreen
wild yam
yerba maté

Asthma
aloe gel
astragalus

borage seed oil
evening primrose oil
feverfew
ginkgo

Astringent
sage
tea
uva ursi
witch hazel
wintergreen

Atherosclerosis
artichoke
cinnamon
garlic
grape

Attention deficit disorder (ADD)
evening primrose oil

Blood clots, herbs that prevent clots or "thin blood"
cinnamon
flaxseed
garlic
ginger
ginkgo
gotu kola
grape
red clover
red pepper

Blood pressure, high
garlic
grape
hawthorn

Bruising
arnica
gotu kola
grape
horse chestnut
turmeric
witch hazel

Burns
aloe gel
chamomile
marshmallow
witch hazel

Cancer
bilberry
chamomile
dandelion
evening primrose oil
flaxseed and oil
garlic
grape
parsley
red clover
tea
turmeric

Cholesterol, high
artichoke
cinnamon
evening primrose oil
flaxseed
garlic
red clover
red pepper
soy
tea
wild yam

Circulatory and blood vessel disorders
ginkgo
gotu kola
grape
horse chestnut
red pepper
tea
witch hazel

Colds
echinacea
garlic
peppermint
red pepper
tea

Cold sores
lemon balm
sage

Constipation
aloe latex
bilberry
cascara
cat's claw
flaxseed
parsley
peppermint
senna

Cough
flaxseed
licorice
marshmallow
sage
saw palmetto
tea
witch hazel

Crohn's disease
cat's claw

Cystic fibrosis
turmeric

Depression
ginkgo
ginseng
kava kava
lemon balm
St. John's wort
tea

Diabetes
aloe gel
bilberry
cinnamon
eleuthero
ginseng
grape
red pepper

Diarrhea
bilberry
catnip
lavender
peppermint

sage
tea

Diuretic
artichoke
astragalus
dandelion
eleuthero
nettle
parsley
tea
uva ursi
yerba maté

Dizziness
ginger
ginkgo

Eczema
borage seed oil
evening primrose oil
saw palmetto
witch hazel

Edema due to circulatory problems
gotu kola
grape
horse chestnut

Eye problems
bilberry
ginkgo
grape

Fatigue
astragalus
eleuthero
ginseng
guarana
lavender
peppermint
red pepper
tea
turmeric
wintergreen
yerba maté
yohimbe

Fever
lemon balm
parsley
peppermint
wintergreen

Flu
 echinacea
 garlic
 peppermint
 red pepper
 tea

Fungal infections
 aloe gel
 garlic
 tea tree oil

Gallbladder problems
 artichoke
 dandelion
 peppermint
 turmeric

Gas
 artichoke
 catnip
 chamomile
 lavender
 lemon balm
 garlic
 ginger
 peppermint
 red pepper
 turmeric
 wintergreen

Graves' disease
 lemon balm

Headache
 feverfew
 guarana
 lemon balm
 peppermint
 red pepper
 tea
 wintergreen

Heart problems
 astragalus
 flaxseed and oil
 ginkgo
 grape
 hawthorn
 red pepper
 tea

Hemorrhoids
 aloe gel

 grape
 horse chestnut
 witch hazel

Herpes
 lemon balm
 tea tree oil

Hot flashes
 black cohosh
 red clover
 soy
 wild yam

Immune stimulation
 astragalus
 cat's claw
 echinacea
 eleuthero
 ginseng

Impotence
 ginkgo
 ginseng
 red pepper
 saw palmetto
 yohimbe

Indigestion
 aloe gel
 artichoke
 bilberry
 catnip
 cat's claw
 chamomile
 cinnamon
 dandelion
 flaxseed
 ginger
 guarana
 hawthorn
 hoodia
 lavender
 lemon balm
 licorice
 marshmallow
 milk thistle
 parsley
 peppermint
 red pepper
 sage
 turmeric

 wild yam

Infection
 astragalus
 echinacea
 eleuthero
 garlic
 lemon balm
 peppermint
 tea tree oil

Infertility
 chaste tree

Inflammation
 cat's claw
 chamomile
 flaxseed oil
 ginger
 ginkgo
 grape
 marshmallow
 milk thistle
 red pepper
 tea
 turmeric
 wintergreen
 witch hazel

Insomnia
 catnip
 chamomile
 gotu kola
 kava kava
 lavender
 St. John's wort
 valerian

**Intermittent claudication
 (limping)**
 ginkgo

Irritable bowel syndrome
 artichoke
 flaxseed
 peppermint

Kidney problems
 cranberry
 tea
 uva ursi

**Leg pain or limping after
 exercise, see "intermit-
 tent claudication"**

Liver problems
  artichoke
  milk thistle
Lupus
  flaxseed
**Memory, see "mental
  performance"**
Menopausal symptoms
  black cohosh
  chaste tree
  evening primrose oil
  red clover
  soy
  wild yam
Menstrual problems
  black cohosh
  chaste tree
  evening primrose oil
  feverfew
  flaxseed and oil
  lemon balm
  parsley
  red clover
  sage
  soy
  St. John's wort
  wild yam
Mental performance
  ginkgo
  ginseng
  guarana
  lemon balm
  sage
  tea
Migraine prevention
  feverfew
Multiple sclerosis
  evening primrose oil
Muscle aches and pains
  feverfew
  kava kava
  peppermint
  ginger
  red pepper
  soy
  turmeric

wintergreen
witch hazel
Nasal congestion
  garlic
  licorice
  peppermint
  red pepper
  tea
Nausea
  ginger
Neuralgia
  ginkgo
  red pepper
Osteoporosis
  evening primrose oil
  flaxseed and oil
  red clover
  soy
  tea
  wild yam
**Parkinson's disease,
  prevention**
  guarana
  tea
  yerba maté
**Premenstrual syndrome
  (PMS)**
  black cohosh
  chaste tree
  evening primrose oil
  feverfew
  lemon balm
  parsley
  peppermint
  red clover
  sage
  soy
  St. John's wort
  wild yam
Prostate, enlarged
  flaxseed
  nettle
  saw palmetto
Psoriasis
  aloe gel
  flaxseed oil

turmeric
Raynaud's syndrome
  evening primrose oil
  ginkgo
Respiratory problems
  borage seed oil
  evening primrose oil
  flaxseed
  licorice
  marshmallow
  peppermint
  red clover
  red pepper
  sage
  tea
Sedative, see "insomnia"
Sjögren's syndrome
  evening primrose oil
Skin problems, acne
  arnica
  tea tree oil
  witch hazel
**Skin problems, dry, rough,
  or inflamed**
  aloe gel
  arnica
  chamomile
  borage seed oil
  evening primrose oil
  flaxseed oil
  marshmallow
  turmeric
  witch hazel
Skin problems, wounds
  aloe gel
  chamomile
  gotu kola
  marshmallow
  St. John's wort
  turmeric
  witch hazel
Sprains
  ginger
  peppermint
  red pepper
  turmeric

wintergreen

witch hazel

Stimulant, see "fatigue"

Stress

borage seed oil

catnip

chamomile

eleuthero

gotu kola

kava kava

lavender

lemon balm

peppermint

Sweating, excess

sage

soy

witch hazel

Throat, sore

flaxseed

licorice

marshmallow

sage

tea

witch hazel

Tinnitus

ginkgo

Tooth decay, prevention

parsley

tea

Ulcers

aloe gel

chamomile

eleuthero

gotu kola

horse chestnut

licorice

marshmallow

red pepper

Urinary tract infections or irritation

bilberry

cranberry

saw palmetto

uva ursi

Varicose veins

gotu kola

grape

horse chestnut

witch hazel

Vomiting

ginger

Warts

lemon balm

tea tree oil

Water retention, see "diuretic" and "edema"

Weight loss

guarana

hoodia

red pepper

soy

tea

yerba maté

The Herbs

Who bends a knee where violets grow,
A hundred secret things shall know.

—*Rachel Field,* A Charm for Spring Flowers

ALOE
Aloe vera, Aloe barbadensis, Aloe capensis

HISTORY AND FOLKLORE

This succulent member of the lily family has distinctive, fleshy, "lanceolate" leaves, which is a botanist's special way of telling you that the leaves are shaped like lances. After accumulating excess experience with their pointy ends, I quarantined my own aloe outdoors from my small apartment. It rapidly grew larger than a toddler. That my own aloe grew to threatening proportions is significant—aloe almost thrives on neglect.

Though aloe flourishes in the most barren soils, it is a native of the wetter tropics of Africa and Southern India. Despite its spiny form, it is not a cactus, nor is it the same as the American agave, which it resembles. It is also confused with an unrelated incense mentioned in the Bible that is more properly called *aloe wood,* or *lignaloe.*

The Bible's reference to aloe is questionable, but the ancient Sumerians, Greeks, Romans, and Egyptians used it. Aloe is frequently noted as the legendary skin treatment for Cleopatra, and aloe gel may indeed help maintain a healthy complexion.

Aloe is one of the most popular herbs. Despite this, most people are not informed that two entirely different products are made from this plant, the gel and the latex, which have considerably different properties. ("Latex," in this context, is a botanical term, and should not be confused with the commercial rubber latex.) The gel is a clear, gooey mucilage, obtained from the insides of the leaves, and is most often used for topical skin repair. The latex, on the other hand, is a bitter yellow liquid secreted by cells just beneath the rind of the leaf, and is often dried to make a product that is also confusingly called aloe, and may be reconstituted with water as aloe "juice." To further obfuscate matters, the gel is also sometimes thinned down with water, which is used as a beverage and is then *also* confusingly called "juice." The latex has quite different properties than the gel, when taken internally. Aloe latex is often called a "natural laxative," and it is—in the same sense that a hurricane is a natural building renovator.

HOW SCIENTISTS THINK
ALOE GEL WORKS

Aloe gel's polysaccharides keep your wounds moist by absorbing water like a sponge. The reason for aloe gel's snotty texture, as well as for many other snotty things in life, lies in its polysaccharides. Polysaccharides are large chains of small, ring-shaped sugars bonded together like beads on a chain. Sugars of all kinds, including those that make up aloe gel's predominant polysaccharide, *acemannan,* attract water.

When sugars are small, simple molecules like those in table sugar crystals, they dissolve in water. When the sugars occur in a polysaccharide's chains, like acemannan, however, the chains are too large to be surrounded and separated by tiny water molecules, so they can't dissolve like table sugar. But water sticks to these chains, and the chains stick to one another, and this network of chains swells with water. This forms a gooey gel. This gel is similar to what you get if you soak rice, potatoes, or paper in water. Starch, found in grains and potatoes, and cellulose, a component of paper, are also polysaccharide chains, and if you soak them in water, they will swell just like acemannan and ultimately form a gooey pulp, too. Aloe gel is like this—a natural water-retaining sponge.

For many simple wounds and light burns, moisture speeds healing. Dry wounds get crusty, and any living cells in them shrivel up and die. That can be all right in some cases, because underlying tissues just seal themselves off from this arid wasteland and continue living. But processes required for repair must take place in a fluid environment, because particles can *move* and do things in a fluid. Dryness prevents particle motion. Water gives a wound's particles mobility. So water's tendency to cling to aloe gel probably helps accelerate wound mending.

Aloe gel recruits your white blood cells; they can help heal you, but can also cause irritating inflammation. If you are allergic to pollen, you already know that plants "stimulate" your immune system. Your troubles are often caused by plant polysaccharides, which can fool your immune system by resembling bacterial polysaccharides. Some people's immune systems are more susceptible to being duped into this inflammatory overreacting. Aloe gel's acemannan does stimulate the immune system, attracting and activating your white blood cells to the site of application.

White blood cells repair and defend your tissues, but can also damage them with inflammation. So the recruitment of white blood cells could be good for some cases but bad for others. This pro-inflammatory action could even account for a few negative reports following the use of aloe gel, like itching, redness, delayed healing, and allergic responses. These negative results are fortunately not as common as positive ones, which include reports of accelerated wound repair after aloe gel is applied. You should be aware that the gel could cause adverse affects, however, so a small test patch might be warranted before committing it to liberal use, especially if you are prone to allergies.

Beta-sitosterol from aloe gel gets your blood vessels to grow faster, which speeds healing. Beta-sitosterol is found in a wide variety of plants and is more commonly regarded by scientists as an effective cholesterol-lowering agent. But a couple of animal studies suggest it also stimulates the growth of new capillaries, a process called *angiogenesis.* Three studies link aloe gel's beta-sitosterol to angiogenesis, and all but your most superficial wounds require angiogenesis to heal. Not only do your preexisting, broken blood vessels need to mend, but also new blood vessels supply nutrients that support cellular mending activities.

One of aloe gel's glycoproteins breaks down your bradykinin, which would otherwise cause swelling, cramps, and enhanced pain perception. Other commonly cited active ingredients of aloe gel are some of its glycoproteins. One glycoprotein from aloe gel apparently breaks down bradykinin. Bradykinin is a chain of amino acids that stimulates the widening of blood vessels, or vasodilation. When blood vessels dilate, they leak fluid, and surrounding tissues become swollen. Bradykinin also causes involuntary muscle contractions that, when painful, are called "cramps." And as if that were not enough, in addition to causing swelling and cramps, bradykinin enhances your perception of pain. Aloe's degradation of bradykinin, then, may explain why aloe gel can reduce your pain and swelling.

Aloe gel inhibits the formation of damaging free radicals. In other research, an aloe gel glycoprotein inhibited the formation of superoxide, a free radical. This positive effect was corroborated by another study, which found that a water-based aloe gel extract inhibits white blood cells' creation of oxygen-containing free radicals. Free radicals damage tissues, and though white blood cells protect us by flinging free radicals at foreign invaders such as bacteria, free radicals can damage your own tissues, too. Aloe gel's inhibition of free radical formation may therefore lessen your own "friendly fire." This could help mitigate the free radicals formed by recruitment of white blood cells mentioned above.

Aloe gel inhibits COX-2, giving it an aspirin-like effect. In one study, a glycoprotein from aloe gel inhibited the cyclooxygenase-2 (COX-2) enzyme, which is how painkillers like aspirin work. A second study confirms that a water-based extract of aloe gel inhibits COX-2. COX-2 accelerates the production of painful molecules called *prostaglandins* during inflammation. Anti-inflammatories like aspirin also work by inhibiting this enzyme.

Aloe gel reduces blood clots. The same glycoprotein that inhibits COX-2 also reduces the concentration of another enzyme (thromboxane A2 synthase), which makes thromboxane. Thromboxanes are made by blood platelets and cause blood clotting. Thromboxane lessens your blood loss, but it can also restrict oxygenated blood flow to damaged tissues, a negative phenomenon called *ischemia.* Although you might conclude that you want thromboxanes to stop your bleeding, thromboxane formation is more commonly thought to cause injury through ischemia. Decreasing thromboxane formation is actually associated with a positive outcome for wound repair. Aloe's anti-thromboxane activity could hasten your healing.

How Scientists Think Aloe Latex Works

Aloe latex contains laxatives. These colorful plant pigments, anthraquinones and anthrones, are collectively called *anthranoid laxatives.* They may remain in some incompletely purified aloe *gel* preparations as well, so if you take the gel internally you still might want to be wary of their effects.

Anthranoid laxatives are found in other, unrelated plants, and act the same way. You can find them in senna, cascara ("sacred bark"), rhubarb root ("rhein"), buckthorn, and frangula. If you take any one of those herbs, you will notice an effect very similar to your taking aloe latex. This discussion therefore applies to these herbs as well.

For the active ingredients to work, they must be liberated from attached sugars by your intestinal bacteria. The anthranoid laxatives in these plants usually have sugars attached to them, and the general term for a molecule that has attached sugar is a *glycoside.* Glycosides are very common in plants. The active ingredients of many plants are often less effective when in the glycoside form, and anthranoid glycosides are no exception. The sugar must be removed by your gut bacteria to liberate the active *aglycone,* the general term for any former glycoside that has had its sugar disconnected. Therefore, if you expect these plant anthranoid laxatives to work, you ought to have working gut bacteria that can free the active ingredient, the aglycone, from its attached sugar. If you are taking antibiotics or some other factor causes you to have compromised gut bacteria, you might not get the same action.

Anthranoid laxatives reverse the normal direction of the flow of water from your colon to your bloodstream. The cells of your colon normally push charged particles called *ions* from the interior of the colon out into your bloodstream, which eventually reach your blood through capillaries surrounding the colon. When things flow in this direction, it is called *absorption.* Water follows this parade of ions, because ions have charges, and water loves anything with a charge. Your absorption of water keeps you hydrated. Anthranoid laxatives reverse this flow.

What's In It

ALOE LATEX, or "juice," contains anthracene derivatives such as antrone-10-C-glycosyls like aloins A and B, hydroxyaloins, and aloe-emodin. The gel contains the hydrated polysaccharide acemannan, which consists primarily of acetylated mannose and other monosaccharides. The gel also contains lipids, amino acids, enzymes, sterols, salicylates, and magnesium lactate and other salts.

Specifically, anthranoid laxatives appear to open chloride ion channels, such that chloride flows into the colon, a direction opposite its normal route. Positively charged sodium ions may be expected to follow the negatively charged chloride ions, as opposite charges attract. Water always follows ions, so the colon fills with water, producing a watery diarrhea.

Anthranoid laxatives also stimulate production of a prostaglandin, causing gut contractions. This speeds your gut's contents on a one-way trip. Overly forceful, involuntary contractions are painful and better known as "cramps." That aloe's action is inhibited by anti-inflammatories (like

indomethacin) suggests some inflammatory process mediates it. The details are not entirely clear, but anthranoid laxatives do cause more nitric oxide to form in the colon. Nitric oxide, in turn, stimulates the synthesis of a prostaglandin, (PGE2), an inflammatory molecule. Although PGE2 can stimulate processes that protect your stomach lining, such as decreasing acid and increasing protective mucous secretion, in your colon it has a different action, making your colon muscles jump around unpleasantly. This gives you cramps and diarrhea.

Aloe latex kills some of your colon cells, but at least they die a clean death. For some reason, chronic use of anthranoid laxatives is associated with colon cells committing suicide, or "apoptosis." Apoptosis is a tidy sort of cell death that does not incite inflammation and is generally benign. Cancer researchers tend to perk their ears up when apoptosis is discussed. Since stimulating apoptosis of cancer cells interests them, aloe latex has been proposed for use against colon cancer, but so far not enough research has been performed to validate this suggestion.

Like aloe gel, aloe latex recruits and activates immune cells. This is both good and bad. Aloe latex increases some of your cytokines, which attract and activate white blood cells. If you take anthranoid laxatives, immune cells will be recruited to your colon. But what do they do there? After people take anthranoid laxatives, these white blood cells are then observed dining on the remains of their suicidal colon cells—that is, the colon cells that have undergone apoptosis. They also eat up and metabolize the colorful anthranoid laxative molecules, too. So on the one hand, these white blood cells seem to be cleaning up some of the mess that the anthranoid laxatives created. On the other hand, immune cells can irritate and damage an area through inflammation if they get overly aggressive.

If you take a lot of anthranoid laxatives, you will get a strangely polka-dotted colon. White blood cells recruited to the colon by aloe latex contain a dark pigment, and chronic abuse of anthranoid laxatives causes "melanosis coli," a condition in which infiltrated white blood cells are seen as dark spots in the colon. The pigment they contain is actually the partially digested remains of the anthranoid laxatives, which are highly colored as well. The term "melanosis" is misleading, because the pigment they contain is lipofuscin, not melanin, so sometimes you will hear the condition called *pseudo*melanosis coli. A polka-dotted colon might raise your gastroenterologist's eyebrows during a colonoscopy, but most researchers say that the condition is benign. Although many have searched for a link between melanosis coli and cancer, the association currently remains ambiguous. Melanosis coli might worsen constipation, if severe. The spots do go away over time if the laxative use is halted.

Anthranoid laxatives generate damaging free radicals. While aloe gel contains free radical scavenging properties, anthranoid laxatives in the latex have the opposite effect: free radical production. Free radicals can damage your DNA, causing cancer, but anthranoid laxatives' epidemiological link to cancer currently remains equivocal. That they cause painful cramps and violent diarrhea probably serves as the best reason to avoid use of plant anthraquinones as laxatives.

Good Effects . . . and Not So Good

Read labels carefully. Do not confuse aloe *latex* with aloe *gel,* as they have different chemical constituents and dramatically different effects. Liquids sold as "aloe juice" are often just watered-down gel, which is far more benign, and are not aloe latex at all. However, some oral gel preparations are incompletely purified and may contain traces of latex. To further obfuscate matters, the aloe latex that you want to avoid is sometimes dried and then merely called "aloe." If you aren't sure what it is, don't take it. If you do consume actual aloe latex, and if you have active gut flora, which can liberate its active anthranoid laxatives from their sugars, you will know.

Aloe latex and other anthranoid laxatives are not recommended. Medical references describe the bitter, yellow latex as a purgative, a pharmacist's euphemism for violent laxative, or what my clinically experienced graduate students indelicately call a "colon blower." Most herbalists generally recommend you take safer products than aloe latex for constipation, like pectin, psyllium, or flaxseed. Aloe's anthranoid constituents "relieve" your constipation in an aggressive way, accompanied by painful cramps. This is the FDA's latest pronouncement on anthranoid laxatives, in May 2002: "The Food and Drug Administration (FDA) is issuing a final rule stating that the stimulant laxative ingredients aloe (including aloe extract and aloe flower extract) and cascara sagrada (including casanthranol, cascara fluid extract aromatic, cascara sagrada bark, cascara sagrada extract, and cascara sagrada fluid extract) in over-the-counter (OTC) drug products are not generally recognized as safe and effective or are misbranded."

The best source of topical aloe gel may be the plant itself. You can readily get the gel commercially, too, but it reportedly works best if fresh. If you must increase the coffers of some herb-selling corporation, however, choose a reputable one. The better-quality gel products contain over 95 percent gel, and terms like "stabilized," "naturalized," or "purified" are not a guarantee of freshness and should be ignored.

These statements could make aloe gel sellers unhappy. Some companies do make an effort to remove all traces of aloe latex from their gel and to concentrate the moisture-retaining polysaccharide acemannan, both of which are sensible actions. Yet some worry that processing the gel can remove unidentified active ingredients. Since no single ingredient is responsible for all the beneficial effects of aloe gel, this provides justification for you to use the whole, fresh gel, rather than an isolated component from it.

If you have an aloe plant, you can obtain aloe gel easily, by snapping a leaf off a plant and spooning out this abundant, inner goo, which has a viscous, snotty texture. Avoid scraping next to the leaf rind itself, where the latex is located. If you have leftover gel, you may want to keep it in a closed container in the refrigerator for a few days to help preserve it, and so you can continue to use it as your burn heals. But don't keep it any longer than necessary—it can go "bad" like any food item. I personally find the gel quite soothing on sunburns and imagine this speeds healing, but officially I do not know if this is true, because I am too impatient to set up a control situation when I am burned. You will find that your plant remains merrily oblivious to your exploitation of it, and as with the mythical Greek hydra monster, chopping it up only stimulates its pointy expansions.

Use aloe gel only on minor injuries or unbroken skin. Clean the area prior to its application. Allergic reactions are rare, but you might want to test a patch of skin first. Deeper wounds may even experience delayed healing if treated with aloe gel.

Aloe gel is also commonly used internally for ulcers, but this use requires more scientific validation. Although anecdotal testimonials for aloe gel's internal benefit for ulcers abound, research substantiating these allegations is scarce. The gel occasionally causes severe stomach cramps. It is not known if some component of the gel causes this, but if anthranoids from the latex contaminate the gel, diarrhea and cramps may be expected.

Evidence of Action

Several studies of people using aloe gel show a positive outcome, but some show no effect, and some even show delayed healing. In one study, thirty female factory workers wore aloe vera gel–treated gloves on one of their dry, irritated hands for eight hours a day, for a month, followed by ten days without the glove, and another thirty days with the glove. The gloved hand was compared to the untreated hand and was reportedly less red and irritated.[1]

The incidence of dry socket (alveolar osteitis) occurrence in 1,064 tooth extractions treated with aloe gel's acemannan was compared to that of 1,031 extractions, which were treated instead with an antibiotic. Dry socket occurs when an extracted tooth loses its blood clot prematurely, and can be quite painful. Those treated with acemannan had significantly less incidence of dry socket.[2]

Tests of aloe gel on irradiated skin have yielded uncertain results. Cancer patients receiving radiation therapy were divided into two groups. One group treated their radiated skin with soap and then treated the area with aloe gel, and the other group used the same soap but did not use aloe gel. For patients receiving higher-dose radiation, the onset of skin injury caused by radiation was delayed in the group using aloe gel. There was no difference in the two groups when a lower dose of radiation was used.[3] Another similar study was more disappointing. The irradiated breast tissue of 225 breast cancer patients was treated with either aloe vera gel or a placebo treatment of aqueous cream three times daily for two weeks after radiation therapy. Aloe vera gel did not improve the breast tissue with respect to the aqueous cream, and the aqueous cream was actually better at relieving dryness and pain. The aloe gel was even associated with redness and itching in some cases.[4] Also, two other large, double-blind trials where irradiated cancer patients were treated either with aloe gel or placebo cream or had no treatment showed that aloe did not protect the irradiated tissue from dermatitis.[5]

Some studies suggest aloe gel may not be the best treatment for deeper or more severe wounds. Thirty patients with bedsores were treated daily with either a commercial aloe gel product or moist bandages. During a ten-week observation period, 63 percent of the patients had completely healed sores, but there was no difference between those treated with aloe and those who used the placebo.[6] Also, women treated with aloe vera gel following cesarean surgery or laparotomy actually experienced significantly *delayed* healing of their surgical wounds with respect to placebo.[7] Since the placebo was considered ineffective, this result implies aloe gel treatment may even be detrimental for severe wounds.

A placebo-controlled, double-blind study suggests aloe gel might reduce psoriasis. Sixty people with psoriasis were given either placebo cream or a cream containing 0.5 percent aloe vera gel. They were instructed to apply the cream three times daily, five times a week, for up to four weeks. The psoriasis disappeared in twenty-five of the thirty people using aloe vera, while only two of the thirty people using placebo were cured. No patients reported any ill effects from the aloe cream.[8]

Commonly Reported Uses for Aloe*

Internally

ALOE GEL: stomach ulcers, ulcerative colitis, gastrointestinal disease, asthma, diabetes
ALOE LATEX: laxative
forms available for internal use:
ALOE GEL: commercial beverages, "aloe juice"
ALOE LATEX: dried capsules and pills
commonly reported dosage:
As a laxative, 0.05 to 0.2 grams of dried latex is taken for short periods only.
Both the liquid juice and gel are taken in doses of one tablespoon up to three times daily.

Externally

ALOE GEL: topical healer, beauty aid, minor cuts and burns, fungal infections
forms available for external use:
fresh from the plant, bottled gel, lotions, moisturizers, creams, hair products
commonly reported dosage:
Apply to affected skin after cleansing the area, or follow product instructions.

*These uses and dosages are from historic use and are not necessarily tested nor recommended.

Many take aloe gel internally for ulcers, yet human studies on this use of aloe gel are scarce. A 1963 study states that aloe gel cured seventeen out of eighteen patients' peptic ulcers, but that study was preliminary in nature and has not yet been reproduced.[9] However, a more recent placebo-controlled, double-blind study did show that aloe gel significantly quelled gastrointestinal inflammation. Forty-four patients with inflammatory bowel disease were given either 100 milliliters of aloe vera gel orally, twice a day for four weeks, or a placebo. Those taking aloe gel significantly improved.[10]

THE BOTTOM LINE

- Aloe gel and aloe latex are not the same product and have different activities.
- Fresh aloe gel may accelerate the healing of minor wounds and burns, but could delay the healing of deeper wounds.
- Moisturizing tissues, white cell activation and recruitment, angiogenesis stimulation, bradykinin breakdown, free radical prevention, COX-2 inhibition, and thromboxane inhibition are mechanisms that could theoretically mediate aloe gel's wound-healing properties.
- Aloe latex is a drastic purgative, causing cramps and diarrhea, and is not recommended.
- Chronic anthranoid laxative abuse can produce melanosis coli, a pigmented colon, which, though abnormal, is reportedly benign. Melanosis coli disappears if the anthranoid use is stopped.

ARNICA

Arnica montana, A. fulgens, A. sororia, A. cordifolia, A. chamissonis

History and Folklore

Arnica is also known as *leopard's bane, wolf's bane, mountain tobacco,* and *mountain daisy,* and its various species grow in mountainous regions of Europe and North America. The plant resembles its cousin, the daisy, as they are both in the same, large family (*Asteraceae,* or *Compositae*). Arnica's bright yellow, daisylike flowers are now its favored therapeutic bits, but internal and external applications of the entire plant were once more common.

You should not eat arnica, however. Although arnica was once historically recommended for heart and nervous system stimulation, some people apparently received more excitement than they anticipated and died. Oral arnica is toxic to the heart, even in small amounts. Besides death, other side effects of arnica ingestion are severe gastrointestinal upset, nervousness, rapid pulse, high blood pressure, and muscle weakness. Therefore, its internal use is now strongly discouraged.

Arnica still remains intensely popular, especially in Europe, in topical preparations for treating bruises, aches, pain, swelling, insect bites, and poor complexion. Curiously, however, many of the popular preparations contain no arnica at all, because they are "homeopathic." For preparations that actually contain arnica, numerous cases of allergy and acquired contact dermatitis have been reported.

How Scientists Think Arnica Works

Arnica shuts off an inflammatory molecule called NF-kappa-B. This should, at least theoretically, decrease your inflammation. Helenalin from arnica keeps a proinflammatory molecule with the unwieldy title "nuclear transcription factor kappa beta," or NF-kappa-B, inactive. When you are subject to oxidative stress, viruses, toxins, or carcinogens, several different kinds of cells in your body produce NF-kappa-B.

This molecule causes your body to make inflammatory proteins, called cytokines. It activates the use of particular genes that instruct your cells how to make these nasty things. NF-kappa-B does this by attaching to the "promoters" of these genes. This causes the genes' instructions to be read, and their inflammatory products are then constructed. So NF-kappa-B is sort of like a foreman who instructs a bunch of different workers to construct an array of weapons. Ideally these weapons are used responsibly—against foreign invaders like bacteria, for example—but they can hurt you, too, and cause damaging inflammation.

NF-kappa-B is normally kept at bay inside your cells, with an *inhibitory* molecule called *I-kappa-B* (the "I" is for inhibitory.) This binds to and disables NF-kappa-B inside cells. When cells are provoked, however, this inhibitor is broken down, and the NF-kappa-B is freed to go about performing its inflammatory business. Helenalin works by preventing the inhibitor's release from NF-kappa-B. This, in theory, should quell your inflammation.

Arnica might also inhibit the complement system. This could also quell your inflammation. One paper suggests that a glycoprotein from arnica strongly inhibits what is known as the *complement system*. After your immune system's antibodies "finger" a target such as a bacterium, your complement system destroys it. This "system" is actually more than thirty-five proteins that interact to protect you from pathogens, but it also creates inflammation. Arnica's possible constraint on the complement system also provides a theoretical anti-inflammatory mechanism.

But arnica also has inflammatory effects as well. It causes you to make an unpleasant molecule called TNF. On the other, pro-inflammatory hand, arnica's polysaccharides stimulate your white cells to produce tumor necrosis factor (TNF). TNF is also called *cachexin,* because it plays a major role in *cachexia,* the horrible wasting state that long-term cancer patients endure.

TNF provokes the division and activation of several types of immune cells and even causes cancer cells to commit suicide in a petri dish. All this sounds good, but researchers more often worry about TNF's dark side. TNF recruits blood vessels to feed tumors. And while TNF plays a role in a normally functioning immune system, excessive TNF inflicts damaging inflammation in many diseases. Rheumatoid arthritis, Crohn's disease, and ankylosing spondylitis are exacerbated by TNF, and *anti*-TNF drugs, in fact, help treat these illnesses. So increasing your TNF does not seem like a good idea.

Arnica hinders blood clot formation, contradicting its traditional application for bleeding and bruising. The first thing you will probably hear herbalists say about arnica is that it is used to prevent and treat bruises. However, arnica may make bleeding, which causes bruising, more likely. Both helenalin and dihydrohelenalin from arnica were shown to inhibit clot formation. They have also been observed hindering the production of thromboxane, and thromboxane causes blood clotting and blood vessel constriction, which stops bleeding. In fact, some researchers advise you not to use arnica prior to surgery or with blood-thinning medications, because it may cause bleeding problems. On the face of things, this mechanism contradicts arnica's use for bruising.

GOOD EFFECTS . . .
AND NOT SO GOOD

You should never take arnica internally, because it can kill you. At one time alcoholic tinctures of arnica were recommended for a wide range of complaints, from heart problems to depression. Fortunately internal preparations are no longer as popular as they once were. As little as one ounce of tincture (alcoholic extract) can cause severe distress, and 70 grams of arnica tincture has been fatal. In a 2003 case report of Uruguayan women who tried to induce abortions using plants, arnica caused multiple organ system failure.[1] The FDA restricts the use of arnica to small amounts for flavoring alcoholic beverages, probably because it is historically considered a required ingredient in the preparation of Benedictine.

Topical application of arnica is more accepted, but not without risks as well. In scientific literature, over thirty-five citations with more than one hundred cases of contact dermatitis with arnica are reported. The same molecules celebrated for their therapeutic activity, helenalin and related molecules, are thought to cause the sensitivity. Because these molecules and their

HOMEOPATHY HAS its pros and cons. Few fields in alternative medicine are more controversial than homeopathy. Here's a detailed look at its pitfalls and promises:

Scientists find homeopathy hard to swallow. If you look at homeopathic preparations, you will see notations on them such as "30x" or "9c." The "x" means that the material on the label was diluted tenfold, so "30x" means the substance was first diluted tenfold, and then this resulting liquid was diluted tenfold again, and so on, until the procedure had been repeated thirty times. Therefore a 30x preparation contains one part in 10^{30}, that is, a 1 followed by 30 zeroes. A "c" means the material was diluted by one-hundred-fold, so "9c" means the material was diluted one-hundred-fold nine times, or one-billion-billion-fold. To create pills, the plant is diluted in lactose (milk sugar) rather than water. Given that 18 milliliters of water contains 6.02×10^{23} water molecules, or that 342 grams of lactose contains 6.02×10^{23} lactose molecules, you can calculate how much of a typical homeopathic extract you would have to take to get a dose of arnica. You literally would have to take either billions of pills, or in the case of liquid extracts, drink planet-sized bodies of water to get one single arnica molecule! Since the purpose of this book is to discuss the effects of plant molecules on your body, the absence of plant molecules in homeopathic remedies renders the topic of their effectiveness outside this book's domain.

Homeopaths have done these calculations as well. They already know that their remedies contain not a single molecule of the diluted substance. In fact, they believe that the more dilute the preparation is, the more potent it is. Homeopathic medicine states that water retains a "memory" of what was once in it. This rests on an eighteenth-century notion of the German Samuel Hahnemann, who spent his life testing natural products on people to see what symptoms they provoked. He then treated people troubled by these symptoms with infinitesimally diluted substances that induce the symptoms. Thus the diluted version of an itch-creating plant like poison ivy was used to treat someone complaining of itchy skin.

But can water really retain a memory of a molecule? It has never been proven by any experiment, although scientists have repeatedly tried.[2]

Yet there is a way that homeopathy could work. Taking homeopathic remedies makes people feel like they are doing something, and sometimes just doing something helps to a surprising degree. As Carl Jung famously noted, rituals and symbols speak to the subconscious mind, and I believe the nourishment of the dreaming parts of our minds should not be neglected. Taking homeopathic remedies may be viewed as a ritual involving symbols. Rituals help us feel like we are doing something, and the symbols used in them can change our state of mind. If it works, we call that the placebo effect, the power of your mind to affect your body, and it is nothing to scoff at. It works.

Homeopathy and the placebo effect work better for some symptoms than others. They can prove astonishingly powerful in treating pain, menopausal hot flashes, and prostate enlargement. Homeopathy may indeed work for some, by the powerful mental mechanism of the placebo effect, so it is no surprise that many regard homeopathy highly, and it is immensely popular.

relations are found in other daisy (*Aster-aceae*) family plants, an allergy to one plant species can confer an allergy to its cousin. If you know you are allergic to plants in the daisy family, you should be careful using arnica and at least before using it perform a test patch to see how you react to it. If do not have an allergy to these plants, repeated contact with arnica can create one. If you are considering using arnica to prevent bruising, keep in mind that in clinical studies other herbs like horse chestnut and gotu kola have established better scientific credibility for treating vascular problems than arnica.

Interesting Facts

Arnica is a damn yellow composite.

ARNICA HAS been called *wolf's bane* and *leopard's bane,* but it is a member of a group of flowers that may as well be called *botanists' bane.* They are hard to identify, particularly if they are yellow.

This troublesome group has lots of members, and they tend to look the same. This is the daisy or sunflower family, which botanists alternately call either *Asteraceae* or *Compositae.* Over twenty thousand species of this family make it the largest plant family (or second largest to orchids, depending on the parameters used). The most common flower color in this family is yellow, so its yellow members are especially difficult to identify and distinguish from one another. A flower in this family is nicknamed a "composite," but yellow ones are frequently called DYCs, or "Damn Yellow Composites," by frustrated botanists trying to identify them. Mexican botanists have their

own term, calling them "PCAs," which condemns their *"Compuestas Amarillas"* with a more colorful adjective.

The reason these flowers are called composites is that what appears to be one flower is actually a composite of two types of flowers. Look at a sunflower—it's the most obvious example. In the center of the flower, where you find the sunflower seeds, each seed arises from a tiny "disk flower."

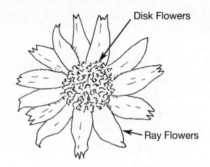

The more obvious petals surrounding the composition arise from outer "ray flowers." The next time you see a DYC, see if you can at least identify the disc flowers and the ray flowers. Identifying individual DYCs is a different—and much more difficult—matter entirely.

Be environmentally caring. If you *still* want to try arnica, be aware that overharvesting threatens the European version, *A. montana,* so it is conscientious to use other species. Also, you should not use arnica on open sores or blisters, because of the dangers of its internal effects.

A great number of arnica products, however, do not have any arnica in them, because they are homeopathic remedies. Arnica is one of the most popular homeopathic plants. Homeopathic remedies are completely safe, because they have no active ingredients (see text box on homeopathy, page 27).

EVIDENCE OF ACTION

Unfortunately, most of the clinical trials on arnica were conducted using homeopathic preparations, which means they did not actually contain any arnica. They are not very exciting. One study on impacted wisdom teeth even showed that the *placebo* group felt significantly less pain than the arnica-treated group![3] Not surprisingly, of the five published clinical trials on *homeopathic* arnica, none of them show any benefit over placebo.[4, 5, 6, 7, 8] Nevertheless, the Web sites of some of these commercial homeopathic products boast that they were "tested in clinical trials" but neglect mentioning their sad outcomes. Yes, they certainly were tested in clinical trials.

What's In It

THE PROFESSED effects of topical formulations, both the therapeutic and allergic ones, are commonly attributed to the plants' helenalin and dihydrohelenalin, which fall into the chemical category of sesquiterpene lactones. The plant also has immune-stimulating polysaccharides and glycoproteins.

There are very few clinical trials using actual arnica, but they are not promising either. One report suggested that, along with a skin-soluble form of aspirin, a commercial arnica spray (containing 100 mg of arnica tincture per mL) demonstrated a "synergistic" effect against the pain of electrical stimulation in healthy volunteers.[9] However,

another study that used fresh arnica plant gel on osteoarthritic volunteers' knees claimed improvement, but they did not use a control group of any kind, so this unfortunately does not mean anything one way or the other. One volunteer suffered an allergic reaction to the plant.[10]

Commonly Reported Uses for Arnica*

Externally
anti-inflammatory, aches, bruising, arthritis, acne, insect bites
forms available for external use:
gel, infusion, ointment, tincture, cosmetic preparations
commonly reported dosage:
Maximum concentrations of either 15 percent arnica oil or 20–25 percent tincture are used in ointments.

*These uses and dosages are from historic use and are not necessarily tested nor recommended.

In a double-blind, randomized, controlled study, nineteen patients were treated for facial spider veins with laser therapy. One group applied arnica to half of their face twice a day for two weeks before laser treatment, and the other group did the same after the treatment. No difference in bruising was seen between the arnica-treated areas and those that were untreated in either group.[11.] Thirty-seven patients undergoing carpal tunnel surgery were randomly assigned either a placebo or arnica ointment. Although no difference in wrist circumference or grip strength was noticed, the group treated with arnica reported significantly less pain.[12]

THE BOTTOM LINE

- Arnica is traditionally used externally for bruises, aches, swelling, pain, acne, and insect bites.
- Components in arnica provoke the immune system, which could exacerbate inflammation. Paradoxically, arnica inhibits an inflammatory mediator called NF-kappa-B, as well as the complement system.
- Arnica may also enhance bleeding, which, contrary to claims for it, may increase bruising.
- Arnica is unsafe for internal use and should never be taken internally.
- Continued application can create an allergy to the plant.
- Homeopathic preparations of arnica are common, and actually contain no arnica. There is no clinical evidence that they work, yet some people may find the placebo effect of homeopathic remedies helpful.

ARTICHOKE

Cynara scolymus

HISTORY AND FOLKLORE

The first thing that comes to your mind when you think of artichoke is probably "vegetable," not "herb." Yet if you take a peek at the herb shelves of most health food stores, you will find encapsulated artichoke extracts being sold everywhere, and research suggests it could actually do good things for you.

Artichokes are actually a type of thistle that ancient Mediterraneans popularized as a delicacy. It remains beloved in Italian cuisine today, along with the related cardoons (*C. cardunculus*), although the concept of eating them disturbed the Roman author and philosopher Pliny: *"Thus we turn into a corrupt feast the earth's monstrosities, those which even the animals instinctively avoid."*

This odd plant is in the daisy family (*Asteraceae* or *Compositaceae*), and you actually eat the immature flower bud. The "choke" consists of undeveloped, prickly flowerets, which you must carefully remove. And if you allow the bud to go unharvested, it will bloom into a magnificent purple flower.

If you know your Greek mythology, you know that the adulterous king of the gods, Zeus (or the Roman Jupiter), at times transiently promoted his woman du jour to goddess status, but she usually just ended up being transformed into some novel object at the end of the tale. The artichoke is supposed to be one of these remnants of women that he seduced. Cynara's particular offense was to grow homesick, so Zeus turned her into an artichoke. This unlucky woman gives the plant its Latin name.

In keeping with this scandalous story, ancient and medieval people considered the artichoke to be an aphrodisiac. In fact, it was considered unseemly for women to eat it, because of this, until the sixteenth century, after Catherine de Medici flaunted tradition by eating them openly. In doing so, she shocked everyone, but the now universally public consumption of artichokes is attributed to her disdain for social mores.

Besides its historic and scientifically doubtful reputation for stimulating sexual desire, artichoke is used as a diuretic, digestive aid, liver protector, choleretic (bile-flow enhancer), and cholesterol-lowering agent.

HOW SCIENTISTS THINK ARTICHOKE WORKS

Artichoke may work like prescription statin drugs to lower your cholesterol. Artichoke's reputed cholesterol-lowering power appears supported by a valid mechanism, at least from the standpoint of animal studies. Something in its extracts may work like the oft-advertised prescription statins now so in vogue for lowering your cholesterol when all else fails. Like statins, artichoke inhibits an enzyme needed to make cholesterol, HMG CoA-reductase, in rodents.

You make cholesterol whether you want to or not; everyone does. This takes several steps, each hastened by its own enzyme, but HMG CoA-reductase is the enzyme that speeds up what is known as the "committed step." That is, once this step takes place, you will make cholesterol and some other important molecules, such as steroid hormones and coenzyme Q, but not other molecules instead, so arresting this particular step is more critical. Statins do this in humans, and artichoke does it in rodents. If artichoke does the same thing in *people,* it could serve as a non-prescription alternative to statin drugs.

If artichoke does work like statins, it could have additional benefits. Prescription statin drugs possibly do even more than lower your cholesterol. Usually the side effects of drugs are negative, and though statins are not entirely without risks, they actually seem to have several *good* side effects. Surprised researchers have uncovered unforeseen side benefits to statins, like reducing inflammation and osteoporosis and decreasing the risk of colon cancer and Alzheimer's disease. That artichoke might work similarly is unknown but worth investigating, so stay tuned.

Or it could have negative side effects. On the other hand, the inhibition of HMG CoA-reductase by both statins and artichoke theoretically prevents a very important molecule called *coenzyme Q* from being made. You may have heard of it—it is sold as a supplement called *CoQ 10.* It is essential in the generation of biochemical energy by mitochondria in your cells and seems defective in the brains of those with Parkinson's disease. Supplementing Parkinson's patients with CoQ seems to help them (but not cure them.) That statins inhibit CoQ synthesis concerns some scientists, and artichoke could very well do the same thing. This potential side effect of artichoke is theoretical and has not been tested, and in theory it would probably be encountered only by taking medicinal quantities of the herb in supplement form.

Artichoke does not act exactly like statins, though. Artichoke inhibits HMG CoA-reductase in a more roundabout way. It is not clear how artichoke extracts inhibit this cholesterol-generating enzyme, but new research points away from the previously suspected agent, cynarin. Though you will find most artichoke supplements standardized to this molecule, you might actually want a different one. Cynaroside, and especially luteolin, which is obtained when cynaroside loses its attached sugar, are in part responsible for artichoke's effect. A statin drug works by parading as the intermediate material that HMG CoA-reductase works on, so it acts like an imposter, competing for the enzyme's attention directly, so to speak. Artichoke extract's inhibitory mechanism is less clear, but apparently it does not work as directly on the enzyme. For example, luteolin seems to work in part by inhibiting insulin's stimulation of this cholesterol-making enzyme. This could be good or bad—how this modifies artichoke's activity with respect to statins is not yet known.

But artichoke engages another cholesterol-lowering mechanism, which may in turn improve your digestion as well. Artichoke stimulates your liver's synthesis of bile. Herbs that stimulate bile production are called *choleretics,* and artichoke is one of the better-documented ones. Bile is bright green fluid made by your liver and stored in your gallbladder, a little bag-shaped organ connected to your liver. After you eat, fat entering your intestines causes this little bag to contract, pushing its bile through a duct into your intestine to join the fat that signaled it. Bile's green color comes from the pigment of broken-down red blood cells, and during its journey through your digestive tract it oxidizes to the brown color bestowed upon ordinary feces. But more significantly, bile also contains cholesterol and cholesterol-derived products. So artichoke encourages your cholesterol to literally merge with your excrement, graphically speaking.

Artichoke helps you make bile, and some of bile's cholesterol-derived ingredients are bile *salts*. Without bile salts, you would have a hard time digesting fats and oils. These salts are technically detergents, because each bile salt has a water-attracting (polar) region and grease-attracting (non-polar) region. Bile salts allow water and grease to mix in your intestines, breaking big fat blobs into smaller ones. Fat blobs are simply clumps of many fat molecules stuck together, and detergents unstick fat molecule from fat molecule, separating them all. This enables your fat-digesting enzymes to work on the individual fat molecules, because they can't get a handle on the big blobs, which are just too big for them to work with. Since artichoke helps your body produce this fat-handling substance, it improves your digestion of greasy meals.

It is not clear yet whether artichoke's choleretic effect could help or hurt those with gallstones. If bile salts are *not* making it into your intestines, you will not be able to digest fat efficiently, and will suffer indigestion and fat-laden diarrhea (steatorrhea). Why might your bile fail to move? Occasionally cholesterol solidifies in your gallbladder, creating gallstones. If you have enough gallstones, they block bile's entrance to your intestines. And when your stone-filled gallbladder contracts after eating a greasy meal, indigestion results, in the form of vague, upper-right-side abdominal pain. If you have liver or gallbladder problems, bile could get released into your blood in excess, making your skin and eyes appear yellow or "jaundiced," and your feces may even lose their classic color. Should you use artichoke to stimulate the production of bile

if your gallbladder is jammed up with stones? The answer depends on which researcher you talk to.

Some researchers reason that choleretics help keep your gallbladder clear, preventing the crystallization of stones. This idea is sort of like running water through your rain gutter to keep it clear of leaves. However, others say that increasing your bile traffic could theoretically cause impaction or buildup of bile, impinging on your already blocked gallbladder. In clinical studies, artichoke seems to relieve indigestion rather than exacerbate it, tentatively supporting its use for those with gallstones. However, if you *do* possess gallstones, you should still remain cautious about using medicinal quantities of artichokes and other choleretics, taking careful note of how you respond if you do.

What's In It

ARTICHOKE CONTAINS about 2 percent phenolic acids, including chlorogenic acid (3-caffeoylquinic acid), as well as cynarin (1,5-di-O-caffeoylquinic acid) and caffeic acid, sesquiterpene lactones, flavonoids like luteolin and luteolin glycosides, sterols, and inulin.

Artichoke improves your HDL/LDL cholesterol ratio. Cholesterol that is targeted for disposal through your bile is associated with HDL (high density lipoprotein) cholesterol, the so-called good cholesterol. If you have high cholesterol, your doctor will be less worried if more of it is in the form of HDL cholesterol. Simplistically speaking, HDL contains cholesterol that is more likely to make it, in one form or another, to the toilet, through bile. On the other hand, your newly made cholesterol ultimately ends up in the bad cholesterol, or LDL (low density lipoprotein), and this cholesterol is more likely to go in a less favorable direction, getting delivered to your cells. LDL cholesterol is also more likely to oxidize, forming artery-choking atherosclerotic plaques. In clinical studies artichoke not only lowered total cholesterol, but it also improved the ratio of good cholesterol to bad.

Artichoke's antioxidants prevent your LDL from turning into atherosclerotic plaques. Artichoke also contains a number of antioxidants. Its extracts contain molecules classified as flavonoids, and related flavonoids are often antioxidant in other plants. One of artichoke's flavonoids, luteolin, inhibits LDL oxidation. This is good, because your oxidized LDL becomes dangerous arterial plaques that can slow your blood down to a rush-hour crawl. How do flavonoids act like antioxidants? There are several mechanisms, but artichoke's flavonoids are thought to bind to metals like iron in your body, a process called *chelation.* Chelation impairs the metals' typical ability to spawn oxidizing free radicals. Artichoke's flavonoids may put other antioxidant mechanisms to work in your body as well.

GOOD EFFECTS . . .
AND NOT SO GOOD

If you are like most people, you can expect no ill effects from eating artichokes and their extracts. But some people have allergies to the plant. The FDA considers the leaves safe for use in foods. However, artichoke is in the daisy family, which usually raises a red flag concerning allergic responses (see also Arnica, Chamomile, Dandelion, Echinacea, Feverfew, and Milk Thistle). Indeed, professional artichoke handlers can develop contact sensitization to the plant over time, and if you know you have an allergy to plants in this family, you might want to be careful approaching it. Most studies in which people consume artichoke leaf extracts suggest it is well tolerated by the volunteers, and it really does seem to be useful for lowering your cholesterol, improving your LDL/HDL cholesterol ratio, and lessening your digestive complaints. It won't rescue you from a night of excess, however. One research article—and you can't help but wonder what inspires such studies—found artichoke of absolutely no use for treating hangovers in volunteers.

It's not clear if artichoke depletes coenzyme Q. If you do take artichoke, keep in mind that if it works like statins, it may theoretically decrease your synthesis of coenzyme Q. Indeed, some scientists are now suggesting that perhaps statins should be formulated with coenzyme Q to limit the loss of this important molecule. But these days you can also take coenzyme Q as a supplement, which could possibly blunt the risk of decreased coenzyme Q. Coenzyme Q has not yet been extensively tested, however, so the amount to take for this purpose, or indeed whether it is even necessary when taking either artichoke or statin drugs, remains unknown.

There is no evidence to suggest artichoke stimulates sexual desire. The plants' libido-stimulating reputation does not have any scientific support at present, though you could always confide to your dinner date the fabled danger of eating them and hope for the placebo effect to kick in. A paper titled "The Action of the Artichoke (*Cynara scolymus*) on the Male Gonads in an experiment" conjures up uncomfortable images, but merely discovered that artichoke extract had no untoward effects on rodent sperm.

The Artichoke Effect

IF YOU have ever noticed that water tastes funny after you eat artichokes, you have encountered the "artichoke effect." Not everyone is susceptible to this, so noticing the strange taste may be genetic. Artichoke eaters throughout history have observed that other foods and drinks taste peculiarly sweet after they have indulged in this vegetable. Serious wine tasters ban artichokes prior to their samplings for this reason.

The reason for the artichoke effect is not known but has historically been attributed to the cynarin in it. Some suggest that it suppresses bitter taste receptors on the tongue, which makes other foods taste overly sweet. Others have proposed that sweet receptors on the tongue are stimulated. There was once excited talk over manufacture of a new artificial sweetener based on this effect in the 1970s, but apparently the prepared food industry has been unable or unwilling to benefit from it, because nothing has come of it.

For those who are vulnerable to this effect, fresh, steamed artichoke produces a dramatic effect, but marinated ones have no noticeable effect. The sweet flavor is most striking upon drinking water afterward, and while not exactly unpleasant, I think it has an odd, "chemical" taste, so I am not convinced any artificial sweetener related to it would be completely pleasing.

If you have gallstones, treat choleretics such as artichoke with caution. While some scientists recommend choleretics to prevent gallstone formation, others worry this could cause impaction, especially on an already blocked gallbladder. If you know you have gallstones or a bile duct obstruction, see a doctor. The German Commission E recommends people with these conditions take artichoke only under a doctor's advice.

EVIDENCE OF ACTION

There is good evidence that artichoke may lower cholesterol. In a placebo-controlled, randomized, double-blind trial of 143 adults whose initial cholesterol was greater than 280 mg/dL, those taking 1.8 grams of dry artichoke extract daily for six weeks significantly decreased their cholesterol, as well as LDL ("bad") cholesterol, with respect to the placebo takers.[1] Although many references loosely attribute this effect to a molecule in artichoke called *cynarin,* research does not clearly support cynarin as the active ingredient. Cynarin administered (250 mg and 750 mg daily) by itself had no effect on cholesterol or triglycerides in seventeen patients with familial cholesterolemia after three months in an older study.[2] However, another older but larger study found that of sixty patients with "various dislipidemic" problems, the thirty treated with cynarin fared better, with a significant reduction in cholesterol, than the thirty patients taking a placebo for fifty days.[3]

Artichoke molecules other than cynarin were found to mediate an effect similar to statin drugs used to lower cholesterol. Like statin drugs, an aqueous artichoke leaf extract inhibits an enzyme called *HMG CoA-reductase,* a liver enzyme that is used to make new cholesterol. However, to my knowledge, this enzymatic effect has not been tested for in humans, but was discovered in cultured rat liver cells. Cynarin itself was not able to inhibit HMG CoA-reductase, but cynaroside and particularly luteolin (the flavonoid obtained when cynaroside loses its attached sugar) did. The inhibition was not a direct effect on the enzyme, but in part resulted from luteolin inhibiting insulin's normal stimulatory effect on the enzyme.[4]

Commonly Reported Uses for Artichoke*

Internally
liver and gallbladder problems, improving bile flow, high cholesterol, indigestion, irritable bowel syndrome, atherosclerosis, diuretic
forms available for internal use:
capsule, tablet, tincture, often standardized to cynarin or caffeoylquinic acids, whole fresh plant
commonly reported dosage:
Two to three 100-milligram capsules daily, standardized to 15 milligrams of caffeoylquinic acids are commonly recommended. The fresh plant is steamed and the bud base is eaten along with the more tender leaves. The German Commission E monographs recommend 6 grams per day of dried cut leaves or pressed juice of the fresh plant.

*These uses and dosages are from historic use and are not necessarily tested nor recommended.

Artichoke also has enjoyed positive results for treating digestive complaints. In a placebo-controlled, randomized, double-blind trial, 129 patients with chronic indigestion significantly rated their indigestion less and their quality of life better after six weeks of taking 230 milligrams of artichoke leaf extract twice daily, compared to 115 dyspeptic patients who took a placebo.[5] Another large trial did not control with a placebo but randomly assigned 454 indigestion sufferers either 320 or 460 milligrams of artichoke leaf extract daily for two months. Both groups reported significantly improved digestion for all parameters measured.[6]

Irritable bowel syndrome (IBS) is a mysterious and nasty complaint, and those who suffer from it usually spend a lifetime cycling back and forth between diarrhea and constipation. Current treatments for IBS, like fiber therapy and intestinal nerve signal attenuators, are of limited effectiveness. A study that unfortunately did not use a control gave 279 IBS patients two capsules of 320 milligrams of artichoke leaf extract three times daily for six weeks, and they rated their IBS as significantly less.[7] Better-controlled studies of artichoke on IBS should be repeated to determine if this effect is worth discussing.

These cholesterol-lowering and indigestion-soothing effects of artichoke have both been attributed to, in part, its well-documented "choleretic" effect, that is, it increases the synthesis of bile. This theoretically could alleviate reduced bile flow, a condition called *cholestasis.* Artichoke's choleretic effect has been repeatedly observed in studies using rats.[8,9,10]

In addition, there is good evidence that some artichoke compounds are antioxidant.[11] Of particular significance is artichoke's ability to prevent the oxidation of LDL ("bad") cholesterol, a process that is part of the generation of atherosclerotic plaque. Researchers noted that a luteolin-rich artichoke extract, as well as luteolin alone, prevented LDL oxidation in vitro. The naturally occurring sugar-bound luteolin is also effective, but less so.[12] Besides preventing LDL oxidation, artichoke extract has reduced protein oxidation, elevated the antioxidant enzyme glutathione peroxidase with respect to controls, but not other antioxidant enzymes measured, in rats.[13] Another study on rats treated with oxidizing agents found that besides decreasing LDL oxidation, artichoke leaf extract prevented lipid peroxidation (a mechanism that oxidizes LDL and other lipids) and prevented depletion of the antioxidant glutathione.[14]

THE BOTTOM LINE

- Artichoke may lower cholesterol by inhibiting the same enzyme that prescription statins inhibit, although by a different mechanism. Like statins, it theoretically could decrease coenzyme Q synthesis, which is not ideal, but this has yet to be tested.
- Although artichoke supplements are most often standardized to cynarin, the active ingredient may be something else, like luteolin.
- Artichoke leaf extract acts as a choleretic, stimulating the flow of bile. It also contains antioxidants.
- Some authorities suggest that people with gallstones could be adversely affected by choleretics, so those with gallstones may find it prudent to avoid the plant and its extracts.
- Allergy to artichoke is not common but can develop, and those possessing allergies to plants in the daisy family should approach it with caution.

ASTRAGALUS

Astragalus membranaceus, Astragalus mongholicus

History and Folklore

This Asian member of the pea family (*Fabaceae* or *Leguminoseae*) is only now grabbing the attention of Western herbalists and doing so in a big way. Known as *milk vetch* in the West, it has been ignored until recently. Perhaps initial lack of interest stemmed from the fact that the western half of the United States harbors several species that are poisonous. The "locoweeds," *A. lentiginosus, A. lusitanicus,* and *A. miser,* menace livestock that dine on them, producing serious neurological disorders and birth defects. But rest assured that the medicinal species, *A. membranaceus* and *A. mongholicus,* do not contain the poisons swainsonine, miserotoxin, or toxic amounts of selenium that the locoweeds possess.

Better known as *haung qi* in China, astragalus root has been used for over two thousand years as food and medicine in Asia. The Chinese unearth four- to five-year old plants to harvest their dark, slightly sweet taproots. These are either cured in honey or sliced into long, thin, tongue depressor–shaped strips.

Traditional Chinese medicine holds that this root stimulates your life energy, or *qi,* and has warming properties. It is usually taken along with a great variety of several other herbs in traditional Asian medicine, which complicates the interpretation of Asian studies on astragalus. Astragalus has been historically used to combat fatigue and for protection against infection. These uses are still heavily promoted, along with a more modern claim that it helps those with heart disease.

How Scientists Think Astragalus Works

Astragalus certainly affects your immune system. This is good for some but bad for others. Studies have shown that astragalus increases the white blood cell count of volunteers consuming it. This could indeed be a boon for those with depressed immune function. If you do *not* have a compromised immune system, be wary of "immune stimulators." A normally functioning immune system protects you from microorganisms and cancer. Yet an overly aggressive immune system can wreak havoc on your body, like an out-of-control army running amok. Paradoxically, a chronically hyper-vigilant immune system generates inflammation and even initiates diseases such as cancer. Where the immune system is concerned, balance is the key.

Astragalus increases the activities of some types of immune cells and decreases the action of others. Though astragalus amplifies the numbers of some of your immune cells, your immune cells are not all identical. As in a hypothetical army, some soldiers may be better at hand-to-hand combat, while others are better at using long-distance weapons. Your immune cells are like this, each possessing various specialties. Astragalus recruits some types and reduces others by altering your cytokine levels.

Cytokines are proteins that dramatically change the numbers and activities of your immune cells. But they are a complicated bunch, because there are dozens of different ones, often with opposing actions, and each typically affects several others. Many studies show that astragalus implements a shift in their balance. Astragalus increases a category of cytokines called *Th-1 cytokines,* and decreases Th-2 cytokines. Both types have their good side and their bad side. A healthy immune system is supposed to use both types and to be flexible switching them.

Astragalus is said to help you regain your Th-1/Th-2 immune system balance if you are Th-2 dominant. Keep in mind that the Th-1/Th-2 concept is now being reevaluated as immunologists eye it more critically. It is an old paradigm that has been oversimplified and does not always hold true. Enough of the theory does work for it to be useful in several circumstances, however. Here is what Th-2 dominance is supposed to do.

A Th-2-stimulated immune system protects you from nasty things that don't make it inside your cells, like certain parasites and bacteria. It also helps you make antibodies against pathogens. The bad side of Th-2 is that it predisposes you toward allergies and asthma. So taking astragalus might theoretically help you with allergies and asthma, though there is little data on this effect: There is only one mouse study suggesting that this might be so.[1]

Most people are normally somewhat "Th-1 dominant." Th-1 cytokines stimulate your immune system to protect you from strange things that get *inside* your cells, like viruses, cancer, and certain types of bacteria (mycoplasma). The bad thing about Th-1 dominance is that it can launch an immune attack against your own body, and you can wind up with autoimmune diseases, organ transplant rejection, or even fetus rejection. Indeed, women normally temporarily switch away from Th-1 dominance to Th-2 dominance during pregnancy. When they do not, they risk miscarriage. Since astragalus stimulates the

Th-1 immune system, some scientists suggest those who have organ transplants or skin grafts should not take it and that pregnant women should be wary of it, too.

Astragalus may thin your blood and lower your blood pressure. Cultured human cells increase a clot-busting substance called *tPA* (tissue plasminogen activator) when exposed to astragalus extract, so astragalus is expected to have some blood-thinning power. In clinical studies astragalus also decreased the synthesis of the blood pressure–raising hormone vasopressin (also called *antidiuretic hormone*) in rats with heart failure. In the same rats, astragalus also increased the sensitivity of their kidneys to a chemical distress call from the heart, atrial natriuretic peptide, by increasing the kidney's receptors for it. This hormone is made when the heart is stretched by high blood pressure, and the kidneys respond to it by increasing urine output. The resultant decrease in blood volume lowers your blood pressure.

GOOD EFFECTS . . .
AND NOT SO GOOD

Astragalus has been valued as a food and medicine for more than two thousand years and has a very good safety record. Also, large doses have been given to rats, and they were none the worse for it. The two medicinal forms, *A. membranaceus* and *A. mongholicus,* do not contain the toxic molecules found in other species, such as those found in the United States ("locoweed"), which devastate livestock that dine on them. But there are still precautions.

If you are pregnant, or if you are a transplant patient or a skin graft recipient, you should not take astragalus. Because astragalus stimulates the branch of the immune system that is implicated in organ transplant rejection, scientists are beginning to worry about transplant patients taking this herb. No studies have assessed this herb's risk of provoking miscarriages. However, this type of immune system stimulation also increases the risk of miscarriage. Therefore it seems wise to avoid astragalus if you are pregnant.

What's In It

ASTRAGALUS CONTAINS several triterpene glycosides (otherwise known as *saponins*), a class of molecules that are frequently prime suspects as active ingredients in other herbs. These include brachyoside A, B, and C, cyclocephaloside II, astrachrysoside A, astragalosides, cyclocanthoside, soyasaponin, and cycloastragenol. It also possesses various isoflavonoids, another class of molecules that are often antioxidant and protective, including astrasieversianin, as well as the phytosterols daucosterol and beta-sitosterol

Avoid astragalus if you have an autoimmune disease or take blood-thinning medication. Immune-stimulating herbs can make autoimmune diseases worse. Also, since astragalus may thin your blood, some scientists worry that you can overdo this effect if you also take astragalus.

If your immune system is chronically weak, or if you have asthma or allergies, astragalus might help you, but the small amount of good evidence for this effect is overblown. Astragalus does stimulate the immune system, but the number of well-designed studies on this effect in humans is distressingly low. Mediocre results from poorly designed cell and animal studies have

been blown out of proportion by—guess who—people trying to sell you the stuff.

Commonly Reported Uses for Astragalus*

Internally
fatigue, infection, heart problems, diuretic, immune stimulation
forms available for internal use:
capsule, concentrated drops, decoction, extract, fresh and cured root, candied root, powder, tea, tincture
commonly reported dosage:
Either 1 to 4 grams of dried root or one dropperful of tincture is usually taken two to three times a day. Traditional Chinese medicine usually prescribes 9 to 15 grams of the dried root, which is simmered in a quart of water until the water is reduced to one-fourth the original volume.

*These uses and dosages are from historic use and are not necessarily tested nor recommended.

Astragalus might mend a damaged heart. Clinical and mechanistic studies support astragalus for lowering blood pressure and thinning the blood. One clinical study showed that heart patients suffered less angina (chest pain) when they were given astragalus, and other studies show improved heart function, too.

Astragalus is still an unknown. There are hundreds of studies on astragalus, but most are done on isolated cells or animals, have no controls, and are poorly designed. This does not mean that astragalus does not work. It means that better-designed studies need to be performed.

EVIDENCE OF ACTION

There are hundreds of published studies on astragalus. However, a majority of these do not use a control group, which is essential in order to determine whether an effect is truly significant. Also, most use mixtures of several different herbs, leaving it impossible for you to sort out which herb is doing what, assuming they don't actually interact with each other. As if that were not enough, most inject the herbs, and injected herbs are metabolized quite differently than those that you eat. Most people around the world take astragalus orally. It is irresponsible to use such studies to make definitive claims for astragalus, yet many people who are trying to sell you astragalus do so anyway.

From the small handful of better-designed human studies in which astragalus alone is taken orally, it seems that astragalus does stimulate your immune system. This lends credibility to its use against pathogen-based diseases and cancer. Increasing doses of pure astragalus preparation were seen to provoke greater elevations in white blood cell counts of 115 patients that originally had low white blood cell counts.[2] Also, a study showed that immune-stimulatory T-cells were significantly increased, while other, immune-suppressing T-cells were decreased with respect to healthy controls when viral myocarditis patients were treated with oral astragalus.[3]

Astragalus might have positive effects on heart function, too, though in general these studies are not well designed. It increased cardiac output of angina patients.[4] It also improved the heart function of those with heart failure.[5] In addition, astragalus improved the water-sodium balance in rats with heart failure.[6]

THE BOTTOM LINE

- Astragalus stimulates the immune system. This increases your defense against pathogenic organisms and cancer, which is good, but it can also increase inflammation, which is not so good.
- Astragalus alters the amounts of different immune-stimulating cytokines that you produce. It stimulates the Th-1 cytokines, which are said to protect against intracellular pathogens, like viruses and certain types of bacteria, yet Th-1 cytokines are implicated in organ transplant rejection and miscarriage. Astragalus inhibits the production of Th-2 cytokines, which are thought to defend against extracellular pathogens, but Th-2 cytokines may exacerbate allergies and asthma.
- Astragalus may have positive effects on the heart. It may increase your clot-busting tPA levels, and decrease a blood pressure–raising hormone called *vasopressin*. It also may lower blood pressure by acting as a diuretic, by increasing your kidneys' sensitivity to your atrial natriuretic peptide hormone.
- Astragalus should not be taken by pregnant women, people with organ transplants or skin grafts, or people with autoimmune diseases, or by those on blood-thinning medication.

BILBERRY

Vaccinium myrtillus

History and Folklore

At first glance you might mistake a bilberry for a blueberry, except closer examination will reveal the bilberry—a smaller relative of the blueberry—is blue throughout, whereas blueberries' skins hide white flesh. And if you were blindfolded and tasted bilberries, you might mistake them for cranberries. All three berries are close relatives, sharing the genus *Vaccinium,* in the family *Ericaceae.* Though not as popular as its cousins, you can run across bilberry-based foods here and there throughout Europe and North America, particularly in colder places like Canada, Washington, Oregon, and Scandinavia.

Historical opinions about bilberry are hard to interpret, because its genus has around 150 different species, including the blueberry and the cranberry, and ancient writings interchange their common names to the extent that you can't tell which one is the subject of the intended reference. Their colorful nicknames persist; in England you call them whortleberries, and traditionally eat them with cream. In Scotland, ask for blaeberries, and in northwestern American states, huckleberries. Bilberry is the name most often used by herbalists, which comes from the Danish *bollebar,* meaning dark berry.

The first thing you will probably hear about bilberries is that they are good for your eyes. But bilberry has also commonly been used for diarrhea, constipation, urinary tract infections, and varicose veins. These uses are frequently submerged amid the more romantic anecdotes of British

Royal Air Force pilots using it, however. World War II pilots ate bilberry jam before flying night missions, and a legend spread that this helped them see in the dark.

How Scientists Think Bilberry Works

If you have diarrhea, bilberries might bring it to a stop. Bilberry's tannins have a historic reputation for ending diarrhea. Many plants make tannins to protect them-selves, but some plants simply have more tannins than others. Bilberry is one of these plants, but many other berrylike plants, such as grapes, blueberries and raspberries, have them as well. You might be familiar with how tannins make your mouth feel strangely dry—a quality called astringency—and they also taste slightly bitter. You can get even more tannins from the leaves and stems of bilberry and other berries. To procure the water-soluble tannins from bilberries, you can make a tea out of the berries, stems, or leaves.

After you consume them, tannins create a temporary, physical barrier lining your diges-tive tract, sort of like a temporary, tough coating. This dries out your gut's secretions and minimizes its contact with irritants that could cause diarrhea. Tannins "tan your hide" by binding to several proteins at once, tying them together and tightening the tissue. This is what gives tannins their skin-tightening astringency. Tannins also hog-tie the proteins of an herbivorous bug or plant pathogen, disabling them and protecting the plant, which is probably why plants bother to make them.

Tannins should be used with caution, however, because some people find them especially irritating. You may find yourself in even more digestive distress than before, should you try to use tannins from bilberry, or any other source for that matter, in excess. Concentrated tannins can chemically aggravate your mucous membranes—use them in moderation.

Paradoxically, you can use bilberry fruit to treat constipation or diarrhea—but you have to use the right form. Bilberries can either speed the transit of your digestive contents or slow them down, depending on whether the berries are dried or fresh. Pectin is the component of bilberry that has the potential to regulate your intestinal traffic speed. You may have some familiarity with pectin if you make jam or jelly. Pectin may be purchased in a dry powder form and is found in most grocery stores. It thickens liquids, turning them into a gel. Fruits already have pectin, but some fruits have more than others. So if you are making a fruit jam or jelly, you might add pectin just to be sure it gels properly. Bilberries are already loaded with the stuff.

Pectin is a linear chain of three hundred to one thousand sugar molecules bonded together, quite a large molecule. Your digestive tract can't break the links of this chain to use its individual sugars for energy, so the chain goes right through you, and thus is classified as "fiber." Pectin's sugars are electrostatically attracted to water, and when consumed in a relatively dry form, pectin will not only attract excess water but will also adsorb or adhere to irritants that might be causing your diarrhea, making the the irritants less irritating. Indeed, pectin is used in some antidiarrheal medicines, such as Kaopectate.

Interesting Facts

To see better in the dark, look away.

It is not officially known if bilberry can help your night vision, but if you really want to see something better in the dark and you don't have time to pop an herb, don't look at what you want to see. You are better off not looking directly at faint objects at night, so use your peripheral vision. Your retinas have two light-gathering types of cells: the rods and the cones. The cones are better at seeing color, but you can't see color at night, so cones do not do you much good then. The rhodopsin-containing rods, however, discern shades of gray and are found in greater numbers around the edges of your retina rather than in the center.

Try looking directly at a faint star, and then look just off to the side of it. This is an old trick used by astronomers everywhere. I found it a little frustrating at first, but it truly works, so it is worth practicing. Stars will always just look like points of light, even through a telescope, because they are so far away. But you will see them better with peripheral vision. If you are viewing objects through a telescope that have more detail than stars, like planets, nebulae, or galaxies, you will see much more detail by not looking directly at them. As a longtime amateur astronomer myself, I swear this works, but it takes a lot of practice. I know astronomers who, for a double whammy, take bilberry regularly, too. It can't hurt.

Which form of bilberry should you use, dried or fresh? Think of pectin as being like a sponge. A wet sponge releases water, but a dry one absorbs it. If you are having watery diarrhea, the dry pectin in a small handful of dried bilberries can suck up excess moisture and slow your food's transit to a reasonable speed. Go easy on the dried berries, though. Even in a normally functioning gut, the presence of too many dried bilberries there will suck water right through your gut lining, filling your digestive tract with water and bulky, slippery, water-filled bilberries, giving you diarrhea again. Moderation is the key.

What's In It

Bilberry contains tannins, pectin, and flavonoid glycosides, including at least fifteen anthocyanins, which provide the fruit its color. When removed from the sugar they are bound to, the anthocyanins are called *anthocyani*dins. The anthocyanins known represent all the possible combinations of five anthocyanidins (cyanidin, delphinidin, peonidin, petunidin, malvidin) with three types of sugars (arabinose, glucose, and galactose) attached by their third oxygen (creating 3-O-arabinosides, 3-O-glucosides, 3-O-galactosides).

If your digestive tract is excessively dry, its contents may crawl through at a pace you find distressingly slow. Wet pectin from fresh bilberry fruits furnishes the moisture needed to speed everything along. Fresh bilberry fruits already have water clinging to pectin, so like wet sponges, they are swollen to their maximum size. Thus they also act as bulking agents, a gentle type of laxative. Bulky things stretch the lining of your digestive tract, activating receptors that are sensitive to this stretching ("stretch receptors"). This stimulates the involuntary muscular contractions that prompt the departure of these gut-stretching items. The effect can be overdone: After quickly gobbling too many delicious, pectin-containing bilberries, you may find yourself a mere vehicle for transporting the fruits to the toilet.

Anthocyanins give bilberry its color, and they can do several good things for you. They might even help your vision. These molecules are what give most fruits and flowers red, blue, or purple hues. Bilberry fruits, which are highly colored throughout, are a good source of them. Anthocyanins (also called *anthocyanosides*) are ubiquitous in nature; they impart their color to a great many fruits, like plums, grapes, and most berries, and are responsible for coloring the majority of red, blue, and purple flower petals. Anthocyanins are classified as flavonoids because of the design of their carbon rings. Flavonoids are a broader category of molecules that come in a wider variety of colors, and are ubiquitous in plant-based foods but are gaining positive reputations for their high concentrations in red wine and chocolate. Like other flavonoids, bilberry's anthocyanins are antioxidant and scavenge free radicals, protecting you from toxins both internally generated and from your environment.

One study on bilberry found its anthocyanin production was increased by increasing the berries' exposure to sunlight, and the authors hypothesized that bilberry makes these molecules to protect itself from radiation damage. This is interesting, because sometimes you can actually eat a plant's radiation-protecting molecules and usurp their protective power, at least to some extent. However, carotenoids, which are different, non-flavonoid pigments found in higher concentrations in *other* plants, such as carrots and tomatoes, currently have a better reputation for this effect. Like eating sunscreen for your eyes, consuming carotenoids shields your eyes from radiation and other sorts of damage. The evidence supporting anthocyanins' ability to defend your eyes in this manner is still sketchy, but theoretically they could help, and they probably can't hurt.

Commonly Reported Uses for Bilberry*

Internally

diarrhea, laxative, vision problems, diabetes

forms available for use:

capsules standardized to either anthocyanin (also called *anthocyanosides*) or anthocyanidin (concentrated extracts are generally standardized to contain 25 percent anthocyanidins, the equivalent of 37 percent anthocyanins), fresh or dried berries, dried berry powder, dried leaf tea

commonly reported dosage:

For vision problems, 500-milligram standardized capsules are often recommended, up to twice a day. For diarrhea, dried berries or tea is consumed. For constipation, fresh berries are eaten.

---

*These uses and dosages are from historic use and are not necessarily tested nor recommended.

If you are like most people, as you get older you typically can't see as well as you used to. Damage to your retinas accumulates over time, from oxidizing agents, free radicals, and radiation (sunlight), which generate these things. Bilberry's reputed vision-aiding effect could simply be a consequence of its anthocyanins slowing the ongoing destruction of your retinas. Besides being antioxidant and free radical–scavenging, anthocyanins induce your synthesis of antioxidant enzymes such as quinone reductase.

Some of bilberry's anthocyanins regenerate rhodopsin, your night vision pigment. Will bilberry help your night vision, like it did for the legendary jam-eating World War II flying aces? One study showed that some anthocyanins accelerate the regeneration of rhodopsin in frogs' retinas. Frog retinas are not human ones, but rhodopsin is at least the same pigment your retinas use for night vision. Also, these anthocyanins were from black currants, not bilberries, but bilberry does contain the same anthocyanins used in the study, so they theoretically could work the same way.

The quercetin in bilberries is antioxidant, free radical–scavenging, plus it inhibits an eye-damaging enzyme. Quercetin is another flavonoid that is present in many plant foods, and people are starting to publicize its possible health benefits. Bilberries are a good source of quercetin, but if you can't get your hands on bilberries, so are apples, onions, raspberries, black and green tea, citrus fruits, red grapes, red wine, cherries, leafy greens, and broccoli. This flavonoid's antioxidant and radical-scavenging potential has created a market for quercetin supplements, which are now growing popular. However, no one is sure how much quercetin to take, and taking too much of certain free radical scavengers like quercetin can theoretically turn them into free radicals and pro-oxidants themselves, which is bad.

Quercetin is still recommended—but from food, not quercetin supplements. The quercetin in bilberries also supports this herb's reputation as an eye protector. Quercetin inhibits an enzyme called *aldose reductase.* This enzyme is normally present in your eyes and in several other body parts. It changes glucose into an alcohol called sorbitol, but too much *sorbitol* in your eyes or nerves causes retinopathy or nerve damage, respectively. This is especially a problem for people with high blood sugar: The excess glucose in their blood is more likely to be altered into eye-damaging sorbitol by aldose reductase. Some diabetics use aldose reductase inhibitors to prevent vision problems associated with the disease. So, theoretically, bilberry could protect your eyes with its quercetin.

Good Effects . . .
and Not So Good

Recommended doses of bilberry are probably quite safe. Large doses of anthocyanins from bilberry have been given to rats, and they did not appear to suffer ill consequences. The leaves, on the other hand, have caused wasting and death when given to animals in high doses over a long period of time. Perhaps because of their tannins, the leaves and fruit can cause distress, so use them in moderation.

Use bilberry fruits in moderation. Too many berries, dried or fresh, can exacerbate digestive problems, so take only a small handful. Too much bilberry tea can irritate your gut with its tannins, so drink one cup slowly and observe how you feel; some people are more sensitive to tannins than others.

If you want to take bilberry anthocyanins for vision, it may or may not work, but it probably will not hurt you.

Just make sure that you find a preparation standardized to anthocyanins, since these are its proposed vision-aiding agents.

Evidence of Action

Although there are around thirty clinical trials testing bilberry constituents on human night vision, most of the studies are quite old and poorly designed. For example, many used no placebo and relied on subjective responses of the subjects rather than instruments that objectively measure dark adaptation. A comprehensive review[1] of the better-designed studies notes that only one of five non-placebo, randomized clinical trials showed better dark adaptation, and though the positive study[2] was old, it did use a higher dose of bilberry (400 mg per day) than the studies that had negative outcomes (12 to 160 mg per day).[3, 4, 5, 6] Seven placebo-controlled trials also used higher doses, except for one, and all of these showed positive effects of bilberry on vision, but lacked a "rigorous design," which means they are still questionable.[7, 8, 9, 10, 11, 12, 13]

Animal studies indicate that there is at least some theoretical basis for bilberry improving night vision. The retinas of rats treated with bilberry extract contained more rhodopsin, the night vision pigment, than those not given the extract.[14] Also, bilberry reportedly gave lab animals faster dark adaptation.[15, 16, 17] Anthocyanins from black currant (cyanidin-3-glycosides) increased rhodopsin regeneration,[18] and these particular molecules are also present in bilberry. In addition, bilberry reduced the damaging oxidation of retina pigment caused by singlet oxygen in cell culture.[19] Human trials using bilberry, however, currently render its effects on vision ambiguous.

There is tentative evidence that anthocyanins from bilberry and related berries have anticancer effects, as they induce cancer cells to "commit suicide" (apoptosis) in cell culture,[20] and a mixed berry extract containing bilberry prevents blood vessel growth,[21] a process tumors stimulate to enhance their survival.

THE BOTTOM LINE

- Tannins in bilberries may "tan" the lining of the digestive tract, protecting it, but they can also irritate it. Dry pectin in dried berries can absorb excess water from diarrhea, and moisture-laden pectin in fresh berries adds bulk to stools, relieving constipation.
- The reddish-purple anthocyanin pigments in bilberries are antioxidant and free radical–scavenging, and theoretically could help eyesight, although that has not been clearly shown.
- When taken in moderation, bilberry is a relatively safe herb.

BLACK COHOSH

Actaea racemosa (formerly *Cimicifuga racemosa*)

History and Folklore

Native Americans regarded this tall, striking, and slightly unpleasant-smelling member of the buttercup family as medicine. Indeed, "cohosh" is a Native American designation for a medicinal plant. The plant's dark, twisted roots produced the nicknames "rattlesnake root" and "black snakeroot," and its alleged bug-repelling odor gave it further appellations of "bugbane" and the Latin genus *Cimicifuga*, which means "bedbug repellant." Native Americans used black cohosh decoctions in a number of ways, such as for snakebite, indigestion, and cold symptoms, and in a steam bath for arthritis pains. However, black cohosh was mainly used for so-called female discomforts.

Perhaps because of this, black cohosh was included as a primary ingredient in Lydia Pinkham's Vegetable Compound, sold to millions of women for a couple of generations, between 1875 and the 1920s. This was claimed to *"cure entirely the worst form of Female Complaints, all Ovarian troubles, Inflammation and Ulceration, Falling and Displacements, and the consequent Spinal Weakness, and is particularly adapted to the Change of Life."* This product contained as much as 20 percent alcohol, greatly enhancing its appeal, if not its affect on "Falling and Displacements." Lydia Pinkham (a member of the temperance movement) defended this ingredient as a required "solvent and preservative."

An apparent reincarnation of black cohosh that is almost as popular as Lydia Pinkham's Compound once was is the non-alcoholic, German *Remifemin,* and other black cohosh products marketed with vague suggestions of doing something mysteriously good for women have emerged as well. It's likely that black cohosh contaminated with other species may have helped spread misinformation that black cohosh acts like estrogen and contains estrogenic ingredients. It apparently does not. Yet it may help some women by other mechanisms.

How Scientists Think Black Cohosh Works

How can black cohosh alleviate "female complaints" when it has no estrogenic activity? Like other scientists, I had taken for granted an idea that I had heard for years: that black cohosh contained some sort of estrogen-like ingredients. This provided a satisfying explanation for why many women claimed black cohosh reduced their hot flashes. Hot flashes are linked with low estrogen—for example, during menopause or while on the breast cancer drug tamoxifen, which blocks estrogen's receptors. So the growing number of scientific publications insisting that black cohosh did not have any obvious estrogenic activity baffled us all.

Where's the phytoestrogen? It isn't there. Previously, respectable scientists observed formononetin, a "phytoestrogen," or plant estrogen, in black cohosh, but this probably resulted from unintentional contamination with other look-alike plants. Dutiful analytical chemists consequently attempted to quantify the formononetin in black cohosh, only to find it missing. One paper reports that after testing thirteen different black cohosh preparations, as well as the popular German treatment *Remifemin,* none contained any of the estrogenic formononetin as was previously believed.[1] Other papers confirm black cohosh's formononetin levels are essentially zero.

Black cohosh just does not act like estrogen. Studies in animals and women further disclosed that black cohosh does not affect their uterine cells, as does estrogen, and previous observations that black cohosh lowered luteinizing hormone (LH) levels, as estrogen does, could not be confirmed in subsequent studies. Female rats without ovaries, deprived of their usual estrogen, could not avoid their rat version of menopause with black cohosh. Black cohosh doesn't affect other sex hormones either, like follicle-stimulating hormone (FSH), prolactin, androgens, or estrogen itself. Black cohosh doesn't have anything that binds in any dramatic way to estrogen receptors either. Although some constituents of the extract weakly cling to at least one subtype of estrogen receptors, this induces very little, if any, estrogenic effect and may even block estrogen, though it's more likely the effect is imperceptible. Nor does black cohosh "up regulate" or increase the number of estrogen receptors.

It's the serotonin, silly. It turns out scientists may have been looking in the wrong place. Lately, it's come out that menopausal women who take antidepressant drugs that boost the hormone serotonin, such as selective serotonin reuptake inhibitor (SSRI) drugs, have fewer and less intense hot flashes. Indeed, these antidepressants are now being prescribed "off label" to treat hot flashes. Their effect on the brain's thermostat should not have been much of a surprise, since it has long been known that serotonin's binding to

subsets of its receptors in the brain's hypothalamus cools you down. Yet it was a surprise for researchers to learn that black cohosh has serotonin-like activity, too. Some as-yet-unidentified ingredients in black cohosh were found to bind to serotonin receptors, in cell cultures, partially activating at least one type of serotonin receptor.[2] Thus there might be something to the rumors that black cohosh reduces hot flashes, after all.

Maybe black cohosh's apparent lack of estrogenic action is a blessing in disguise. You have probably heard that the 2002 Women's Health Initiative study discovered that the once fabulously popular hormone replacement therapy for menopausal women is risky, increasing the likelihood of heart disease and stroke, and thus recommended only for severe menopausal symptoms and for short time periods only. Also, estrogen stimulates cell division in certain tissues, increasing the risk of forming breast, uterine, or ovarian tumors.

What's In It

BLACK COHOSH has none of the phytoestrogen formononetin, as was formerly reported. Its active ingredients are not known but are often presumed to be in its triterpene glycosides, including actein, 27-deoxyactein, and cimifugoside, typically bonded to xylose or arabinose. It also contains caffeic acid derivatives, including caffeic acid, ferulic acid, isoferulic acid, fukinolic acid, cimicifugic acid A, and cimicifugic acid B. The root also possesses the quinolizidine alkaloids cystisine and methyl cytisine.

Now menopausal women jumping off the hormone replacement therapy boat are in a bind: What can they take? The problem with estrogenic alternative herbs is that they may theoretically be just as bad as synthetic hormones, since both synthetic and herbal molecules can activate estrogen receptors in the same way, and scientists are sincerely worried about this. The good news for all of black cohosh's lack of estrogenic action is that black cohosh is unlikely to stimulate estrogen-sensitive diseases, like endometriosis, uterine fibroids, or cancers of the breast, uterus, or ovaries. Indeed, animal studies show that black cohosh extracts do not stimulate estrogen-sensitive tumors.[3] In fact, these extracts inhibited the growth of tested breast cancer cell lines,[4, 5] and one prostate cancer cell line,[6] at least in cell culture studies.

Commonly Reported Uses for Black Cohosh*

Internally

    so-called female discomforts:
    menopause, premenstrual syndrome,
    painful menstruation
    forms available for internal use:
    capsules, decoction, dried or powdered
    root, tincture
    commonly reported dosage:
    Most studies have used black cohosh
    standardized to 1 milligram of triterpene
    glycosides per 20-milligram tablet; one
    to three of these are taken daily for up
    to six months.

*These uses and dosages are from historic use and are not necessarily tested nor recommended.

The bone mystery remains. Unfortunately, estrogen is good in that it helps you build bone, so given black cohosh's dubious estrogenic power, it's debatable whether black cohosh can help limit osteoporosis. Doctors are now being advised to warn their patients that because black cohosh doesn't act like estrogen, you shouldn't expect it to prevent osteoporosis.[7] Nonetheless, some preliminary studies suggest black cohosh could have a positive influence on bone growth. If this is true, we don't yet know how black cohosh does this.

Black cohosh may be anti-inflammatory, at least in theory. In a limited number of cell studies, black cohosh extracts scavenge damaging free radicals, and its fukinolic acid proved to be a potent elastase inhibitor. Elastase is important in the generation of inflammatory responses, and it breaks down various proteins, such as elastin, a structural protein that helps your tissues stay young and springy. Whether this means that black cohosh helps preserve your own tissues requires further investigation.

Good Effects . . . and Not So Good

Long-term use of black cohosh has unknown effects. Other members of the buttercup family (*Ranunculaceae*) are toxic, and the safety of black cohosh has not been thoroughly investigated. Because of this, most herb experts recommend you do not take black cohosh for a prolonged period of time. Since most clinical studies have lasted no longer than six months, the consensus medical opinion is that you should not take it for longer than six months.

Watch out for the following. Most people taking black cohosh in moderate doses don't suffer side effects. Stomach upset is an occasional complaint, but nausea and vomiting have also been reported. Pregnant and nursing women should always check with their doctor first before taking any herb or supplement, and black cohosh is no exception. Large doses have been linked with miscarriage, so don't take this herb if you are pregnant. Because its hormonal effects are still being investigated, don't take it if you are nursing either. One case report associated a woman's serious liver inflammation with her taking black cohosh, yet it remains unknown whether her product was contaminated or adulterated, or if in fact other factors contributed to her hepatitis[8]. Older literature cautions anyone with estrogen-sensitive diseases to avoid the herb, because it was once assumed to be estrogenic, though that now appears less likely to be true.

Black cohosh may relieve your hot flashes, but if you are worried about osteoporosis, let a doctor monitor your progress. There is moderately good evidence that black cohosh may reduce hot flashes. However, it's not clear whether it can help prevent osteoporosis. If you are taking black cohosh and are vulnerable to osteoporosis, your doctor should be monitoring your diet, exercise, medications, and bone density on a regular basis anyway.

As always, seek a quality product. Most clinical studies have used products standardized to black cohosh's triterpene glycosides, although we don't yet know if those are the active ingredients. Standardized ingredients are not a guarantee of quality, but they are probably a better indication of quality than unstandardized ones. Do not confuse black cohosh with blue cohosh, an unrelated, toxic plant.

Evidence of Action

All though there are over half a dozen studies of black cohosh for treating menopausal symptoms, many are not well designed; for example, some do not use a placebo group, or they are not blinded as to who is taking what, which reduces the effectiveness of a placebo.[9] The omission of an effective placebo group is serious when testing menopausal treatments, because hot flashes, while very measurably real and at times agonizing, are more vulnerable to the amazing power of mind over body, than other problems, like bone loss. The placebo group in studies examining treatments for hot flashes often tends to fare surprisingly well, for example.

Though to some extent these studies are flawed, some do suggest black cohosh is comparable to estrogen in reducing hot flashes. Yet biochemical tests on the women taking black cohosh reveal no obvious estrogenic effects of the herb, such as any change in the vaginal or uterine lining. Theoretically, interaction with serotonin receptors could explain black cohosh's hot flash–abating action, yet this still requires more study. One study showed breast cancer survivors on or off of tamoxifen fared no better than the placebo group for reduction of hot flashes, yet both groups did in fact suffer fewer hot flashes.[10]

While black cohosh may well reduce hot flashes, you might guess it is theoretically less likely to prevent osteoporosis, given its lack of obvious estrogenic action. However, a study of rats that had had their ovaries removed demonstrated that black cohosh extract was comparable to the prescription anti-osteoporotic, estrogenic drug raloxifene in reducing bone degradation.[11] Also, a large double-blind, randomized study of menopausal women showed that bone metabolism markers in their blood were improved by taking black cohosh compared to placebo, to levels almost comparable to those women who were taking estrogen.[12]

Although black cohosh is often suggested for treating premenstrual syndrome (PMS) and menstrual problems, there are only a few, isolated case reports supporting this. There are no trials investigating this use, so the value of black cohosh for treating menstrual problems remains an unknown.

THE BOTTOM LINE

- For women undergoing menopause, black cohosh may reduce the occurrence of hot flashes. It is less clear that it can prevent osteoporosis.
- Black cohosh probably does not work by an estrogenic mechanism, as was previously thought, nor does it contain the phytoestrogen formononetin. It may work by targeting serotonin receptors in the brain's hypothalamus that control body temperature.
- Don't take black cohosh for longer than six months, and let your doctor know you are taking it. Avoid it if you are nursing or pregnant.

BORAGE
Borago officinalis

History and Folklore

Borage is a very pretty European native plant. Its star-shaped flowers are strikingly blue and often said to be the inspiration for artists painting the blue robe of the Virgin Mary. Some references say the word "borage" stems from a Gaelic term *borrach,* or "proud man," suggesting the herb gives you courage. The *bor* in borage could also be derived from "burr," referring to its hairy stem.

Borage is most often associated with bringing courage and gladness. It was once a more common comestible, with cool, pleasant, cucumber-tasting leaves that I confess I've enjoyed, on occasion, in salads. The flowers are also edible and were once more often used as a food decoration, sometimes candied, or included in ice cubes to make drinks more festive. Borage was often included in alcoholic drinks, particularly the claret cup, and something called a "stirrup cup," a farewell drink given to embolden a mounted rider preparing to depart on a journey.

It may be for the best, however, that eating borage is no longer so popular. A charmingly outdated and desperately optimistic 1971 herb book that wowed me as a child—this book had nothing but good things to say about *every* herb—enthused that "its vitamin content, still to be explored, is probably substantial."[1] I don't know about its vitamin content, but I do know it contains traces of toxic pyrrolizidine alkaloids, which can damage your liver. Thus you probably shouldn't eat it on a regular basis.

Historic references abound with borage's ability to make one glad or courageous, such as the cute little couplet *"Ego Borago, Gaudia semper ago,"* or "I, borage, always bring courage." Its modern use, however, has been refined toward its seed oil, which is an uncommonly good natural source of gammalinolenic acid, otherwise known as *GLA.* Most plants don't have such high concentrations of GLA; black currant seeds and evening primrose seeds are the only other places in nature where you can find a lot of it. GLA is also a central fatty acid in human and animal metabolism, so many have hoped GLA supplementation confers health benefits.

How Scientists Think Borage Works

Borage seed oil is one of only a few good sources of dietary gammalinolenic acid (GLA), but this does not mean you need it. GLA is a fatty acid, and you make it from an *essential* fatty acid (that is, one that you need in your diet because you can't synthesize it on your own) called *linoleic acid.* However, your diet is probably not deficient in this essential fatty acid. Linoleic acid is abundant—many nutritionists are saying far *too* abundant—in the diets of people living in developed countries. On one hand, it's far better for you to have essential fatty acids than nonessential ones, such as the notorious heart-stopping saturated fatty acids found in animal fats, and the even scarier trans fats created by partially hydrogenating oils that are now drenching many fast and processed foods. On the other hand, not all essential fatty acids are created equal.

Borage seed oil is loaded with both GLA and linoleic acid, and both are omega-6 fatty acids. Omega-3 fatty acids are far better, although both are essential. Fatty acids are characterized by the lengths of their chains of carbons and how these carbons are linked together; they are joined with either single bonds, making a fatty acid more "saturated," or double bonds, making a fatty acid "unsaturated." Like most animals, we make mainly saturated fatty acids—the ones without double bonds. We can make a limited number of unsaturated fatty acids, too. Although our enzymes can place double bonds in the middle of the chains, they just can't put a double bond close to the end—called the "omega" position—of a long chain. Unfortunately, we need both omega-6 fatty acids (which have a double bond located six carbons from the end) and omega-3 fatty acid (which have a double bond three carbons from the end) in order to live, making these two classes of fatty acids essential in our diet.

Authorities now are raising an alarm, saying that the modern diet contains too much omega-6 fatty acids and too few omega-3 fatty acids. Experts speculate that our diets once possessed a 1:1 ratio of omega-6 to omega-3 fatty acids, which now is skewed as high as 10:1 or 20:1, depending on who you talk to, in favor of omega-6s. This is because the vegetable oils that modern society has recently become so skillful at harvesting and using in processed foods—corn oil, safflower oil, soybean oil, and sunflower oil—are loaded with the omega-6 fatty acid linoleic acid (not to be confused with the popular and dubious weight loss supplement *conjugated* linoleic acid, or CLA, which is completely different).

Also, feeding livestock corn, a source of omega-6 oil, rather than their preferred grass enables even our commercial meat supply to be loaded with omega-6s. Grass-fed livestock has more omega-3s.

What's wrong with omega-6 fatty acids? The linoleic acid abundant in borage seed oil, as well as in the modern diet, gets concentrated in the "bad" cholesterol carrier, LDL, and goes on to get oxidized to form harmful free radicals and atherosclerotic plaque. It is also associated with the formation of cancer and tumor growth. There is also a problem with the hormone-like molecules it generates: Both classes of essential fatty acids, the omega-3s and the omega-6s, are used to make 20-carbon fatty acids, which can go on to make short-lived, hormone-like molecules called *eicosanoids*. These have dramatic and various contrasting effects on blood pressure, blood clotting, pain and inflammation, allergic and immune responses, uterine and gastrointestinal cramps, digestion, brain development and mental state, even tumor development and growth. To say the least, they have many powerful effects! The omega-6 fatty acids tend to make pro-inflammatory, damaging eicosanoids. The eicosanoids made from omega-3 fatty acids are more anti-inflammatory and protective in general. Therefore, long-term supplementation with borage oil, which contains a fatty acid that you already get plenty of and is associated with negative health risks, seems questionable.

You probably have adequate linoleic acid, but certain people could have trouble turning it into GLA. Low GLA is sometimes associated with skin problems, and possibly even mental disorders, like depression and schizophrenia. Here is how you make GLA: GLA looks almost like linoleic acid except that it has a double bond where linoleic acid has a single bond. Your body can convert the 18-carbon linoleic acid from your diet, which has two double bonds, to the 18-carbon GLA, which has three double bonds, by changing a single bond to a double bond using an enzyme called *delta-6 desaturase.* Low GLA could thus result from inefficient delta-6 desaturase activity, and there are factors that appear to negatively affect this enzyme, such as age, alcohol, insulin, zinc deficiency, and trans fats. There are not many dietary sources of GLA other than uncommon ones like borage seed oil, evening primrose oil, black currant seed oil, and some fungal oils. Thus supplementation with borage seed oil could, in theory, help boost low GLA.

What's In It

BORAGE SEED oil contains triglycerides that, when hydrolyzed into glycerol and fatty acids, yield 17–25 percent gammalinolenic acid (usually esterified to the middle or second hydroxyl position of glycerol) and the rest of the fatty acids are mainly linoleic acid. The oil could have minute trace amounts of pyrrolizidine alkaloids. The leaves and flowers have slightly more pyrrolizidine alkaloids, along with silicic acid, tannin, and mucilage.

Scientists are listening to nature's hints that GLA might be good for the skin. Infants with low GLA do not grow as readily and tend to get dry, thickened skin. This is why you now see more commercial infant formulas including GLA. Infants don't make GLA well on their own. Breast milk is a good source of GLA, but unsupplemented infant formula is not. Also, some animals studies show that some of the GLA

that animals eat eventually gets secreted onto their skin and fur, where some scientists theorize it plays an anti-infective or protective function there.

GLA from borage seed oil is converted to dihomogamma-linolenic acid (DGLA), which is both good and bad. Your enzymes make DGLA, a 20-carbon fatty acid, by elongating the 18-carbon GLA by two carbons. Remember that the 20-carbon fatty acids are precursors to those very biologically active eicosanoids, and DGLA is no exception.

The good news about DGLA is that it can be turned into an eicosanoid called *prostaglandin E1.* Prostaglandin E1, or PGE1 for short, is one of the more benign eicosanoids. It relaxes blood vessel linings, lowers blood pressure, prevents blood clot formation, and is "antiproliferative," meaning that it can halt the runaway cell growth that leads to tumors. PGE1 is also a potent anti-inflammatory. Another positive effect of DGLA is to inhibit the production of a less benign eicosanoid called *leukotriene B4* in both animal and human studies. Since leukotriene B4 is associated with asthmatic and allergic responses, scientists have considered GLA in treating allergy and asthma and have obtained variable and sometimes positive results in human studies.

DGLA can unfortunately also be turned into another 20-carbon omega-6 fatty acid called *arachidonic acid,* the major precursor to inflammatory prostaglandins. This fact is something scientists have lost sleep over and have occasionally tried to prevent by supplementing volunteers with omega-3 fatty acids along with borage seed oil. The reason aspirin is associated with so many health benefits, such as reduced risk of stroke, heart disease, and cancer, is thought to be a result of its blocking arachidonic acid from being turned into certain eicosanoids. Also, a lot of the scientific consternation over our superabundant dietary omega-6 fatty acids stems from the knowledge that they are precursors to arachidonic acid. Arachidonic acid is not something you want to have a lot of. Some studies attempt to reassure you that borage does not raise arachidonic acid levels, which could simply mean that arachidonic acid is converted into other substances more quickly than they can detect it. At least one human study shows that borage oil does in fact raise arachidonic acid,[2] but it also discovered that the effect was reduced by taking borage oil with an omega-3 fatty acid from fish oil.

GOOD EFFECTS . . . AND NOT SO GOOD

Use only "UPA-free" borage products, and limit your consumption of the plant as a food. Borage leaves and flowers are edible but contain pyrrolizidine alkaloids. These are also called *unsaturated pyrrolizidine alkaloids,* or *UPAs* in herbal literature. These molecules damage your liver, and in other plants, like comfrey, long-term ingestion is associated with liver cancer. Borage is related to comfrey, and its leaves and flowers also possess low amounts of these toxins. This is a shame, because I think borage leaves taste quite lovely and somewhat like cucumber in a salad. If you do eat borage leaves, don't do it very often. Borage seed oil has even less of the toxin, but long-term use of borage seed oil might lead to increased risk of liver problems. Several health authorities advise buying pyrrolizidine-free borage seed oil. Look for "UPA-free" or some other certification on the label indicating the manufacturers removed this toxin from their product.

If you want to take borage seed oil, consider taking it with fish oil or flaxseed oil to reduce arachidonic acid formation. Some people believe borage seed oil helps them combat their rheumatoid arthritis or skin problems. However, one of the main problems with borage seed oil is its potential to feed your pool of the inflammatory arachidonic acid. The fatty acids you eat can sit in your body a long time, as they get incorporated into larger fats and cell membrane molecules.

Commonly Reported Uses for Borage*

Internally

    rheumatoid arthritis, allergy, stress, dermatitis, respiratory problems

    forms available for internal use:

    seed oil capsules, fresh herb, tea, extracts

    commonly reported dosage:

    In most human studies, 1 to 2 grams of borage seed oil is taken daily.

*These uses and dosages are from historic use and are not necessarily tested nor recommended

Studies where people take borage oil along with fish oil, a source of the omega-3 fatty acids docosahexaenoic acid (DHA) and eicosapentaenoic acid (EPA), generally have a more positive outcome than when borage seed oil is taken alone, and fish oil could theoretically limit borage oil's transformation into arachidonic acid. If you don't care to take fish oil, try flaxseed oil instead, which contains the omega-3 fatty acid alpha-linolenic acid (ALA). In either case, follow dose instructions—most products have you take 1 to 3 grams of fish oil or flaxseed oil daily. ALA is converted by enzymes in your body to the fish oils DHA and EPA, although slowly and often inefficiently. Even so, ALA theoretically could compete for the same enzymes that convert the fatty acids in borage seed oil to arachidonic acid, thus limiting arachidonic acid formation.

EVIDENCE OF ACTION

On paper, borage oil's high GLA content makes it appear theoretically useful for several things, like skin problems, allergies, and asthma. When tested on people, it tentatively looks promising for rheumatoid arthritis, but results for using it for other conditions are disappointing. This could well be because not only is GLA converted to helpful molecules, but it is also converted to unhelpful inflammatory agents as well, complicating the picture. If you want to learn more about the effects of GLA supplementation, take a peek at the chapter on evening primrose oil (see page 110). It is also used in clinical studies of GLA.

The most promising studies indicate borage seed oil's usefulness in treating rheumatoid arthritis. Taken for six weeks or longer, when compared to placebo (cottonseed oil[3] or sunflower oil[4]), borage oil significantly reduced the number of painful joints, swelling, and pain. Studies using borage oil for other problems are more disappointing.

Although people with dermatitis or eczema often have low GLA, it isn't clear whether borage seed oil can relieve their skin problems. Borage oil produces either no effects or subtle ones in human studies. When pitted against a placebo oil, half a gram of borage oil daily for twenty-four weeks in 160 people with atopic eczema slightly reduced symptoms and their use of steroid ointment, but not significantly so.[5]

The authors claimed, however, that the more compliant patients were the only ones who did significantly improve, which could be true: they had measurably higher levels of GLA metabolites than the allegedly noncompliant volunteers. Adults and children with atopic eczema were randomly placed in groups taking either borage seed oil or placebo, and neither they nor the researchers knew what they were taking. The placebo (paraffin or olive oil) worked slightly better than borage oil, however![6] Another study found borage oil compared favorably to sunflower oil in reducing the development of atopic dermatitis in infants with a family history of the problem, but did not do so significantly,[7] nor did the treated infants have lower immunoglobulin E (IgE), an antibody associated with allergic dermatitis.

The effect of borage oil on asthma is also inconclusive, yet intriguing. Although 2 grams of GLA daily from borage oil did not significantly reduce the measured symptoms of asthmatic patients relative to corn oil placebo, it did, however, decrease their synthesis of the inflammatory leukotriene B4, which is classically associated with asthma symptoms, indicating this effect should be studied further.[8]

One of the problems with the GLA in borage oil, not to mention its high linoleic acid content, is that both fatty acids can be turned into arachidonic acid, a precursor to inflammatory and potentially damaging molecules. Theoretically, taking borage oil with fish oil could limit this conversion, and the most promising studies of borage use a combination of borage oil plus fish oil. For example, borage oil plus fish oil helps patients with acute respiratory distress syndrome (ARDS),[9] growth in preterm infants and nerve and motor development in preterm boys,[10] and atopic dermatitis in dogs.[11] Scientists are now discovering that the omega-3 fatty acids in fish oil are helpful in treating a surprising number of conditions, so it is unfortunate that these studies did not test borage oil alone. We are thus left scratching our heads over whether or not the fish oil, rather than the borage oil, is entirely responsible for these positive outcomes.

THE BOTTOM LINE

- Borage seed oil is a good source of gammalinolenic acid, or GLA, as well as the essential fatty acid linoleic acid, which most people efficiently convert to GLA. Linoleic acid is abundant in the typical modern diet, so it is debatable whether you need either fatty acid from borage oil. Both fatty acids are omega-6 fatty acids, which can be pro-inflammatory.

- GLA is converted in your body to dihomo-GLA, which potentially generates either positive or negative effects. Your body can either turn dihomo-GLA into the beneficial, anti-inflammatory prostaglandin E1 and shut off inflammatory leukotriene B4 production, or it can turn dihomo-GLA into arachidonic acid, a major precursor of inflammatory and potentially damaging molecules.

- The best indication for use of borage seed oil is rheumatoid arthritis. Its usefulness in treating atopic dermatitis remains questionable. Better results have appeared in studies when borage seed oil is taken along with fish oil, which limits inflammatory arachidonic acid formation.

- Although the liver-damaging pyrrolizidine alkaloid content of borage seed oil is minute, long-term use of the oil requires you find a refined, pyrrolizidine-free product. The leaves and flowers are edible but should not be eaten often, as they have higher levels of these toxins.

CASCARA SAGRADA
Rhamnus purshiana

HISTORY AND FOLKLORE

After Native Americans of Mendocino, California, introduced the laxative effects from the bark of this small tree to sixteenth-century Spanish priests, the priests christened it with the suggestively thankful name "sacred bark," or cascara sagrada. And in 1878 the Parke-Davis company sold an over-the-counter formulation of cascara extract as laxatives to Americans. World War II soldiers in the U.S. Army were issued a descendant of this medication, which they called *CC pills.* Cascara sagrada is also called *chittam* or *shittamwood,* and some herbalists suggest these sound like slang names for what the herb does.

Cascara is in the buckthorn family (*Rhamnaceae*), and grows from Northern California to British Columbia, almost reaching the Alaskan panhandle. It also grows in Montana and the Idaho Rockies, and Native Americans in all of these regions have used it medicinally. Europeans have their own cathartic cousins, alder buckthorn, or "frangula" (*Rhamnus frangula*), and common buckthorn (*Rhamnus catharticus*). The European buckthorns contain similar assortments of the same active ingredients as cascara but are described as more gastrointestinally savage.

Every summer, "cascara barkers" from Northern California to British Columbia remove cascara bark with sharp knives to earn a bit of cash. Overharvesting has encouraged regulation of the annual removal of millions of pounds of cascara bark from wild trees.

HOW SCIENTISTS THINK CASCARA WORKS

Cascara owes its properties to anthranoid laxatives, which are also found in other purgative plants. Aloe latex, rhubarb root, and senna, as well as other buckthorn trees contain the same smorgasbord of chemically related molecules in varying proportions. Because cascara has more of the milder anthraquinones and anthraquinone *dimers*—that is, two molecules bonded together to make the chemical equivalent of conjoined twins—than the harsher anthrones, some say that cascara is the mildest intestinal irritant among these plants, but most sources still warn of cascara's ability to cause sharp abdominal pains and diarrhea.

You need gut flora to activate the ingredients. Six to eight hours after ingestion, cascara reaches the colon, where your bacterial enzymes must liberate its active ingredients from attached sugars in order for them to work. Freed from their sugars, these anthranoid laxatives reverse the normal flow of ions and water through the lining of the colon. Aggressive gut contractions are also triggered, mediated by the anthranoid's stimulation of the synthesis of a prostaglandin, reducing fecal transit time. Such contractions can be painful and are typically described as abdominal "cramps."

Cascara and other anthranoid laxative herbs can give you melanosis coli. Chronic use of anthranoid laxatives like cascara leads to colon cell death and white cell infiltration of the colon. Because recruited immune cells gobble up deceased colon cells, which in turn

---

CASCARA'S MANY QUESTIONABLE USES: IRRITATING FURNITURE AND SUN-SCREENS, PURGATIVE COFFEE SUBSTITUTES, AND INFURIATING BEAR FOOD.

Although cascara's purgative and vomit-inducing powers dominate the literature about it, the yellow-white wood historically was converted into furniture. You might want to think twice about building a comfy chair out of it, however. Cascara sap is irritating, and one occupational exposure report describes cascara's induction of asthma and allergies in workers who process it.[1] Also, some "natural" sunscreen lotions contain cascara extracts, which could give you a rash if you have sensitive skin.

Cascara has berries, too, which some people eat and have dubbed "coffee berry" because of the bitter taste of the glossy, black berries. They have never caught on in any big way as a coffee substitute, however, as they make some people vomit. Though tougher folks boast no damage after eating a few berries, most references advise avoiding them, and some call them outright poisonous. Naturalists report that birds are oblivious to this effect and love the berries, but mammals are different. Because of their cathartic effect, the seeds in the berries are distributed well by animals, in their own exclusive manure. If you are camping, avoid bears that are dining on cascara berries (if you're able to determine such a thing!), as naturalists say the bears will subsequently become cantankerous, presumably from gastrointestinal distress.

---

contain half-digested anthraquinone dyes, the colon assumes a spotted appearance. This reversible condition, called *melanosis coli,* is reportedly benign but has concerned enough researchers for them to propose an equivocal link with cancer. The mechanisms by which anthranoid laxatives like senna work are described in even greater detail in the chapter on aloe, under aloe latex (see page 19)—not to be confused with aloe gel.

Good Effects . . . and Not So Good

Only you can tone your gut, not an herb. Pay no attention to advertisers who talk about cascara—or any other irritant laxative, for that matter—"toning the gut," or "restoring tone to the gut," thereby enabling you to overcome laxative dependence. It is more likely that such irritants will cause laxative dependence. The theory that irritant stimulation of gut muscles "trains" or "tones" them

is similar to the optimistic hope that vibrating belts strapped around your middle jiggles off fat. Unless you perform the work yourself, no toning is going on.

What's In It

CASCARA CONTAINS anthracene derivatives, chiefly cascarosides A and B (aloin-8-glucosides), C and D (11-deoxy-aloin-8-glucosides), and E and F (C-glucosyl-emodin-anthron-8-glucosides) as well as aloin and 11-deoxy-aloin.

Cascara, like other anthranoid laxatives, causes painful cramps, and its toxicity is in debate. Because of these concerns, most reputable doctors and herbalists suggest trying more accepted methods of relieving constipation, like exercise, and increasing fiber and water intake. Cascara is sometimes recommended for pets, especially dogs, but the same concerns that make professionals hesitate before prescribing it for humans should prevent you from giving it to your animal companion.

Commonly Reported Uses for Cascara*

Internally
 laxative
 forms available for internal use:
 capsule, decoction, liquid extract, powdered bark, tablet, tincture, powder, as ingredient in several over-the-counter laxatives
 commonly reported dosage:
 The average dose of powdered, aged bark is 1 gram, or one-half teaspoonful.

*These uses and dosages are from historic use and are not necessarily tested nor recommended.

Don't expect it to taste nice. Germans call cascara's European relative *Rhamnus frangula* "faulbaum," which means "rotten tree." A tea of the bark is unpopular due to its foul smell and bitter taste, so aromatic herbs like cinnamon and cloves are traditionally taken with it.

If you still want to use it, use only aged bark. Fresh cascara bark causes violent spasms and vomiting, and must be aged for at least one year so that its active ingredients can oxidize to less poisonous versions. Some companies accelerate its oxidation by heating it. Find a standardized commercial formula, do not use more than the directed dose, and do not use it for longer than two or three days. It's notable that the *Physician's Desk Reference* for herbal medicine says, "The individually correct dosage is the smallest dosage necessary to maintain a soft stool."

EVIDENCE OF ACTION

Anthranoid laxatives found in cascara and other plants are effective,[2] but can cause painful cramps. A greater concern is the toxicity of cascara and other anthranoid laxatives. A liver toxin is formed in the intestines after anthranoid laxative use, and a few cases of liver inflammation after their ingestion are reported.[3, 4, 5, 6] Chronic anthranoid laxative ingestion may be linked with the development of cancer, but more evidence is required to validate these studies.[7, 8, 9]

THE BOTTOM LINE

- Cascara is an effective laxative but can cause cramps and diarrhea. The active ingredients in cascara are anthranoid laxatives, which are also found in aloe latex, senna, and rhubarb root.
- The laxative effect of anthranoid laxatives is induced by a reversal of the flow of ions and water in the colon that is caused by chloride channel opening. Increased nitric oxide may stimulate synthesis of a particular prostaglandin (PGE2), which initiates peristaltic contractions in the colon.
- Melanosis coli, a pigmented colon, can result from chronic anthranoid laxative abuse. This is reportedly benign, though abnormal. The condition disappears if the anthranoid use is stopped.
- Long-term use of anthranoid laxatives like cascara is discouraged.

CATNIP
Nepeta cataria

History and Folklore

Catnep, catmint, and catswort are alternate titles for catnip. Despite these obvious references to some cat-related property, its ability to amuse cats was strangely regarded with skepticism by the 1834 drug authority, *The United States Dispensatory.* Expert opinions often change sluggishly, and it took more than fifty years for the reference to admit, "Cats are very fond of it." People have historically been fond of it, too.

In the ancient Roman city of Nepete, which gives the herb its Latin name, catnip was cultivated for cooking. European gardeners later popularized the herb, which was used in salads, stews, and on meat. Catnip has a minty, sweet, lemony smell, and resembles mint, with its square stem, opposite leaves, and white or purple flowers. A member of the mint family (*Labiatae* or *Lamiaceae*), it shares mint's ability to propagate, and now this Mediterranean import grows wild in most parts of the United States.

Catnip's ability to launch cats into a euphoric frenzy is due to a molecule called *nepetalactone.* Cats have a receptor—or docking port, if you will—for this molecule, in their noses. Whether catnip has any effect in people as well is a mystery that remains unsolved. Humans do not possess the nepetalactone receptor and don't seem to be overly affected by the scent of catnip—at least they typically do not go wild over small plush mice filled with the stuff. While catnip excites cats, it reputedly sedates humans when they ingest it. According to worldwide folk wisdom, catnip relieves insomnia, calms rattled nerves, and soothes an upset stomach.

A frustrating aspect of science is that once an authority pronounces an error, retracting it from popular culture becomes practically impossible. A 1969 *Journal of the American Medical Association* article mistakenly labeled catnip as marijuana, confusing the effects of the two plants. Despite 1,612 letters to the beleaguered editor pointing out the error, the retraction failed to sway members of the 1970s drug counterculture, who enthusiastically commenced smoking catnip. This must have been anticlimactic for them, because it does *not* have any effect like marijuana. However, there may be something behind its renown as a mild sedative.

How Scientists Think Catnip Works

To be vulnerable to catnip's effects, you need two things. But humans don't have either of these things, as far as scientists know. The first is a functional vomeronasal organ, or VNO for short. The VNO, also called *Jacobson's organ,* is in the noses of vertebrates, with the exception of birds and fish, picking up chemical *pheromones,* which are often associated with signaling mating readiness and arousal. Catnip contains a pheromone that cats respond to called *nepetalactone.* Although humans have a rudimentary VNO, it may have degraded through lack of evolutionary use, thanks to our ability to communicate arousal using words and quite a variety of other means. Nerves from our VNO appear to dead-end, failing to reach the brain. There is some controversy about how well we respond to pheromones. Some scientists say that if we *do* respond to them, receptors in your everyday sniffer, the olfactory bulb, may have taken over the job of the VNO to a slight extent.

What's In It

THE LION'S share of the volatile oil is nepetalactone (80–90 percent). The oil also contains epinepetalactone, caryophyllene, camphor, thymol, carvacrol, and pulegone.

The second thing you need is a nepetalactone receptor in your VNO. We don't have this either, but about 80 percent of cats do, which explains why they need only smell the plant to become engrossed. When nepetalactone binds to its receptor, sensual pleasure areas in the cat brain are stimulated. If you are a cat lover like myself, you can testify that cats try to saturate their entire bodies with the plant, rubbing and licking it ecstatically. We can only look upon our aroused cats' behavior with amusement and perhaps some envy, however, because we do not have a nepetalactone receptor. Nevertheless, catnip may affect a different receptor in our own brains.

Nepetalactone resembles ingredients in valerian that, according to popular lore, are sedative. Human studies testing valerian as a sedative are currently inconclusive, but there are at least some good theories for how it might work. Some of these theories presume valerian's sedative ingredients are molecules called *valepotriates*. A few scientists note that nepetalactone's structure resembles the valepotriates

in valerian,[1] and molecules with similar structures often produce similar effects. Cats at least act as though catnip and valerian are similar. Some cats even prefer valerian to catnip, to their owners' surprise. In humans, valerian is said to have a mild sedative or antianxiety effect. Some scientists postulate that valerian's valepotriates enhance the action of GABA, an inhibitory, sedating brain neurotransmitter. Is it merely a coincidence that cultures around the world have used both valerian and catnip as sedatives? It is a shame that no research has yet attempted to determine whether nepetalactone has an effect on your brain's GABA, because it very well could.

Commonly Reported Uses for Catnip*

Internally
insomnia, anxiety, upset stomach
forms available for internal use:
capsule, dried leaves, leaf infusion (tea), tincture
commonly reported dosage:
An infusion or tea is made from two or more teaspoons of dried leaves steeped five to twenty minutes in either cool or hot water and is drunk up to three times per day. One reference suggests that boiling water should not be used.[4]

*These uses and dosages are from historic use and are not necessarily tested nor recommended.

Catnip is usually taken in the form of an herbal tea. But warm tea is usually relaxing anyway. In the absence of better research, and because humans lack the cat nepetalactone receptor, most scientific references state that catnip has *no* known physiological activity in humans. The relaxing effects of catnip tea are attributed to the warmth of the beverage and its pleasant aroma. As anyone who has taken a warm bath knows, heat helps you relax. We have yet to learn whether or not nepetalactone acts upon our brains as a sedative. This would provide a whole new meaning to the term "cat nap."

Safe Storage

ENTERPRISING CATS can go to great lengths to obtain catnip. A determined neighbor's cat once broke into my apartment and opened an elevated kitchen cabinet to steal catnip-containing tea bags. Seeing the cabinet open and things awry, I first thought I was the victim of a burglary, yet realized the intruder left muddy paw prints around a broken window screen, and half-chewed tea bags were scattered on the kitchen floor. If you have similar opportunist cats around you, you may want to store the leaves in a more impregnable location, like a refrigerator or freezer. This helps keep the herb's volatile oil from evaporating away in any case.

Good Effects . . . and Not So Good

Catnip is quite safe to ingest. Unlike many herbs, catnip has an almost completely unblemished safety record. There is only one documented negative report—that of a one-year-old boy who was taken to an emergency room after eating some questionable, old, fermenting food he had discovered, in addition to what his mother claimed was catnip tea. (Whether or not it was really catnip was questioned.) He "looked drugged" but recovered quickly.[2] Catnip's relatively untarnished safety record allows most herbalists to unreservedly recommend a tea made from the leaves. This is either sipped to ease jangled nerves, or drunk before bedtime to ensure sleep. The tea is even given to infants to ease colic.

Catnip Attracts Cats but Bugs Some Bugs

ABOUT 80 percent of cats are attracted to catnip. The trait is inherited. The gene for it is autosomal—that is, not located on a sex chromosome—and dominant, which means that only one copy, either from the tom or the queen, is required for the kitten to express the trait whereby they develop nepetalactone receptors. Kittens take a few weeks for this to occur and may even avoid catnip before then. Other catnip lovers include lions, pumas, and leopards, but not tigers. In cats (as well as people) it is non-addicting, nontoxic, and causes no hangover. Cats generally sleep off the effects. Curiously, some cats also love the herb valerian in the same ridiculous manner. Valerian contains similar molecules.

Researchers from Iowa State University have recently discovered that although catnip arouses cats, it is a big turn-off for mosquitoes and roaches.[3] Nepetalactone was ten times more effective at repelling mosquitoes than the commercial repellent DEET. As concern over mosquito-borne West Nile virus rises, mosquito-repelling catnip products are being tested. At a concentration of only one-hundredth the amount of DEET normally used, nepetalactone warded off roaches as well. Why these bugs don't like catnip remains a mystery: "It might be just an irritant," said one researcher, "or they just don't like the smell."

Don't smoke catnip. If you want catnip to make you "high," you will be disappointed. There is not even a trace of evidence that it has any marijuana-like action. Smoking the leaves is said to cause a sore throat, but inhaling smoke from anything causes a sore throat, and neither doctors nor firefighters advise it.

Evidence of Action

There are regrettably no well-designed published, scientific, clinical trials assessing the effects of catnip on humans.

THE BOTTOM LINE

- Catnip might calm and sedate people, but science has not yet verified this.
- Catnip is relatively safe.
- Catnip contains nepetalactone, which resembles the theoretically sedative molecules in another herb, valerian.

CAT'S CLAW
Uncaria guianensis, Uncaria tomentosa

History and Folklore

Cat's claw is a tropical vine in the coffee family (*Rubiaceae*) that can climb up to an impressive one hundred feet. Dozens of species are found in South America and Asia, but *U. guianensis* and *U. tomentosa* are the most popular exports. The vine's curved, hooklike thorns resemble cat's claws and provide its name.

South American Indian culture's high regard for cat's claw has attracted the attention of ethnopharmacologists. The Indians use the inner bark of the vine to treat numerous conditions, including arthritis, indigestion, infections, and also as defense against infection.

How Scientists Think Cat's Claw Works

Cat's claw is commonly said to stimulate your immune system. However, its suppression of one actor in your immune system might explain why it helps treat arthritis pain. One of the hottest new therapies for rheumatoid arthritis these days is "anti-TNF" drugs. These are injectable antibodies that irreversibly stick to a protein called *tumor necrosis factor,* or *TNF,* rendering it disabled. What is tumor necrosis factor? Anything with a name that sounds like it necrotizes, or kills, tumors *seems* like a lovely thing, but it isn't—it was named prematurely, based on initial, test tube experiments. It actually is in part responsible for the devastating wasting seen in advanced cancers. TNF is a primary mediator in certain types of damaging inflammation, and people with illnesses such as rheumatoid arthritis or Crohn's disease probably have elevated amounts of it. Something in cat's claw potently inhibits the ability of cells to make TNF.[1] A couple of human trials support taking cat's claw for both rheumatoid arthritis and osteoarthritis.

Cat's claw's anti-TNF action might calm inflamed bowels as well as your aching joints. Like rheumatoid arthritis, Crohn's disease is a devastating autoimmune disease, except it attacks the colon instead of the joints. Anti-TNF drugs are also helpful for those with Crohn's disease, and perhaps it is not coincidental that traditional Peruvian medicine enlists cat's claw for treating both arthritis and indigestion. However, evidence for its effectiveness in Crohn's disease has not yet been scientifically tested.

It may not be the alkaloids that are anti-inflammatory. A whole lot has been written about which types of alkaloids from cat's claw should be taken, since there are different kinds. But cat's claw alkaloids don't seem particularly responsible for this anti-TNF effect. There is evidence that cat's claw extracts of all sorts, both standardized to various types of alkaloids and not, also suppress the action of another immune system stimulator, interferon-gamma, which can spur TNF production. But just how cat's claw stops your TNF production, and what is in it that does that, is not yet clearly known.

Contributing to cat's claw's anti-inflammatory activity are some nice yet moderate free-radical scavenging properties, as well as weak anti-cyclooxygenase (COX) enzyme-1 and -2 activities. COX enzymes produce inflammatory prostaglandins, and cat's claw does indeed stop the production of an inflammatory prostaglandin called *E2.* But cat's claw's TNF-stopping action remains the most exciting of these anti-inflammatory bonuses, because even small amounts of the extract do this, at least in test tube studies.

Stopping TNF can stop HIV replication, but no one knows if cat's claw helps those with AIDS. HIV, the virus that causes AIDS, is particularly insidious because its genetic code becomes part of your own DNA. There the viral DNA lingers unless inflammatory triggers spur its use to produce more viruses. Since one of these triggers is TNF, people infected with HIV are understandably excited to try cat's claw. Cat's claw also decreases nuclear factor kappa beta (NF-kappa-B) in cell studies, which binds to infected DNA strands, causing them to create more viruses. Unfortunately there are no well-documented trials telling us whether cat's claw makes people infected with HIV better or worse, so if you are infected with HIV, trying cat's claw is a gamble.

One cat's claw plant is not like the other. Imagine what it would be like to be given a bottle of aspirin, only to find that some pills in it had no aspirin and others had far too much, and they all looked the same. This is a common problem with herbal remedies, in general. Plants that are the same species, growing even in identical environments, can have varying levels of active ingredients in them. Some plants are more subject to this variability than others, and cat's claw is one of them. In fact, cat's claw has varying amounts of two active ingredients with opposing activities. Pentacyclic oxindole alkaloids (POAs) in cat's claw stimulate your immune system, but tetracyclic oxindole alkaloids (TOAs) found in some apparently identical cat's claw

plants stop the POAs from working. In cell studies, POAs from cat's claw stimulate human endothelial cells—the cells lining your blood vessels—to release a substance that stimulates the production of lymphocytes, a type of immune cell. POAs also stimulate the "cell eating" behavior of white blood cells called *phagocytosis.*

However, TOAs do not have immune-stimulating activity and seem to keep the POAs from working. TOAs may also have unrelated effects on the central nervous system, because they block NMDA, or glutamate receptors, in cell culture studies. Exactly what these effects translate into, in human brains, is not known. TOAs are less commonly found in cat's claw, and in lower concentrations than POAs. Even within the same species of cat's claw, two apparently identical plants can actually be two different "chemotypes," each possessing the different types of alkaloids, with opposite activities. This is why chemical analysis and standardization of supplements from herbs is so important.

GOOD EFFECTS . . . AND NOT SO GOOD

Neither POAs nor TOAs inhibit TNF. Older literature refers to the two "chemotypes" of *U. tomentosa,* suggesting you should get the kind with immune-stimulatory pentacyclic oxindole alkaloids (POAs) rather than the kind with tetracyclic oxindole alkaloids (TOAs), which inhibit the POAs. Some products are labeled for their POA or TOA content, and consumers will be faced with choosing between the two. But the anti-inflammatory, anti-TNF activity of cat's claw that everyone is now excited about occurs in both *U. tomentosa* and *U. guianensis* species, and neither type of alkaloid seems particularly good at inhibiting TNF. The bottom line is that the anti-TNF agent has yet to be identified, so no one knows what type of cat's claw supplement is best, at least for now. Cat's claw is often standardized to the POAs, but this information does not do you much good, since they are no longer considered the active ingredient.

Immune stimulation by herbs can sometimes make you worse. Cat's claw may sound appealing to people with weak immune systems, because it is purported to stimulate the body's defenses. But you should avoid cat's claw if you have had an organ transplant or skin graft. You may be increasing your odds of transplant rejection. Also, some scientists worry (I think rightfully so) about people with autoimmune disorders taking immune stimulating herbs. More common autoimmune diseases include type I diabetes, Crohn's disease, thyroid disease, lupus, myasthenia gravis, multiple sclerosis, ankylosing spondylitis, and rheumatoid arthritis. If you have the more common, age-related form of arthritis, osteoarthritis, which is not caused by an overactive immune system, cat's claw probably won't hurt you, and it might even help.

If you have rheumatoid arthritis, Crohn's disease, or are infected with HIV, cat's claw is still a gamble. Cat's claw's anti-inflammatory, TNF-suppressing action makes it different from other "immune-stimulating" herbs. On the one hand, its potent anti-TNF property really does support its use for these conditions. But its immune stimulating action could theoretically make you worse, especially if you have an autoimmune disease, and Crohn's disease and rheumatoid arthritis are autoimmune diseases. Only one small, short-duration study showed it did not adversely affect those with rheumatoid

arthritis, and it hasn't been tested in those with Crohn's disease. Support for its use for rheumatoid arthritis, Crohn's disease, and AIDS, for that matter, are still on the fence.

CAT'S CLAW contains immune-stimulating pentacyclic oxindole alkaloids. It occasionally also contains tetracyclic oxindole alkaloids, which allegedly suppress the action of the immune-stimulatory ones. Cat's claw's anti-inflammatory components are not known, but it also contains oleanolic acid, ursolic acid, quinovic acid glycosides, procyanidins, and plant steroids such as beta-sitosterol, stigmasterol, and campesterol.

Cat's claw may cause mild diarrhea. Cat's claw can cause mild abdominal pain and loose, tarry stools, probably because of its tannins. Perhaps this is why one herb promoter dubs cat's claw with the dreamy phrase "the Opening of the Way." Another herb marketer enthuses that it "cleanses the entire intestinal tract!" These claims might not sound so positive, however, if the herb opens your "Way" excessively. Some people are more sensitive to tannins than others, but if you use cat's claw for indigestion, go easy on it until you can determine how it affects you personally.

Cat's claw is still an unknown. As popular as it has become, cat's claw has not been tested enough. Cat's claw is nontoxic to cells in culture, but a human being is more complicated than a petri dish. The American Herbal Products Association gives it a class 4 safety rating, meaning its safety and efficacy is still largely unknown. For this reason it should not be taken by children or by pregnant or nursing women.

EVIDENCE OF ACTION

If you look at advertisements for cat's claw, you will find it is most often sold for treating viral diseases like AIDS, herpes, and shingles, and for defense against infection. However, studies on this sort of use are extremely preliminary at this point. AIDS patients are now experimenting with cat's claw supplements, and though *theoretically* there exist mechanisms for it to limit HIV replication, sadly, claims concerning prolonged survival of HIV infected patients taking it are premature. At present, the few small studies of HIV-infected people taking cat's claw have not been published in mainstream scientific journals for scientists like myself to critique, but they are reportedly inconclusive and have not been duplicated.

Commonly Reported Uses for Cat's Claw*

Internally

arthritis, intestinal disorders, weakened immune system

forms available for internal use:

dried root bark, capsule, extract, infusion, tincture

commonly reported dosage:

Three times daily, one to two 500-milligram bark capsules are taken.

*These uses and dosages are from historic use and are not necessarily tested nor recommended.

Cat's claw does stimulate, or provoke, depending on your point of view, your immune system. Several studies, including one with humans, have noted a significantly increased number of lymphocytes upon taking cat's claw.[2] Also, people who took cat's claw supplements daily apparently significantly prolonged the activity of a vaccine, compared to those who did not.[3]

There is slightly hopeful evidence that cat's claw might help those with arthritis—both the ordinary osteoarthritis type and the less common rheumatoid sort. Forty-five people with osteoarthritis of the knee took part in a four-week trial where neither they nor the experimenter's knew who was taking cat's claw and who was taking placebo. Though the thirty who took cat's claw had significantly less knee pain when they were active, knee pain was not lessened when they were resting, and their knee circumference remained unchanged.[4] The study's authors suggest that a longer period of treatment with cat's claw might have afforded the experimental group better results.

Another similarly designed trial enlisted forty people with rheumatoid arthritis. Those taking cat's claw had a slightly significant reduction in the number of painful joints.[5] This study used one of two types of cat's claw: the kind with pentacyclic (five-ringed) oxindole alkaloids. The other type, which contains tetracyclic (four-ringed) oxindole alkaloids, is thought by some scientists to have the opposite activity. However, recent studies suggest that neither type of alkaloid is responsible for cat's claw's anti-inflammatory activity and that as-yet-unidentified components are responsible.[6]

The potential benefit of taking cat's claw for indigestion is only tentatively indicated in one study, where cat's claw reduced the stomach damage in rats caused by indomethacin, a pain-relieving anti-inflammatory known for causing harsh side effects on the gut.[7]

THE BOTTOM LINE

- Cat's claw contains some unknown component that potently inhibits the production of TNF (tumor necrosis factor) in cell cultures. For this reason, cat's claw may be a valuable anti-inflammatory herb, but it remains largely untested in people.
- Because cat's claw's pentacyclic oxindole alkaloids (POAs) stimulate lymphocyte proliferation and phagocytosis by granulocytes, it should be avoided or used cautiously by those with autoimmune diseases, organ transplants, or skin grafts.
- Cat's claw may reduce osteoarthritis pain.
- In theory, cat's claw might limit HIV replication, but the few small studies of HIV-infected patients taking cat's claw have not been published and are reportedly inconclusive.
- Although there is a little evidence that it does not hurt those with rheumatoid arthritis, and may help them, it *theoretically* could make these people worse. Similarly, those with Crohn's disease could either theoretically be assisted or hurt by cat's claw.
- Cat's claw can cause diarrhea.
- Because cat's claw is an unknown, it should be avoided by children, and pregnant or nursing women.

CHAMOMILE

Matricaria recutita (also known as *M. chamomilla* or *Chamomilla recutita*)

History and Folklore

Ancient Egyptians, Romans, and Greeks used this small, daisylike flower, referring to it in their medical writings. Its apple-scented fragrance inspired Greeks to call it *kamai melon,* or *ground apple.* Anglo-Saxons believed it was one of nine sacred herbs given to them by their god Woden. It remains intensely used and cultivated in Germany today.

If you want to try chamomile, you will find it has a bewildering excess of common names. Of the two species most often referenced, German chamomile, also called *Hungarian chamomile,* is far more popular. The "common" chamomile, also called *Roman* or *English chamomile,* does not have all the same active ingredients (it is low on the azulene derivatives discussed below and tastes somewhat bitter).

If you have ever read Beatrix Potter's *Peter Rabbit,* you learned that chamomile tea calmed him down after a traumatic night of eating in Mr. MacGregor's garden. (Incidentally, Potter was actually quite a scientist, but her gender frustrated her attempts at acceptance into scientific societies in the late 1800s, so all most people know of her are her children's stories.) Beatrix Potter's implicit trust in the pacifying property of chamomile tea is not merely historical, but probably has a molecular basis as well.

Chamomile flower extracts are also used to calm indigestion. Chamomile is thought to speed wound healing and is used in every conceivable cosmetic application. Its flowers' luteolin dyes fabrics yellow, therefore chamomile is also used to lighten skin and hair.

How Scientists Think Chamomile Works

Chamomile has for ages been used to quiet nerves, and its Valium-like molecules literally do just that. What Valium, Halcyon, and other relaxing benzodiazepine drugs do is bind to your nerve cell's GABA (gamma amino butyric acid) receptors. Chamomile contains molecules that do the same thing, at least in rodents. Studies of how chamomile affects *human* benzodiazepine receptors have not yet been done, but humans have long regarded chamomile as a calming herb.

The molecules from chamomile that are responsible for interacting with benzodiazepine receptors are apigenin and chrysin, two flavonoids that are very common in the plant kingdom. For example, you can also get them from parsley, celery and carrots, cherries, hot peppers . . . and this list goes on. Although apigenin and chrysin are not very water-soluble, you do get a good dose of their water-soluble counterparts that have attached sugars when you drink chamomile tea. Gut bacteria release apigenin and chysin from attached sugars, allowing these flavonoids to be absorbed into your system. Apigenin and chrysin temporarily stick to rodent benzodiazepine receptors on nerve cells possessing these docking ports. This causes the nerves to transmit signals more sluggishly, slowing them down. Not all benzodiazepine receptors are the same, and not all work the same way. This is why different benzodiazepine drugs have diverse activities, and chamomile should be expected to be unique, too. If humans are anything like the mice and rats that have been given chamomile, chamomile probably will calm you and may, to a lesser degree, relax your muscles and make you sleepy.

What's In It

THE MORE interesting ingredients of chamomile's flower heads include flavonoids such as chrysin, apigenin, and luteolin. Its volatile oils possess alpha-bisabolol and bisabolol oxides, and matricin, which degrades upon steaming to the blue chamazulene and other azulene derivatives. It also has coumarins, some of which are newly discovered.

The sedative effects of benzodiazepines, and thus theoretically chamomile, involve benzodiazepines receptors in the brain and spinal cord—the central nervous system. (Benzodiazepine receptors called *peripheral benzodiazepine receptors* do exist outside the central nervous system but serve different purposes.) Whenever a plant molecule is theorized to affect the central nervous system, you should ask whether the molecule can get to there in the first place. It's all very well to find plant molecules that stick to benzodiazepine receptors in a test tube, but your body doesn't admit molecules that you eat into your central nervous system very easily. A lot of herbal research is guilty of extrapolating test tube studies to people, so it's good to watch out for that pitfall. So can apigenin and chrysin get into your brain

after you eat them? Very little research exists on whether molecules of this class, flavonoids, can get into your brain, but a recent study lends support to the idea. A related plant molecule that greatly resembles apigenin and chrysin (hispidulin) was found able to cross the blood-brain barrier of gerbils that were fed the flavonoid.[1] This supports the notion that apigenin and chrysin can do the same.

In a screening of 200 plant extracts, chamomile pollen was singled out for containing a substance that blocks nerve cells' pain receptors. Both Roman and German chamomile possess this previously undiscovered tetracoumaroyl spermine, which is an "NK1 antagonist."[2] This means it clings to receptors especially designed to sense pain. It blocks substance P—the P is for pain, of course—from binding there. Substance P is also reportedly elevated in the brains of some people with depression and fibromyalgia. Does this mean chamomile will lessen your sadness and pain? The scientists who discovered this new molecule suspect that although tetracoumaroyl spermine is plentiful in commercial chamomile extracts, it will stick unhelpfully to proteins in your blood, making it less available to do its job. Nonetheless, this newly discovered natural product is worth keeping an eye on.

Chamomile reduces inflammation by several means. Inflammation is usually your immune defense system spun off into the weeds, turning normally protective molecules into bad guys that, in general, slow wound healing and cause swelling, pain, cramps, indigestion, and other unpleasantness. Multiple anti-inflammatory mechanisms of chamomile combat this process, at least according to cell and animal studies. It's likely it should work for you, too.

First, the apigenin mentioned above that

slows down your nerve cells also won something like an experimental challenge[3] to see which plant flavonoid best inhibited the production of two inflammatory bad actors called *COX-2* and *i-NOS* in cell cultures. COX-2, or cyclooxygenase-2, is an enzyme that makes several damaging inflammatory substances and makes you more sensitive to pain. Aspirin works by stopping COX-2 once it is already made, but apigenin keeps COX-2 from being made in the first place.

The enzyme i-NOS, or *inducible nitric oxide synthase*, makes nitric oxide, which has valuable functions in moderate amounts, such as lowering blood pressure and increasing blood circulation, but it is rebellious when in excess. Nitric oxide enhances the activity of the COX enzymes mentioned above and is a damaging free radical. In fact, activated white blood cells lob nitric oxide as a chemical weapon at pathogenic bacteria, but nitric oxide can hurt our own tissues as well. There are different nitric oxide–making enzymes, but the i-NOS one is particularly implicated in inflammation. Chamomile's apigenin keeps this nitric oxide manufacturer from getting out of hand.

How does apigenin prevent these inflammation factories from being made? It is thought to prevent something called NF-kappa-B (nuclear factor kappa beta) from unsticking to its inhibitor in cells. Once NF-kappa-B gets loose, it triggers an inflammatory cascade that triggers the production of these enzymes.

Apigenin has also grabbed scientists' attention for its power to inhibit something called *MAP (mitogen activated protein) kinase*. Once this enzyme gets activated, a cascade of events occurs in a cell that can trigger a variety of different events, like cell growth and division, and yes, inflammation. Indeed, some scientists are trying to design new MAP kinase–inhibiting drugs as anti-inflammatories. Chamomile has beaten them to it.

Commonly Reported Uses for Chamomile*

Internally
sedative, spasmolytic, anti-inflammatory, vulnerary (wound healing), anticancer
forms available for internal use:
capsule, extract, infusion, tincture, all made from dried or fresh flowers
commonly reported dosage:
Commonly, a tea of 2 to 3 teaspoons of dried flowers per cup of water is drunk, or one-half to 1 teaspoon of tincture is taken, up to three times daily. Capsules are taken according to package label or when indigestion occurs.

Externally
anti-inflammatory, wounds, lightening agent for hair and skin spots
forms available for external use:
compress, lotion, ointment, cosmetic products, bath additives
commonly reported dosage:
Cooled chamomile tea, or a teaspoon of tincture in a cup of water, is used in a compress or gargle.

*These uses and dosages are from historic use and are not necessarily tested nor recommended.

But there are other anti-inflammatories in chamomile besides apigenin that do not mimic apigenin's flavonoid structure. Chamomile's oil is bright blue due to the presence of azulene and molecules related to it, like chamazulene and matricin. Some of these azulenes are thought to chemically resemble "profens," that is, anti-inflammatory drugs like naproxen, ibuprofen, and ketoprofen. These, like aspirin, inhibit the COX enzymes, and chamomile's azulene derivatives work similarly.[4] So if apigenin can't entirely stop the production of COX enzymes, the azulene derivatives can block COX once it is already present.

Good Effects . . . and Not So Good

Chamomile is quite safe, unless you are allergic to it. Allergies to chamomile are uncommon, but they do occur. If you are already allergic to plants in the daisy or ragweed family (*Asteraceae*), you are more likely to become allergic to chamomile, so use it with care. Other *Asteraceae* herbs that might provoke an allergic response are arnica (page 25), dandelion (page 92), echinacea (page 97), feverfew (page 119), and milk thistle (page 230).

To harness chamomile's calming flavonoids, you can use a water extract, like tea. Chamomile's allegedly sedative flavonoids, chrysin and apigenin, often have attached sugars and as such are water soluble, so you can either take encapsulated dried flowers and rely on your gut to extract these flavonoids from them, or you can extract them yourself with some hot water from a teakettle.

Both water-soluble extracts and oil extracts contain anti-inflammatory molecules, so experiment and find the form that works best for you. These anti-inflammatories could well be responsible for ages of rumors concerning chamomile's anti-spasmodic, wound-healing, and pain-relieving properties, but since they work by several different possible mechanisms, you need to find a formulation that works for you. Be sure to use good quality preparations made entirely from chamomile flower heads rather than stems and leaves, which contain fewer active ingredients and are thus less effective.

Evidence of Action

The legendary calming power of chamomile has not been carefully assessed in people, but it will definitely relax any stressed rodents that you might know. Plenty of studies confirm that chamomile best works as an *anxiolytic,* or anxiety-reducing, agent and mildly works as a sedative, muscle relaxant, and anticonvulsant in mice and rats.[5, 6, 7, 8] Chamomile's calming ingredients in rats appear to be its flavonoids apigenin and chrysin. One study observed that these nerve-soothers worked without impairing rats' memories.[9] Another experiment showed that rats given chamomile were less likely to become dependent on morphine and less likely to suffer withdrawal symptoms from it.[10] Chemical alteration of chamomile's mild sedatives has increased their receptor stickiness and their soothing potential.[11] This suggests chamomile's natural, milder versions of these drugs really do work, only more gently.

Mechanistically, chamomile has several anti-inflammatory properties, according to cell and animal studies. But how does this action play out in human clinical trials? One of the oldest studies addressing this question used only fourteen patients, but the credibility of the data is strengthened in that neither they nor their experimenters knew who was getting the chamomile and who was getting a placebo. Those who used chamomile extracts on their dermabraded tattoos enjoyed faster healing than those who did not.[12] Chamomile creams have also held their own when compared to anti-inflammatory hydrocortisone and other steroid creams, in treating eczema and general skin inflammation. Chamomile proved comparable to steroid creams with 0.5 and 0.25 hydrocortisone, and a commercial chamomile cream was moderately superior to the nonsteroidal anti-inflammatory 5 percent bufexamac and the steroidal anti-inflammatory 0.75 percent fluocortin butyl ester.[13, 14]

Less exciting results developed for two of three studies where an oral chamomile spray or rinse was used to prevent inflamed tissue and sore throats. In one trial it did not prevent postoperative sore throats caused by intubation.[15] Short-term treatment of a chamomile spray also made no difference for patients undergoing head and neck chemotherapy or radiation therapy,[16] but this study has been criticized for being too short in duration, as the mucositis that results from these cancer treatments usually takes more time to develop. In a similar, older trial, cancer patients who did develop oral mucositis found a chamomile rinse sped resolution of their inflammation.[17]

Chamomile is quite often used as a digestive aid, which certainly could be attributed to its calming and anti-inflammatory actions, but experimentally this effect hasn't been explored to any satisfactory degree. The only controlled, human study of chamomile's digestive attributes showed that an apple pectin and chamomile combination significantly helped stop diarrhea in children, compared to a placebo,[18] but it's impossible to say how much the chamomile helped, since pectin is already known to be a moderately effective antidiarrheal medicine.

Anticancer properties of chamomile have been found in both cell and animal studies. Its extracts reduced skin cancer development in UV light–treated[19] and carcinogen-treated[20] mice. Other studies show apigenin stops cells from dividing.[21, 22] Apigenin can also get cancer cells in culture to neatly commit suicide,[23] something unhealthy cells are normally, and conveniently, good at, but cancer cells sometimes resist this natural process. Cancer cells also become troublesome when they send out chemical signals recruiting the growth of new blood vessels to feed them. New research shows apigenin is particularly good at switching off a molecular switch called *HIF-1* that activates this blood vessel–recruiting process in cancer cells, and it can thus theoretically starve tumors of their blood supply.[24, 25] However, anticancer studies using chamomile or apigenin have not yet been expanded to human clinical trials.

THE BOTTOM LINE

- Chamomile probably works as a calming agent. It has molecules that, like Valium, interact with GABA receptors on nerve cells, slowing them down.
- Chamomile has several different anti-inflammatory mechanisms and may work as a topical anti-inflammatory.
- Chamomile contains a substance that blocks pain receptors, but it is not known if and how this works in people.
- Chamomile's anti-inflammatory and relaxing properties probably enable it to act as a good digestive aid, though it has not been extensively tested as such in human clinical studies.
- A few people develop an allergic response to chamomile, but this is rare. If you are allergic to plants in the daisy or ragweed family, you are more likely to become allergic to chamomile.

CHASTEBERRY
Vitex agnus-castus

HISTORY AND FOLKLORE

If the term "chaste" in the common name were not enough, both "agnus" and "castus" in this plant's Latin name refer to purity or chastity. ("Vitex," on the other hand, has little to do with abstinence, and is thought to refer to the viticultural employment of its stems to stake wine grapes.) This Mediterranean shrub's nickname, "monks pepper," also hints at its former use by medieval monks. The berries reportedly have a pepperminty smell and a warm, peppery taste. Monks are said to have liberally sprinkled these upon their food, which was thought to have the added benefit of ensuring their chaste condition. Virgins and wives who wanted to impress upon others their chastity or faithfulness strew chaste tree leaves upon their beds.

An association between its benefit to women during painful menstruation and for treating other "women's problems" developed, and these uses remain popular today. Whether or not chasteberry truly acts as an antiaphrodiasiac has not appeared obvious from today's research, but it does appear to exert some hormonal action.

HOW SCIENTISTS THINK CHASTEBERRY WORKS

Some of chasteberry's constituents behave like dopamine. Dopamine is a hormone-like substance that occurs naturally in the brain, transmitting signals from certain nerve cells to others—that is, it is a neurotransmitter. Not all nerve cells are sensitive to dopamine; they must possess a dopamine receptor, and there are different sorts of dopamine receptors with various activities. Something in chasteberry extracts binds specifically to pituitary dopamine D2 receptors and act almost as well as dopamine itself. These ingredients were tentatively identified as some of its diterpenes known as *clerodadienols*. (Diterpenes are a class of molecules found in a majority of plants, but clerodadienols are more specific to chasteberries.) This was determined in cell studies of isolated rat pituitary cells, so you should be suspicious that a petri dish of cells is *not* a human brain. Although a lot of the extract was dumped upon these isolated cells, and injected into rats in order to notice this effect,[1] oral chasteberry nonetheless appears active in its relatively dilute form when taken by people.

Dopamine inhibits prolactin, and women who take chasteberry lower excess prolactin. Prolactin is a major female hormone produced mainly by a part of the brain called the *anterior pituitary,* and, to a much lesser extent, a variety of other cells in the body. Its most obvious effect is stimulating breast development and breast milk production. (Men make prolactin, too, but less of it, and its role in men remains mysterious.) Menstrual problems and infertility can arise if your prolactin is overactive. You can have it measured by your doctor, but the numbers are sometimes misleading. Even if your prolactin is in the normal range, this hormone may be overactive. This is because there are three forms of prolactin with different potencies. Endearingly termed "little," "big," and "big-big" prolactin, these can be further modified by the cells that make them, causing them to become either more or less active, so your total prolactin can at times be less important that your percentage of active prolactin. People with rare forms of brain damage that prevents the hypothalamus from conveying its dopamine to the adjacent pituitary have excess prolactin. Thus we know that the dopamine in healthy people helps tame prolactin secretion, and without dopamine doing its job, you will make too much prolactin. Medications such as estrogen, breast stimulation such as suckling, stress, and some tumors can also increase prolactin to varying degrees.

Normalizing prolactin may reduce breast soreness and stabilize menstrual patterns, increasing female fertility in certain cases. Excessive prolactin is associated with breast swelling and pain, especially before menstruation. For reasons that are unknown, some women just make a lot of prolactin during this time, and suffer. Excess prolactin sometimes causes a bit of lactation, too, a startling discovery for any woman who has not recently had a baby. There are indications that chasteberry may help with this type of breast soreness.

Also, excess prolactin can interfere with a woman's menstrual cycle, decreasing estrogen, which can stop her menstrual cycles completely or at least throw them out of whack. Although chasteberry does not clearly have *direct* effects on the major menstruation-affecting hormones—estrogen, progesterone, FSH (follicle stimulating hormone) and LH (luteinizing hormone)—its ability to normalize prolactin may indirectly get the rhythm of these hormones and menstruation back in order.

Menstrual cycles that aren't regular can

be more than an irritation. In some cases the result can be infertility. Some women are infertile because the luteal phase, the approximately ten-day period after ovulation (the release of an egg), is too short. During this phase, the intrepid egg's old resting place becomes a transient structure called the *corpus luteum,* which secretes progesterone. The hormone progesterone is required at this stage for fertility. A fleeting luteal phase results in insufficient progesterone, and progesterone is needed to maintain the uterine lining for implantation of an embryo. There are some preliminary yet intriguing results suggesting that some infertile women have lengthened their luteal phase to the normal ten-day period using chasteberry and consequently succeeded in getting pregnant.

What's In It

COMMERCIAL PREPARATIONS are sometimes standardized to its iridoid glycosides, agnuside (hydroxybenzoylaucubin) and aucubin, but dopamine-like agents are more likely to be in its terpenes, present in its volatile oil. Its oil includes 1,8-cineol, camphor, alpha- and beta-pinene, vitexilactone, limonene, p-cymol, and sabinene. It's flavonoids include casticin, orientin, isovitexin, chrysosplenol D, cynaroside, 5-hydroxy-3,4,6,7-tetramethoxyflavone, 6-hydroxykaempferol, isorhamnetin, luteolin, and luteolin glycosides.

The apparent estrogenic activity of chasteberry in test tube studies requires further investigation—in people. Again, you have to be cautious interpreting the results of these sorts of isolated cell culture studies and relating them to actual people. Although components of alcoholic chasteberry extracts bind to various types of estrogen receptors in isolated cell cultures, and induce some effects there, the ingredients allegedly responsible for this are already known to be prevalent in our diets.

For example, one study found linoleic acid from chasteberry was clinging to estrogen receptors and getting them to do their estrogenic jobs, in cell cultures.[2] Linoleic acid is not some rare, esoteric plant molecule, but very much abundant—some think *too* abundant—in our modern diets, being a major constituent of our most commonly used vegetable oils: corn, safflower, sunflower, and soybean oils. So it seems silly to suggest using chaste tree berries as a source of linoleic acid, given it is already prevalent in our diets. (Its possible stimulation of estrogen-sensitive tumors is perking up the ears of some scientists; see the chapters on borage and evening primrose oil for more information on this common plant molecule.) Another study attributed the effect to apigenin,[3] which also abounds in the plant kingdom and is not unique to chasteberry either. These preliminary findings demand further investigation of chasteberry's power to induce estrogenic actions in people.

Good Effects . . . and Not So Good

Chasteberry is generally safe. No major untoward effects are associated with taking chasteberry, including its historic antilibidinous one. However, some people who take it get mild stomach upset or a rash, both of which go away when they stop using the herb.

Certain people may want to avoid using it, however. Although the herb is used in some cases to assist female fertility, you should stop taking it if you do become pregnant, because its influence on fetal development is not known and it does appear to have hormonal effects. Also, since it seems to affect dopamine and prolactin, it could interfere with other medications you are taking, like dopamine agonists, which are commonly taken for neurological and movement disorders such as Parkinson's disease, nervous tics, restless leg syndrome, and cerebral palsy.

The best form of chasteberry to take is not yet known. That's because we don't know the active ingredients. Although it is commonly standardized to its flavonoids, agnuside and aucubin, there is no obvious evidence that these are the active ingredients. Some scientists think the chasteberry ingredient that acts like dopamine may be one of its diterpenes, and if that is true, you might want to look for an alcoholic extract, which is more likely to possess this molecule than an aqueous one.

Evidence of Action

Human studies of chasteberry for treating particular female hormonal irregularities look tentatively promising. Some symptoms of premenstrual syndrome (PMS) may be improved, plus certain types of female infertility could be treated. Although chasteberry is sometimes recommended for menopausal symptoms, there is insufficient data from human studies to evaluate it for this purpose. Adverse effects are mild and reversible. Despite its folkloric reputation, people taking chasteberry in modern studies had no obvious deviations in their libidos.

Though there aren't a lot of well-designed studies, the best indications for treatment so far appear to involve problems arising from excess prolactin (prolactinemia), from decreased luteinizing hormone (LH), decreased progesterone, and from having an overly brief luteal phase. A short-lived luteal phase is called a *luteal phase defect,* and it's one of several possible causes of female infertility, since during this phase progesterone is secreted, which helps maintain the uterine lining for implantation of an embryo.

An older German study suggests a luteal phase defect may be normalized by chasteberry, and also that earlier test tube studies indicating that chasteberry decreases prolactin secretion may have been on to something. Fifty-three women with prolactinemia and related luteal phase defects were enlisted in a double-blind, placebo-controlled trial.[4] For those taking 20 milligrams of chasteberry extract daily for three months, prolactin was decreased significantly. Also significant was an increase in duration of their previously too-brief luteal phase of ovulation, which increased their progesterone secretion to normal during this phase. This could have improved their fertility; indeed, two of the women taking chasteberry got pregnant during the study.

These results were later echoed by a 2004 pilot study of infertile women at Stanford University.[5] Their double-blind, placebo-controlled investigation involved thirty women who had trouble conceiving. Half took a placebo, and half took a mixture of chasteberry and green tea, along with vitamins and minerals. After three months, those taking the chasteberry compound significantly increased their luteal phase and showed a trend toward increasing progesterone secretion during that phase. The presence of green tea and vitamins makes it impossible to interpret whether chasteberry alone helped or had any effect. There was a dramatic effect, however. Notably, five of the fifteen women taking the chasteberry mixture got pregnant, while none of the fifteen in the placebo group did.

Commonly Reported Uses for Chasteberry*

Internally
female reproductive problems, absent or irregular menstruation, premenstrual symptoms, breast swelling and pain
forms available for internal use:
dried berries, capsule, decoction, extract, tincture
commonly reported dosage:
In some human studies, 20 milligrams of chasteberry in tablet form has been taken daily.

*These uses and dosages are from historic use and are not necessarily tested nor recommended.

The studies evaluating chasteberry's power to treat PMS appear good on the surface, but perhaps because researchers have trouble quantifying PMS, many rely on less reliable subjective measures, like self-assessment and questionnaires. Also, several of these studies lack control groups. One study with only a positive control that was considered, at least by the authors, to be effective pitted chasteberry against an antidepressant of the SSRI (selective serotonin reuptake inhibitor) class called *fluoxetine,* better known as Prozac. Both were evaluated for their ability to relieve PMS and associated depression. Chasteberry held its own. Those rating the women's progress were blinded as to whether the study participants were taking fluoxetine or chasteberry, yet regarded both to have improved similarly. Fluoxetine was considered somewhat better at relieving psychological distress, while chasteberry had slightly better success in treating physical symptoms.[6]

One of the few randomized, placebo-controlled trials of women who were deemed regularly vulnerable to PMS symptoms noted that chasteberry provided significant improvement in both self-assessment and clinical assessment of symptoms.[7] A couple of other studies concluded that chasteberry reduced PMS symptoms, yet these studies had no controls, so their results remain equivocal.[8, 9] Another investigation examined only breast soreness, or mastodynia, and they did use a placebo, noting that those taking chasteberry had significantly less intense breast pain after two months and decreased yet not quite statistically significantly reduced pain at three months.[10]

Men are more reluctant to try chasteberry these days, perhaps for obvious reasons. Yet a couple of publications observed the effects of different doses of chasteberry taken by twenty male volunteers over fourteen days compared to a placebo. The lowest dose of chasteberry (120 mg) increased their ability to secrete prolactin, while the highest dose (480 mg) decreased prolactin secretion, both significantly.[11] A negative feedback mechanism for secreting prolactin could have kicked in when a maximum threshold level was reached, shutting down prolactin secretion; this phenomenon is common with hormones. When repeated, chasteberry was found to increase the men's melatonin in a dose-dependent manner: The greatest dose of chasteberry caused them to make the most melatonin.[12] Although melatonin classically helps initiate sleep, and you make melatonin when less light gets to your retinas, the volunteers' circadian and sleeping rhythms did not appear affected during the short duration of the study. No mention of adverse effects, such as decreased libido, was noted.

THE BOTTOM LINE

- Chasteberry may exert hormonal actions by acting like dopamine, which in turn suppresses prolactin. This has been attributed to some of its diterpenes. (Diterpenes are a large class of molecules found in many plants, and chasteberries possess diterpenes called *clerodadienols,* which are currently the presumed active ingredients.)
- Although chasteberry is not obviously estrogenic in human studies, test tube studies suggest that an alcoholic extract of chasteberries could be.
- Chasteberry may be useful for treating excess prolactin, breast soreness, premenstrual symptoms, absent menses or menstrual irregularities, and some cases of female infertility.
- Chasteberry seems relatively safe and side effects are uncommon but include mild stomach upset and rash. Pregnant women should avoid it, and it could theoretically interfere with the hormonal effects of some medications. It has not been found to act as an antiaphrodisiac in modern human studies.

CINNAMON

Cinnamonium verum (C. zeylanicum), Cinnamonium cassia (C. aromaticum)

HISTORY AND FOLKLORE

Cinnamon is one of the prized Oriental spices of the ancient world, and in the middle ages, cinnamon was second in popularity only to the costly black pepper. The familiar barklike rolls are, in fact, the inner bark of a tropical evergreen in the laurel family. Although there are many cinnamon species, usually you hear finicky cooks discussing just two forms: "true" cinnamon, or *C. verum,* which is native to Sri Lanka, and the reportedly harsher-tasting and cheaper "bastard," or "Chinese," cinnamon, *C. cassia,* also called "cassia."

Supposedly you can distinguish them with an iodine drop, which stains starch dark blue. The cheaper cassia cinnamon possesses more starch, turning bluer when exposed to iodine than so-called true cinnamon. Or, with a good eye, you can differentiate them just by looking at them: cassia is reddish-brown, while its more expensive sibling is tan. In the United States both can be called "cinnamon" legally, so what you buy in the American stores is mostly cassia. Other countries are required to have more discriminating labels. Both cinnamons contain a similar array of molecules, at any rate, and are likely to have similar therapeutic activities. It's unlikely you will, but don't confuse the species *cassia* with the genus *Cassia,* containing the unrelated, nauseatingly distasteful and laxative species *senna,* also in this book (see page 278). Oddly enough, cassia (cinnamon) is often used to disguise the taste of *Cassia senna* (the nasty-tasting laxative.)

Besides its value as a spice and as incense, cinnamon has traditionally been used therapeutically to treat digestive upset, gas, arthritis pain, bleeding, and menstrual cramps. Its oil is usually regarded with ambivalence, as the herbalist Mrs. M. Grieve notes in her 1931 *A Modern Herbal:* "The oil is a powerful germicide, but being very irritant is rarely used in medicine for this purpose."

HOW SCIENTISTS THINK CINNAMON WORKS

An ingredient in cinnamon potentiates the activity of insulin, at least in cell and animal studies. This was accidentally discovered by Richard Anderson at the U.S. Department of Agriculture's Human Nutrition Research Center in Beltsville, Maryland, when he screened dozens of foods for their power to lower blood glucose, what most people call their "blood sugar." He realized that something in apple pie seemed to lower blood glucose, and although he did not expect it to be the seasoning, he ultimately traced the effect to a water-soluble component of cinnamon called *methylhydroxy chalcone polymer (MHCP).*

MHCP from cinnamon helps activate the insulin receptor, with or without insulin. After insulin is released into the blood by the pancreas, it travels about, eventually sticking to insulin receptors on cells. The bound receptor then triggers a complex chain of events inside the cell. The insulin receptor not only protrudes outside a cell like a flag, but like so many other receptors, it has a long shaft that penetrates through the cell membrane into the cell, where it can activate various processes inside the cell like an on-off switch. The binding of insulin to its receptor flips the switch, so to speak, and the intracellular portion of the receptor gets "phosphorylated." This means that nearby molecules in the cell temporarily decorate the insulin receptor with phosphate molecules. This, in turn, activates a complicated signaling mechanism with many intracellular messengers involved, ultimately triggering various blood sugar–lowering events.

What's In It

BOTH C. cassia and *verum* bark contain varying proportions of cinnamaldehyde, cinnamylacetate, cinnamyl alcohol, o-methoxycinnamaldehyde, coumarin, and condensed tannins, and flavonoid derivatives (proanthocyanidins) as well as mucilage. True cinnamon may contain more eugenol, which is also found in clove oil.

One of these is the movement and fusion of otherwise useless internal glucose-carrying channels with the cell's external membrane, allowing the cell to import glucose from the blood and use it. This is important, because glucose can't enter a cell without being transported by a special glucose-recognizing channel, and insulin increases the number of these channels present on muscle and fat cells. This lowers blood sugar. In test tube studies, phosphorylation of the insulin receptor, a key step in this process, is stimulated by MHCP from cinnamon, even in the absence of insulin.[1] When insulin is around, the effect is enhanced. Thus MHCP does not compete with insulin—it does not bind where insulin binds—but synergistically enhances insulin's effect.

Indeed, in a separate test tube assay, MHCP, albeit in rather concentrated form (0.1 mg/ml), enhanced insulin's ability to get fat cells to remove sugar from their surroundings. MHCP alone also got the fat cells to take in sugar, although more slowly and less dramatically than insulin.

Like insulin, MHCP stimulates the conversion of glucose to its storage form, glycogen. Insulin not only allows your fat and muscle cells to take up glucose from the blood more efficiently, but it also kicks into action the enzymes that are involved with glucose storage. After you eat a meal, a lot of the resultant excess blood glucose is normally strung together into chains of glucose, creating a polymer called *glycogen.* This is stored, mainly by your liver, which generously releases glucose from it when you have haven't eaten for a while, and your blood sugar dips again, plus glycogen is stored in and used by your muscles. Glycogen synthase, as the name implies, is a major enzyme involved in synthesizing glycogen (it strings glucoses into chains of glycogen), thus its activation lowers blood sugar. Now hang on for some double-negative logic: Like insulin, MHCP inhibits an enzyme that inhibits glycogen synthase. To inhibit the inhibitor of a process means that you activate the process. In other words, MHCP indirectly activates glycogen synthase, which lowers blood sugar.

MHCP from cinnamon may help insulin regulate an enzyme that is central to metabolism. Insulin and MHCP both inhibit glycogen synthase kinase, or GSK for short. GSK plays a role in an almost bewildering number of metabolic functions that we are only now learning about. GSK is defined as a kinase, a very common sort of enzyme. Kinases normally transfer phosphates from one molecule to another, like those that decorate a newly bound insulin receptor (insulin receptor

THERE ARE two general ways for insulin to fail, and possibly a third way, as well. Are you at risk?

The less common way is called *type 1 diabetes,* where insulin-producing cells in the pancreas don't make enough insulin, usually because they are attacked by the friendly fire of the diabetic's own immune system. Type 1 diabetics must carefully monitor their blood sugar and inject insulin for the rest of their life. Thus type 1 diabetes is occasionally called *insulin-dependent diabetes.* It used to be called *juvenile onset diabetes,* except this term has become confusing: Adults can get type 1, and, sadly, more and more kids are getting type 2 diabetes, along with adults, as type 2 diabetes is increasing at an alarming rate. Type 2 diabetics make insulin but have lost sensitivity to it. Even seemingly healthy people can get type 2 diabetes, but obesity and lack of exercise increase the risk. MHCP from cinnamon could theoretically help both types of diabetics to an extent. This is because MHCP not only enhances the action of insulin, but it can also mimic insulin somewhat if insulin is absent.

In both kinds of diabetes, either absent or ineffective insulin results in excess blood sugar. The superfluous sugar causes multiple forms of damage. It sucks water out of adjacent tissues osmotically, increasing thirst and urination. It bonds to blood vessel proteins, damaging capillaries, decreasing blood flow, and harming organs. Excess glucose is also reduced to eye-damaging molecules. While there is too much glucose in the blood, ironically some cells starve for glucose, because they require the action of insulin to take in glucose from the blood. This kicks in odd metabolic problems not unlike those found in starvation, such as muscle wasting.

There is hope, however, if you can catch the problem. And there are many new ways to manage diabetes. If you think you have symptoms of diabetes, like excess thirst, urination, blurry vision, sudden weight gain or loss, or fatigue, see a doctor; the test for diabetes is simple and can save you a lot of pain down the road.

A possible "type 3" diabetes may exist, although it does not affect blood sugar. Very recently, researchers have discovered the pancreas is not the only organ to produce insulin. The brain makes insulin as well, and abnormally low brain insulin is associated with poor maintenance of the brain's nerve cells, and the development of Alzheimer's disease. Curiously, people with type 2 diabetes are known to have a greatly enhanced risk for acquiring Alzheimer's disease. This newly discovered link between insulin and Alzheimer's disease requires further exploration.

kinases). Phosphorylation is an important regulatory phenomenon you see all the time in biochemistry, and it typically turns the phosphorylated molecule's activity either on or off, depending on the molecule. GSK phosphorylates its namesake, glycogen synthase, and this inhibits it. This inhibition of glycogen synthase can raise your blood sugar to undesirable levels, because you need glycogen synthase to turn blood sugar into glycogen. Insulin normally keeps GSK in control and keeps this from happening. However, if insulin is less active, as in diabetes, it might be helpful to have MHCP around, which also keeps GSK in check, although more slowly and less potently than insulin.

Commonly Reported Uses for Cinnamon*

Internally

indigestion, gas, arthritis, bleeding, hyperglycemia, diabetes, dislipidemia

forms available for internal use:

bark, powder, oil, capsules, tea, extracts, tincture

commonly reported dosage:

In one clinical study, 1 to 6 grams of encapsulated cinnamon was taken daily for no longer than forty days.

*These uses and dosages are from historic use and are not necessarily tested nor recommended.

The enzyme that MHCP inhibits is the target of both old and new wannabe pharmaceuticals. Policing GSK activity does more than allow glycogen synthase to string glucoses into glycogen. Researchers were surprised to learn that lithium, the classic treatment for bipolar disorder, inhibits it, too. It has come out that GSK possesses many important regulatory functions, having implications in several disorders in addition to diabetes, such as Alzheimer's disease and cancer. Thus drug makers are now trying to come up with new ways to inhibit GSK. The trick is to find ways of messing with such an involved enzyme that leads to more benefits than side effects.

Speaking of side effects, cinnamon contains coumarin, a blood thinner, and its cinnamaldehyde can be irritating. Coumarin, the sweet, vanilla-scented molecule that lends new-mown hay its odor, interferes with vitamin K's ability to help you clot your blood. Also, anyone sucking on "hot" cinnamon candy can tell you that too much can hurt—molecules like cinnamaldehyde in cinnamon oil may not only be responsible for cinnamon's reputed antimicrobial activity, but can be harsh to your own cells upon its application, too.

Good Effects . . . and Not So Good

Don't overdose on cinnamon, and don't ingest the pure oil. Overdose symptoms, reportedly from the oil, include rapid heartbeat and breathing, sweating, and central nervous system shutdown. Consuming an inordinate amount of cinnamon herb may do the same.

It may be too soon to take tons of cinnamon every day for medicinal purposes. Some experts worry about people taking massive amounts of cinnamon because of cinnamon's coumarin content. Coumarin is a blood thinner and could interfere with other blood-thinning medications. Fortunately, you shouldn't need to take massive amounts for it to help control blood sugar. Only a little bit is needed to see an effect, or so the principal investigator of the study of cinnamon on blood sugar claims. Of course, it won't lower your blood sugar if you pile it on top of sweets and cinnamon rolls. It seems sensible to enjoy it in normally consumed amounts, however, and a little extra now and then can't hurt.

Cinnamon can be irritating. It's fun to play with herbal oils, but they can hurt. After getting cinnamon oil on my skin, I regretted it for hours later: It burns. It can irritate mucous membranes especially, and cause dermatitis on skin. Some people can develop an allergic reaction to the cinnamaldehyde in it as well.

Evidence of Action

Cinnamon would probably be absent from this book, except for a single study that recently captured headlines. One reason the study raised heads is because it indicated cinnamon's use to treat type 2 diabetes, which is growing in our society at an epidemic rate. True, there are other popular antidiabetic herbs out there, like bitter melon, but so far none of the human studies performed with it were placebo-controlled, as was the one study with cinnamon, so bitter melon remains an unknown, scientifically. In my book (literally!), one placebo-controlled study is worth more than ten uncontrolled ones.

In this 2003 study,[2] sixty men and women with type 2 diabetes were divided randomly into six groups. For forty days, groups 1, 2, and 3 consumed either 1, 3, or 6 grams of encapsulated cinnamon (*C. cassia*), respectively, daily. The other three groups took similarly escalating doses of wheat flour placebo. You might guess that it's probably hard to disguise cinnamon's pungent taste and smell, even if encapsulated, so the experimental group could have guessed that they were taking something. It's important to use a placebo for studies on blood sugar, because stress can easily elevate blood sugar, and if people think they are getting the "good" treatment, the cinnamon, they are more likely to be calmed. But at least there was a placebo group, which helps validate the outcome.

Only those in the group taking the heftiest dose of cinnamon had significantly reduced blood glucose (18 to 29 percent) and triglyceride (23 to 30 percent) levels after twenty days, and all the cinnamon eaters eventually had the same positive effect after forty days. All those taking cinnamon also lowered their cholesterol, and significantly so for those taking the larger doses of 3 and 6 grams of cinnamon. They lowered their LDL ("bad") cholesterol (10 to 24 percent) without affecting their HDL ("good") cholesterol after forty days. None of the placebo groups enjoyed any of these positive effects on blood sugar and lipids.

Although cinnamon has traditionally more often been regarded as an antimicrobial, antifungal agent, such conclusions were reached with test tube–type studies. There is almost nothing in the way of human studies published on this effect. One small preliminary study found that 80 milligrams of cinnamon daily had no effect compared to placebo in reducing *Helicobacter pylori,* a bacterium linked to stomach ulcers, in infected people.[3] Application of cinnamon to skin in the treatment of topical or oral infections is limited to some extent by cinnamon's irritating nature, which may be why it is antimicrobial to begin with.

THE BOTTOM LINE

- There is one human study that indicates cinnamon may lower blood sugar, triglycerides, and LDL cholesterol. In test tube studies it enhances the action of insulin. More studies must be performed to better characterize this effect and to prove that it is reproducible.
- Toxicity of long-term, high doses of cinnamon are unknown. Some professionals worry about cinnamon's coumarin content. Coumarin is a blood thinner and may interfere with blood-thinning medication.
- Topical cinnamon has antimicrobial properties but can be irritating, initiating allergic responses.

CRANBERRY

Vaccinium macrocarpon, Vaccinium oxycoccos

HISTORY AND FOLKLORE

Though cranberry grows in the cold, northern parts of Europe and America, the larger-berried, American *Vaccinium macrocarpon* has stolen the agricultural and culinary show since the complexities of cultivating this swamp dweller were finally surmounted in the late 1800s. Massachusetts and Wisconsin remain the primary world producers today.

Early American settlers first dubbed this plant "craneberry." Depending on whom you ask, this was either for the crane's appetite for them or for the resemblance of its tiny pink flowers to cranes' heads. American settlers purportedly found the Native Americans' traditional use for them strange—they were typically incorporated into pemmican cakes along with dried deer meat and fat. Nonetheless, the colonists' adoption of this locally abundant food gave birth to a maple syrup–sweetened sauce that became a routine accompaniment to meat on colonial New England tables. Native Americans used the berries extensively as well, as food, dye, and medicine. They made cranberry poultices to draw poisons out of arrow wounds, some tribes used it for urinary ailments, and others ascribed calming and fever reducing properties to the fruits.

In the early 1920s, women, who are more likely to suffer urinary tract infections than men, spread a rumor that cranberry juice prevented their chronic urinary tract infections. They reasoned that the tart acidity of the berries kills bacteria, and this rumor remains active today. Perhaps based upon the assumption that what's good for one urinary ailment might work for another, cranberry is often also taken with the hope of preventing and treating kidney stones.

HOW SCIENTISTS THINK CRANBERRY WORKS

Cranberry's proanthocyanidins keep pathogenic bacteria from sticking to your cells. This is the best explanation, so far, for why cranberry prevents urinary tract infections. For decades, scientists have been trying to find out what cranberries do to your urine. This is because there is good evidence that consuming cranberry juice, tablets, and concentrates lowers the risk of urinary tract infections (UTIs). At first, cranberry was thought to simply acidify your urine, making your urinary tract an unwelcome home for troublesome bacteria. This seemed a reasonable hypothesis to the 1920s housewives who first tried the remedy and suggested this mechanism. Surely, they reasoned, this mouth-puckeringly tart beverage bestows its sourness to the fluid into which it is transformed. But there is more going on than that.

Many studies have shown that if you drink a great deal of cranberry juice, like one glass with each meal, your urine will be more acidic. However, you will also be more prone to want to *stop* drinking cranberry juice, as did several of the volunteers, who dropped out of these studies because they were so weary of drinking cranberry juice. Fortunately, you do not have to saturate yourself with as much cranberry as these volunteers did, because the acidification of urine does not seem necessary for prevention of UTIs. As a matter of fact, several studies say cranberry does *not* reliably acidify urine, so this mechanism is now disputed.

UTIs are usually caused by *E. coli,* and these and other similar bacteria often have a hairy exterior. These hairs, called *pili* or *fimbriae,* can stick to cells and take up residence there. This sticking is required for infection, so anything that prevents the sticking thus prevents infection—the killing of bacteria isn't even necessary. Thus the studies that disputed cranberry's effectiveness because it did not act like an antibiotic nor reduce the amount of bacteria in urine may have been on the wrong track.

What's In It

CRANBERRY IS a close relative of blueberries, currants, and bilberries, and possesses the same blue-red anthocyanidin flavonoids. It is notably the most sour of the lot, owing to its acids, notably, vitamin C, quinic, malic, and citric acids. Cranberries' astringent tannins assist in puckering your mouth, and its red-colored anthocyanidins bond into various proanthocyanidins.

Not all sticky bacteria are bad. More benign bacteria have fimbriae that stick to a sugar called *mannose,* which is on the exterior of your cells. While this connection is prevented by fructose, a sugar abundant in all fruits and fruit juices, preventing the adhesion of benign sticky bacteria does not have any effect on UTIs. This is because the more pathogenic bacteria have different sorts of fimbriae that stick to galactose sugars on your cells instead. Most fruit juices tested

did not prevent this more insidious sort of adhesion, except for cranberry and blueberry juice, although cranberry reportedly works better.[1] So what is it about cranberry juice that helps prevent urinary tract infections? The active antistick agents are in a class of plant molecules called *proanthocyanidins,* which are common in plants. It may be that the proanthocyanidins prevent the pathogenic bacteria from adhering to cells.

Whether proanthocyanidins get absorbed into the blood after you eat them is an important issue. They must first get to the blood to gain access to the urinary tract in order to work to prevent infections there. Scientists have raised the valid criticism that proanthocyanidins' especially large structures may prevent them from getting absorbed through the gut lining into the blood stream. So just because some studies show that cranberry pigments prevent bacteria from sticking to urinary tract cells in a test tube does not prove they can do this in your body. Clinical studies do suggest cranberry works, though, and models of the gut lining suggest that smaller proanthocyanidins can indeed traverse the gut lining to enter the blood.

Cranberry's proanthocyanidins might make your dentist happy, too. These proanthocyanidins are one of those scientific words with an annoying number of synonyms. You will also see them called *oligomeric proanthocyanidins, OPCs,* and *condensed tannins* on herb labels. Many papers have not only reported that the ones in cranberry prevent E. coli adhesion, but they also keep other troublesome bacteria from sticking. In cell cultures, cranberry prevents plaque-forming bacteria from sticking to actual and simulated teeth. No tests of any new cranberry spiked toothpastes or mouthwashes have been published, however.

If you or anyone you know has had

kidney stones, cranberry juice is often one of the first things recommended. However, it might actually make things worse, at least theoretically. You might be surprised to learn that no well-designed studies of cranberry's ability to affect stone formation have been performed. All we have to go on are a few studies that examined the changes in urine chemistry after a small sample of healthy, *non*–kidney stone–prone male volunteers drank cranberry juice, which suggested cranberry *might* acidify urine. If cranberry *does* acidify urine (and some say it does not, at least not reliably), this would help those who make calcium oxalate stones (see sidebar on Calcium Oxalate and Kidney Stones, below), but hurt those who make uric acid stones. But don't go gulping cranberry juice for preventing calcium oxalate stones just yet. Cranberry has a lot of oxalate, which can make calcium oxalate stones more likely to form.

white hard water deposits, or "lime," you get on your sink fixtures. If you have ever tried to clean this gunk off your sinks and coffee pots, you may have learned that acids like vinegar and lemon juice work. Acid does the same for calcium oxalate kidney stones. Here's why:

Acid renders one of the kidney stone ions uncharged and thus unsticky. Acidifying a fluid simply means adding lots of hydrogen ions. These are positively charged particles that stick to the negatively charged oxalate, rendering it uncharged and less interested in sticking to the positive calcium ions. Thus fewer calcium oxalate stones will form in acidic urine, plus acid can dissolve an existing calcium oxalate stone. More reliable urine acidifiers than cranberry exist, however, which is why your doctor might prescribe vitamin C or citric acid for calcium oxalate stones instead.

Urine Acidity and Calcium Oxalate Kidney Stones

IF YOU have kidney stones, your doctor can give you a device to catch the stones as they pass so you can have their composition analyzed. This is an important step in determining what treatment will work for you. Calcium oxalate stones are far more common than uric acid stones and are made of two things: calcium ions, which are positively charged, and oxalate ions, which are negatively charged. Since opposite charges attract, and these two ions stick together with bonds that water can't squeeze between and break, they will not break up and dissolve in even the most watery urine. This water insolubility is typical of several calcium-containing salts, like the insoluble,

Despite its debated urinary acidification, cranberry may create more calcium oxalate stones. This is because cranberry has a lot of oxalate ions, itself, and in two of three studies an abundance of oxalate ions were found in the urine of those who consumed cranberry. Oxalate is not recommended for people with kidney stones.

On the face of things, it seems prudent to avoid foods and drinks that contain a lot of kidney stone ingredients if you are one of those people who get frequent calcium oxalate kidney stones. But this is just theory, and you have a right to be suspicious of theory alone. Experimental data is far better, but we don't have that for cranberry and kidney stones just yet. In the face of uncertainty, it's best for people who chronically make calcium oxalate kidney stones to avoid cranberry juice until we know better how it affects stone formation.

Commonly Reported Uses for Cranberry*

Internally
urinary tract infections, kidney stones
forms available for internal use:
fresh, frozen, and dried berries, juice, capsules, tablets, dried cranberry powder
commonly reported dosage:
For preventing urinary tract infections, 3 fluid ounces (a half glass or juice glass) of juice are recommended, and the dose is increased to 12 to 32 ounces for treating an existing infection. Some supplement labels give the dose, which is equivalent to 3 fluid ounces.

*These uses and dosages are from historic use and are not necessarily tested nor recommended.

If you make uric acid stones, cranberry could cause you to make more. A surplus of uric acid, a waste product derived primarily from meat, is found in some people, usually men, with a genetic predisposition for metabolizing it poorly, so it accumulates. Excess uric acid can turn into kidney stones and also predisposes you to gout. Uric acid crystals, unlike the calcium oxalate ones, are not made of positive and negative ions, but are usually pure uric acid, which sticks to itself so ardently that it forms a relatively pure rock. The growth of these stones can be slowed by making the urine less acidic. Making urine less acidic means *removing* hydrogen ions from the urine—in such a hydrogen ion–deficient environment, hydrogen ions naturally fall off of the uric acid in order to replenish those that are not present in the urine. Uric acid is then no longer uric acid, but a negatively charged ion called *urate,* which does not find itself attractive, does not form rocks and can be washed away by water. Since cranberry acidifies your urine, it won't help this situation, and it might make things worse. More alkalinizing beverages, such as black currant juice, might help,[2] but you should see your doctor for advice if you have any sort of kidney stone.

GOOD EFFECTS . . . AND NOT SO GOOD

Try taking cranberry regularly if you suffer from chronic urinary tract infections. The best thing for a urinary tract infection is an antibiotic, so please see a doctor if you suspect you have this sort of infection. An antibiotic will banish the pain and infection faster than any herbal treatment. In addition to this, take cranberry for treatment, and for prevention when you are not infected. According to a couple of clinical studies, it may not matter whether you take the juice or concentrated tablets. If you do take a supplement form, however, make sure it is standardized to the active ingredients, the proanthocyanidins. This are also called oligomeric proanthocyanidins, OPCs, and condensed tannins. Also, note that some cranberry juices are better than others. Avoid cranberry juice that is sweetened with high fructose corn syrup, "HFCS," sugar, or corn syrup. Dietitians agree the added sugar is bad for you. Most "no sugar added" juices are cranberry diluted with other juices, which is still caloric but more nutritious. The bravest palates can now buy *pure* cranberry juice, which is *terribly* tart but can be made more palatable with additions of your own favorite juices.

Don't use "white" cranberry juice for

urinary tract infections. White cranberry juice is popular because it is less sour, and is made from immature cranberries, which have not yet developed their classic red color. Despite what the cranberry juice companies tell you, it is less likely to contain the active ingredient in a therapeutically useful dose. Their own funded research says otherwise, but their claim requires independent verification.

What does color have to do with it? The proanthocyanidins that you want are made from several red-colored molecules called *anthocyanidins,* and these get stuck together in a variety of ways to make the desired *pro*anthocyanidins (hence the alternate term "oligomeric" proanthocyanidins; "oligomeric" is a scientist's way of saying "a few things stuck together"). If the juice is missing its red color, it is less likely to contain the active ingredients that the colorful anthocyanidins form.

Don't try cranberry yet for kidney stones until better studies have been done. See a doctor for the best treatment for you. There are too many theoretical risks, which have not yet been experimentally verified, for you to try preventing or treating kidney stones with cranberry juice at the present time. There are other things you can do, like drinking more water, which helps prevent all sorts of kidney stones. Don't try treatment without guidance, because what helps one person can hurt another! Certainly, you must see a doctor if you have kidney stones. The doctor might recommend urinary acidifiers such as citric acid or vitamin C if you have calcium oxalate stones, but conversely he or she might recommend you *avoid* acids, reduce your meat intake, and possibly take medications like allopurinol if you have uric acid stones.

Roses are Red and Violets are Blue. But Why?

THE SAME anthocyanidins that make cranberries red are found all over the plant kingdom, making red, blue, and purple colors. In fact, before World War II a scientist named R. M. Willstätter concluded that almost *every* fruit or flower that is bright red, blue, or purple contains anthocyanidins. Anthocyanidins are generally thought to be good for you, as they are antioxidant, and they are in the category of molecules called *flavonoids.* (Sometimes they are attached to sugars and are then called *anthocyan*ins.) When a handful of anthocyanidins link to each other, they make a larger, more complex *pro*anthocyanidin. They can link to each other in many different ways, so there are many different proanthocyanidins, and they are common in the plant kingdom, too. Proanthocyanidins are the active ingredients in cranberry that prevent urinary tract infections.

But are anthocyanidins red, or blue? They can be both: It depends on the pH. Actually, they range from pink in acids, reddish-purple in neutral solutions, and can even be green in base. The differences between these types of solutions—acid, neutral, and base—are the number of protons in each. (Low pH has excess protons and is called "acidic," and high pH has a deficiency of protons and is called "basic.") The extra protons in acidic solution stick to the proanthocyanidin molecules, changing their structure and their color. And this difference in proton concentration is enough to affect the color of a flower, fruit, or leaf.

Some anthocyanidins are better at changing color than others. Red cabbages and onions contain anthocyanidins, and their color depends on the proton concentration of the soil in which they grow. You can turn red cabbages or red onions green by subjecting either to basic solutions like baking soda in water, or to deep red by putting them in acidic solutions like lemon juice or vinegar. Their color is affected by the pH of the soil in which they are grown, too.

EVIDENCE OF ACTION

Cranberry seems to help women who have chronic urinary tract infections. Two independent reviewers analyzed randomized, clinical tests of cranberry for preventing urinary tract infections (UTIs). They picked only two of seven possessing a more rigorous design and concluded that cranberry did indeed reduce the risk of UTIs, though the volunteers were exclusively women, and they had to take either cranberry juice or tablets for a year before the results became statistically significant.[3] Both cranberry juice and tablets had statistically equivalent results. In another study, cranberry-lingonberry juice also significantly reduced UTIs in women.[4]

Surprisingly, there are no well-designed studies of whether cranberry increases or decreases kidney stone formation. Instead, there are only a few very small studies noting the change in urine chemistry for healthy men who drank cranberry juice. Each of these three studies showed that cranberry increased urine acidity, but several studies contradict this.

Two of these studies showed oxalate is increased in the urine of those taking cranberry.[5, 6] The other actually showed decreased oxalate in the urine, but this study had volunteers on a less controlled diet.[7]

THE BOTTOM LINE

- There is good evidence that the proanthocyanidins in cranberry help prevent and treat urinary tract infections. The active ingredients, proanthocyanidins, prevent infectious bacteria from adhering to the lining of the urinary tract.
- For preventing urinary tract infections, either red cranberry juice or supplements standardized to proanthocyanidins (also called oligomeric proanthocyanidins, OPCs, and condensed tannins) are recommended.
- Though many people take cranberry for kidney stones, cranberry might actually make matters worse. Although this is based on theory and has not yet been verified clinically, avoid cranberry if you have kidney stones, see a doctor, and drink lots of water.

DANDELION

Taraxacum officinale

History and Folklore

You probably require no assistance identifying this herb. The bane of gardeners and the beloved toy of children, its serrated leaf margins caused the French to dub it *dents de lion,* or "tooth of the lion." The lesser-known French label, *pis en lit,* or "pee in bed," suggests that consuming it causes you to urinate more than usual. It has also variously been called *blowball, lion's tooth, Irish daisy,* and *wild endive.* But the name I like best is *fairy clock,* which alludes to a method of telling time once used by English children. The number of puffs needed to blow the seeds off the seed head is supposed to equal the hour. (Results, however, are variable.)

As you might guess, based on a casual survey of your neighborhood lawns, dandelion grows everywhere in temperate areas of the world. Historically, both Asian and European cultures used all parts of the dandelion medicinally and as food. It's a shame that we religiously poison this common lawn weed every spring, because its leaves are edible and nutritious, as long as you are not allergic to them (and as long as they haven't been treated with pesticides or weed killers). The root is sometimes roasted to make a nonstimulating, bitter, coffee-like beverage. The yellow flower was once commonly used to make yellow-tinted dandelion wine. Although one of my hobbies is home winemaking, I confess I have not tried this one, so am not familiar with its taste. However, the herbalist Varro Tyler once suggested that its flavor had the power to suddenly make you find cheap jug wines more compelling. Winemakers repeatedly inform that if you use any of dandelion's green parts in the wine, the wine will become bitter and nasty.

As a medicinal herb, dandelion is associated with bile production. This may be due to the fact that dandelion's flower is yellow. Ancient and medieval herbalists noted that jaundice caused yellowed skin, so they superstitiously looked around for anything yellow to treat it. (This could also be why it was regarded as a diuretic, though this is just my hypothesis.) The bitterness of the greens is thought to stimulate various secretions in addition to bile, such as gastric juices, and thus the greens are traditionally used as an appetite stimulant and digestive aid. The roots and leaves are also commonly regarded as a diuretic.

How Scientists Think Dandelion Works

What you will first hear about dandelion has not been supported, but it hasn't been contradicted either. Dandelion is frequently said to act as a diuretic, reducing your water retention, and perhaps blood pressure, by making you urinate more than usual. You will also hear that it stimulates your secretion of bile. Neither of these actions has yet been validated, because well-designed experiments have simply not been done. But stay tuned.

Dandelion does share some molecules (luteolin and luteolin glycosides) with artichoke (see page 31) that are known to increase your bile output. Though an old paper once linked dandelion's diuretic effect to its potassium content, its potassium is not remarkably high, compared to other herbs, nor is it low—most plants have a good share of potassium. However, other dandelion constituents, such as vitamin C, luteolin, and caffeic acids, are diuretic, supporting anecdotal reports of dandelion's diuretic power.

What's In It

FIRST OF all, it's not at all clear what dandelion really does, but most sources suggest dandelion's active ingredients are its bitter compounds. Its flavonoids (such as apigenin and luteolin) are bitter to more sensitive tongues and are known to be active ingredients in other plants. Dandelion's bitterness also comes from its sesquiterpene lactones, such as taraxacin (lactucopicrin), eudesmanolides and germacranolides. Its inulin content varies greatly between spring and fall, and according to the German Commission E, pharmacopial-grade dandelion root must come from roots collected in the fall, when its inulin content is the highest (40 percent). Besides its antioxidant flavonoids, dandelion leaves have vitamin A and other nutritious carotenoids, such as lutein. It also has phytosterols and triterpenes, such as taraxasterol and beta-sitosterol.

Dandelion is said to stimulate your appetite, like other classic "bitter herbs." For ages, bitter-tasting herbs like dandelion have been used to stimulate the appetite. The theory says that the bitter taste on your tongue—which requires that the herb not be taken in encapsulated form—supposedly jabs your cranial nerves into reflexive stimulation of your gastric juices, whetting your appetite. The bitter taste is supposed to act like some sort of neurological Pavlovian bell, making you salivate, though you could argue that you are more inclined to salivate over tastier sensations. But some bitter herbs, like wormwood, actually seem to do this. Scientists don't know if the bitter components in dandelion, classified as sesquiterpene lactones, do the same thing, because they have not attached a high priority to performing the studies to find out.

More recent studies contradict the notion that all bitter herbs whet your appetite. Putting almost anything, bitter or not, in your mouth stimulates a normal gastric response. Some scientists suggest that bitter herbs work better for people whose gastric secretions are abnormally low, but not for those whose gastric response to food is relatively normal.[1] Of course, putting *anything* bitter in your mouth might simply make you want to eat something different, just to get the taste out of your mouth.

The inulin in dandelion feeds your beneficial intestinal flora. One of the few strikingly concentrated constituents in dandelion is inulin, although its presence in dandelion is not usually discussed in herb books. Inulin-containing foods are now being recommended by nutritionists. If you collect dandelion roots in the fall, they will be full of inulin. In the spring they have only a negligible amount, however, because its concentration varies seasonally. Inulin is really a collection of different oligosaccharides—that is, small handfuls of sugars tied together. They contain mostly fructose sugar rings, with a few other sugars, tied together into chains of varying lengths, and your beneficial colon bacteria love to eat them. (Don't confuse inulin with the similar-sounding *insulin,* which is totally different.) You don't digest inulin very well yourself, so it is technically fiber.

Inulin is sold in supplement form as a "prebiotic." Prebiotics are thought to enhance your beneficial gut bacteria by feeding them. *Bifidobacteria,* a type of beneficial gut bacteria that you can get from yogurt, particularly enjoy dining on inulin. Feeding your personal gut bifidobacteria with inulin is thought to increase their numbers, and the presence of these bacteria is thought to crowd out the growth of unwanted pathogenic bacteria.

Commonly Reported Uses for Dandelion*

Internally
> diuretic, choleretic (bile stimulating), appetite stimulant, digestive aid
> **forms available for internal use:**
> capsule, fresh leaves, dried leaves, dried root, root juice, decoction, tincture
> **commonly reported dosage:**
> Three to 5 grams a day of dried root is commonly taken three times daily, or 1 to 2 teaspoons of tincture of root taken three times daily.

*These uses and dosages are from historic use and are not necessarily tested nor recommended.

Feeding helpful gut bacteria inulin may decrease your risk of tumors, too. When your intestinal bacteria eat inulin, they make a very small, or "short chain," fatty acid called *butyrate* that is also found in milk fat and butter. (Milk fat and butter also contain cholesterol and less healthy saturated fat, however, so it may be healthier to make your own butyrate with inulin.) Butyrate may help

protect you from cancer. Some studies show that this inulin by-product arrests cell growth, causes cancer cells to self-destruct, and prods cells' differentiation into a normal cell rather than a cancer cell. Many other plants have high concentrations of inulin, too, including onions, garlic, bananas, asparagus, and artichokes. Inulin is water soluble, so aqueous dandelion extracts, like dandelion tea, are a good source of it.

Dandelion is a nutritious salad herb— as long as you are not allergic to it. It's not at all clear what the dandelion in commercial supplements does for you, simply because the studies have not been done. But why not eat the leaves in a salad? If you enjoy the pizzazz of bitter greens like arugula, you might like dandelion, too. It isn't a bad idea, as long as you don't have allergies to it.

In fact, this common lawn weed has gained popularity as an exotic salad green. The produce sections of natural health stores are now selling pesticide-free versions of dandelions whose agricultural histories are trustworthier than your neighborhood weeds. Dandelion greens are absolutely loaded with vitamin A, have 50 percent more vitamin C than a tomato, and have as much iron as spinach. They also contain antioxidant flavonoids that have been shown to help stabilize your cell membranes against attack by oxygen and free radicals. Allergies to dandelion are relatively common, however, so treat this herb with caution if you have an allergy to the related ragweed or to other plants in the daisy family.

GOOD EFFECTS . . . AND NOT SO GOOD

It is not clear what dandelion supplements do, because they have not been thoroughly tested. It's quite possible that the claims for dandelion's diuretic and bile-stimulating actions are justified, because dandelion contains some ingredients that could theoretically stimulate bile and urine production. Many sources simply *assume* that dandelion stimulates bile, regardless of the lack of evidence, and based on this assumption such sources advise you not to take it if you have gallstones or a bile duct obstruction, for fear of causing impaction. But there are better-documented bile stimulators, like artichoke (see page 31), and more reliable diuretics, like guarana and tea (see pages 179 and 301, respectively).

Allergies to dandelion are common. Most scientific papers on dandelion simply document the unfortunate people who got a rash from dandelion, or worse, went into life-threatening anaphylactic shock after taking it. If you know you have an allergy to ragweed pollen or other plants in the daisy family, treat dandelion with caution! Even some allergy-prone dogs can develop a skin rash from this common lawn weed.[2]

As long as you are not allergic to them, dandelion greens are quite nutritious. If you want to try dandelion greens, get pesticide-free ones from your produce section. Don't pick your own unless you are certain they are pesticide-free. Scientific papers document dandelion's ability to accumulate environmental toxins such as carcinogenic PCBs[3] and heavy metals.[4] Most natural foods grocery stores stock dandelion greens, and some mainstream stores are catching the wave, too. Raw in salads, they may be too bitter for some, but lightly boiling them like spinach washes out some of their bitter components. Like spinach, they are full of iron, vitamin A, plus antioxidant flavonoids and fiber.

Some dandelion supplements are standardized to vitexin, a flavonoid that can affect your thyroid adversely. Many plants besides dandelion contain vitexin, but consuming a lot of vitexin over time could prevent your thyroid gland from working properly. The vitexin in millet grain was fingered as the dietary culprit for thyroid disorders in peasants in western India.[5] If you have a thyroid disorder, you should steer clear of dandelion or other supplements that are standardized to vitexin. Eating dandelion greens on occasion, however, is unlikely to adversely affect your thyroid.

EVIDENCE OF ACTION

For such a ubiquitous herb, well-designed human clinical studies using dandelion are surprisingly rare. Other than several reports of allergic responses in sensitive people, there aren't any.

One frequently cited yet scientifically antique (1959) study noted that an alcoholic extract of dandelion increased rats' bile secretion by more than 40 percent.[6] But this study later gained some critics, and it should be repeated to see if it is reproducible. Dandelion's bile-stimulating (choleretic) activity is usually associated with its bitter sesquiterpene lactones, perhaps superstitiously, because bile is also bitter. So far there is no data on this supposition. You might want to note, however, that a fellow *Asteraceae*, artichoke, is a known choleretic. Some assign this activity to its bitter flavonoids (luteolin and luteolin glycosides),[7] which are also in dandelion. So there may very well be something to this claim, after all, but more research is needed to support it.

Dandelion very well may make you urinate more, but there are hardly any studies examining this simple effect. Thus there is as of yet not much in the way of supporting this most noted property of dandelion experimentally, except that some scientists thought it might be linked to its potassium content, which is not remarkable compared to other greens.[8] Dandelion does at least contain additional ingredients that may be diuretic, including luteolin, vitamin C, and caffeic acid.

THE BOTTOM LINE

- It's not clear what dandelion does, because good experiments have not been done yet.
- Dandelion is most commonly sold as a diuretic and choleretic (bile secretion stimulator). Though these actions have not been experimentally proven, they have not been disproved either, and dandelion does contain ingredients that may validate both of these claims.
- The inulin in dandelion root encourages the growth of beneficial intestinal bacteria and is associated with halting tumor development.
- Dandelion greens are nutritious, containing vitamin A, carotenoids, and antioxidant flavonoids.
- Allergies to dandelion are common, and it should not be taken by those with gallbladder or bile duct obstructions such as gallstones, just in case it really is choleretic.
- Some commercial dandelion products are standardized to vitexin, which can interfere with the thyroid gland's function when taken in large quantities. People with thyroid problems should probably avoid regular consumption of vitexin, but they are unlikely to be adversely affected by occasional dandelion greens.

ECHINACEA

Echinacea augustifolia, E. purpurea, E. pallida

History and Folklore

You can recognize echinacea fairly easily; it is a common garden addition with a distinctive appearance. This tall plant sports a single, big purple flower surrounding an orange, cone-shaped center, hence the common title "coneflower." It's native to the American plains, and archeological excavations have unearthed evidence of its use by Lakota Sioux four hundred years ago. Native Americans chewed the root, drank its tea, or applied it topically, for colds, toothache, arthritis, wounds, stings, and bites, including snakebite.

In the 1870s, Native Americans revealed this remedy to a Nebraskan doctor, H. C. F. Meyer. Meyer was so eager to prove its worth to the medical establishment that he offered to be bitten by a snake to prove that it cured rattlesnake bite. Understandably, they refused. However, he eventually grabbed enough attention to allow the herb's inclusion in the American *Materia Medica*, the passages of which sang its praises for use against infection. Meyer promoted his echinacea-based formulas as a cure for a broad list of complaints and touted it as a "blood purifier."

You might be surprised to learn what he meant by that. These days many modern herb books still unquestioningly copy and paste phrases from old texts, recommending herbs as "blood cleansers," ignorant of the term's original meaning. Scientists don't have any definition for the term and don't use it. If asked about blood purifiers, we will just look befuddled and say we don't know what you are talking about. That's because although today's society feels free to speak the word syphilis out loud, in the past, mentioning venereal disease was grossly impolite, so people daintily said it was a problem with impure blood. "Blood purifiers" were cures for venereal diseases, which were rampant before antibiotics appeared in the 1940s. "Meyer's Blood Purifier" was both popular and accepted by conventional medicine until antibiotics stole the show, and its popularity then subsided for a while. Resurfacing over the past few decades, its employment as an infection fighter has intensified to the point that it is now one of the top sellers in the world's herbal market.

How Scientists Think Echinacea Works

Echinacea stimulates your immune system—and so do allergies. If you put echinacea in a test tube with bacteria to fight it out, nothing happens. Echinacea itself has no obvious, direct bactericidal properties, yet is said to work by activating the immune systems of those who expose themselves to it. This places echinacea in the category of an *immunomodulator*, an immune system stimulator.

Echinacea does appear to rev up some mediators of the immune system, at least in certain tests, and it obviously affects the immune systems of people who are allergic to it. Echinacea is related to ragweed (both plants are in the *Asteraceae,* or daisy, family), and ragweed certainly excites a lot of people's immune systems. Like other members of this family, ragweed pollen is a common allergen. If you have allergies, you can testify that having your immune system stimulated in such a manner is not necessarily the most pleasant phenomenon. Indeed, echinacea is also known for giving people rashes, or allergic atopic dermatitis, further evidence of a stimulated immune system. When considering an immune-stimulating agent, you should always keep in mind that the immune system is a double-edged sword, and you don't want to overdo it.

Echinacea's immune-stimulating effects are hard to pin down. Once one immune cell is stimulated, it releases factors to produce a cascade of immunological effects, which makes it difficult to identify the direct cause of all these effects by echinacea and other immunomodulators. Scientists report that echinacea's effects are "nonspecific." The term "specific" means that a drug or herb's molecules bind to either our receptors or enzymes in a lock-and-key type fashion, initiating an effect. Thus echinacea's "nonspecific" action implies that no similar lock-and-key type binding has been identified. Echinacea ingredients may instead exert an indirect change in your body's environment, alerting the immune system that something isn't right.

Echinacea's immune-stimulating effects are observed in both *in vitro* (in test tube studies of isolated cells) and *in vivo* (in live animal studies). Bear in mind, however, that several *in vitro* and *in vivo* studies have also completely failed to show these effects. Rather than throw the echinacea baby out with the bathwater entirely, some researchers assume that the variability in both the types of echinacea preparations used and the methods of administration could account for this inconsistency in experimental results.

What's In It

ECHINACEA'S POLYSACCHARIDES include 4-O-methylglucuronylarabinoxylans and acidic arabinorhamnogalactans. Other therapeutic molecular candidates evaluated for activity include alkylamides and caffeic acid derivatives, such as chicoric acid and echinacoside.

Echinacea extracts in cultures of immune cells makes them hungry, perhaps because echinacea's polysaccharides fool them into acting as though bacteria are present. In the presence of echinacea extracts, immune cells start undergoing phagocytosis in the test tube. Phagocytosis literally means *cell eating*. A phagocytosing immune cell completely engulfs foreign cells and debris, and then digests the invader or merely imprisons it within the body of the cell. Phagocytosis appears to be stimulated by echinacea's polysaccharides. These large carbohydrates are strings of smaller ring-shaped sugar molecules linked together to make one long chain, and are found in all plants and animals but in different forms. They are all made of similar building blocks, but like Tinker Toys or Legos, they can be stuck together in a tremendous variety of different forms. Most cells are in fact sugarcoated with polysaccharides. Bacteria and cancer cells often exhibit polysaccharides that our bodies detect as foreign, and the presence of these alien carbohydrates is often enough to activate our immune system. Indeed, certain odd carbohydrates are injected medically as *adjuvants,* typically along with a vaccine—that is, a substance administered in order to help the vaccine provoke an immune response. The polysaccharides from echinacea are apparently strange enough to stimulate immune cells to start eating potential invaders.

The problem with echinacea's polysaccharides mediating this activity in your bloodstream after you eat it is that you digest polysaccharides, breaking them down, or else they go right through you. So unless you want to inject them, they may only work topically, in theory. In other studies, the more absorbable alkylamides and chicoric acid from echinacea enhance phagocytosis as well, so eating the stuff may still initiate this phagocytic response.

Echinacea's chicoric acid might keep some bacteria from breaking and entering topically. Chicoric acid is thought to be at least one echinacea active ingredient that hampers a bacterial chemical weapon called *hyaluronidase.* Some invading bacteria like *Streptococcus, Staphylococcus,* and *Clostridium* use hyaluronidase, also known as the "spreading factor," to break down a structural tissue molecule called *hyaluronic acid.* Hyaluronic acid is a polysaccharide that is found in the tissues of animals, and this large molecule forms scaffolding networks around cells, attracting water to form a gel that helps provide cushioning and strength. Inhibiting the breakdown of this tissue-supporting network prevents microbes from invading, and may also accelerate wound healing. The concentrations needed to perform this trick in a test tube may not be achieved in your body when you take it internally. The mechanism is more likely to work topically.

Some cell studies suggest echinacea primes your defense against viruses by increasing interferon, but there are con- cerns. Virally infected cells are known to produce proteins called *interferon,* sort of like a chemical warning beacon. Echinacea stimulates the cellular manufacture and export of interferon as well. The released interferon then binds to uninfected cells, eliciting a broad-spectrum (nonspecific) antiviral state in them. Interferon-stimulated cells produce two enzymes that work by different mechanisms to inhibit protein synthesis. Protein synthesis is significant where viruses are concerned, because viruses require a cell's protein-making machinery to make more virus copies, and this is the only way that a virus can reproduce. If echinacea shuts down protein-making machinery through interferon, it could prevent virus production and infection of other cells.

One study attributes increased interferon production to echinacea's melanin. This is surprising, since melanin is the dark pigment that colors our skin and hair. But it is also common in plants, in various forms. (It is not one molecule but a collection of molecular subunits bonded together in various ways.) The reason melanin hadn't been pinpointed before is that it requires just the right solvent to extract it. The melanin from echinacea not only increased interferon but also boosted an inflammatory mediator called *NF-kappa-B (nuclear factor kappa beta),* which turns on genes involved in creating inflammatory proteins. However, because inflammation is not something most people want, scientists are more interested in *decreasing* NF-kappa-B for therapeutic purposes. It seems unlikely that the low amounts of melanin in echinacea supplements would have much effect, anyway.

According to cell studies, echinacea increases TNF, but in most people it's better to decrease it. Tumor necrosis factor, or TNF, enhances the proliferation and activation of several types of immune cells.

TNF's name sounds great, and it does cause tumor cells to commit suicide in a petri dish, but its dark side now appears more clinically relevant. It stimulates the growth of blood vessels that feed tumors *in vivo* and is the major mediator of the classic patient wasting (cachexia) seen in advanced cancers and possibly some patients with AIDS (hence its alternate name, *cachexin*). It's definitely not something a cancer or AIDS patient wants. Although TNF is required for the normal function of the immune system, its overabundance orchestrates injurious inflammation, and inflammation predisposes you to disease. TNF is particularly evident in several diseases, such as rheumatoid arthritis, Crohn's disease, and ankylosing spondylitis. *Anti*-TNF drugs, in fact, are very popular and have proven very useful in treating these illnesses. The potential negative effects of TNF should make anyone with a chronic, inflammatory disease or autoimmune disease think twice about taking echinacea. (Some of the more common diseases of this type include type I diabetes, Crohn's disease, thyroid disease, lupus, myasthenia gravis, multiple sclerosis, ankylosing spondylitis, and rheumatoid arthritis.)

GOOD EFFECTS . . .
AND NOT SO GOOD

Ask yourself if stimulating your immune system is a wise thing to do. Echinacea remains tremendously popular, especially in Europe, as an agent to prevent or shorten illnesses. But popularity doesn't mean something works, or that it's even safe. Scientists are now realizing that an overly stimulated immune system *causes* a surprisingly large number of diseases. This dawning revelation is now revolutionizing the medical field.

Enough studies do show enough consistent immune-stimulating effects to indicate that this plant has rightfully earned a reputation as an immune stimulator. It hasn't proven itself in clinical studies for preventing the contraction or severity of infections, however. Since it theoretically could boost certain immune agents in people with deficits in them, it could still have some use in specialized cases that have not yet been clearly outlined. However, bear in mind that "enhancing the immune system" is sort of like "giving even more power to an existing army"—sometimes that is helpful, but sometimes the army runs amok and does damage.

Some people develop allergic or other adverse reactions to echinacea. Most don't, but some people are sensitive. One of the more common complaints about echinacea use is the development of an itchy rash with red bumps.[1, 2] Itchy, red eyes, diarrhea, vomiting, dizziness, or a runny nose may also occur. More serious echinacea-associated problems include trouble breathing, respiratory system swelling, and even life-threatening anaphylactic shutdown of the respiratory system,[3] though these problems are rare. If you know you have an allergy to plants in the ragweed family, like daisies or sunflowers, you should avoid echinacea. Even people with no such allergy can develop one on exposure to echinacea, however.

Don't take echinacea if you have one of these problems. People with autoimmune diseases suffer from an overly aggressive immune system and should definitely not provoke their immune system any further with echinacea. If it really does rile the immune system, it will make your autoimmune disease worse. More common autoimmune diseases include type I diabetes, Crohn's disease, thyroid disease, lupus, myasthenia gravis, multiple sclerosis, ankylosing spondylitis, and rheumatoid arthritis.

Anyone with a chronic inflammatory disease should avoid it, too, for the same reason. Echinacea is not recommended for those with HIV infections, as it might exacerbate the symptoms of AIDS.[4] Cancer patients' symptoms are made worse by TNF, which is something that echinacea is supposed to increase. Also, overly stimulated immune systems engage mechanisms that allow cancer cells to chew their way through tissues with enzymes, enter the bloodstream, reattach themselves to inflamed blood vessels, and chew through more tissue to implant themselves in a new location. Thus an overly stimulated immune system can spread tumors to other parts of the body.

Echinacea comes in a bewildering number of forms. One thing that makes echinacea difficult for anyone to use is the occurrence of nine different species, and debate regarding which species works best continues. To further complicate matters, another completely unrelated plant (*Parthenium integrifolium*) was discovered as a common contaminant in preparations made prior to the 1980s, rendering older studies questionable. The most frequently used commercial formulas today employ the more easily cultivated *Echinacea augustifolia* and *E. purpurea*, which commonly decorate gardens with their attractive flowers.

In an attempt to reassure consumers that they are getting one of these more thoroughly researched species, *E. augustifolia,* standardized preparations that are guaranteed to contain a particular *augustifolia*-derived molecule, echinacoside, are sold. But echinacoside has been found in other species of echinacea, and this ingredient does not have impressive biological activity on its own. There is still debate over which echinacea ingredient to use for standardization, because no one is precisely sure what the active ingredient or ingredients are.

Commonly Reported Uses for Echinacea*

Internally
immunostimulant, colds, infections, protection from disease and cancer
forms available for internal use:
capsule, concentrated drops, dried leaves, leaf infusion (tea), tincture, extracts, dried root
commonly reported dosages:
Two teaspoons of root per cup of water is used to make a tea that is taken three times daily. The tincture or concentrate is taken by one or two dropperfuls per day. The solid extract is recommended at 300 to 400 milligrams per day. Two or three 400-milligram root capsules are taken per day. It is usually recommended that echinacea not be taken for an extended period of time; after taking it for six to eight weeks, a break of one to four weeks is advised.

*These uses and dosages are from historic use and are not necessarily tested nor recommended.

If you take a commercial formula these days, you are probably taking either *Echinacea augustifolia* or *E. purpurea*. There isn't much known about which is least likely to cause side effects, unfortunately, but you certainly should avoid either if you have an inflammatory condition or one of the autoimmune diseases listed above. If you are already healthy, neither species is likely to cause undue harm, other than the occasional rash, which goes away when you stop using the herb. A more pertinent question is whether or not echinacea really works to prevent or cure illness. If you look at the

"Evidence of Action" section below, you'll see that most human studies suggest it does not.

Don't get suckered by testimonials, because most people do eventually recover from colds.

THE EVOLUTION of cold remedies' reputations teaches valuable lessons in data interpretation. Since most people do not die from colds, whether you take a cold remedy or not, you will probably get better sooner or later. If you are just one person conducting a self-experiment with a cold remedy, realize there is no control group. That is not to say it's a bad thing to try to shorten the period and severity of your illness! Just be discriminating when listening to anecdotal testimonies of those who claim that this or that agent helped their cold. How do they know how long their cold would have lasted *without* the remedy? For all they know, what they took might have lengthened the duration of their cold and increased the severity of its symptoms, since they have nothing to compare it to. A previous illness was likely caused by a different organism. There really is no way to tell if a cold remedy shortens the duration of one person's illness, unless they are in a clinical trial with a control group. When weighing a possible treatment, look for reports of publications of large clinical trials testing what you want to try, with the terms "double-blind," "placebo controlled," and "randomized."

An injectable form of echinacea is available in Europe but has not been legally approved in the United States, because ques-

tions remain concerning its effectiveness. Drugs act very differently depending on how they are administered. In the United States the aerial parts, or rootstock, of *E. purpurea, pallida,* or *augustifolia,* or water/alcohol extracts thereof, are taken orally. Echinacea is also applied externally to wounds with the hope of accelerating healing.

Some people use a tingle test. The famous herb pharmacologist Varro Tyler observed that Midwestern farmers regularly mailed him samples of some newly "discovered" root that produced a tingling sensation on their tongues. This tingling root turned out to be echinacea, and the sensation is attributed to the anesthetic effect of the alkylamides in the root. Since the alkylamides are often cited as one of the active ingredients in the plant, perhaps it's not unreasonable for people to qualitatively "test" the root for this tingling ingredient by chewing on it. Since alkylamides aren't clearly known to be active or effective agents, however, a tingle is no guarantee that it will work.

Most herbalists advise you not to take echinacea continuously. The effects are said to wear off, but perhaps more importantly, it's not a good idea to continually provoke your immune system, assuming its effects do *not* wear off. The German Commission E health authority advises that echinacea should not be used longer than eight continuous weeks.

EVIDENCE OF ACTION

While some cell culture assays and rodent studies look promising, most of the recent human clinical trials using echinacea are disappointing. A few have positive results, but most that do use a mixture of different herbs, including echinacea, and since there is no way to sort out which herb is doing what, they are not covered here. The lion's share of clinical trials using echinacea by itself are not promising. In a 1998 study of 302 volunteers, twelve-week oral consumption of alcoholic extracts of E. purpurea or augustifolia failed to prevent or delay the onset of upper respiratory tract infections relative to placebo.[5] A 1999 trial involving 108 volunteers taking four milliliters of E. purpurea extract also failed to decrease the incidence or severity of colds.[6] Another similar study a year later yielded the same conclusions.[7] Forty healthy males received freshly pressed E. purpurea juice or placebo for two fourteen-day periods, and no increase in phagocytic activity nor changes in the immune mediators interferon or TNF were found.[8] One hundred and forty-eight college students taking either dried, encapsulated, or whole-plant E. purpurea and augustifolia or placebo failed to show any difference in severity or incidence of colds.[9] E. purpurea also failed to decrease the severity and duration of upper respiratory infections relative to placebo in one very large study involving more than four hundred children, but the poor kids taking echinacea did acquire a statistically significant increase in the number of skin rashes.[10]

The newest studies also look unpromising for echinacea. Forty-eight subjects taking E. purpurea or placebo for seven days were then intentionally infected with a rhinovirus, but there was no statistical difference in the number of people developing a cold.[11] Also, 128 people who had just contracted a cold used either freeze-dried E. purpurea juice or a sugar pill, and their symptoms were clinically assessed in a double-blinded manner.[12] No difference was seen between the groups in their symptoms or duration of illness.

If all this bad news for echinacea is not enough, just recently news organizations across the world are avidly reporting the results of the New England Journal of Medicine's study, which is hailed as the most rigorous—that is, double-blind, randomized, placebo-controlled, and large—study of echinacea so far.[13] "Echinacea Ineffective," say the headlines. This most recent study is another nail in the coffin of echinacea studies: 399 volunteers were given either a placebo or one of three different standard preparations of E. augustifolia after an influenza virus was introduced into their nostrils. There was no difference in infection rates or symptoms expressed by either group.

It's always easy to be the critic. Echinacea supporters complain that this study should have also tested the other popular species of Echinacea, E. purpurea, and that the dose in this study was too low, even though it was a standard dose recommended by the German Commission E. People advocating (and in some cases benefiting from) echinacea sales—a healthy 300 million a year—protest that it isn't dead yet. They point out that there are still some positive studies, although relatively few.

Eighty volunteers using a commercial preparation of fresh juice from the aboveground parts of E. purpurea (Echinacin) reportedly had colds that lasted a median time of six days, as compared to nine days for the placebo.[14] When 128 subjects in another study got a common cold,[15] they were split into groups receiving either another commercial echinacea product (Echinilin) or a placebo, and the echinacea group self-rated their symptoms as significantly better than the placebo group. While these studies may be perfectly valid, keep in mind that studies on commercial products are often funded by the company selling the products (sometimes in a very roundabout way), which has a tendency to bias the experimenter's opinion of it. Taken as a whole, the overwhelming evidence for echinacea in treating and preventing colds appears poor, or at best inconclusive.

Although echinacea was originally promoted to ameliorate venereal diseases, herpes is one of the few venereal diseases that has been clinically studied for treatment with echinacea. While effective against the virus in the test tube, *E. purpurea* extract failed to show any activity against herpes in fifty people with the virus.[16]

There is limited evidence that external application of echinacea can aid wound healing. The antihyaluronidase effect of echinacea's echinacoside molecule was thought to be responsible for enhanced wound healing in rats.[17]

THE BOTTOM LINE

- Echinacea has a reputation for immunomodulation—that is, enhancing the activity of the immune system. Clinical evidence for its ability to prevent infection or delay the period of infection is weak.
- In some animal and cell studies, echinacea shows signs of stimulating the immune system. Other cell and animal studies are inconclusive.
- Echinacea should not be taken for an extended period of time.
- Those with allergies to plants in the daisy or ragweed family, and people with autoimmune diseases or chronic inflammatory diseases should avoid echinacea.
- Echinacea can cause rashes and allergic anaphylaxis.

ELEUTHERO

Eleutherococcus senticosus (Acanthopanax senticosus)

HISTORY AND FOLKLORE

If you have heard of eleuthero, or "Siberian ginseng," the former Soviet Union's marketing campaign paid off. Despite the current lack of decent data on this herb, eleuthero sales are booming, making it one of the top-selling herbs. No one paid much attention to it until the 1970s, when it was given a new name and advertised as "Siberian ginseng." This imbued it with the glamour of the popular, expensive, and revered Asian (*Panax ginseng*) and American (*Panax quinquefolius*) ginsengs. Eleuthero is cheaper and more abundant than ginseng, however, growing in Siberia, Korea, and the Shansi and Hopei provinces of China.

Soviet studies of questionable design boasted of similar properties for the root and root bark of this spiny shrub as ginseng—that it combated fatigue, stress, made you more productive, athletic, and resistant to disease. In China, where it is called *ci wu jia,* eleuthero is used traditionally for similar purposes, as well as for bronchitis, heart ailments, and rheumatism.

However, eleuthero is not so closely related to ginseng. It's in the same family (*Araliaceae*) but in a different genus. It also does not possess the same molecules as ginseng, which are collectively called *ginsenosides.* Ginsenosides are supposedly responsible for ginseng's alleged properties. Some herbal literature incorrectly states that ginseng and eleuthero contain the same constituents, but that is not true. The Soviets cleverly called the unrelated constituents of eleuthero *eleutherosides,* however, making them sound

similar. Yet many of the eleutherosides are not unique to eleuthero and are found in other plants. If the goal was to confuse eleuthero with ginseng, it was successful; older scientific studies confused the two genera to the point that now, according to the U.S. Farm Security and Rural Investment Act of 2002, commercial products can't legally use the term "Siberian ginseng" or "ginseng" unless they contain the *Panax* species. No thanks to former deceptive marketing practices and biased studies, eleuthero still requires investigation with a more objective, scientific eye.

HOW SCIENTISTS THINK ELEUTHERO WORKS

Cell and animal studies offer tentative evidence that eleuthero could exert anti-inflammatory, DNA-protective, and limited antiviral effects. Mice that were fed water-soluble polysaccharides from eleuthero stem showed better biochemical resistance to liver toxins.[1] For example, they had less liver damage as measured by liver enzymes, and less of an inflammatory mediator called *tumor necrosis factor (TNF).* Eleuthero additionally prevented TNF release from a type of immune cell commonly involved in allergic responses known as a *mast cell,* after these cells were provoked into a state of inflammation in culture.[2] Also, eleuthero root contains coniferyl aldehyde, and this molecule (when isolated from cloves) protected cells from mutating by various chemicals and ultraviolet light.[3] Eleuthero root extracts were able to inhibit the replication of some RNA-containing viruses (human rhinovirus, respiratory syncytial virus, and influenza A), but not DNA-based viruses (adenovirus or herpes simplex type 1).[4] The mechanisms underlying these effects have not been thoroughly investigated as of yet.

What's In It

ALTHOUGH THEY are glamorously titled "eleutherosides" when derived from eleuthero, these ingredients aren't unique to eleuthero. Nor does eleuthero contain the ginsenosides present in *Panax* species (ginseng). Eleuthero root contains chiefly caffeic acid derivatives like chlorogenic acid and the lignans, (+)-sesamin (eleutheroside B4), (+)-syringaresinol and its monoglucoside (eleutheroside E1) and diglucosides (eleutherosides D and E). It also contains syringenin and its monoglucoside (eleutheroside B), and coumarins such as isofraxidin and its monoglucoside (eleutheroside B1). Sterols include beta-sitosterol and daucosterol (eleutheroside A).

Some of the major ingredients in eleuthero resemble the blood thinner coumarin. Syringin and isofraxidin from eleuthero structurally bear a resemblance to a sweet, vanilla-scented plant molecule called *coumarin,* which you can smell in mown clover. In higher doses, coumarin is known to interfere with vitamin K's ability to help clot your blood and in excess is used in rat poison as a rather revolting and painful way to kill rats. Coumarin-like drugs like warfarin are used therapeutically as blood thinners. Eleuthero's blood-thinning activity has been touched upon only slightly in various older publications but not rigor-

ously studied. Theoretically, however, any blood-thinning action of eleuthero should not come as a surprise.

If eleuthero binds to steroid hormone receptors, we don't know what it does there. An older Japanese study suggested that eleuthero interacts with steroid hormone receptors.[5] However, they used a crude extract of 44 percent saponins, a common class of plant molecules that all share a steroidlike structure, so it isn't surprising that they might stick to steroid receptors when dumped upon them in test tubes. In current research we now have better ways of telling whether or not receptor binding produces any effect, like the increased production of certain types of proteins, a typical result of steroid hormone–receptor interactions. Using more modern techniques, a recent extensive assay of plant extracts for estrogenic or progesterone-like action turned up negative results for eleuthero.[6] Other steroid receptors besides these remain untested, so its effect on other steroid hormones and their receptors requires further investigation.

Eleuthero's effect on catechols, or "stress hormones," isn't clear. Some older and more poorly designed studies suggest eleuthero combats so-called stress, and leap to the conclusion that they decrease stress-associated catecholamines. Yet a few newer, better-designed studies show that, if anything, eleuthero may have a *very* slight stress hormone–raising effect. For example, cortisol was slightly raised with respect to testosterone in a study in which athletes partook of eleuthero.[7] Other studies showing animals injected with eleuthero experience elevated cortisol, but these are more suspect, as either no control was used or eleuthero was compared to other active drugs, and the act of injecting anything into an animal is likely to stress them out a bit.

Some scientists regard the old and new studies as conflicting data and have perhaps too diplomatically sought to explain it by postulating that eleuthero interacts with stress hormone–metabolizing enzymes like catechol-O-methyl transferase.[8] There is no evidence that it does or does not do this, at this point, and yet these scientists are now merrily being misquoted by others in herbal literature, saying that it does. Perhaps this action isn't worth postulating about until we have better data.

GOOD EFFECTS . . . AND NOT SO GOOD

Eleuthero seems relatively safe. The herb is not associated with obvious side effects when used as directed. However, less commonly, higher doses have been associated with drowsiness, anxiety, and irritability, and long-term use has been associated with inflamed nerves and muscle spasms.[9]

Watch out for interactions with other drugs, such as blood-thinning medications. Eleuthero could theoretically thin your blood. Keep in mind that eleuthero's properties remain relatively unknown and could interact with other drugs as well. There have been lots of studies on it, but very few are well-designed ones.

Watch out for contamination. Like ginseng, eleuthero products carry a notorious reputation for being adulterated with fillers or spiked with active drugs. For example, in order to preserve resources, Japanese sources may mix eleuthero, which they call "*ezoukogi*," with *Eucommia ulmoides* stem bark ("*du zhong*") or leaves ("*tochu*"). According to preliminary Japanese studies with animals and a few with people, *Eucommia* is believed to lower blood pressure and has antioxidant properties.

Commonly Reported Uses for Eleuthero*

Internally
"tonic," used to fight fatigue, stress, diabetes, boosting resistance to infection, arthritis, appetite stimulant, diuretic, anti-ulcer
forms available for internal use:
capsule, concentrate, extracts, powder, tablet, tincture, tea
commonly reported dosage:
Between 250 to 500 milligrams per day, standardized to eleutherosides, is commonly taken.

*These uses and dosages are from historic use and are not necessarily tested nor recommended.

More alarming is the story of a pregnant woman taking "Siberian ginseng," who had a child with hirsutism—that is, it was excessively hairy. A contamination with the unrelated silk vine (*Periploca sepium*) was found in her eleuthero product, another herb used in Chinese medicine. Since this contaminant was unlikely to have caused the birth defect, the product was investigated further. Three lots of the product labeled "Siberian ginseng" revealed no eleuthero in any except one, which was further spiked with undeclared caffeine. A mixture of other undeclared herbs added to the products may have been responsible for the birth defect.

Another case report of a man taking "Siberian ginseng" along with digitalis medication found his digitalis was far too high every time he took the herb. Some herbs do affect drug metabolism, generating plasma concentrations of medications higher or lower than their intended doses. Eleuthero is unlikely to have caused this effect, and unfortunately the product was not analyzed to uncover any possible contaminating culprit, but based on the data it appears likely that his product was spiked with digitalis.

The lesson in these true stories is that popular, expensive herbs like eleuthero are vulnerable to adulteration and illegal drug spiking. Needless to say, if you want to take eleuthero, find a company whose source is traceable and preferably has hired an independent third party, like Consumerlab, to label their product for standardization to eleutherosides, marking the presence of eleuthero.

EVIDENCE OF ACTION

Most of the human studies on eleuthero are older, Russian ones. Keep in mind, the former Soviet Union had a stake in creating a so-called Siberian ginseng market, and they succeeded. On the surface these studies appear intriguing, indicating that groups of people collectively taking eleuthero improved work performance, athletic ability, and resistance to adverse conditions. However, upon closer examination they can't tell you anything one way or the other, because they were not designed properly according to current standards—that is, they were not placebo-controlled nor double-blinded. If you tell a group of people that they will be taking something that might help them feel better and ask them to note their condition, chances are they will refer positively to how they feel. That is called the *placebo effect,* and there is no way to judge whether the herb was effective, since there was no control group taking a placebo or "dummy" pill. Furthermore, these older studies are being contradicted by newer, more carefully constructed studies, which generally show no

difference between placebo groups and those taking eleuthero.

For example, nine highly trained cyclists on controlled diets participated in a more rigorously constructed study, (that is, a double-blind, placebo-controlled, randomized, crossover design) and 1.2 grams per day of eleuthero did not have any effect on their cycling performance, self-assessed exertion, blood sugar, lactate, oxygen consumption, breathing, or standard heart parameters.[10]

This echoes an older double-blind study with twenty highly trained distance runners who were randomly assigned to a placebo or a daily dose of 3.4 milliliters of eleuthero extract for six weeks of training. Every two weeks, treadmill tests showed no significant difference between eleuthero and the placebo on heart rate, oxygen consumption, other standard breathing measurements, and perceived exertion.[11]

Also, in a placebo-controlled, randomized, double-blind trial, twenty elderly hypertensive patients felt no difference in quality of life with or without eleuthero, nor did it alter their blood levels of digitalis medication.[12] This lessens former concerns of eleuthero interacting with digitalis medications; the one case report of this happening probably involved eleuthero that was adulterated with another herb or digitalis.

For the two well-designed studies where eleuthero is associated with a statistically significant effect, the effects were just *barely* significant and nothing to write home about. For example, testosterone dropped and the stress hormone cortisol rose when endurance athletes took 8 milliliters per day of an alcoholic extract of eleuthero. Neither hormone alone was altered significantly with respect to placebo, but the ratio of testosterone over cortisol dropped significantly.[13] Noteworthy in this study is the lack of impact of eleuthero on any immunological parameter (such as T-cells, T-helper cells, T-suppressor cells, natural killer cells, and B lymphocytes). This contradicts an older Soviet study stating that "drastic" changes in numbers of immunocompetent cells occurred when volunteers took eleuthero.[14]

In another investigation, there was no difference for ninety-six people with chronic fatigue syndrome taking either eleuthero or a placebo for two months.[15] A subgroup of people with less severe fatigue had a just barely statistically significant decrease in fatigue by three months, but this could have been a chance occurrence, given the size of the effect.

The good news is that eleuthero, when it was not adulterated with undeclared ingredients, doesn't seem associated with obvious side effects in these studies. A preliminary human study indicates eleuthero (or at least doses of 485 milligrams twice daily for fourteen days) doesn't interfere with major drug-metabolizing liver enzymes either.[16]

THE BOTTOM LINE

- Eleuthero is not a ginseng and contains none of the presumed therapeutic constituents of ginseng, yet is often compared to it, as an advertising gimmick dreamed up by the former Soviet Union. It has thereafter become enormously popular, commercially.
- Eleuthero is a relative unknown. The many studies done on it in the past were poorly designed, and results from them are questionable. The evidence for its ability to boost athletic performance and stamina and to defeat fatigue has been contradicted by more rigorous, modern clinical studies.
- Eleuthero may have antioxidant and anti-inflammatory action. It may also protect against cancer cell formation and RNA viruses. These claims are tentative, based on cell or animal studies, and require further investigation.
- Eleuthero appears relatively safe when used in moderation, but commercial products are sometimes contaminated with adulterants and may even be spiked with undeclared drugs, such as caffeine.

EVENING PRIMROSE

Oenothera biennis, Oenothera spp.

HISTORY AND FOLKLORE

Evening primrose is not a rose, but a lovely flower with delicate yellow petals. These, as the name implies, open in the evening and remain open until dawn, making it good for an "evening" garden. Another way you can recognize them is by finding their distinctive X-shaped stigmas sitting atop the pistils, in the center of the flower. This flower is very hardy and grows in dry conditions. I once was astonished by the results of my randomly flinging some native seeds upon one of my gardens in Utah. So many evening primroses triumphantly burst forth that my housemate eventually complained, "There's just too much yellow here!"

Native to North America, Europeans took a liking to the plant. The French liked to boil the roots and eat them. Some people say the roots taste peppery, while others liken them to sweet parsnips. The shoots were used as a salad green.

For its therapeutic properties, evening primrose was dubbed "king's cure-all." The stems and leaves were cooked in lard to make a lotion for skin problems afflicting both infants and adults. Its leaves were bruised and applied to wounds. Internally, the plant was said to treat indigestion and insomnia, and according to the 1898 *King's American Dispensatory,* "Dr. Scudder points out as the indications for it, a sallow, dirty skin, with full and expressionless tissues, an expressionless face, an unnatural and large tongue, having the sallow, dirty hue of the skin, and the patient's mentality is of a gloomy and despondent character."

Whether or not the plant can aid these people has not been determined. No one pays much attention to its roots, leaves, and shoots anymore. Today, everyone appears focused on the uses of the oil from evening primrose seeds.

HOW SCIENTISTS THINK EVENING PRIMROSE WORKS

Evening primrose seed oil is one of only a few good sources of dietary gammalinolenic acid (GLA), but this does not mean that you need it. Many references state the GLA in evening primrose oil is "rare," but this is misleading. Saying that something is rare suddenly makes you feel like you need it, right? But everyone's bodies make GLA, and most appear to make it without difficulty. So it isn't "rare" at all. What is meant by calling it "rare" is that it isn't found in most dietary oils. Another oil that has lots of GLA is borage seed oil (see page 53), which mirrors the properties of evening primrose oil, although it is less researched.

You make GLA from linoleic acid, a fatty acid that is plentiful not only in evening primrose oil, but also abundant—experts are saying too abundant—in our modern diet. What's wrong with linoleic acid? You do need *some* linoleic acid, because your body can't make it. This puts it in the class of "essential" fatty acids. Obviously it's better to have essential fatty acids than the nonessential ones that we already make, like saturated fatty acids.

These are the infamous artery-clogging agents found in animal fats. Possibly even more menacing are the relatively unnatural trans fats created by partially hydrogenating oils that many fast and processed foods are now dripping with and, like saturated fats, are also tied to health problems. On the one hand, people who have more essential fatty acids than nonessential ones generally fare better, healthwise. On the other hand, some essential fatty acids are healthier than others. The proportion of linoleic acid in our diet is disproportionate compared to other essential fatty acids. A glut of one type of essential fatty acid drowns out the beneficial actions of the others.

The GLA and linoleic acid from evening primrose oil are both omega-6 fatty acids, and unless you use them for energy, these can only be turned into other omega-6 fatty acids. We can use fatty acids for energy; in fact your body regards their energy content so highly that, disregarding your own opinion of them, it merrily stashes fatty acids away in your fat cells. Fatty acids also become incorporated into the phospholipids that comprise your cell's outer boundaries, the cell membranes. They are either used for energy and "burned" to become carbon dioxide, or transformed into other, bioactive molecules. In the latter case, it matters whether they are omega-3s or omega-6s.

What does it mean for a fatty acid to be an "omega-6" or an "omega-3"? Essential fatty acids are categorized by their chemical structures. They are chains of carbons that may be linked by either double bonds or single bonds. The saturated fatty acids do not have carbons linked by double bonds, only by the more common single bonds, and they are not essential, because our bodies already make them. We can turn these into fatty acids with double bonds only to a limited extent. We have

enzymes (desaturases) that insert some double bonds into the chain, and other enzymes (elongases) that can even lengthen the chains by tacking on two carbons, but we just can't put a double bond in certain places. Fatty acids with double bonds in these locations are thus essential in our diet.

Fatty acids with a double bond situated three carbons from the end or "omega" carbon (linking the third to the fourth carbon from the end) of the chain are called *omega-3s* and those with double bonds at the sixth carbon from the end (linking the sixth to the seventh carbon from the end) are *omega-6s*. This is a very useful classification system, because even after a fatty acid is transformed by your body, this critical double bond designating the fatty acid as omega-3 or omega-6 tends to stay in one place. Thus omega-3 fatty acids are transformed into *other* omega-3 fatty acids, and omega-6s are transformed into *other* omega-6s. The omega-6 fatty acid linoleic acid, which is already abundant in our diets and also present in evening primrose oil, is transformed in our bodies to another omega-6, GLA. This goes on to make even more omega-6s—some good, some bad.

What is the problem with omega-6s? I admit that it's really an oversimplification for me to classify all omega-6s as "bad" and all omega-3s as "good." The problem is their ratio in our diets. If you look at the assortment of fatty acids in the modern diet, the *real* "rare" essential fatty acids are the omega-3s, and this has some health experts worried. They argue that although our diets once possessed a 1:1 ratio of omega-6 to omega-3 fatty acids, that ratio is now skewed in favor of omega-6s as high as either 10:1 or 20:1, depending on which expert you talk to. Modern society has recently become so adept at harvesting and using certain vegetable oils—corn oil, safflower oil, soybean oil, and sunflower oil—and these are all loaded with the omega-6 fatty acid linoleic acid. We feed our livestock in the form of corn, a source of omega-6 oil, rather than their preferred grass, enabling even our commercial meat supply to be unbalanced with omega-6s. Grass-fed livestock has more omega-3s. Omega-3s are abundant in fish oils and flaxseed oil (see page 123), and present to a lesser extent in other vegetable oils, such as canola and soybean oil, and some nut oils, like walnut oil.

Atherosclerosis, cancer, inflammation . . . the list goes on. Besides being incorporated into the usual fatty acid resting grounds—fat and cell membranes—linoleic acid makes its rounds in your body in the "bad" cholesterol, LDL, where it is vulnerable to being oxidized. This creates harmful free radicals and atherosclerotic plaque. Linoleic acid may also stimulate the formation of certain cancers as well as their growth. But wait, there's more: some of the hormone-like molecules it generates are troubling.

Both classes of essential fatty acids, the omega-3s and the omega-6s, are used to make 20-carbon fatty acids, which are transformed to hormone-like molecules called *eicosanoids* (from "eikosi," Greek for 20). The types of essential fatty acids your body has stored influence what types of eicosanoids you tend to make. Eicosanoids, classified as prostaglandins, thromboxanes, and leukotrienes, work only briefly in tissues nearby where they are generated, and are thus called "local" hormones. Nonetheless they have powerful and often opposing actions on blood pressure, blood clotting, pain and inflammation, allergic and immune responses, uterine and gastrointestinal cramps, digestion, brain development and mood, even tumor development and growth . . . in other words, just about everything you can think of! At the risk of oversimplification, I'll come to the punch

line: The omega-6 fatty acids *generally* make more pro-inflammatory, damaging eicosanoids. Eicosanoids derived from the omega-3 fatty acids are more anti-inflammatory and protective.

What's In It

THE SEED oil is mainly triglycerides, which, when hydrolyzed into their constituent glycerol and fatty acids, yield 65–85 percent linoleic acid, and gammalinolenic acid (8–14 percent), as well as some oleic acid (6–11 percent) and palmitic acid (7–10 percent).

Omega-3 fatty acids from flaxseed oil (see page 123), fish oils, or certain nut oils have now grabbed the attention of health officials for treating several health problems. Besides making the more helpful eicosanoids, they compete with omega-6 fatty acids for enzymes that make the 20-carbon fatty acids precursors of eicosanoids, diminishing the more negative effects of the omega-6s. Too many omega-6s, on the other hand, will negate the action of what little omega-3s you may have in your diet. So why would anyone want to take *more* omega-6s from evening primrose oil?

Evening primrose oil could theoretically help you, if you have trouble making GLA. It hasn't proven itself in clinical studies, but GLA supplementation could help some conditions, according to a reasonable theory. You make GLA from linoleic acid, which modern diets are now brimming with because of our enthusiastic use of corn, cottonseed, safflower, sunflower, and soybean oil. This requires an enzyme called *delta-6 desaturase,* but this enzyme is sometimes limited by certain factors. For example, delta-6 desaturase needs zinc to function, and trans fatty acids, alcohol, smoking, diseases like diabetes, and just plain age may diminish its action.

Evening primrose oil could thus help people with low GLA. So researchers have dutifully gone out to look for people with low GLA. But it's difficult to say what low GLA means. Just because you are low in GLA doesn't mean you need it; the problem could alternatively lie in your body's over-enthusiastic conversion of it to other less desirable things, for example, in which case GLA supplementation would make you worse. Infants are reportedly low in GLA, yet mother's milk possesses it, and cow's milk doesn't. Infants with low GLA tend to have dry skin and slow development, so some infant formulas are now being supplemented with it. Animal studies show that they may secrete GLA through skin glands onto their fur, where it may serve as a moisturizing or protective molecule; some have proposed it even has antibiotic functions. Because of these findings, researchers have energetically tested oral evening primrose oil for its ability to treat skin problems in general. (The results are disappointing; see below.) Topical evening primrose oil, like any oil, is moisturizing on skin, but beyond acting as a physical barrier to water loss, it doesn't seem to do any more than other plant oils.

You do need GLA, but it can be turned into either helpful or unhelpful eicosanoids. Your body needs GLA to make the 20-carbon eicosanoid precursor dihomo-gammalinolenic acid (DGLA), which is both good and bad. On the positive side, DGLA may be converted to an eicosanoid called *prostaglandin E1,* or *PGE1* for short. PGE1 opens up blood vessels, lowers blood pressure, and prevents blood clots. PGE1 is also

Linoleic . . . Linolenic . . . Agh!

IF ALL this piques your curiosity about dietary omega-3 and omega-6 fatty acids and you want to read more—and they *are* an important, hot health topic—watch out. Many of these fatty acids sound the same but aren't, and the scientific literature on them is rife with spelling errors! *Linoleic* ("lin-oh-LAY-ic") acid is an omega-6 fatty acid, but *linolenic* ("lin-oh-LEEN-ic") acid is an omega-3, and well-meaning authors often use the wrong term. It drives me nuts, so I don't know how people with less technical backgrounds can stomach it. Sometimes linolenic acid is called *alpha*-linolenic acid, or "ALA," to help distinguish it from linoleic acid. I personally keep my fatty acids straight by remembering that the "LEEN" syllable in linolenic acid has a long "E" sound, as in the number thrEE. (This trick doesn't work for *all* fatty acids, however; the gamma-linolenic acid derived from linoleic acid is an omega-6.)

Also, don't confuse linoleic acid with the popular and dubious weight loss supplement *conjugated* linoleic acid, or CLA, which is completely different. What people selling it will not tell you is that CLA is a collection of different fatty omega-6 acids; people aren't sure which is one best, if any, and the CLA sellers don't tell you which one their product contains. "Conjugated" in chemistry means having an alternating pattern of double, single, double-single, etc. . . . bonds linking the carbons in the chain, which ordinary linoleic acid does not have, and CLA is unusual in that it is a naturally occurring trans fatty acid, which is relatively uncommon.

a powerful anti-inflammatory and can tame tumor growth. Another benefit of DGLA lies in its ability to inhibit formation of leukotriene B4. Leukotriene B4 triggers inflammation, more specifically symptoms of asthma and allergies, so you can see why scientists have been curious to test evening primrose oil for its ability to quell inflammatory diseases.

On the negative side, DGLA may be turned into another 20-carbon omega-6 fatty acid called *arachidonic acid.* You do not want to have a lot of arachidonic acid. This is the major precursor to several inflammatory eicosanoids. Although not everything arachidonic acid makes is harmful, it is the basis of much of the scientific anxiety over our glut of dietary omega-6 fatty acids, since they are precursors to arachidonic acid, which can subsequently be turned into these inflammatory eicosanoids. Now you may wonder whether the inflammatory effects of arachidonic acid might not cancel out the former anti-inflammatory ones. We don't know the answer to that question.

Evening primrose oil, in some studies, raises arachidonic acid levels. This is a concern, but you may be able to prevent it. Not all studies show increased arachidonic acid after taking evening primrose oil. Curiously, increased arachidonic acid in one study was associated more with taking linoleic acid alone (from safflower oil) than GLA from evening primrose oil.[1] The researchers argued that if you consume linoleic acid, it might be first converted to GLA, then to DGLA, and finally to arachidonic acid by a "tightly linked enzyme sequence," but that the dietary GLA is more likely to be turned into the more benign DGLA and then just persists as DGLA. Unfortunately, evening primrose oil has *both* GLA and linoleic acid, so if this is true, the risks of the large amount of linoleic acid in it could negate the benefits of its smaller GLA content. In studies of borage seed oil, which is very similar in composition to evening primrose oil, additional supplementation with an omega-3 fatty acid, like fish oil, is often taken with the hope of limiting arachidonic acid formation. This is at least hypothetically sound.

Good Effects . . . and Not So Good

Evening primrose oil is probably very safe. Years of use and testing show no obvious side effects from eating moderate amounts of it regularly. There is one precaution in the *Physician's Desk Reference* for herbal medicine noting that it could lower the seizure threshold for people vulnerable to seizures; it appears that in the one documented case where this happened a woman was taking other herbs and medications as well. Like other plant oils, large doses may cause indigestion and loose stools.

The question remains, what is it good for? Evening primrose has been described as a remedy in search of a disease. Theoretically, it may help those who can't easily make GLA, although we are not sure who those people are. Since evening primrose oil seems relatively safe, if you think it helps you, maybe that's a good thing.

You may want to take it with omega-3 fatty acids. Some nutritionists worry about the pro-inflammatory arachidonic acid that evening primrose can elevate. Theoretically, taking evening primrose oil with a source of omega-3 fatty acids will help moderate arachidonic acid formation. Good sources of omega-3 fatty acids are fish oil and flaxseed oil.

Evidence of Action

Human clinical studies using evening primrose oil are bountiful, and most of those cited below appear trustworthy, boasting scrupulous (placebo-controlled, double-blind) designs. Evening primrose oil is a source not only of linoleic acid, which is already abundant in most diets, but also of its normal metabolite, gammalinolenic acid (GLA), which is *not* common in our diets. Therefore, researchers have been busy trying to learn what happens when we eat more GLA from evening primrose oil, even though most people make it from dietary linoleic acid with no problem.

Several studies measure changes in cell membrane fatty acid composition and plasma fatty acids for people taking evening primrose oil compared to placebos like paraffin, which ought to go right through you and have no effect, or to non-GLA–containing oils, which includes most oils. They repeatedly show that evening primrose oil supplementation causes significant changes in your fatty acids, which isn't surprising: The oils and fats that you eat become part of your cell membranes and fat.

Oral evening primrose oil is almost always associated with significant increases in both GLA and a metabolite of GLA, dihomo-GLA (DGLA). This is tantalizing because DGLA is a precursor to more anti-inflammatory eicosanoids, such as PGE1, and PGE1 is decreased in certain disorders like rheumatoid arthritis, atopic dermatitis, and lupus. Researchers have thus reasonably hoped evening primrose oil may aid people with these disorders. In several animal studies, evening primrose oil increased various types of rodents' PGE1. Yet PGE1 was not often tested for in these human studies, and when it was, it wasn't altered by taking evening primrose oil.[2]

Unfortunately, DGLA is also a precursor to arachidonic acid. This is troubling, because arachidonic acid itself is a precursor to less benign, pro-inflammatory eicosanoids. People who take evening primrose oil occasionally, but not always, endure increases in arachidonic acid as well, according to well-designed studies. The authors of one paper that investigated people taking evening primrose oil for their rheumatoid arthritis noted this increase with some alarm and penned in the conclusion that evening primrose oil could in theory make those with rheumatoid arthritis worse.[3] The issue remains unsettled as to whether the benefits of using evening primrose oil to make more PGE1 can outweigh the costs of also elevating arachidonic acid.

How do all these intriguing biochemical alterations translate into observable changes in health? They don't, really. Perhaps the studies needed to be longer—the longest ones lasted up to a year—for shifts in eicosanoid expression to be manifest as changes in clinical status. Or perhaps beneficial eicosanoids made from DGLA were cancelled out by the negative ones derived from arachidonic acid.

Most clinical research on evening primrose oil evaluates its use for skin problems, and these studies are for the most part disappointing or inconclusive. Though earlier studies on atopic dermatitis initially looked promising,[4] some of these were funded by people trying to sell evening primrose products, making them more suspect. Eventually even the researchers financially connected with the product were forced to admit that five scrupulously designed (double-blind, placebo-controlled crossover) trials showed no significant improvement when using it.[5] Most well-designed independent trials also show no significant clinical improvement for atopic dermatitis,[6] as well as non-atopic dermatitis,[7, 8] although many do show the curious changes in fatty acid profiles noted above.

Commonly Reported Uses for Evening Primrose Oil*

Internally
skin problems, rheumatoid arthritis, premenstrual syndrome, endometriosis, menopausal symptoms, breast pain, osteoporosis, Raynaud's syndrome, multiple sclerosis, Sjögren's syndrome, attention deficit disorder, gastrointestinal problems, high cholesterol, Alzheimer's disease, cancer
forms available for internal use:
oil-filled capsules, oil, tablet
commonly reported dosage:
Two to 4 grams of oil is commonly taken daily, sometimes combined with fish or flaxseed oil.
Externally
skin problems, sore breasts
forms available for external use:
oil, ointments, lotions
commonly reported dosage:
Oil is applied daily for moisturizing.

*These uses and dosages are from historic use and are not necessarily tested nor recommended.

What about putting the oil directly on your skin? Most oils applied to the skin are excellent moisturizing agents, and are certainly more moisturizing than leaving skin bare, so evening primrose oil probably doesn't hurt dry skin, and may help—as any type of inert vegetable oil should. However, evening

THE BOTTOM LINE

- Evening primrose oil is a source of linoleic acid, an omega-6 fatty acid that some health authorities worry we already have too much of compared to omega-3 fatty acids.
- Evening primrose oil is also a source of gammalinolenic acid (GLA), which humans usually make from linoleic acid. Although we make GLA normally, natural sources of GLA are uncommon. Theoretically, GLA-containing oils like evening primrose oil and borage oil should help those who are compromised in converting dietary linoleic acid to GLA.
- Clinical studies show significant changes in plasma and membrane lipid composition when people consume evening primrose oil, with increases in GLA and its metabolite, dihomo-GLA, a precursor to more beneficial, anti-inflammatory agents. Unfortunately, dihomo-GLA also makes pro-inflammatory arachidonic acid, which may be increased by evening primrose as well.
- There is no evidence that evening primrose oil causes any harm, despite concern over it supposedly increasing the pro-inflammatory arachidonic acid.
- In most human studies the presumed benefit of increasing dihomo-GLA by using evening primrose oil is not mirrored by any significant changes in clinical outcomes, for better or worse. It may help those with Raynaud's phenomenon and ulcerative colitis, but more research is needed to substantiate initial findings.
- Evening primrose oil, like other inert vegetable oils, probably makes a satisfactory moisturizing agent when applied to skin.
- Evening primrose oil is probably quite safe.

primrose oil didn't go beyond the call of moisturizing duty when applied to dermatitis caused by side effects of steroid creams.[9]

Evening primrose oil is also commonly taken for so-called women's problems, but results in this category are equally unsatisfying. For example, no significant effect of was noted in for topical[10] or oral[11] evening primrose oil in treating sore breast pain, nor did it affect women using oral evening primrose oil to lessen breast cyst formation.[12] There was also no significant impact of evening primrose oil for treating symptoms of premenstrual syndrome.[13] Evening primrose oil offered no protection against the development of preeclampsia in pregnancy,[14] although when pregnant women took fish oil with evening primrose oil in a second study,[15] they suffered less water retention than the placebo group. Evening primrose oil also failed to abate menopausal hot flashes,[16] and did nothing to perk up increases in bone density from taking calcium, compared to women taking calcium by itself.[17] As if all that were not enough, obese women who consumed evening primrose oil were not able to reduce weight any better than those taking a placebo.[18]

For rheumatoid arthritis, two studies give evening primrose oil a thumbs-down,[19, 20] although a third study observed significant improvement for those who took it for at least three months.[21] However, the study lasted for six months, which makes you suspicious about just what happened to this positive effect by month six. By this time, the olive oil "placebo" was working better than the evening primrose oil, and the authors ended up recommending the placebo as well, which makes you scratch your head over their definition of "placebo" in the first place, since a placebo is supposed to be inert. Another autoimmune disease, Sjögren's syndrome, was similarly not aided by patients taking evening primrose oil in two separate studies.[22, 23] In two other trials, a collection of patients with hepatitis B[24] and others with liver cancer[25] volunteered to suffer additional ineffectual results from evening primrose oil.

Children with attention deficit hyperactivity disorder (ADHD) were not helped by taking evening primrose oil either,[26] but a retrospective analysis looked at the kids' zinc status and optimistically speculated that the oil may have had a better influence on a subset of kids who were zinc deficient.[27]

If this is true, it is intriguing, since zinc is required for conversion of linoleic acid to GLA, thus evening primrose's high GLA content could hypothetically compensate for a zinc deficiency. More research is required to see if this idea is correct; but if a problem stems from zinc deficiency, wouldn't zinc itself be a better solution?

Slightly more promising are a couple of small preliminary studies that showed evening primrose oil may have significantly lessened the number of attacks for those afflicted with Raynaud's phenomenon,[28] and in another trial, those with ulcerative colitis who took evening primrose oil had significantly improved stool consistency but no recovery in several other symptoms caused by their colitis.[29]

FEVERFEW
Tanacetum parthenium

HISTORY AND FOLKLORE

Feverfew is a daisylike white flower, with aromatic, lobed leaves. It is native to the Balkan Peninsula, but since it spreads easily, and was popular for ages in adornments and remedies, it is now found throughout much of the European and North American continents.

As a decoration it was supposed to have the added benefit of warding off noxious insects. According to Maud Grieve's 1931 oft-quoted botanical journal, *A Modern Herbal,* bees are particularly repelled by its bitter smell. However, enough gardeners have observed bees pollinating feverfew flowers to put this theory on the fence.

Feverfew is derived from *febrifuge,* or "fever-driving-away," yet most historic references to this flower don't even mention fevers. Most go on almost exclusively about using feverfew for vaguely termed "female complaints." Nicholas Culpeper's medieval, midwife-berating *Complete Herbal* reports: "Venus has commended this herb to succour her sisters, to be a general strengthener of the wombs, and to remedy such infirmities as a careless midwife has there caused." Poor midwife! Only recently, though, rumors of some Europeans' habitual munching of fresh feverfew leaves to ward off recurrent migraines has transformed into a few intriguing clinical trials. Yet the herb is historically not connected to its use to prevent headaches, except for this fleeting reference, again from Culpeper: "It is very effectual for all pains in the head coming of a cold cause, the herb being bruised and applied to the crown of the head."

HOW SCIENTISTS THINK FEVERFEW WORKS

Feverfew could prevent migraines by regulating your platelets' release of the hormone serotonin. There are several theories for the causes of migraine, which are probably not mutually exclusive and interconnect to some extent. Feverfew's alleged mechanism concerns itself with the serotonin theory of migraines. Just before the onset of a migraine headache, platelets appear to dump serotonin off into the surrounding blood. Feverfew leaf extracts, on the other hand, prevent this serotonin dumping, at least in several test tube experiments.

Serotonin dumped by platelets causes nearby blood vessels to tighten and enhances nerve cell's response to pain. It may even causes migraine sufferers' reported heightened sensitivity to light and sound. Following this surge in serotonin release, serotonin levels plummet, causing cranial arteries to widen and swell. This brain vasodilation accompanies migraine pain. The serotonin theory of migraines does not entirely explain all aspects of migraines, like why migraines are often felt on one side of the head in particular. Nonetheless, serotonin probably has something to do with these debilitating headaches.

The active ingredient responsible for feverfew's effect on serotonin is often thought to be one of its sesquiterpene lactones. These are a common class of oily molecules found in a great number of plants, and the one that most scientists have studied while examining the properties of feverfew is called *parthenolide.* Feverfew's parthenolide appears to prevent this unwanted serotonin discharge by platelets, but it might not be the active ingredient, or the only one. Other sesquiterpene lactones from feverfew do this trick as well.[1]

What's In It

FEVERFEW'S AROMATIC oil contains camphor, camphene, para-cymene, gamma-terpinene, germacrene, linalool, and other terpenes. Its sesquiterpene lactones, in particular, are being regarded as possible migraine reducers and include parthenolide, 3-beta-hydroxyparthenolide, costunolide, reynosin, and others. It also provides flavonoid glycosides containing apigenin, chrysoeriol, luteolin, and tanetin.

Feverfew might have aspirin-like ingredients, too. That feverfew extracts stop inflammatory prostaglandin production, in a manner similar to aspirin, could also explain why people with headaches like this herb. This activity is found in test tube–type experiments. However, feverfew was not shown to help those with rheumatoid arthritis, and none of their blood's inflammation markers seemed affected by their taking the herb. Therefore, feverfew may not be as anti-inflammatory as we might like, or perhaps the volunteers used an inadequate herbal preparation.

GOOD EFFECTS . . . AND NOT SO GOOD

There are several reports in the United States of feverfew preparations containing insufficient feverfew or inadequate active ingredients. The classic manner of

Interesting Facts

Here are some additional ways to prevent migraines.

GET PLENTY of rest. Dreaming regulates your brain's serotonin levels too, and migraine sufferers who are sleep deprived suffer more migraines. If you take estrogen for any reason, see your doctor for an alternative. Estrogen can make serotonin levels jump about, causing nasty migraines in some sensitive people. (If you *have* to take estrogen, consider asking your doctor for a non-oral form, such as a patch, which provides the same effective dose as the larger oral dose. The larger oral dose can wallop your system first into a migraine-prone status before the estrogen gets metabolized down to the desired therapeutic dose.) Keep a migraine diary to help figure out what your personal migraine triggers might be. Common triggers include alcohol, aged cheeses, monosodium glutamate (MSG), aspartame, caffeine, nitrates (a meat preservative), and extreme emotional or sensory stimuli. Of course, if you think you are susceptible to migraines, you should be under a doctor's care in order to rule out more serious, underlying causes. A doctor can also offer recently developed migraine medications.

taking feverfew to ward off migraines is to chew two to three fresh leaves every day. Some migraine sufferers stick the leaves in a sandwich, or salad, but others find its taste so bitter they can't swallow it. It is at least easy enough to grow in most gardens, as its weedlike, self-seeding nature requires very little tending. Since gardeners commonly enjoy planting feverfew, your local plant nursery is likely to carry some feverfew plants, or they can order some for you. If you can't find fresh feverfew in this manner, try to get a high-quality commercial preparation standardized to at least 0.2 percent parthenolide.

Chewing feverfew leaves can cause numbness and ulcers in your mouth. This happens in about 10 percent of feverfew chewers. Perhaps this is why some people take it between bread slices—to reduce its contact with the mouth. Feverfew appears relatively safe, despite this side effect. Since its effects in pregnant and nursing women are unknown, they should probably avoid it.

If you have allergies to plants in the daisy family, watch out. Feverfew is an *Asteraceae*, which always raises a red flag for allergies. If you are allergic to other plants in this family, like ragweed or daisies, you are more likely to develop an allergy to feverfew.

EVIDENCE OF ACTION

Feverfew might not have any effect on fevers, but it could prevent some nasty headaches. A couple of randomized, placebo-controlled, double-blind studies suggest that feverfew leaves, taken regularly, can prevent migraines and lessen their severity but perhaps not their duration.[2, 3] A third, more rigorous study got mixed results. This more recent phase II clinical trial gave 147 chronic migraine sufferers either a placebo, or various doses of encapsulated feverfew leaves (2.08 mg; 6.25 mg; or 18.75 mg, three times daily) with correspondingly increased doses of feverfew's putative active ingredient, parthenolide.[4] Instead of finding that the highest dose worked the best, as is usually hoped for in these dose-response studies, the middle dose won out, affording the best protection from migraines.

Commonly Reported Uses for Feverfew*

Internally
headaches, arthritis, asthma, menstrual problems, aches and pains
forms available for internal use:
tablet, capsule, fresh and dried leaf, liquid extract, tea
commonly reported dosage:
Two or three fresh leaves a day are commonly eaten to prevent migraines, often with food to mask its bitter taste. Alternatively, a 250-milligrams capsule standardized to 0.2 percent parthenolide is taken daily.

*These uses and dosages are from historic use and are not necessarily tested nor recommended.

That the highest dose did not work so well suggests parthenolide may not be the active ingredient after all. Those participants with the most intense migraines received the most benefit from feverfew. Though the latter study shows we don't understand feverfew as well as we would like, it did not strictly contradict feverfew's use for preventing migraines either. This study also showed the herb causes no obvious adverse effects.

In contrast, another study shows that feverfew won't help you if you have rheumatoid arthritis.[5] This is disappointing, in light of occasional research references to feverfew's alleged ability to reduce inflammatory prostaglandins, in a manner similar to aspirin's action. Yet when forty-one women with rheumatoid arthritis took either feverfew (70–86 mg) or a placebo daily for six months, no change in symptoms, biochemical measures of inflammation, or other blood chemistry variables arose between the two groups. Volunteers continued to take standard anti-inflammatories like aspirin throughout the trial, which may have obfuscated the results.

THE BOTTOM LINE

- Feverfew leaf extracts taken regularly might help prevent migraines, possibly by inhibiting serotonin release by platelets.
- Parthenolide, a molecule from feverfew, inhibits serotonin release from platelets, but so do other similar molecules from feverfew. It is not longer clear that parthenolide is the active ingredient. Commercial preparations that are standardized to parthenolide are thus of unknown effectiveness. However, standardized preparations are at least usually higher quality preparations than nonstandardized ones.
- Whether feverfew helps other conditions, such as arthritis, is not clearly known.
- Feverfew appears relatively safe, but prolonged chewing of fresh leaves can cause oral numbness and ulcers in some people. People with allergies to plants in the daisy family should be cautious with it, and nursing and pregnant women should avoid using it.

FLAX

Linum usitatissimum

HISTORY AND FOLKLORE

Flax is a small, graceful, blue-flowered plant of great use since antiquity. Though it demanded a lot of the soil—Pliny said flax "scorched" the earth—it was worth it, for its fibrous stalks were used to make linen. Besides the obvious clothing, linen helped people travel faster. Pliny marveled that linen sails enabled you to get from Egypt to Italy in a record five days: "What department is there to be found of active life in which flax is not employed? . . . To think that here is a plant which brings Egypt to close proximity to Italy! . . . What audacity in man! What criminal perverseness! Thus to sow a thing in the ground for the purpose of catching the winds and tempests; it being not enough for him, forsooth, to be borne upon the waves alone." If you want to know how to make linen from flax, Mrs. Maud Grieve's 1931 *A Modern Herbal* includes a medieval passage on the making of linen, possessing a delightfully dizzy array of lost verbs. Dried flax was *"knockyd, beten and brayd and carflyd, rodded and gnodded; ribbyd and heklyd, and at the last sponne."* There you go.

Flaxseeds were also long recognized for their medicinal qualities, and certainly remarked upon often enough for their laxative effect, but also were wet and ground to make a mucilaginous poultice. The seeds were employed in cough syrups and teas for respiratory ailments; the seeds' mucilage probably coated inflamed membranes. Crude flaxseed oil, known as *linseed oil,* is unstable and goes rancid quickly but was recommended externally for burns as well as more chronic skin afflictions. In 1931 the seed's incorporation into food was less well regarded than it is today, according to Mrs. Grieve: "Linseed has occasionally been employed as human food—we hear of the seeds being mixed with corn by the ancient Greeks and Romans for making bread—but it affords little actual nourishment and is apparently unwholesome, being difficult of digestion and provoking flatulence." The current popular opinion on flaxseeds' virtues has improved considerably.

HOW SCIENTISTS THINK FLAX WORKS

Whole flaxseeds are the kindest type of laxative. Stick a flaxseed in some water and watch how it grows. It doubles its size in swelling with water, and the fibrous hairs on its shell also inflate, coating the seed with a soft, lubricating gel. They do this in your gut, too, adding bulk, and their slippery coating moves everything along. Unlike harsh chemical stimulant laxatives that may deaden the nerve endings of your gut, worsening constipation in the long run, flaxseeds can be consumed regularly ad libitum. This also helps you feel full and less hungry—for a while. Just go very easy on them if you are new to using fiber, and drink lots of water, the second ingredient required for them to work; otherwise they will have the opposite effect and form a temporary traffic jam.

Drive down your cholesterol by taking it on a one-way trip. Fiber lowers cholesterol by sticking to it in your gut, preventing you from absorbing it. Most of the studies that measure cholesterol of flaxseed eaters also show they significantly lower their cholesterol.

What's In It

THE SEED coat has 3–10 percent polysaccharide mucilage, made of galactose, arabinose, rhamnose, xylose, and galacturonic and mannuronic acids. The main lignan is secoisolariciresinol diglycoside, and phenylpropanoid precursors include linusitamarine. The seed contains trace cyanogenic glycosides (0.05–0.1 percent) linustatin and neolinustatin. The seed oil is mainly triglycerides, which, when hydrolyzed into their constituent glycerol and fatty acids, yield mainly alpha-linolenic acid (40–70 percent), as well as linoleic acid (10–25 percent) and oleic acid (13–30 percent).

Flaxseeds are one of the richest dietary sources of lignans and lignan precursors, and these are attracting the attention of nutritionists. Lignan precursors are common to plants, and all have a similar structure: a six-sided carbon ring known as a *phenyl,* bonded to a short chain of three carbons. When two of these lignan precursors stick together, they create a lignan. Lignan precursors can pair up and bond in quite a variety of different ways, so the plant kingdom abounds with a large number of different lignans with different structures. Plants use them as building blocks; they bond multiple lignans together into long chains to create a type of plant fiber called *lign*in. The fibrous seed coat of a flaxseed is therefore where you will find the lignans and lignan precursors.

Flax's lignans could prevent blood clots and allergic responses. Lignans from many plants block the action of a substance called *platelet activating factor,* or *PAF.* PAF is made by certain immune cells and blood platelets when they are provoked, and it causes platelets to clump up and form a clot. This implies that flax could help prevent blood clots, and indeed, studies of people taking flaxseeds demonstrate their platelets are less sticky. PAF also causes constriction of the airways and causes allergy symptoms, so in theory flax might also ameliorate such symptoms. Studies on this effect have not yet been performed, however.

Fight cancer by making your own estrogens—with flax's lignan precursors. The secoisolariciresinol diglucoside (SDG) is the major flax lignan precursor, and your colon bacteria convert it to the weakly estrogenic lignans enterolactone and enterodiol, which then circulate in your plasma. But don't expect this to increase the activity of estrogen. These plant-derived estrogens, or "phytoestrogens," are not as potent as the estrogens that people normally make on their own ("endogenous estrogens"). Because enterolactone and enterodiolare weak estrogens, they theoretically dampen overactive estrogen. Plus, studies show they shift the proportion of estrogens that people make from more active to less active forms. This estrogen-taming activity serves a role in fighting cancer, since overactive estrogen accelerates the growth of both normal sex gland cells and cancerous ones, too. In test tube studies, enterolactone and enterodiol inhibit growth of colon cancer, too. Thankfully, no decrease in bone growth has been seen in clinical studies, which is always a concern when you are messing with estrogen as estrogen helps bone form.

Flaxseed oil is a winner for high omega-3 content. Flaxseed oil beats other plants hands down for high omega-3 content (see table below). We need more omega-3 fatty acids in our diet, according to a growing consensus of health experts. The omega-3 fatty acid's beneficial effects are drowned out by the far more abundant omega-6 fatty acids present in oils from corn, safflower, sunflower, and soybean oils that are now dominating our diet since modern agricultural techniques have become so adept at generating them (see the chapters on borage and evening primrose for even more information on omega-6 oils.) Now that livestock are supplemented with these grains, they too now contain more omega-6 fatty acids than they would normally, if they ate their usual grass.

Both omega-3 and omega-6 fatty acids are used to make biologically active molecules called *eicosanoids,* but they make different types of eicosanoids. We need both omega-3-derived and omega-6-derived eicosanoids for life, but the current dietary imbalance favoring omega-6 fatty acids predisposes a body toward making too many omega-6 derived eicosanoids, and some experts think that phenomenon underlies the root of several modern health woes, like heart disease, arthritis, diabetes, and cancer, to name a few. It's an oversimplification to say all omega-6s are "bad" and all omega-3s are "good." But in *general,* omega-6 derived eicosanoids stimulate the immune system, and in excess they are inflammatory. They may also spawn blood clots and high blood pressure, and their inflammatory and oxidizing potential stimulates cancer-generating processes. On the other hand, omega-3 derived eicosanoids are either less inflammatory than the omega-6 ones or anti-inflammatory, plus they are more antithrombotic, antiatherogenic, and anticancer. Omega-3 fatty acids compete for the enzymes used to turn

omega-6 fatty acids into eicosanoid precursors, so their eicosanoids not only oppose the omega-6 derived eicosanoids in action, but their very presence also diminishes the formation of omega-6 derived eicosanoids in the first place.

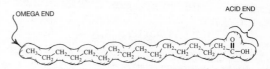

Saturated Fatty Acid with 16 Carbons
(Palmitic Acid)

Humans can make saturated fatty acids like palmitic acid. Saturated fatty acids have only single bonds joining carbons. Palmitic acid has 16 carbons.

We can lengthen fatty acids by adding two carbons with our elongase enzymes.

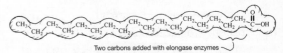

Saturated Fatty Acid with 18 Carbons
(Stearic Acid)

A different saturated fatty acid, with 18 carbons.

We can turn single bonds into double bonds with our desaturase enzymes, but only for the bonds closer to the acid end. Putting a double bond between the 9th and 10th carbon from the acid end is as close to the omega end as we can get with this process.

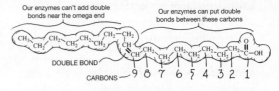

Unsaturated Fatty Acid
(Oleic Acid)

However, starting from the omega end, omega-3 fatty acids have a double bond that is in between the 3rd and 4th carbon from the omega end, and omega-6 fatty acids have a double bond that starts at the 6th carbon from the omega end. That is why we need omega-3 and omega-6 fatty acids in our diet:

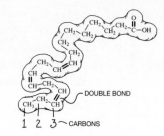

Omega-3 Fatty Acid
(Linolenic Acid)

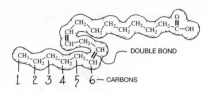

Omega-6 Fatty Acid
(Linoleic Acid)

Alpha-linolenic acid, also called linolenic acid or ALA, is the main omega-3 fatty acid in flaxseed oil, and you can turn it into one valuable fatty acid found in fish oil. ALA gets incorporated into your cell membranes and fat after you eat it, so your body stores it. Ignoring minor pathways, ALA has two general fates: It can either be "burned" for energy or turned into another omega-3 fatty acid. This is typical: Omega-3 fatty acids, when metabolized by your enzymes, are turned into other fatty acids of the omega-3 class, and omega-6s can only get turned into other fatty acids of the omega-6 class. Humans can turn ALA into the omega-3 fatty acid eicosapentaenoic acid, or EPA. This is the same as a fatty acid found in fish oil, which has been noted for its health benefits.

EPA is one of the two essential fatty acids in fish oil that everyone is now raving about for its health benefits. If you haven't heard lately that nutritionists want you to eat more fish oil because of its omega-3 fatty acids, you've been living on another planet.

How to Turn Flax Oil into Fish Oil

FIRST, EAT the flax oil. This gives you the 18-carbon ALA. Making the fish oil EPA (eicosapentaenoic acid) from ALA requires two steps. "*Eicosa-*" is Greek and refers to EPA's length, of twenty carbons, so the 18-carbon ALA must be first lengthened. Our elongase enzymes lengthen the ALA by adding two carbons to give it the required twenty carbons. And "-pentaen-" comes from the Greek *penta-* for "five" and refers to the number of double bonds ("-*en-*" means double bond in chemistry) in eicosapentaenoic acid's chain, which is five. Since ALA starts out with three double bonds, our desaturase enzymes insert two more double bonds into the 20-carbon chain to get five double bonds. This creates EPA, one of the two major fatty acids from fish oil.

We also have all we need to then turn this EPA into a second valuable fish oil, DHA (docosahexaenoic acid). "*Docosa-*" means that it has twenty-two carbons, so the former 20-carbon EPA must be lengthened. We have enzymes that can lengthen the 20-carbon EPA to the 22-carbon DPA (docosa*penta*enoic acid), which still has the five double bonds that EPA had. DHA, however, has six double bonds, and then add yet one more double bond to finally make DHA (docosa*hexa*enoic acid). Clinical studies show, however, that for unknown reasons, although people can turn flaxseed oil into EPA, we don't readily turn EPA into DHA.

But overfishing and fish farming harms fish, and many fish species are notoriously tainted with mercury, so you have to be

Percent Mass of the Major Omega-3 and Omega-6 Fatty Acids In Common Vegetable Oils

	alpha-linolenic acid (omega-3)	linoleic acid (omega-6)
Almond oil	0	17.4
Avocado oil	0.8	13.1
Canola oil	10	26
Coconut oil	0	1.8
Corn oil	0.5-1.5	39.4-65.6
Cottonseed oil	<0.4	46.7-58.2
Flaxseed oil	47-55	17-30
Grape seed oil	<0.1	58-78
Macadamia nut oil	0	1.8
Olive oil	0-1.5	3.5-20
Palm oil	<0.5	6.5-12
Peanut oil	<0.1	14-43
Safflower oil	0.4	74.1
Sesame oil	0.3-0.4	41.5-47.9
Soy bean oil	5.5-9.5	49.8-57.1
Sunflower oil	0.2	39.8
Walnut oil	6.1-11.6	52.9-62.1
Wheat germ oil	6.9	54.8

Data from the 2001 IUPAC (International Union of Pure and Applied Chemistry)

careful about what types of fish or fish oil to take. If you don't eat fish, you can make at least one fish fatty acid, EPA, by taking flaxseed oil. Why is EPA so exciting?

Medical professionals are rewriting the textbooks, literally. We are only now becoming aware of how important EPA-derived eicosanoids are. In fact, if you look at even relatively recent medical textbooks, they only discuss eicosanoids derived from the omega-6 fatty acid, arachidonic acid, and barely mention those derived from EPA. Fortunately, most texts are now being revised to include discussions of EPA-derived eicosanoids' activities.

EPA-derived eicosanoids perform the following healthy tasks. Remember, EPA is an omega-3 fatty acid, and to make a long story short, omega-3-derived eicosanoids generally lessen the negative effects of the omega-6-derived eicosanoids. If you want more detail about EPA's progeny of eicosanoids and their benefits, read on.

EPA is used to make the following menu of eicosanoids: prostaglandin E3 (PGE3), prostacyclin I3 (PGI3), thromboxane A3 (TXA3), and leukotriene B5 (LTB5). Now here is what they do: PGE3 has an anti-inflammatory mode of action similar to that of steroids like hydrocortisone—it prevents the omega-6 eicosanoid precursor arachidonic acid from being liberated from cell membranes, thus halting its conversion into inflammatory omega-6 derived eicosanoids. In addition, PGE3 reduces intraocular pressure, so scientists are now looking at it as a possible glaucoma treatment. PGI3 is anti-inflammatory by the same mechanism—it prevents arachidonic acid release, plus it potently inhibits blood clot formation.

While the omega-6 arachidonic acid derived thromboxane, TXA2, makes platelets sticky, potently forming blood clots and narrowing blood vessels, the EPA-derived TXA3 is relatively inactive and competes with it. Similarly, the leukotrienes derived from omega-6 arachidonic acid are countered by the leukotrienes made by EPA. The leukotrienes made from arachidonic acid (such as LTB4) mediate the distressing bronchoconstriction in asthma, as well as chronic asthmatic hypersensitivity and acute asthma attacks. They are also involved in the inflammatory processes seen in disorders like cystic fibrosis, inflammatory bowel disease, and psoriasis. Although the leukotriene B5 derived from EPA also signals the immune system, it does so more weakly by an order of magnitude, and competes with formation of the more inflammatory leukotrienes. Thus it tames the immune system's response, without shutting it down. In theory, all this could help combat the negative effects of the omega-6-derived eicosanoids.

You can't turn flaxseed oil's alpha-linolenic acid (ALA) into the second valuable fatty acid in fish oil, at least not very well. I write this to correct a common misperception still bandied about in the nutritional literature. Fish oil's other valuable omega-3 fatty acid is the 22-carbon long docosahexaenoic acid, or DHA. Although humans have enzymes capable of turning ALA into DHA, human studies repeatedly show that we just don't do it very well, though some sources (often associated with flax oil sellers) glibly say that you can. This is frustrating if you realize how important DHA is, and if you don't eat fish oil.

DHA is not used to make eicosanoids (it doesn't have the prerequisite 20-carbon-length chain for that), but it is of startling importance in the brain's growth, development, and signaling, as well as retinal function. Because of the growing awareness of our requirement for DHA and our limitations in making it, some are now suggesting this fatty acid is essential on its own, because ALA isn't a very good precursor to it. For strict vegetarians, it's possible to make *some* DHA from flaxseed oil, but unfortunately not a large amount.

GOOD EFFECTS . . .
AND NOT SO GOOD

Go easy on the seeds to see how your body handles them at first. If you aren't used to fiber, or if you have digestive problems, more is not better. You can create minor impaction in your digestive tract with too many flaxseeds and too little water to go with them. After your body gets used to the seeds, you can increase your dose over time, and many people notice their predictably "regulating" effect on digestion.

Unless all you want is a laxative, grind the seeds. Whole seeds will pass right through you, although they may take a bit of cholesterol with them. With the ground seeds, you get all three purportedly therapeutic components of flaxseed; the seed's coat possesses the fiber and lignans, and its innards harbor the omega-3 containing oil. Many people recommend using an old, clean coffee grinder. Grinding or at least chewing the seeds will release more of the oil and lignans.

There are many types of flaxseed oil products, but they are best used cold. Flaxseed oil does not contain lignans, or fiber, although there are now products in which the lignan is intentionally added back to the oil and the label says something like "high lignan" on it. Some boast a higher alpha-linolenic acid content. If you do take the oil for its omega-3 content, keep in mind that a high concentration of omega-6 fatty acids in your diet theoretically competes against their therapeutic effects.

The omega-3 fatty acid in flaxseed oil is vulnerable to heat and light, so although you can cook with the oil, its stability is questionable. To preserve the omega-3 fatty acid in it, put it on a salad or other room-temperature foods. It doesn't taste bad, but that's because it doesn't have much of a taste: It's not something that gourmet chefs rave about, as they do with other oils like olive. One study's authors wrote that baking the therapeutic groups' ground flaxseed-laden muffins didn't decrease their omega-3 content, and there are occasional rumors that the oil is tougher than reported. Still, err on the safe side and treat it as if it is heat-fragile: You don't want to fry with it, for example.

Store all flaxseed products in a cold dark place: the refrigerator. By the way, this is where you find the oil, and sometimes the seeds, in the more knowledgeable health food stores. If you grind the seeds, store those in the refrigerator as well, to sprinkle on foods later.

Use products for human consumption only, and follow these precautions. Never take a flaxseed preparation, such as the linseed oil that is mixed with oil paints, unless it is labeled for human use. There are other flax species that, fortunately, are not on the commercial food or supplement market, because they could make you sick. Thus it's probably not a good idea to pick your own wild flaxseed unless you are a botanist who knows his or her flax species. Also, the plant contains cyanogenic glycosides that, under certain conditions, can release hydrogen cyanide. Don't panic, though, flax's cyanogenic glycosides haven't killed anyone yet, because their quantity in the seed and oil is so low. Grazing livestock that eat the stems and leaves of the plant have suffered from it, however.

Don't take flaxseed if you have any sort of bowel obstruction, because this could cause an impaction. The seeds, because of their laxative effect, may reduce absorption of oral medications if you take them together. Because flax is supposed to prevent blood clots, it might excessively enhance the effects of any blood thinners you are on. Also, the estrogen-moderating lignans have unknown effects on fetuses or nursing mothers, and some sources thus prudently warn pregnant and nursing women to limit flax consumption, although no such complications have been reported. Consuming too much of any vegetable oil, including flax, may cause loose stools and indigestion.

EVIDENCE OF ACTION

There are quite a lot of studies on both flaxseed and its oil. Because of scientists' growing interest in omega-3 fatty acids, there will probably be a lot more in the future, so this information below, based on relatively well-designed studies, is not likely the end of the flax story.

There is more data on flax*seed,* usually ground and sometimes baked into muffins aside non-flaxseed wheat germ or wheat bran–containing placebo muffins, than there is on the flaxseed *oil.* Some of these hint at anticancer potential. In two preliminary studies,[1,2] men awaiting surgery for prostate cancer ate a low-fat diet and flaxseed. Prostate biopsies later proved significantly better biochemical markers, such as more cancer cell death and less proliferation, and decreased prostate specific antigen (PSA). These positive indications could have resulted from flaxseed's ability to affect estrogen.

For example, four separate studies observe increases in plant-derived estrogen-like molecules called *enterolactone* and *enterodiol* in people who were eating flaxseed preparations.[3,4,5,6] This doesn't mean these flaxseed eaters had more estrogenic activity. On the contrary, although one study found no changes in serum hormones,[7] a number of studies indicated that the ratio of a less active form of estrogen, 2-hydroxyestrone, to a more active

one, 16-alpha-hydroxyestrone, was significantly increased by the flaxseed lignans.[8,9] An augmented "2/16-alpha ratio" is commonly regarded as a marker for protection against the development and progression of estrogen-sensitive cancers such as breast and prostate cancer. Flaxseed was significantly better able to swing this ratio into more protective zone than soy, which did not budge it.[10]

In theory, flaxseed's shunting the estrogens you make toward its less active forms could diminish bone growth, which estrogen aids. However, more data from flaxseed studies may reassure you that no decreases in bone growth were seen.[11,12,13] No increases were seen either, so based on that, you shouldn't expect it to help treat osteoporosis.

Flaxseed's estrogenic lignans could affect menopausal women, according to a couple of studies, but it's too soon to say exactly how. Menopausal women taking flaxseed increased their prolactin slightly, which is interesting, since this hormone tends to drop during menopause.[14] Flaxseed also significantly decreased their 17-beta estradiol, a more active estrogen, which in theory would exacerbate those menopausal symptoms caused by low estrogen. However, when pitted against traditional estrogen plus progesterone hormone therapy in another trial, both treatments offered similar decreases in menopausal symptoms and in glucose and insulin levels. Nonetheless, those women who were getting the hormones still achieved a better cholesterol profile than those taking flaxseed.[15]

The estrogen-affecting action of the seed's lignans may have played a role in normalizing the periods of a few menstruating women.[16] Some women may believe they menstruate normally, but in fact experience a shortened luteal phase (the period of time following ovulation). This is one possible cause of infertility if it is chronic, because during this time insufficient progesterone may be secreted, and progesterone helps prepare the uterine lining for an embryo's implantation. Women taking flaxseed, compared to those taking a placebo, had a significantly longer luteal phase, with significantly increased progesterone secretion during that time. While the placebo group had three abnormal periods lacking ovulation (out of thirty-six cycles) the flaxseed group had none (out of thirty-six).

Flaxseed affects chicken's eggs as well. When shopping, have you run across eggs boasting of their omega-3 content? They result from adding flaxseed to a chicken's ordinary diet. One study addresses these eggs, offering ordinary eggs as controls, and found that eating them does increase your omega-3s.[17] First they examined the eggs, finding that chickens that were fed flaxseed significantly increased their omega-3 alpha-linolenic acid, one of the main fatty acids in flaxseed oil, and incorporated it into their eggs, but the eggs had the same cholesterol content as ordinary eggs. The eggs from flax-fed chickens also possessed a significant amount of the beneficial essential fatty acid docosahexaenoic acid, one of the darlings of omega-3 researchers. This is exciting, since humans aren't very good at this trick of turning flaxseed oil into DHA.

Second, researchers examined volunteers. When volunteers ate four flaxseed-based eggs a day for two weeks, they significantly increased their omega-3 fatty acids compared to those eating the same number of ordinary eggs. While there was no difference between the cholesterol levels of those who ate the flaxseed-based eggs and those who ate the placebo, how this egg-eating adventure impacted their cholesterol from the start of the study wasn't mentioned, so it's still probably not a good idea to eat four eggs a day if you are worried about it. On

the other hand, eating flaxseed without the chicken intermediaries probably will help lower your cholesterol.

Flaxseed significantly reduces both blood clot formation and cholesterol, say most studies that measure it,[18, 19, 20] and usually just the "bad" LDL cholesterol, although one experiment found "good" HDL cholesterol dropped as well.[21] One study noted significantly lowered blood glucose after eating as well.[22] Cholesterol reduction isn't surprising. Fiber pulls cholesterol through your digestive tract on a one-way trip, and flaxseed is an excellent source of fiber. In keeping with this theme, flaxseed's laxative power is something you can count on. Some people literally did count, and found flaxseed not only lowered their cholesterol but also significantly increased their number of bowel movements.[23]

A couple of human studies with lupus patients appear to bear out the original rodent models indicating that flaxseed reduces lupus-related kidney problems.[24, 25] Lupus patients who consumed ground flaxseed had better kidney function, as well as decreased cholesterol and platelet aggregation and better immune parameters.

You can increase your omega-3 fatty acids by eating ground flaxseed as well as the oil. The formerly mentioned studies, when they bothered to measure it, typically found that people eating ground flaxseed have significantly increased alpha-linolenic acid (ALA) incorporated into their cell membranes. ALA is a component of flaxseed oil, so this demonstrates that the seeds are to some extent a source of the oil as well. But what about taking just the oil?

Consuming the oil without the seeds reliably boosts your supply of the omega-3 ALA, as you might expect. The common assumption persists that you can make the two valuable omega-3 fish oils from flaxseed oils, too, but the data show that's only half right. Many studies prove that people who take flaxseed oil reliably boost their eicosapentaenoic acid (EPA) but not their docosahexaenoic acid (DHA), and we aren't sure why.[26, 27] Nursing women who take flaxseed oil are able to give their babies more ALA, EPA, and something called *docosapentaenoic acid,* or *DPA,* which is a potential precursor to DHA. DPA has just one less double bond than DHA. Theoretically, human enzymes should be able to add an extra double bond to DPA, turning it into DHA, but the study showed that these women did not do that.[28]

Flaxseed oil's ALA is an omega-3 precursor to less inflammatory eicosanoids. In theory this could alter immune status, but most studies of people taking flaxseed oil show no change in most immune parameters, like numbers of circulating immune cells and a variety of their defensive activities (like phagocytic activity and respiratory burst, as well as no change in the numbers of immune-stimulating cytokines like interleukins and tumor necrosis factor).[29, 30] Ideally, scientists would like to see these immune activities decreased by flaxseed oil, as this would indicate lessening inflammation. However, one study found some hopeful anti-inflammatory evidence: flaxseed oil decreased expression of cell adhesion molecule-1 and E-selectin on blood vessel walls. These normally jut out from blood vessels like flags into the blood during inflammation. They grab some of the immune cells flowing past them, activating the immune cells to further provoke the immune response. But the display of cell adhesion molecule-1 and E-selectin is overdone in inflammation, exacerbating inflammatory symptoms. Flaxseed oil decreased this white cell–grabbing activity by blood vessels and thus decreased inflammation.[31] This anti-inflammatory action perhaps wasn't powerful enough to help people with rheumatoid arthritis who took flaxseed oil, yet were not clinically changed for better or worse compared to those taking placebo oil.[32]

THE BOTTOM LINE

- Flaxseed is a bulk-forming, non-habit-forming laxative associated with cholesterol reduction. Its seed coat lignans may exert anticancer activity by modulating estrogen activity, and the lignans may also prevent blood clots by antagonizing platelet-activating factor receptors.
- Flaxseed oil is an unusually good source of the omega-3 fatty acid alpha-linolenic acid. Humans can convert this to another omega-3, eicosapentaenoic acid (EPA), also found in fish oil, which serves as a precursor to eicosanoids, which are anti-inflammatory, antiatherogenic and prevent blood clots.
- Contrary to popular belief, humans have difficulty making the beneficial omega-3 fish oil docosahexaenoic acid (DHA) from flaxseed oil, according to clinical studies.
- Preliminary studies indicate ground flaxseed may help people with breast or prostate cancer, as well as those with lupus. Rheumatoid arthritis was not helped by flaxseed oil, in one study, however.
- Only flaxseed products labeled for human use should be consumed, and certain people may want to limit them (see above, "Good Effects and Not So Good"). The seeds may interfere with absorbing other medications if taken together.

Finally, there are a couple of epidemiological studies reviewing the effects of dietary alpha-linolenic acid (ALA) from various sources, including flaxseed oil, that are worth mentioning. Flaxseed has one of the record highest percentages of ALA, but it is found in much smaller quantities in other plants and there are trace amounts in some meats, too. ALA consumption from all of these sources worldwide was tabulated and found to be associated with lower coronary heart disease. However, increased prostate cancer risk was also noted.[33] The authors questioned their own finding for increased prostate cancer risk, suggesting confounding factors: Those who had increased prostate cancer risk tended to obtain the ALA from meat, which increases saturated fat intake, and this may have been the real cancer-causing culprit. In light of the clinical studies showing a benefit for prostate cancer patients this seems reasonable, and other scientists have published critiques of anomalous association of prostate cancer with ALA consumption as well.[34] Another meta-analysis showed that for case-control studies, ALA in the diet provided "borderline significant" prevention of breast cancer.[35]

GARLIC
Allium sativum

HISTORY AND FOLKLORE

That garlic is a lily surprises some. Yet if you garden, you know that garlic and lily plants are similar. Both have bulbs, and some lily bulbs smell garlicky. Other more or less smelly so-called allies in its *Allium* genus are onion, chives, shallots, and leeks, and they all contain similar and sometimes identical molecules. Breaking these plants' cells by chopping or cooking initiates a reaction that turns a nonsmelly molecule into a tremendous progeny of smelly, sulfurous ones. Some of these liberated molecules become airborne, fly up into your eyes, and sting them. You can taste garlic in your mouth if you get enough of it on your skin, since its sulfurous pong is so penetrating. This has never stopped us from loving it.

One of my good friends, a former student and professional gourmet chef–turned–doctor of pharmacy, frequently pronounces the garlic family as the one family of plants he could least do without in his four-star kitchen. Saying this, his face reliably twists with dread as he contemplates the horror of his imaginary garlic-free world. Fortunately for Fred, these plants are found all over the world and remain one of the most prized herbs, by both chefs like himself and herbalists.

For more than five thousand years garlic has been cultivated and revered by humans. Egyptian slaves were strengthened with a daily garlic ration, and Chinese emperors prized it as well. Garlic is said to have maintained the stamina of Greek athletes during the original Olympics, and soldiers in both world wars nicknamed garlic "Russian penicillin" and treated their wounds with it. Garlic is a folk remedy for ailments as varied as athlete's foot and intestinal worms.

Of course, you know from the movies that vampires detest you if you wear it. This stems from medieval beliefs that garlic wards off all sorts of evil beings that cause sickness, and it is still associated with warding off illness today. Household cold cures are usually incomplete without it. Its use in preventing illness commonly engenders the joke that your subsequent reek isolates you socially, lowering your risk of contracting others' infections. Garlic remains one of the most valued medicinal herbs today.

HOW SCIENTISTS THINK GARLIC WORKS

The best-documented effect of garlic remains its ability to hinder blood clot formation. Like aspirin, garlic messes with the COX enzyme, preventing its manufacture of clotting agents called *thromboxanes*. And like aspirin, it does so in an irreversible manner.[1] This would explain the prolongation of garlic's blood-thinning effect seen in clinical studies; platelets can't make COX enzymes, so it takes time to make more platelets with active COX enzymes. It also may also work by altering the distribution of calcium in platelets, which modifies their ability to stick together.[2] Some components in garlic do this better than others, thus justifying taking real garlic rather than purified components from it.

Garlic might lower blood your pressure by relaxing blood vessels in various ways. Garlic opens up both animal and human blood vessels, lowering blood pressure. This is often associated with increased synthesis of nitric oxide, a molecule that dilates vessels.[3] Some scientists attribute this effect solely to the extra nitric oxide, but other things are going on, too, because garlic extracts still work even when you prevent nitric oxide from being made.[4] Garlic's inhibition of thromboxane production helps, because thromboxanes not only clot platelets but also close down blood vessels.

Garlic's vasodilating effect explains why it makes your nose run. Dilated blood vessels become more leaky, and garlic can thus help clear objectionable blockages in your sinuses when you are sick. Decongestants work the opposite way, narrowing blood vessels in the nose and keeping them from leaking, but this dries out the sinuses. Garlic clears sinuses by a wetter and messier method.

Garlic inhibits various fat- and cholesterol-constructing enzymes. *Fatty acid synthase,* as the name suggests, is an enzyme used in the synthesis of fatty acids. Fatty acids eventually bond in threes to glycerol, to become triglycerides, which your body merrily stashes away as fat. They are transported through your blood, and when triglycerides are chronically high in blood, doctors worry. The construction of this unwelcome fat is increased after a meal by the consequent rise in insulin, which increases the activity of this enzyme, for example. S-allyl cysteine and S-propyl cysteine are sulfurous molecules from garlic that apparently have the opposite effect, as they decreased the activity of fatty acid synthase in isolated rat liver cells.[5]

Also, fatty acid synthesis cannot occur without an electron-donating molecule that is abbreviated NADPH, and much of the NADPH needed for this process is manufactured by two enzymes that garlic also inhibits, malic enzyme and glucose-6 phosphate dehydrogenase. Like fatty acid synthase, insulin drums these enzymes into action as well. Dried garlic fed to rats decreased the activities of these two enzymes, however, and decreased the blood triglyceride levels of rats that were fed lard, compared to lard-eating rats whose chow was not spiced with garlic.[6]

What's In It

INTACT GARLIC cells contain the odorless alliin (S-allyl-L-cysteine sulfoxide), and when crushed the cell's alliinase enzyme turns it into the smelly allicin (diallyl thiosulfinate). Allicin is considered antibiotic but is unstable, and age turns it into mainly diallyl trisulfide and disulfide. Aging, heat, crushing, or fermentation also turns allicin into a wide variety of other sulfurous products, like derivatives of diallyl sulfides, methyl allyl sulfides, and dimethylsulfides. Oils derived from allicin are oligosulfides, the antithrombotic ajoenes, and vinyl dithiins.

The synthesis of cholesterol requires an enzyme that garlic inhibits, at least in the test tube. Trials so far indicate that the cholesterol reduction in humans taking garlic has been unimpressive. There is at least theoretical evidence from cell and animal studies supporting a mechanism behind the small reduction.

Like the statin drugs (Lipitor, Crestor, Zocor, and Pravachol) that are now splashing their way across television advertisements as cholesterol reducers for those for whom all else has failed, garlic inhibits the same cholesterol-generating enzyme, HMG CoA-reductase. Sulfurous constituents of garlic applied to cultured rat liver oxidizes a sulfurous portion of this enzyme, rendering the enzyme less effective.

Other sulfur-containing garlic molecules also decreased the cholesterol-making enzyme's power, by a different enzyme-modifying mechanism: They allowed the enzyme to get decorated with phosphate, a regulatory mechanism known to slow it down.[7] Isolated, purified garlic components do not seem to work as well as the natural mix of them.[8]

Garlic is undeniably antioxidant and free radical–scavenging. Loads of articles testify that the sulfurous molecules from garlic are good at preventing oxidizing agents and free radicals from performing vandalism on your precious molecules. In this manner, garlic may limit their gene-mutating actions that initiate cancer. Although garlic may not lower cholesterol much, according to clinical studies, people who take garlic are less likely to have "bad" (LDL) cholesterol and are also less likely to oxidize LDL. Oxidation of LDL creates atherosclerotic plaques, which increase the likelihood of heart disease, heart attacks, and stroke. Some garlic molecules work by tangling one-on-one with the bad guys; other garlic molecules do it more indirectly, such as by the inhibition of inflammatory enzymes like cyclooxygenase.

Good Effects . . .
and Not So Good

Use your favorite form of garlic. However, supplements may not work as well as the real thing. The question herbalists are asked most about garlic is, "what type of garlic should I take?" because it comes in so many different kinds: raw, cooked, aged, powdered, aqueous or oily extracts, and supplements. If you examine the types taken in successful trials under "Evidence of Action," below, you will see that most all of these forms work to some degree, for different applications, so take the version you find most palatable. However, supplemental garlic may be the least effective of these. These are concerns that many supplements do not generate enough allicin, one of the most important sulfurous garlic molecules. Allicin is needed in order for the garlic to be effective, because besides being antimicrobial and antioxidant itself, allicin degrades into many other different, beneficial, active components. Grocery store garlic is lot cheaper than garlic supplements anyway.

When it comes to buying real garlic, find unblemished cloves with paper skin tightly adhering to them, and discard any with mold. Most bottled garlic is fine, too, but it can have a high salt content. Some of the more alkaline garlic in oil preparations have given people botulism, although this is quite rare.

In order to be effective, it might have to smell. In order to make the smelly all*icin* mentioned in the preceding paragraph, you first need all*iin*. Alliin is a nonsmelly sulfur-containing molecule in whole garlic cloves that remains stable until the clove is mashed or cut, and then it comes into contact with alliinase enzyme. Ideally, we want the alliinase enzyme to do its job, which is to turn the nonsmelly alliin into the garlicky smelling allicin. Since this enzyme is destroyed by heat, some researchers suggest letting the enzyme work a few minutes in chopped or mashed garlic on your cutting board before tossing it into the fray of cooking. The alliinase enzyme breaks alliin down into allicin, which is antioxidant and

antimicrobial. Additionally, allicin spontaneously falls apart over time (and more
quickly when heated) into several other
stinky molecules, and it is allicin's odorous
offspring that are most often cited as garlic's
medicinal ones.

The garlic supplements advertised as
"odor free" or "deodorized" are usually surrounded by an "enteric coating." Enteric
coatings allow pills to pass intact through
the stomach to the small intestine, where
the coating is dissolved, mediating the
release of the pill's active ingredients into
the small intestine. Unfortunately, the
enteric coating of garlic pills interferes with
the activity of the alliinase enzyme in the
pills, and even if they don't, your digestive
juices ultimately will destroy the enzyme.[9]
This means that the alliin in the pills is
unlikely to get converted to allicin. Unfortunately, this means that "deodorized" or
"odor free" garlic supplements may not do
the job.

**Garlic could lower your blood pres-
sure, but watch out for excess blood
thinning.** There is good evidence that garlic
lowers blood pressure, but the most consistently verified effect of garlic is its ability to
prevent blood clots. Blood clots can lodge in
coronary arteries and cause a heart attack, or
travel to the brain and cause stroke. Thus
blood thinning is generally a good thing, but
you should not take garlic if you are already
on blood-thinning medication. Also, sur-
geons are beginning to issue their patients
alerts that, like aspirin, no garlic be consumed for a week prior to surgery, in order
to minimize the risk of excessive bleeding.

**Garlic probably won't lower your cho-
lesterol much.** Clinical studies show it only
makes a small dent in cholesterol. Lowering
cholesterol for better health requires more
extreme measures on your part in the form
of regular exercise and eating more fiber

Interesting Facts

Is garlic safe for dogs and cats?

THERE IS a lot of debate on this question,
and it's not settled. Vets warn that onions are
dangerous for pets, but garlic's molecules
are similar, and some are identical. One of
the more dangerous molecules in onions for
pets to consume is a small, inorganic, sulfur-
containing ion called *thiosulfate.* (This is the
same substance that Europeans term "thio-
sulphate.") Thiosulfate causes pets' red
blood cells to rupture if they have enough of
it, inducing a dangerous crisis known as
hemolytic anemia. A few days after a dog
eats enough onion, he may start vomiting
and having diarrhea. The dog becomes
breathless, and red hemoglobin from burst
red blood cells appears in the urine. Circulating blood cells burst, giving way to a life-
threatening crisis. The toxicity can result
from either a single large meal of onion or
repeated smaller doses. Garlic contains thiosulfate, too, but less of it. Of course, a dog
might scarf down a ton of garlic while your
back's turned, upping the dose. Perhaps
because dogs are notorious for possessing
less discriminating palates, cats get poisoned less often, but scattered reports suggest all sorts of pets that are fed table scraps
tainted with these vegetables could be
adversely affected by them.

Many processed meat products, like
broth and baby food, contain onion and garlic powder, so watch out if you treat your pet
to them. Some popular "natural" pet foods
contain garlic, perhaps to convince pet owners of some kind of extra "herbal" benefit.
The makers of these products assure their
customers that the amount of garlic in their
pet food is too small to harm pets and provides the same benefits humans enjoy. They

could be right, but its toxicity to pets remains an unknown, and perhaps because of this some pet owners insist on using garlic- and onion-free pet foods. Please see appendix C for more information on herbs and animals.

---

and less animal products. No matter how much garlic you eat, if you are also sedentary, eat unhealthily, drink excessively, and smoke, you will not be doing yourself much good if all you do is take garlic.

Garlic is unreliable as an antibiotic substitute, but taking it regularly might keep you from getting sick. Growing up reading wonderful legends of World War I and II soldiers putting garlic powder on their wounds to prevent infection, I was deeply disappointed to later learn that while it can kill some germs, it really is not that remarkable an antibiotic. Applied topically and placed in the ring directly with microorganisms to duke it out, it may or may not win, though it shows moderate promise for treating certain fungal skin infections. However, garlic can be attacked by fungi, too: Just look at the more questionable cloves in your local grocery store and ask yourself how well garlic resists pathogens. In fact, bottled garlic itself can harbor botulism if stored in alkaline conditions, and it has caused a few botulism outbreaks. Garlic should *never* be used as a substitute for an antibiotic, because as such it is too unreliable.

On the other hand, people who take garlic regularly are less likely to get certain cancers, such as stomach and colorectal cancer, and possibly others as well. Also, those who eat garlic regularly could be less likely to get a cold. If you already have a cold or flu and want to pull out all the stops, there is nothing wrong with dosing yourself up with the stuff, because it can't hurt.

EVIDENCE OF ACTION

Garlic's folkloric and scientific fame has catapulted it into a mind-blowing number of studies. The more comprehensive scientific databases list more than two thousand published research papers on the subject, and as usual, some studies are trustworthier than others. Since you don't have time to sift through all these, statisticians have kindly performed meta-analyses to review batches of the most well designed trials.

One the whole, several meta-analyses for garlic show it is unlikely to harm you, though its blood-thinning potential is powerful enough make doctors worry about it causing drug interactions and surgical complications. According to a 2002 meta-analysis,[10] they are justified in doing so, for most studies affirm that garlic prevents blood clots. Your clot-forming tendency is ideally balanced by your blood's *fibrinolytic* or clot-breaking activity. Of the twelve published studies of garlic on human's fibrinolytic activity reviewed in the meta-analysis, ten report increased fibrinolytic activity. Seven of these used garlic oil ranging from an acute, single dose to daily dosing for up to four weeks. Other forms of garlic, either fresh or fried, also worked, showing either a 72 percent or 63 percent increase in fibrinolytic activity, respectively, within six hours of volunteers first taking it, and the blood-thinning effect persisted at least twelve hours. The other two positive studies used either garlic powder or an ethyl acetate garlic extract. The two negative studies both used garlic powder.

Garlic probably lowers blood pressure, too. This is apparent in most animal studies. Of twelve trials investigating garlic's influence on human blood pressure, only three found no effect, and the rest linked a gamut of various garlic products (garlic powder, aged garlic extract, alcoholic extract, garlic tablets, commercial garlic supplements, and dietary garlic) to lowered blood pressure. The three studies that found no effect all used a commercial garlic tablet ("Kwai"), which at the time of the studies, was criticized as not releasing garlic molecules efficiently.[11] Still, some of the positive studies also used the same brand, but they were older studies performed prior to the product's reformulation in 1992.

Careful reviewers of many good trials conclude that garlic may lower cholesterol, but only slightly. A meta-analysis of garlic's influence on cholesterol published in the *Annals of Internal Medicine* in 2000 restricted their gaze to the most carefully designed studies (that is, randomized, double-blind, and placebo-controlled trials).[12] These studies employed people using garlic alone, without additional ingredients complicating the picture. The studies also involved only people with elevated cholesterol, above 200 milligrams per deciliter. Of the thirteen trials reviewed, ten used garlic powder and three used garlic oil. Pooling the data together, they found a slight but significant 5.8 percent cholesterol decrease in the garlic takers. Subsets of the trials pooled together under categories of highest methodological quality and standardization to alliin did not show a difference with respect to placebo, however. The subset of studies that measured "good" cholesterol (HDL) to "bad" cholesterol (LDL) found a slight improvement in the garlic takers' LDL/HDL ratio, but this latter improvement wasn't great enough to become statistically significant. Their conclusion was positive but guarded: "The available data suggest that garlic is superior to placebo in reducing total cholesterol levels. However, the size of the effect is modest, and the

robustness of the effect is debatable. The use of garlic for hypercholesterolemia is therefore of questionable value."

Commonly Reported Uses for Garlic*

Internally
blood clots, high blood pressure, high cholesterol, infection, antioxidant, antimicrobial, anticancer
forms available for external use:
fresh and dried bulb, capsule, extract, infusion, juice, oil, syrup, tablet, tincture, aged garlic extract, garlic powder
commonly reported dosage:
If the inactive alliin from garlic is consumed, allinase enzyme from the garlic, which is liberated by chopping it, should be present to generate the active allicin. Supplements containing alliin should similarly also include allinase enzyme to enable allicin production. One to five fresh cloves per day, or the equivalent, are commonly recommended. One clove, about 4 grams of garlic, contains approximately 10 to 40 milligrams of alliin, which can disassemble into about 4 milligrams of allicin when chopped. For aged garlic extract, a daily dose of 10 to 20 grams is recommended.

*These uses and dosages are from historic use and are not necessarily tested nor recommended.

An anticancer role for garlic is implied by comprehensive analyses of several trials.[13] The National Cancer Institute funded a meta-analysis in 2000, which took in a whopping three hundred trials testing garlic's effect on cancer and tossed out all but twenty-two of the best-designed ones for examination. Both raw and cooked dietary garlic, as well as garlic supplements, were used. Because stomach and colorectal cancers risk were examined most often, these types of cancers gained the spotlight, and garlic's effect on other cancers is less known, as they are less thoroughly tested. The authors concluded that a high intake of garlic may indeed protect against stomach and colorectal cancers. They reported "promising effects" for protection against prostate, laryngeal, and breast cancers, and "divergent evidence" for esophageal cancer, because one study showed protection against this, but two others showed none. According to the meta-analysis statistics, eating raw or cooked garlic could decrease colorectal and stomach cancer risk an eyebrow-raising percentage (10 to 50 percent), but the authors quickly and prudently caution that their conclusions may well have been thrown off by such factors as the diversity of the studies and the bias of the researchers who performed them. They also note the data is confounded in that those volunteers who consumed the most dietary garlic were also likely to eat more vegetables, and a high-vegetable intake is certainly associated with a reduced risk of cancer. Still, using garlic for cancer protection probably won't hurt you. They also reported no risk for garlic *causing* cancer.

Garlic's legendary antimicrobial power has received mixed reviews in the lab. Garlic may confer a better anti-infective status upon those who eat it, but pitted one-to-one against pathogens in the test tube, its antibiotic action is limited to particular pathogens under ideal conditions.

Garlic's direct action when applied to pathogens shows a mixed bag of results. Although fresh garlic was found to have bacteriostatic action against *Listeria* in cheese cultures in one study,[14] it could not prevent the growth of *Salmonella, Listeria,* or *E. coli* in butter in another.[15] All of these bacteria are known to cause potentially serious food poisoning, so you can't trust garlic to protect you from food poisoning. In other test tube studies, disulfides from garlic had activity against *Staphylococcus aureus* (*S. aureus*), methicillin-resistant *S. aureus* (MRSA), and three *Candida* species and three *Aspergillus* species, however.[16] *S. aureus* causes both superficial skin problems like pimples, and the eye infections known as styes, and more serious internal infections like food poisoning, pneumonia, meningitis, and several other nasty diseases. It's promising that garlic also interfered with the antibiotic-resistant version of *S. aureus* (MSRA), too, which is becoming an ever-increasing threat. *Candida* and *Aspergillus* are fungi that can sometimes cause opportunistic infections in people whose immune systems are weakened.

Preliminary test tube evidence also suggests some action for garlic against viruses like herpes, rhinovirus, and parainfluenza.[17] Yet when promising action appears in the petri dish, it may not pan out in people as well. For example, raw garlic in cell cultures provided activity against *Helicobacter pylori,*[18] a bacterium that is commonly linked to gastric ulcers, but two clinical studies revealed that people infected with the pesky bacterium couldn't rid themselves of it by taking garlic.[19, 20] On the other hand, the ajoene (pronounced "Ah-hoe-ENE," from the Spanish *ajo*, for garlic), an oily molecule abundant in chopped garlic, was tested in a cream and was found as effective as the prescription antifungal medication terbinafine when applied to tinea fungal infections such as athlete's foot,[21] jock itch, and ringworm.[22] Another investigation used what could be the sales marketer's worst nightmare, and had volunteers grumbling, but showed that a garlic mouthwash was able to defeat *Mutans streptococci,* but not other microorganisms.[23]

Studies where garlic is consumed, digested, and absorbed look modestly hopeful in certain cases. When 146 volunteers took either a placebo or an alliin-standardized garlic supplement daily for three months, those taking garlic contracted significantly fewer colds and spent signifi-cantly less time being sick when they did.[24] On the other hand, garlic has caused illness, although it is rare. Since garlic occasionally rots, it is obviously vulnerable to microbial offensives. In fact, three separate outbreaks of botulism, affecting a total of forty people, were traced to different companies' bottled garlic-in-oil products.[25, 26, 27] Botulism bacteria survive better in basic pH, so governmental health organizations now request such products be made more acidic.

THE BOTTOM LINE

- Garlic's best-documented effect is as a blood thinner. It may prevent arachidonic acid's release from cell membranes and may also prevent this molecule from turning into clot-forming agents. It may also work by altering the distribution of calcium in platelets.
- Because of garlic's blood-thinning activity, it may interfere with blood-thinning medication. People who are about to undergo surgery should abstain from garlic for a week before their procedure.
- Garlic dilates blood vessels, lowering blood pressure and briefly initiating runny noses. It seems to do this in part by increasing nitric oxide, which widens blood vessels.
- Although garlic has inhibitory effects on several fat- and cholesterol-synthesizing enzymes, including the one that prescription statins inhibit, it only moderately lowers cholesterol in people.
- Garlic can kill some microorganisms, but does not do so reliably or exceptionally well and should not be used in place of prescription antibiotics.
- Garlic is antioxidant and free radical–scavenging. This could explain why diets containing more garlic are thought to prevent cancer and disease in general.

GINGER
Zingiber officinale

HISTORY AND FOLKLORE

Ginger is one of the ancient treasured spices. For thousands of years, Asians have employed ginger not only as a pungent spice but also as a medicine. It was most often taken for stomachache, diarrhea, nausea, and pain.

From BCE 3000 to 200, Arabian traders delivered ginger from its native Asia. Marco Polo aided ginger's importation westward and wrote that one Venetian goat could buy you forty pounds of it. Mediterraneans incorporated it into their cuisines and medicines in an almost exclusively dried form, which is how it was preserved during its long journey over trading routes. Dried ginger is more traditional than fresh: Food historians suggest that even when fresh ginger was available, it was usually dried before adding it to food, so don't feel too discouraged by chefs admonishing their fans to use only fresh spices.

Asian cuisines demanded ginger in savory main dishes, but Europeans fancied its sweetened form in desserts such as candied ginger, ginger snaps, and gingerbread. Among the wealthy English classes, gingerbread evolved into a new artistic medium. Shaped into extravagant houses and men, and even decorated with real gold, it became a status symbol at social gatherings. One of Shakespeare's characters in *Love's Labor's Lost* insists, "An I had but one penny in the world, thou shouldst have it to buy gingerbread."

In the sixteenth century, Spaniards exploited the tropical climates of the Caribbean and South America to provide more of this valuable commodity to the New World. Early American colonists experimented with ginger in "small beers"—herbal and occasionally alcoholic beverages, and developed ginger beer and ginger ale. (Another small beer, root beer, may or may not have originally had ginger in it, but retains a hint of ginger today amid a hodgepodge of other flavors.) Ginger *beer* was originally dark, pungent, and alcoholic, but its use during Prohibition in alcoholic mixers popularized its lightly flavored, alcohol-free version, so-called dry ginger ale. Like ginger, ginger ale is still traditionally used for calming an upset stomach. You can make your own ginger ale easily. Just add ginger powder or sliced ginger root to carbonated water and, if desired, some form of sweetener.

Ginger continues to be cultivated in almost all tropical and subtropical climates. Major importers are China, India, Nigeria, Australia, and the best is said to come from Jamaica. Though what you buy is called a "root," a fussy botanist may insist you call it a "rhizome," a thickened underground stem. In Europe this "root" was called a "race" and may be the origin of the term "racy." The plant is in the *Zingiberaceae* family, along with turmeric (see page 310) and cardamom, which have similar molecules and, not surprisingly, similar medicinal profiles.

How Scientists Think
Ginger Works

Ginger helps some forms of nausea. If your tummy is rebelling, ginger can help. You might think all nausea is the same, but it comes in different flavors. There is the dizziness associated with inner-ear malfunction—specifically the vestibulum of the ear, a small chamber literally full of little rocks that roll around in a gooey fluid as you move your head around. The rocks land on nerve endings in the chamber, telling your brain how your head is oriented and how fast you are moving. If you have a problem with this mechanism, the resulting vertigo gives you the impression that your surroundings are moving when they aren't. Problems with your brain or eyes can also cause vertigo. Ginger does not counteract these mechanisms. But if this vertigo or some other noxious stimulus is making your stomach do flip-flops, ginger is your friend.

It's not your imagination. Your stomach really is capable of lurching around. Gingerols and shogaols are thought be some of ginger's active stomach-quelling agents. Ginger does not actually inhibit your stomach's mobility; rather, it stimulates stomach movements. You might think rousing up your stomach movements is the last thing you would want if you were queasy. But there are normal stomach motions and abnormal ones. Ginger activates your normal ones.

Stomach activity can be measured with something like an electrocardiogram for the stomach, called an *electrogastrogram (EGG)*. Normal stomach motions, such as a normally beating heart, are rhythmic and do not attract your attention. What does attract your notice are your stomachs' more jazzy, syncopated rhythms. These more erratic,

What's In It

ℓℓ

GINGER CONTAINS pungent phenols such as gingerols and their chemically related shogaols, (produced when gingerols lose a water molecule). Ginger's volatile oils are 30–70 percent sesquiterpenes, mainly b-bisabolene, (-)-zingiberene, b-sesquiphellandrene, and (+)-ar-curcumene. Its monoterpenes are mostly geranial and neral and this mixture of geranial and neral is sometimes termed *citral*.

violent motions make you feel sick. This gastric dysrhythmia (or tachygastria) is usually present in people complaining of motion sickness. Ginger gets your stomach rhythms back in step so you can resume ignoring them.

Ginger may act by binding to red pepper–sensing receptors, or by other mechanisms. Ginger's gut-activating mechanism hasn't been outlined clearly yet. Recent tests have determined that some of its components bind to the same heat-sensing receptors that red pepper does, although one report says this activates gut activity,[1] and another says it quells it.[2] This isn't as contradictory as it sounds; the dose of one ginger component may be inhibitory at one level and activating at another, and different ginger ingredients may have opposite effects.

Some older papers suggest that ginger's terpenes, oily molecules that are common to most plants but differ in structure from plant to plant, may help prevent nausea. Ginger's terpenes prevent the hormone serotonin from binding to serotonin receptors in the small intestine. When serotonin is allowed to bind to its receptors in the digestive tract, it causes stomach emptying, diarrhea, and it may even make you throw up. So ginger's potential to block serotonin's action may quell unwanted stomach spasms and nausea. In fact, prescription antinausea medications used by chemotherapy patients (dolasetron, granisetron, and ondansetron) do the same thing; they block serotonin receptors in the gut.

Commonly Reported Uses for Ginger*

Internally

nausea, vomiting, indigestion, arthritis, inflammatory pain, inflammation, blood clots

forms available for internal use:

capsule, decoction, extract, fresh and dried root, candied root, powder, tea, tincture

commonly reported dosage:

Daily doses of 3 to 10 grams of fresh ginger or 2 to 4 grams of dried ginger are commonly used. For motion sickness, about 1 gram of fresh or dried ginger is taken an hour before travel, or one or two 500-milligram doses are taken when required. To aid digestion, 2 teaspoons of powdered or grated root in a cup of water is reportedly taken.

*These uses and dosages are from historic use and are not necessarily tested nor recommended.

Ginger was shown to decrease the gastric dysrhythmia normally induced by the hormone vasopressin. Vasopressin (also called *antidiuretic hormone*) is known to help your kidneys retain water, but its spiking up is also associated with nausea. In volunteers,

both nausea and vasopressin were decreased by taking ginger. Ginger probably prevents vasopressin's release, rather than inhibiting vasopressin directly, since intravenous vasopressin infusions caused nausea that could not similarly be suppressed by ginger.[3] Your body can also make short-lived hormone-like substances called prostaglandins, and some of these cause gastric giddiness, disrupting your stomach's regular beat. Since ginger could not prevent human gastric dysrhythmia caused by a synthetic prostaglandin, researchers guessed that ginger might inhibit your ability to *make* the sickening prostaglandins rather than blunt their activity *after* they are made.[4]

Treat your pain and blood clots gingerly: Ginger's constituents resemble aspirin and have aspirin-like effects. Several of ginger's ingredients have chemical structures that resemble aspirin and other similar nonsteroidal anti-inflammatory (NSAID) drugs. Aspirin inhibits both forms of an enzyme called cyclooxygenase (COX), known as *COX-1* and *COX-2*. Some of ginger's ingredients also inhibit both enzymes and may even prevent COX-2 from getting made in the first place. Both forms of this enzyme make prostaglandins. Theoretically, then, ginger should hinder your prostaglandin-making abilities.

Some prostaglandins cause the classic "heat, pain, redness, and swelling" of inflammation. Others cause involuntary muscle contractions, which can lead to cramps. And at least in human cell culture, ginger behaves like aspirin, inhibiting the cells' ability to make these prostaglandins. Though the enzyme-inhibiting mechanism has been tested only in test tube studies and not in intact people, clinical studies support ginger's use for arthritis of the knee.

Aspirin is also used as a blood thinner, because some of the prostaglandins it makes turn into thromboxanes, which make your blood clot and your blood vessels constrict. This stops the bleeding, but if you are not bleeding, excess blood clots can land in your brain's or heart's blood vessels, jamming them and causing a stroke or heart attack. Indeed, ginger has been shown to work as a blood thinner in humans.

Ginger's inhibition of COX-1 might upset your stomach, too. Some people are more sensitive to this than others. COX-1 also makes stomach-protecting prostaglandins. These prostaglandins limit your production of stomach acid and help your stomach make protective mucous. So ginger's hindrance of this enzyme might theoretically upset your stomach the way aspirin does. Indeed, ginger has been shown to stimulate production of gastric juices. While aspirin is a no-no for those with ulcers, ginger was shown in some older Chinese studies to protect rats from ulcers. A more recent study suggests ginger's ability to reduce the growth of ulcer-associated bacteria might explain this paradox.

Because it has effects similar to aspirin, ginger might upset your stomach like aspirin, although it has been used for ages as a stomach soother. Yet some swear the herb reduces their indigestion, and there could be a mechanism supporting that claim, too. If you want to try ginger to treat indigestion, try just a little bit at first, either raw or fresh, and note how you respond to it to see if it works for you.

Ginger is safe, with some precautions. Ginger's long-time use as a spice worldwide attests its safety. The United States FDA includes the herb on its "generally recognized as safe" (GRAS) list. However, large quantities of ginger have occasionally caused heart arrhythmia and depression of the central nervous system, so use it in moderation. Modern physician's references conservatively suggest you take no more than 4 grams of dried ginger or 10 grams of fresh ginger daily. Also, ginger's blood-thinning effects are well documented, so don't take ginger if you are already on blood-thinning medication, have a bleeding disorder, or are about to have surgery.

Good Effects . . . and Not So Good

Ginger really could reduce your nausea, but only if you have the right kind of nausea. If you feel queasy, ginger may or may not help. Ginger can't prevent the room-spinning vertigo that results from inner-ear imbalance, or from neurological or eye problems. But these problems and many others may cause your stomach to lurch about wildly, giving you the urge to vomit. Therefore, if you feel your lunch going in an unplanned direction, it is appropriate to chase it with ginger.

Some people find ginger helps their stomach; others find the opposite is true.

Evidence of Action

A now-classic antinausea study of ginger is relatively old (1982), but first established the herb as a serious contender against over-the-counter motion sickness medicines like Dramamine. Envision rotating in a computer-powered chair for *six minutes* and imagine how this would make you feel. Most of the thirty-six volunteers could not take the full six-minute period and had to stop and perhaps vomit. These daring men and women were given either a placebo, 100 milligrams of dimenhydrinate (as found in medications like Dramamine), or 940 milligrams of ginger powder beforehand. None of the placebo or dimenhydrinate groups could take the full six minutes, while half of the ginger group remained for their full spinning treatment. In all, those taking ginger tolerated the rotation 57 percent longer than those who took dimenhydrinate.[5]

Because more and more women are using ginger during pregnancy for nausea, its effect on fetal development has rightfully raised concern. Most herbs have not been tested for their safety during pregnancy, and their effects on a fetus are simply unknown. Therefore, health authorities usually recommend that women avoid experimenting with regular doses of obviously large "medicinal" quantities of herbs or herbal supplements during pregnancy, but add that consuming herbs in amounts normally used in food and cooking is probably safe during pregnancy. Only one study, performed by the Canadian Motherisk Program, has addressed this question with a relatively large number (187) of women so far, and it found ginger relatively safe for fetuses whose mothers were taking it.[6] No significant risk of birth defects was found when they were compared to women taking other medications known to be safe. The only difference was a slight tendency of the non-ginger, medication-taking women to bear low birth-weight babies. But this study examined only obvious birth defects; developmental abnormalities that become apparent only later during the child's growth must also be investigated before ginger is proclaimed completely safe for developing fetuses. Additionally, in lab tests ginger has not been shown to interfere with sex differentiation in the fetal brains of animals. This was a concern, because there is new evidence that some thromboxane-inhibiting medicines may also prevent the sexual development of a male fetus, and ginger inhibits thromboxanes.

Several studies have shown ginger effective in treating nausea in pregnant women. Ginger extract (125 mg) or a placebo was given four times daily for four days to 120 Australian women who were less than twenty weeks pregnant and had complained of chronic morning sickness. Nausea was significantly less in the ginger takers compared to the placebo, and though retching was reduced somewhat, vomiting was not significantly reduced.[7] Another Australian study showed that daily doses of 1.05 grams of ginger was as effective as 75 milligrams of vitamin B6 for reducing nausea in pregnant women, though it is impossible to say if the effect was noteworthy, since no placebo was used.[8]

Another trial enlisted seventy queasy, pregnant women to take either one gram of ginger or a placebo daily for four days. Episodes of vomiting were significantly reduced in those taking ginger, and they also enjoyed less nausea.[9] A rarer form of pregnancy sickness (*hyperemesis gravidarum*) characterized by severe, persistent vomiting often requires hospitalization. This was also treated with some success using ginger. Twenty-seven women with the condition took either 250 milligrams of ginger or a lactose placebo. The ginger-consuming women scored significantly greater relief of symptoms than those taking the placebo.[10]

Ginger syrup has also been tried on vertiginous moms-to-be, as the authors of the study believed for some reason that a beverage would be easier to swallow than a capsule. In a study of twenty-six pregnant women, commercial syrup alone or mixed with one gram of ginger was dissolved in a glass of water and taken four times daily for two weeks. After nine days, ten of thirteen ginger drinkers reported less nausea, compared to only two out of ten placebo drinkers. Also, 67 percent of the ginger

THE BOTTOM LINE

- Ginger is taken to prevent nausea, inflammation, arthritis pain, and blood clots.
- Ginger reduces your synthesis of prostaglandins and thromboxanes, which would otherwise cause pain, inflammation, and blood clotting.
- Although ginger actually increases stomach mobility, its antinausea effect is thought to arise from its ability to stop your more erratic or intense stomach motions. Because ginger acts on the stomach to reduce queasiness, it may not work for all forms of nausea, like that experienced during ear infections.
- Although ginger is popular among pregnant women for treating nausea, its effect on fetal development has not been thoroughly tested.

consumers stopped vomiting by day six, compared to 20 percent of the placebo drinkers.[11]

It seems that not all forms of nausea respond to ginger. Although a couple of studies performed in the early 1990s suggested that ginger helped postoperative queasiness, several studies performed more recently show no effect. A recent review of several such studies concluded that the ginger effect was too small to recommend it be taken after surgery. Six controlled trials, with a total of 538 patients testing ginger's efficacy in reducing nausea following surgery, were pooled. Some reduction in nausea and vomiting by ginger was noted but was not judged significant.[12]

The reason why ginger works on some forms of nausea but not on others has been better elucidated by researchers who found that ginger acts primarily on the stomach. Nausea induced either by visual stimuli, or by disturbing patients' inner-ear function, was not affected by ginger.[13] Twenty-two volunteers allowed themselves to be made ill in another study, which discovered that ginger prevented their stomach "dysrhythmias," which are extreme and erratic stomach motions. Because ginger did not prevent the stomach-lurching activities caused by a prostaglandin, the authors concluded that ginger works by inhibiting

prostaglandin *synthesis* rather than by hampering already-made prostaglandins.[14] Ginger was also capable of reducing the gastric dysrhythmias caused by the hormone vasopressin (antidiuretic hormone) in human volunteers and prevented the stimulated release of this hormone.[15]

The ability of ginger to prevent the creation of inflammatory prostaglandins could explain why it reportedly reduces arthritis pain. Twenty older patients with arthritis of the knee were given either 250 milligrams of ginger extract four times daily or the same amount of placebo pills. Those taking ginger had significantly better movement of their knee joints and significantly less pain than those taking the placebo.[16] A larger study performed previously reached a similar conclusion. Two hundred and forty-seven people with arthritic knees took ginger or a placebo for six weeks and found a moderate but statistically significant ability of ginger to reduce their symptoms.[17]

If ginger reduces prostaglandins, it may also reduce blood's ability to clot. After thirty healthy adults each bravely gulped down 50 grams of fat, their blood, as was expected, became more likely to clot. This is a known effect of fatty meals. However, those who took 5 grams of ginger powder along with the fat not only prevented this effect but also significantly increased their anticlot potential (fibrinolytic activity).[18] The same research group had earlier learned that just one hefty dose of ten grams of ginger powder given to patients with coronary artery disease significantly prevented their blood platelets from clumping together. This acute dose was more effective than a lower dose of 4 grams daily for three months, which did not demonstrate this effect.[19] Animal and cell studies confirm an anticlotting of gingerols from ginger.

GINKGO
Ginkgo biloba

HISTORY AND FOLKLORE

The ginkgo tree is a remarkable survivor. There are no other trees like it; it is the only surviving member of an ancient division of prehistoric trees, the Ginkgoales. Ginkgo is related to the more primitive cycads and cone-bearing trees and thrived during the age of dinosaurs. Paleobotanists believe large forests of ginkgoes were wiped out by various catastrophes such as floods, volcanic activity, and glaciation. All but one species of ginkgo became extinct, and according to fossils, it has not changed much in 200 million years.

Fossils of ginkgo's distinctive leaves were known in Europe, but since no living trees had ever been seen, it was thought long extinct. In fact, Western culture thought all ginkgoes were as dead as the dinosaur, until 1691, when an intrepid German botanist, Engelbert Kaempfer, discovered living plants in Japan. While Europe was oblivious to the ginkgoes' survival, Buddhist priests in China had considered them sacred and planted them on temple grounds and monasteries. Their seeds had spread to Japan and Korea.

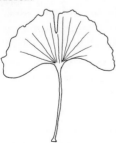

ginkgo leaf

In the service of the Dutch East-India Company, Kaempfer took some of the precious ginkgo seeds to Holland, where they were planted. A ginkgo planted in 1730 in Utrecht can still be admired today. Today, there are no wild ginkgo forests, but because they are so attractive and resistant to pollution they are extremely popular in landscaping. It is marvelous that a tree once thought extinct can be seen today in parks and malls everywhere.

You can recognize a Ginkgo in a second, because of their distinctive, fan-shaped, double-lobed leaves. Because the leaves somewhat resemble those of the maidenhair fern, it is also called the maidenhair tree. A tree with such a romantic history can't escape the attention of herbalists. Indeed, it has been used in ancient Chinese medicine for centuries, and now it is one of the most popular herbs. Its leaf extract is recommended by herbalists for quite a variety of things: vascular dementia, Alzheimer's disease, tinnitus, intermittent claudication (pain in the legs during exercise), dizziness, depression, heart disease, asthma, impotence, eye disorders, Raynaud's disease, poor memory, and neuralgia.

HOW SCIENTISTS THINK GINKGO WORKS

If your brain isn't getting enough oxygen, ginkgo might help. Ischemia (Is-KE-mee-uh) is impaired blood flow, and since blood carries oxygen, ischemia cuts off oxygen to some region of your body that is not getting enough blood. Sometimes ischemia is caused by a feebly beating heart, or by blood clots, blood vessel injury, or atherosclerosis. Different areas of your body can suffer ischemia, but your brain is particularly vulnerable to it. This is because your brain cells are exquisitely sensitive to oxygen loss and will die within minutes if they don't get it.

What's In It

THE ACTIVE ingredients of ginkgo leaf extract are mainly thought to be flavonone glycosides and terpenes. The flavonones include quercetin, isorhamnetin, and kaempferol (named after the German botanist who "discovered" ginkgo). The terpenes include the diterpenes ginkgolides A, B, and C, and J, and the sesquiterpene bilobalide. Ginkgo also contains flavones such as luteolin and tricetin; and biflavones, principally bilobetin, ginkgetin, isoginkgetin.

Depending on the brain area affected and the degree of severity, brain ischemia causes a variety of problems. Less severe symptoms are more often seen in the elderly and range from dizziness, depression, tinnitus (chronic ringing in the ear), and short-term memory loss. More severe ischemia causes vascular dementia, cerebral edema (swelling in the brain), and the third leading cause of death in the United States—stroke. Treating brain ischemia is simple—just get more oxygenated blood to your brain. There is good evidence that ginkgo encourages this. There is also confirmation that ginkgo can diminish the problems that brain ischemia causes, at least a little bit.

Ginkgo makes your blood less sticky, so it flows more freely. One way ginkgo does this is by inhibiting a substance called platelet-activating factor. This inhibition is usually attributed to molecules in ginkgo known collectively as ginkgolides (which, based on their structures, belong to a much larger class of common plant molecules known as *terpenoids*). These ginkgolides (particularly ginkgolide B) have repeatedly been shown to inhibit the activity of a substance called platelet-activating factor, also known as *PAF.* Some of your cells make PAF when they are provoked, and though PAF stimulates your immune system and stops your bleeding, excess PAF injures you. PAF causes blood platelets to clump together, forming clots, and clots can cause heart attacks and stroke. Sticky platelets also make your blood more syrupy in consistency, slowing its flow. By inhibiting PAF, ginkgo makes your platelets less sticky, so your blood flows more freely.

How does ginkgo stop PAF from working? PAF can't work unless it binds to its receptors on cells. Ginkgo's ginkgolides appear to inhibit PAF by sitting inside these receptors, blocking PAF from binding there. Ginkgolides may even put on a poor imitation of PAF, slightly *activating* PAF's receptors, but they do it so inadequately that they mostly end up just sitting in PAF's receptor, preventing PAF from docking there.[1]

Ginkgo's power to inhibit PAF also gives it an anti-inflammatory kick. Another potential benefit of blocking PAF's activity is an anti-inflammatory effect. PAF not only attracts defending immune cells, but also switches them on or "activates" them, causing them to release their chemical weapons to kill any wayfaring pathogens. However, this can cause friendly fire, injuring your tissues and blood vessels and making them fragile. The swelling and damage that ensues is inflammation. Ginkgo shuts down this inflammatory pathway by inhibiting PAF. Shutting down inflammation is particularly valuable in inadequate blood flow to an organ, technically known as *ischemia.* This is because inflammation instigates much of the damage seen in areas not receiving blood. In ischemic strokes, for example, inflammation is thought to play a major role in the brain damage that results.

Ginkgo launches a two-pronged attack against inflammation. Not only do its ginkgolides inhibit the inflammatory PAF, but ginkgo's flavonoids are great antioxidants and free radical scavengers, too. A big part of treating ischemia is treating the inflammation that results from it. Inflammation in the brain is particularly nasty, because the brain is especially vulnerable to the most common mediators of inflammation: free radicals and oxidizing agents. This is because the brain has a higher percentage of polyunsaturated fatty acids. Polyunsaturated fatty acids have a structure that makes them especially fragile when confronted with free radicals and oxidizing agents. The cell death that ischemia causes generates free radicals and oxidizing agents, and these generate even more damaging inflammation. White blood cells investigate the cellular debris and get activated by the leaked contents of dead cells. This causes the white blood cells to go on the attack, releasing even more damaging free radicals, which kills more cells in the area. As you can see, this causes a vicious circle. Ginkgo's free radical–scavenging and antioxidant flavonoids can put a stop to the vicious circle of cell death and inflammation.

These flavonoids neutralize free radicals and oxidizing agents, turning them into less toxic things. Ginkgo's flavonoids protect the polyunsaturated fatty acids in the brain against breakage. Because a brain cells' outer boundaries and internal compartments are made in large part from these fatty acids,

this maintains cellular structural integrity. Flavonoids have been observed to prevent cells from rupturing in otherwise harmful environments. Ginkgo's flavonoids, rutin and quercetin, also decrease the risk of hemorrhage, because they strengthen capillaries, which would otherwise be made frail by free radicals and oxidizing agents.

Nitric Oxide: From Cellular Waste Product to Nobel Prize Material

DESPITE NITROGLYCERIN'S long history of use, the biological activity of the nitric oxide that it releases was unknown until relatively recently, and it astonished scientists. Nitric oxide was dismissed for decades as an inactive cellular waste product. Maybe it was ignored because it is so small compared to other molecules: It has just one atom of nitrogen and one atom of oxygen and that's it. (This is *not* the same thing as *nitrous* oxide, laughing gas, which has *two* nitrogens and one oxygen.) But we now know that nitric oxide has powerful effects on your body, and one of the most dramatic things it does is widen blood vessels. The guy who figured this out was awarded a Nobel Prize in 1998, and scientific journals that year all gleefully proclaimed, "Just Say NO!" (NO is the chemical formula of this simple molecule). Unlike nitroglycerin, though, ginkgo does not *release* this blood vessel opener. It simply stimulates you to make more of it yourself.

Ginkgo is known to widen your blood vessels, which also improves your circulation. It may do this by working somewhat like the old-fashioned blood

pressure medication nitroglycerin. Both ginkgo biloba extract and the quercetin in it appear to alter the calcium concentration in cells lining your blood vessels. This in turn stimulates an enzyme (nitric oxide synthase) to make a tiny gas molecule called nitric oxide.[2,3] Several prescription medications function by increasing nitric oxide, too. Nitroglycerin, a blood pressure–lowering medication that has been used for over a hundred years, also works through nitric oxide—it releases nitric oxide as it breaks down. Nitric oxide relaxes blood vessels, allowing your blood to flow through less constricted pathways, improving blood flow.

Ironically, the free radical–scavenging flavonoids of ginkgo probably help keep nitric oxide levels in check. For all the good nitric oxide can do, it is actually a free radical, and excess nitric oxide damages nearby tissues, just like other free radicals. So on the one hand, ginkgo increases nitric oxide, which widens your blood vessels, but ginkgo also scavenges *excess* nitric oxide, which can do damage.

Finally, ginkgo may affect levels of several neurotransmitters. According to research so far, these effects are tentatively labeled positive. At least in animal and cell studies, ginkgo changes the amounts of different neurotransmitters— the chemicals that nerve cells use to communicate to each other. Now, you are right to feel hesitant about messing with your nerve cells' chemical messenger systems. But researchers so far cautiously suggest that ginkgo's effects on neurotransmitters seem relatively benign, blunting the harmful action of neurotransmitters than can do damage when it is used in excess.

The ginkgolide known as *bilobalide* from ginkgo may blunt the action of "excitotoxic" neurotransmitters like glutamate. Excitotoxic neurotransmitters are needed in

their usual amounts, but in excess they can excite a nerve cell to death. For example, glutamate is an essential neurotransmitter, but in excess it can "excite" or stimulate a nerve cell in your brain literally to death, hence the term "excitotoxic." (Don't panic about eating foods with glutamate or monosodium glutamate; they can't make it into your brain after you eat them.) Ginkgo appears to block the excitotoxic action of your brain's natural supply of glutamate. Some researchers think this is a way that ginkgo can protect your brain cells.

But ginkgo affects several other neurotransmitters as well, at least in animal and cell studies. It does this through the kaempferol, a flavonoid that is found in many other plants besides ginkgo, such as apples, onions, leeks, citrus fruits, red wines, tea, and St. John's wort, to name a few. Kaempferol, besides being a decent antioxidant and free radical scavenger, acts like a monoamine oxidase inhibitor, or "MAO" inhibitor. This is interesting, because people take prescription MAO inhibitors as antidepressants. So this might explain some of the anecdotal reports of ginkgo alleviating depression, but it has yet to be seen whether ginkgo acts as an MAO inhibitor in people, as it does in mice.

MAO inhibitors hinder an enzyme (monoamine oxidase) that breaks down several different types of neurotransmitters (serotonin, norepinephrine, and dopamine). Without this enzyme to mop up these residual neurotransmitters in your brain, their concentrations increase. Since depression is sometimes associated with low levels of these neurotransmitters, it makes sense that letting them build up in the brain a bit alleviates certain types of depression. MAO inhibitors have some side effects, though, like raising blood pressure. Although ginkgo has not been associated with any remarkable side effects in its numerous clinical studies, its proposed MAO-inhibiting effect explains why you will see warnings that people who are already taking an MAO inhibitor for depression should avoid ginkgo.

Good Effects . . . and Not So Good

Ginkgo does seem to help those with vascular dementia, Alzheimer's disease, tinnitus, and intermittent claudication (pain in the legs during exercise). It might help other vascular conditions, too. But don't expect dramatic results. According to clinical studies, ginkgo does seem to work to some extent. But the size of the effect may be small, and some wonder if it is worth taking because of that. You might be an exception and receive an effect that is large enough to please you. Since ginkgo is relatively safe, it might be worth a try. But see the precautions below, and get the right type of extract.

There are only isolated cases of sporadic side effects, but some are severe. In multiple clinical studies, prepared ginkgo products have not been associated with obvious side effects. Ginkgo does seem fairly safe, according to several clinical studies. However, doctors are concerned about cases of subdural hematoma and spontaneous bleeding associated with its use. Because of its blood-thinning effect, it seems prudent to avoid it if you are already on blood-thinning medication. Also, be wary of using it if you have a bleeding disorder, or if you are about to have surgery. Doctor's handbooks recommend physicians tell their patients to discontinue ginkgo two weeks prior to surgery. Prepared ginkgo products ought to have ginkgotoxin removed, but if

not, it could cause seizures. Some herbalists recommend you don't take ginkgo if you are prone to seizures.

Ginkgo could mess with your medicines. Ginkgo's actions have been observed to interfere with some blood pressure medications, such as thiazide diuretics, causing blood pressure to rise. Also, if you are already on an MAO-inhibitor drug, ginkgo might overdo the MAO-inhibiting effect, hypothetically causing side effects, however, these effects are theoretical and have not been observed in humans.

If it isn't working, stop using it. Some doctors suggest that if ginkgo does not cure your tinnitus after three months, stop taking it, because it won't work for you, and they worry about your taking unnecessary herbs that alter your biochemistry.

If you want to try ginkgo, get a high-quality product containing EBG 761 or LI 1370. EBG 761 and LI 1370 are proprietary leaf extracts that were originally produced in Germany, and essentially all of the scientific research on ginkgo has used these products. Other ginkgo extracts have not proven equivalent or have not been tested as thoroughly. Also, buy from a reputable, high-profile company. You might want to check for the latest information on who has been naughty and who has been nice from consumer watchdog groups like Consumerlab (www.consumerlab.com), which reports that not all of the ginkgo products claiming to be standardized contained the percentages of ginkgo constituents that they claimed.

Don't make your own ginkgo preparation. Find a commercial one that has had its ginkgolic acids removed. These constituents of ginkgo have been associated with allergic and toxic responses. If you try to make your own ginkgo tea, for example, it may contain an unacceptable amount of these toxic substances. The above extracts should fulfill this criterion, but you should be reassured to see something on the label about the product being free of ginkgolic acids. Ginkgo supplements are commonly available as tablets, pills, or extracts, but all forms should clearly indicate they are free of ginkgolic acids.

Interesting Facts

Rancid butter-scented seeds, anyone?

GINKGO TREES are either male or female, a reproductive arrangement that is pretty common in the plant kingdom. Though ginkgoes are attractive and popular in landscaping, you will not see many female ones planted. That's because their seeds stink.

The female ginkgo tree makes a hard-shelled seed that reeks of butyric acid—the same smell of rancid butter and sour milk. This has stopped Western cultures from eating them. But Asian cooks know they do not taste as bad as they smell and commonly roast or grill them. Because ginkgoes are considered sacred and thought to bring good fortune, the shells of the seeds are strung, dyed red, and then offered at weddings. The seeds are then cracked and eaten.

EVIDENCE OF ACTION

Ginkgo does not lack investigation. More than four hundred scientific articles on the therapeutic uses of ginkgo and its extracts have been published in the past couple of decades. While many of the older studies have been criticized for poor design, enough modern ones have withstood criticism such that even the more discriminating herbal

pharmacologists, like Varro Tyler, have declared these experiments are on to something. According to these studies, ginkgo works and it usually does not cause side effects. The most nagging question raised by the authors of these studies is whether ginkgo's effects are too slight to be useful.

Ginkgo studies most commonly cover its use for age-related dementia and Alzheimer's disease, pain and limping caused by poor circulation ("intermittent claudication"), and tinnitus. In addition, newer trials are now probing its reportedly helpful effects on asthma, altitude sickness, macular degeneration, asthma, and sexual dysfunction resulting from the use of anti-depressants known as *SSRIs* (*selective serotonin reuptake inhibitors*). Although results from the latter investigations are more variable and require further investigation, ginkgo's effects on vascular (circulation-associated) dementia and Alzheimer's disease have its researchers feeling more hopeful.

A published appraisal of thirty-three of the best (placebo-controlled, nonconfounded, randomized) clinical trials for treating mental impairment with ginkgo concluded that the herb shows promise for improving reasoning and mental function. (Placebo-controlled studies use a dummy pill, or placebo, on some participants to ensure that the results are less likely due to the brain fooling itself by the placebo effect. Randomized trials require that participants taking either ginkgo or the placebo are randomly chosen, and nonconfounded studies take into account additional lifestyle factors that might throw off the data; for instance, people taking ginkgo might also be more concerned about their health and tend to live healthier lifestyles.) The participants in these trials had various types of "acquired" cognitive dysfunction—that is, mental problems not resulting from childhood birth defects or genetic disorders. These most commonly included volunteers with age-related dementia or memory loss. The review states that mentally impaired subjects taking greater than 200 milligrams of ginkgo daily could expect benefits in reasoning ability by twelve weeks, and any of the doses of ginkgo examined also provided similar improvement by twenty-four weeks. Doses of less than 200 milligrams of ginkgo daily also produced an improvement in "activities of daily living" and emotional state by twelve weeks. This study also made the noteworthy observation that ginkgo caused no obvious adverse effects, compared to the placebos.[4]

However, the three modern trials included in this review had more inconsistent results, suggesting that larger trials with better methodology should be carried out. For example, one study included not just people with dementia but also many people with normal age-associated memory loss, and the results were not as positive.[5] Many studies have suggested that ginkgo best aids those with vascular (circulation-associated) mental disorders. The results of an ongoing, six-year ginkgo trial including two thousand people, funded by the National Institutes of Health and the National Center for Complementary and Alternative Medicine, that commenced in 2001 should help address these questions.

Ginkgo compared favorably to the state-of-the-art modern cholinesterase inhibitor drugs currently used for Alzheimer's, according to a review of trials comparing them.[6] This review was initiated because in test tube studies, ginkgo seems to reduce the buildup and toxicity of beta-amyloid, a protein that exacerbates Alzheimer's by accumulating and physically gumming up the brain. It also could enhance the activity of acetylcholine, a neurotransmitter that becomes less active in the disease. These

mechanisms have not been demonstrated in animal studies, however.

Commonly Reported Uses for Ginkgo*

Internally
vascular dementia, Alzheimer's disease, tinnitus, intermittent claudication (pain in the legs during exercise), dizziness, depression, heart disease, asthma, impotence, eye disorders, Raynaud's disease, poor memory, neuralgia
forms available for internal use:
standardized capsules, tablets, or extracts
commonly reported dosage:
Leaf extracts should be standardized to 22–27 percent flavonone glycosides and 5–7 percent terpenes, and ginkgolic acids should be removed. Typically, products suggest that 40 milligrams be taken up to three times a day. If a liquid extract is taken, 10 to 30 drops of extract standardized to 0.5 percent flavonone glycosides are taken three times daily.

*These uses and dosages are from historic use and are not necessarily tested nor recommended.

One review of fifty trials of Alzheimer's patients taking ginkgo applied stringent rules for scientific methodology and cast out all but four that met their approval. Their conclusion was moderately optimistic: "Based on a quantitative analysis of the literature there is a small but significant effect of 3- to 6-month treatment with 120 to 240 milligrams of G. biloba extract on objective measures of cognitive function in AD (Alzheimer's disease)."[7] Again, they noted that ginkgo produced no remarkable side effects, except in two instances where it may have been associated with bleeding complications.

Intermittent claudication is leg pain that arises during exercise, and is usually caused by blocking of blood flow through the femoral artery due to atherosclerosis. Because ginkgo increases circulation, its investigation for the use of intermittent claudication makes sense. One reviewer analyzed eight scrupulously designed (randomized, double-blind, placebo-controlled) trials of ginkgo used for this condition and found that the results were positive and statistically significant, but as with its use for Alzheimer's, ginkgo's positive effects were small. According to some of these trials, those people taking ginkgo were statistically more likely to increase the distance of their pain-free walking. Again, no adverse effects of ginkgo were noted.[8]

People who are driven nuts by incessant ringing in their ears, or tinnitus, might add ginkgo to their list of remedies to try, but the results so far are mixed. Questionnaires and telephone interviews of 1,121 subjects did not show ginkgo helped their tinnitus,[9] but such surveys, while easier to perform, lack the rigor of audiometric testing using standard medical equipment. A more encouraging randomized, placebo-controlled trial of 103 patients with new-onset tinnitus demonstrated that half of the participants enjoyed improvement or abolished the tinnitus within 70 days, compared to 119 days for the placebo takers (unfortunately the article doesn't state whether those who banished their tinnitus did so permanently).[10] In addition, reviewers of five randomized controlled trials came to the conclusion that ginkgo is moderately effective in treating tinnitus.[11]

THE BOTTOM LINE

- Ginkgo increases blood circulation, particularly to certain areas of the brain.
- Ginkgo may aid those with vascular dementia, Alzheimer's disease, tinnitus, and intermittent claudication (pain in the legs during exercise), theoretically. Clinical tests suggest these effects may be small, however.
- Ginkgo theoretically works by several mechanisms: It inhibits platelet-activating factor and increases nitric oxide. Both of these actions increase circulation. It also has excellent free radical–scavenging and antioxidant principles. It might also inhibit glutamate toxicity in the brain, and could function like the antidepressant MAO-inhibitor drugs.
- If you take ginkgo, you should take either EBG 761 or LI 1370, proprietary extracts that have been used in most ginkgo experiments. Also be sure that the toxic ginkgolic acids have been removed.
- Ginkgo seems quite safe according to clinical studies, but it could interfere with certain medications and cause bleeding problems.

GINSENG

Panax ginseng, Panax quinquefolius

History and Folklore

Ginseng's genus *Panax* originates from the Greek *pan* (all) *akos* (cure), which gives you an idea of how folklore regards it. Though ginseng usually brings to mind an ancient and revered Asian herb, an American species (*Panax quinquefolius*) is gaining notice, though it is not as well characterized as its Asian relative (*Panax ginseng*). Ginseng's root was extolled by ancient herbalists at least in part because of its remarkable shape.

Unlike your basic carrot-shaped root, ginseng root bifurcates into what resembles leglike appendages, topped with knobby bits that could easily be interpreted as a torso and head: The root looks like a crudely sculpted man. The ancient and completely unscientific Doctrine of Signatures was not a written document, as the phrase suggests, but simply a once-prevalent belief that plants that resembled a body part were thought by ancient and medieval herbalists to be good for that body part. (This would be like eating potato "eyes" for your eyes, or cabbage heads to treat your head, etc.) On the rare occasion when a plant resembled an entire *man,* well, *then* the root was imagined to be something special indeed and good for a man in all cases. The most anthropomorphic and oldest roots can sell for hundreds of dollars per pound or more. Its value has fueled two negative consequences: frequent adulteration with other, cheaper herbs, and overharvesting of wild ginseng roots.

What about Siberian Ginseng?

IF THE presence of two ginsengs isn't complicated enough for you, you can read about another. Formerly called "Siberian ginseng," it is less related, sharing the same family as American and Asian ginseng (*Araliaceae*) but not the same genus (*Eleutherococcus senticosus*). Herbalists claim it acts like the official ginsengs but is conveniently less expensive although slightly less esteemed as well. However, the presence of three different "ginsengs" has confused former research, and most researchers did not clearly know or state which one they used. The confusion is clearing somewhat now, as you can no longer legally market Siberian ginseng as a *ginseng,* and "eleuthero" is now its official, commercial title.[1] Some references mistakenly state that eleuthero has some of the same active ingredients as ginseng, but it does not. Eleuthero has no ginsenosides. Eleuthero is therefore treated separately from American and Asian ginseng in this book (see page 105).

Ginseng roots are infamously troublesome to grow, taking up to six years to develop. The wild American root is native to the northeastern United States and Appalachia, and is scarce due to overenthusiastic harvesting, which is now restricted. Native Americans used American ginseng, though exactly how they used it is, like a lot of tribal lore, tragically sketchy. They may have used it for treating nosebleeds and female infertility. Americans first turned up their noses to their resident ginseng but are now noticing it. Much of it is still exported to Asia, where it is exalted and used in traditional healing along with Asian ginseng.

In traditional Asian medicine ginseng is thought to restore your life force, or *chi*. Asian herbalists describe Asian ginseng as "hot" and American ginseng as "cold," and they are applied to different tasks. Chinese medicine uses "cold" herbs like American ginseng to treat such ailments as digestive and respiratory complaints, excessive thirst, and fever. "Hot" herbs are used to raise the body temperature, but traditionally Asian ginseng has been used for almost every ailment imaginable, either by itself, or in combination with other herbs.

How Scientists Think Ginseng Works

Ginseng's ingredients have their own yin and yang—many oppose each other's actions. But do they cancel each other out? Some say that ginseng doesn't do anything, but don't give up on it yet. Ginseng's actions are complicated, because several of the ginsenosides (the active compounds in ginseng) oppose each other's activity. Just when a researcher reports that an ingredient in ginseng does one thing, another paper comes out to say that another ingredient in ginseng opposes this activity. But isolated ginsenosides *do* affect your body. The real trick is to know *which* ginsenosides you are getting. Ginseng preparations can have around thirty different ginsenosides, but different species and preparations have high levels of some ginsenosides and low levels of others. Unfortunately, only "total ginsenosides" are so far reported on commercial products, so you don't know which ones you are really taking. Perhaps someday the types of ginsenosides present, and their quantity, will also be included on herb labels. We will have to wait, however, until better characterization and labeling of herbal ingredients occurs.

Some ginsenosides decrease your cells' ability to make nitric oxide. Nitric oxide is an important hormone-like molecule, but a damaging free radical when present in excess. When stimulated, ideally your immune cells lob this chemical weapon at harmful pathogens. Less ideally, nitric oxide builds up during inflammation and hurts your own tissues. Several ginsenosides reportedly inhibit the production of enzymes that make nitric oxide. They hamper the creation of i-NOS, or *inducible nitric oxide synthase,* a little chemical weapon factory that turns on extra nitric oxide production when cells are injured or under attack. This enzyme is made when your tissues are stressed. These ginsenosides that prevent its creation are Rg1 and Rh1, but there may be more that have yet to be identified.

Others do the opposite. The ginsenoside Rg3 has the opposite effect and causes more of this chemical weapon factory to be made. So if you want an anti-inflammatory effect, you might want more Rg1 and Rh1 and less Rg3.

Although excess nitric oxide kills your cells, you still need moderate amounts of it. Some ginsenosides facilitate this. Nitric oxide alleviates male sexual impotence, lowers blood pressure, and increases the flow of oxygenated blood. It widens your blood vessels, increases the flow of oxygenated blood, and is the natural cause of an erection. There are gentler nitric oxide

What's In It

AMERICAN AND Asian ginseng contain similar ingredients, each with around twenty-five or more "ginsenosides," which are in a chemical class called triterpene saponins, or just "saponins." They are not identical, however. Some ginsenosides are present in one species but not the other, and those that are in both occur in differing concentrations.

The ginsenosides are divided into three categories, the panaxadiols, the panaxatriols, and oleanolic acid derivatives. The panaxadiols include Ra1, Ra2, Ra3, Rb1, Rb2, Rb3, Rc, Rc2, Rd, Rd2, Rh2, and Rg3, and the panaxatriols include Re2, Re3, Rf, Rg1, Rg2, and Rh1. Ro is an oleanolic acid derivative. Asian ginseng root has at least thirty ginsenosides, which make up around 2–3 percent of the root, most of which are Rg1, Rc, Rd, Rb1, Rb2, and Rbo. Cultivated American ginseng's predominant ginsenosides include Rc, Rd, Re, Rg1 (0.15 percent), Rb 1, Rb2, Rb3 (0.03 percent), R92 (0.008 percent), Ro, and F2, but *wild* American ginseng has differing concentrations of these and may have higher total ginsenosides.

factories than i-NOS, the enzyme that Rg3 helps create. The enzyme i-NOS is only made under duress, but there are other versions of it that are around all the time and make smaller, less hurtful amounts of nitric oxide. The ginsenoside Rg1 causes more of these nitric oxide generators to be made, in both your blood vessels (in the form of e-NOS, endothelial nitric oxide synthase) and your nerve cells (in the form of n-NOS, neuronal nitric oxide synthase.) Perhaps not

coincidentally, in one small study Rg1 was the only ginsenoside of four tested (against Rb1, Rb2, and Ro) that cured male mice of their impotence. This lends slight credibility to the very few, limited studies that tentatively suggest that ginseng can treat erectile dysfunction.

Some ginsenosides decrease your production of stress-associated catecholamines. At least in isolated cow cells, and theoretically in people, some ginsenosides limit the adrenal glands' ability to release stress molecules, known as *catecholamines.* They do this by blocking the acetylcholine receptor, which normally stimulates release of catecholamines after it binds to acetylcholine. You are probably most familiar with the catecholamine called adrenalin (also called epinephrine), but dopamine and noradrenalin are catecholamines that are decreased, too. These fight-or-flight chemicals increase your heart rate, constrict blood flow to your skin and increase it in your muscles, open your airways, and flood your blood with energy-packed glucose. They are decreased by some ginsenosides, according to animal studies, with Rg2 listed as the most potent, followed in order of potency by Rf, Re, Rh1, Rb2, Rg1, Rb1, and Rc. Theoretically, the more active of these ginsenosides should lower heart rate and blood pressure. Their anticatecholamine action may explain why in clinical studies ginseng sometimes lowers blood sugar.

Sometimes ginseng lowers blood sugar. Sometimes it raises it. This must certainly result from the varying concentrations of different ginsenosides in different types and preparations of ginseng. One paper suggests that the higher the panaxadiol concentration relative to panaxatriol concentration, the better the blood sugar–lowering effect. The cause of the blood sugar—elevating phenomenon is not known.

Good Effects . . . and Not So Good

Ginseng has been used for thousands of years without serious side effects being reported. Some people may be especially sensitive to it, though. Rarely, reports have been made of people taking ginseng and consequently suffering agitation, insomnia, digestive upset, or skin rash. The existence of a "ginseng abuse syndrome" resulting from excess ginseng consumption, causing nervousness, insomnia, high blood pressure, and other problems, is no longer considered valid. The 1979 paper that presented the idea of this theoretical syndrome is now widely discredited for poor quality.[2]

Don't use ginseng to control your blood sugar. Some studies show that ginseng increases blood sugar, and others show it decreases it. Different ginseng preparations may have varying concentrations of either blood sugar—lowering or —raising ingredients. Until these ingredients are better characterized by researchers and quantified on herb product labels, trying to control blood sugar with ginseng could backfire on you.

Ginseng might prevent warfarin from working. One small clinical study showed that people taking both ginseng and the blood thinner warfarin had reduced amounts of warfarin in their blood, compared to those not taking ginseng. Ginseng might accelerate the clearance or breakdown of this drug, so if you are on warfarin, it seems prudent to avoid ginseng.

Ginseng might treat male impotence, but the evidence for this is sketchier than herb vendors would have you believe. Ginseng is not another Viagra. It does not inhibit the same enzyme that Viagra inhibits (phosphodiesterase-5). It also can't "donate nitric oxide" as several labels suggest, because its ginsenosides have no nitrogen, making this physically impossible. However, some of its ginsenosides might increase your own nitric oxide—making factories, specifically in blood vessels and nerve cells, which could theoretically lead to an erection. Unfortunately, other ginsenosides have the opposite action. The claims for ginseng's ability to treat erectile dysfunction are overblown as yet, since only a few small studies have suggested it helps, but only modestly.

Commonly Reported Uses for Ginseng*

Internally
fatigue, depression, immune stimulation, impotence, diabetes
forms available for internal use:
aged, peeled root ("white" ginseng); aged, steamed root ("red" ginseng); standardized capsules, tablets, extracts, decoction, powder, tea, athletic beverages, chewing gum
commonly reported dosage:
0.5 to 2 grams of ginseng root per day is usually taken, though traditional Asian medicine suggests up to 9 grams per day. Around a half teaspoon dried, powdered root per cup of water is taken as a tea twice daily.

*These uses and dosages are from historic use and are not necessarily tested nor recommended.

Science doesn't classify herbs as "tonics" or "adaptogens." Ginseng is historically regarded as a "tonic"—that is, something like an herbal vitamin pill that simply keeps you in good health in general. The modern herbalist's term for tonic is "adaptogen," so you will see this attribute applied to ginseng in newer literature. Adaptogens are thought to "stimulate"—or aggravate, depending on your opinion—the immune system and are taken with the hope of protecting yourself in advance from any wandering pathogens. Be aware that neither label is accepted by the scientific mainstream, as they are simply too vague for us to quantify, so if you query most scientists whether something is a tonic, we will look blank-faced and shrug our shoulders helplessly. This does not necessarily mean these herbs do not help—it just means that you are on your own, scientifically speaking.

Interesting Facts

I'm 252 years old . . . no, really I am.

THE CLAIMS for ginseng can be fairly outlandish, in fact, including extreme life-prolongation. In the 1934 book *Nature's Remedies, Early History of Botanic Drugs*, the author, Joseph E. Meyer, attests with awe that daily ginseng enabled a man to live 252 years. Meyer discovered this man making his living by wowing audiences with unbelievable stories of his great age. But the last sentence of the book unintentionally gives away the man's real secret: "He has married and outlived twenty-three wives and is now living with his twenty-fourth at the age of 252 years. . . . For two hundred years ginseng was part of his diet every day. . . . He seems not older than a man of 52, according to those who have met him."

Ginseng would be an even better herb if it were more carefully standardized by those who sell it to you. Because of its cost, ginseng products are notoriously contaminated with cheaper herbs and fillers. Also, some undeclared ingredients, such as caffeine, have been found in some ginseng products.

When ginseng is pure, you still don't know which ginsenosides you are getting. This is important, since many oppose each other's action. Unfortunately, products are only standardized to "total ginsenosides," which does not help. The fight to get herb companies to assume more legal responsibility for their products' labels continues. In the future, perhaps some herb companies will go the extra mile for their customers and report the percentages of each of the *different* ginsenosides in their product. These vary widely from product to product, and even from lot to lot within one product line. Such standardization would generate a more expensive product, yet a more reliable one.

High levels of carcinogenic pesticides have been found in some ginseng products. The consumer watchdog laboratories of Consumerlab reported the following: "A high amount of the pesticide hexachlorobenzene—a potential human carcinogen—was found in one of five products labeled as containing 'Korean Ginseng.' Levels of two other pesticides, quintozene and lindane, were also above acceptable levels. Another product that failed the new testing was a liquid 'Chinese Ginseng' sold in single-dose bottles. Despite being labeled 'EXTRA STRENGTH' this product contained less than 10% of the expected ginsenosides." Buying ginseng from a highly reputable company may help you avoid these scary pesticides. Some herbalists advise buying ginseng as an intact root from Oriental herb shops, so you at least know that you are getting ginseng.

You then have to trust that the root was grown without pesticides dumped on it.

Evidence of Action

Though there are mountains of scientific articles and books on ginseng (one herb expert suggested it is *the* most researched herb[3]), older studies are troublesome to interpret because of poor design and inadequate documentation of the species used. Overall, clinical studies do not confirm the more astonishing testimonial claims made for ginseng. The most common use for the herb is to improve mood, energy, and athletic performance. According to the better-designed studies, ginseng's effects on mood are unclear; some show no effect, others show positive effects, and other studies show a mixture of both.

For example, in a well-designed (double-blind, placebo-controlled) trial, 112 volunteers over the age of 40 who took 400 milligrams of a commercial, standardized Asian ginseng product daily for eight weeks showed no improvement in concentration, memory, or subjective experience, but did show faster and improved reaction times and improved abstract thinking.[4] There is also concern that ginseng's effects wear off. After taking 200 milligrams of Asian ginseng for four weeks, fifteen volunteers in another similarly rigorously designed study found that their subjective perception of improved social functioning and mental health wore off after an additional four weeks of the same treatment.[5]

Menopausal women apparently felt psychologically but not physically better while taking ginseng, according to another double-blind, placebo-controlled study. Of the 382 symptomatic women, the roughly half that took ginseng reported better psychological symptoms but no improvement in typical menopausal physical complaints such as hot flashes after sixteen weeks of treatment. Ginseng also had no effect on several hormonal variables that were also measured in these women.[6] On the other hand, 83 healthy men and women took either a placebo, 200 milligrams, or 400 milligrams of standardized Asian ginseng daily for eight weeks, yet their moods did not change one way or the other.[7]

The results for ginseng's power to improve energy and physical performance are even more disappointing. One research group failed repeatedly in four separate placebo-controlled attempts to show that 400 milligrams of standardized Asian ginseng daily had any effect on athletic performance or fatigue as measured by standard means such as exercise and stress tests, recovery from exercise, oxygen uptake, heart measurements, and other metabolic parameters affected by exercise and fatigue.[8, 9, 10, 11] Other research groups' placebo-controlled studies also show no change whatsoever [12, 13, 14] in these and other exercise variables with similar doses of ginseng, though one did show that volunteers' reaction times on multiple-choice tests during and after exercise improved slightly with ginseng.[15]

Ginseng's power to aid your immune function with respect to fighting various infections and cancer looks somewhat more promising, but some studies still show it has no effect.[16] Oral (100 mg) ginseng perked up the potency of an injected flu vaccine and significantly enhanced natural killer cell (a type of immune cell) activity in a controlled study of 227 healthy volunteers.[17] Other placebo-controlled studies have shown that ginseng increases immune cell numbers, activities, bacterial clearance, and antibody titers.[18, 19, 20]

An intriguing placebo-controlled preliminary investigation of 4,364 older adults revealed that ginseng apparently significantly lowered the risk of several types of cancer (lip, oral cavity, pharynx, esophagus, stomach, colorectal, liver, pancreas, larynx, lung and ovary).[21] Older ginseng worked, and the longer it was taken, the greater the effect appeared to be. Fresh ("white") ginseng did not produce this effect. However, because the study was performed using questionnaires, confounding factors, such as the fact that people who take ginseng regularly are more likely to have a healthy lifestyle, were not considered, so the results may not be as exciting as they appear on the surface. Nonetheless, ginseng also improved the outcome of patients receiving radiation therapy for nasopharyngeal carcinoma in a controlled trial of 131 patients.[22]

Ginseng has an after-dinner blood sugar–lowering reputation, but it may well depend on what kind you use. Almost all the recent human clinical trials investigating this claim have used American ginseng rather than Asian ginseng, and most, but not all, support the theory. The sole study on the more traditional Asian ginseng, performed by the same people who for the most part noted blood sugar–lowering properties for American ginseng, reported that Asian ginseng had either an opposite or no effect on blood sugar. This is probably because of the different quantities of unknown blood sugar–lowering ingredients in the different species.

A well-designed (randomized, placebo-controlled) trial on the effects of ginseng on both type II diabetic and nondiabetic volunteers found that 3 grams of ginseng taken forty minutes before a standard blood glucose challenge test significantly reduced blood sugar for both. However, while the effect also worked for diabetics who took the ginseng *along with* the overload of glucose, it did not for the nondiabetics.[23] The investigators then decided to see whether increasing the dose of ginseng increased the hypoglycemic effect for type II diabetics in another placebo-controlled trial, and though such "dose dependent" effects are often seen for both drugs and herbs, ginseng may be an exception. Higher doses of 6 or 9 grams of ginseng had similar but not greater effects. Several different time delays between taking the ginseng prior to the glucose load were tried, up to two hours beforehand, but all showed comparable glucose-lowering effects.[24] This suggests that no more than 3 grams of American ginseng is required, taken for up to two hours before a meal, to keep a type II diabetic's blood sugar from spiking. But not all American ginseng does this.

Herbs vary from harvest to harvest and from product to product. The same investigators tried the same design of experiment to test blood sugar lowering on diabetics but found no effect at all for a different "batch" of American ginseng.[25] *Asian* ginseng failed to work, too. In fact, it *elevated* blood glucose when the same investigators tried it on both type II diabetics and nondiabetics in two different trials, again with varying doses and times taken.[26] To unearth the cause of all this frustrating variability, they finally performed similar tests with eight different types of ginseng, including Siberian ginseng. Some tended to raise blood sugar (Asian ginseng, American-wild ginseng, and Siberian ginseng), but others lowered it (American ginseng and Vietnamese ginseng). Total ginsenoside content did not predict this trend, but the ginsengs with more of a type of ginsenoside called a panaxadiol, rather than those with high panaxatriol ginsenosides were the most reliable blood sugar–lowering agents.[27] Unfortunately, the labels of most commercial ginseng products don't currently state how much panaxatriol they contain.

It's difficult to say whether or not the claims for ginseng's ability to treat erectile dysfunction are overblown. There just is not enough data yet. Most herb peddlers trying to sell ginseng for impotence will try to persuade you that it increases nitric oxide, which *would* work (Viagra works by preventing the breakdown of the active molecule that is generated by nitric oxide), but some of ginseng's components actually do the opposite and *decrease* nitric oxide production. One article's badly phrased title, quoted with annoying frequency on ginseng labels, even suggests that ginseng is a "nitric oxide donor,"[28] which is completely impossible, because ginsenosides do not have any nitrogen, so they can't release a molecule that has nitrogen in it. However, ginseng could theoretically increase *a cell's* ability to make nitric oxide. Here's what the data really say: Some ginsenosides inhibit nitric oxide production,[29, 30] while others enhance it.[31, 32] Therefore, as of yet, claims for ginsengs' increasing nitric oxide are inappropriate.

However, what little data there is on ginseng and impotence looks provocative. Researchers noticed that after male mice spent prolonged periods on their own, the mice lost interest in sex when finally presented with the opportunity. They injected either crude ginseng extract, various purified ginseng saponins, or ginseng-free saline solution as a control into such mice to see if anything made them less apathetic. Although the saline had no effect, the crude ginseng extract worked, and the more that was

THE BOTTOM LINE

- Ginseng root seems relatively safe, but its claims appear overblown.
- Some of ginseng's components raise blood sugar, while others lower blood sugar, so it should not be taken for diabetes. It may also interfere with blood-thinning medications such as warfarin.
- Many of ginseng's active ginsenosides have opposing activities, and different types of ginseng have varying amounts of ginsenosides. This is why different preparations of ginseng, even in the same species, can have opposite activities.
- There is a little evidence that ginseng might improve mood, but it may also wear off over time. It may do this by lowering stress hormones called catecholamines.
- The persistent marketing claims that ginseng improves athletic performance have not been substantiated in human tests.
- There is some evidence that red Korean (steamed Asian) ginseng might treat male impotence. Some of ginseng's components increase nitric oxide, which lends credibility to the claim. Other ingredients in ginseng decrease the excess nitric oxide that is produced during inflammation, but this should mainly have an anti-inflammatory effect.
- Ginseng may have a stimulating effect on the immune system. This theoretically could prevent infection, but may aggravate autoimmune disorders and inflammation.
- Products labeled "ginseng" are notoriously adulterated with cheaper fillers, and some products have been found spiked with drugs, like caffeine, not mentioned on the label.

injected, the greater its effect. What was most revealing was that only one of the ginseng saponins, Rg1, had the same effect.[33] Unfortunately, mice are not men, and injected substances can at times produce different effects than the same substance taken orally, which is how most people take ginseng. So it's difficult to extrapolate this study to humans.

As for actual *human* studies of ginseng on impotence, there are only two, and they both use Korean red ginseng (steam processed Asian *Panax ginseng*). An older placebo-controlled study of ninety impotent male volunteers found that ginseng did not have any effect on frequency of intercourse, premature ejaculation, or morning erections, nor did it cure anyone's impotence. It also had no effect on the readings of an AVS-penogram, which records changes during erection after audiovisual erotic stimulation. Nonetheless, the authors still reported that ginseng significantly improved other parameters, such as the duration and quality of erections and "patient satisfaction." A more recent placebo-controlled trial employing forty-five older impotent men measured only the more promising variables as measured from the previous study (subjective sense of improvement and penile rigidity) and confirmed a statistically significant improvement for those who took 900 milligrams of Korean red ginseng three times daily. They noted the ginseng had no effect on testosterone and postulated that nitric oxide might be responsible instead.[34]

GOTU KOLA

Centella asiatica, syn. *Hydrocotyle asiatica*

History and Folklore

You can find this member of the parsley (*Umbelliferae*) family's round, fan-shaped leaves creeping along swampy ground in tropical Asia, South Africa, South America, and the southern United States. Despite the "kola" in its name, it is not related to the kola nut, and it does not have caffeine or stimulants in it. That's a common misperception about this herb. In fact, it may act as a sedative. It is also called *hydrocotyle, Indian penny, Indian pennywort,* and *water penny.* Ayurvedic medicine calls it *brahmi.*

Indian elephants like to snack on gotu kola leaves and seem none the worse for it. Like the gotu kola–eating elephants, humans use the aboveground portion of gotu kola—the stem and leaves. Perhaps because elephants have a reputation for long lives and good memories, ancient Indian Ayurvedic medicine has revered this herb for hundreds of years as a memory-enhancing and longevity agent. But modern research is turning up better evidence for its action as a tissue-regenerating and blood vessel–strengthening agent.

How Scientists Think Gotu Kola Works

Gotu kola extract increases synthesis of collagen. Collagen strengthens your blood vessels and speeds wound healing. Both cells and animal wounds exposed to gotu kola extracts make more collagen. Gotu kola extracts seem to do this by acting at the level of cells' DNA, causing the collagen-making information in collagen genes to be "read" to construct more collagen protein. Not all of the constituents of gotu kola extract do this. Two ingredients, asiatic acid and asiaticoside, were most effective at achieving this beneficial effect in test tube (*in vitro*) studies with isolated cells.

Gotu kola promotes renewal of other tissue-reinforcing materials, too, and stimulates the division of cells that produce it. Human cells called *fibroblasts* divide more rapidly in cell cultures after they are exposed to asiaticoside from gotu kola. Your own fibroblast cells are not always active, but when they are, they churn out scaffolding material that your cells adhere to, and this material includes collagen. This material, called *extracellular matrix material,* reinforces and cushions your tissues. Asiaticoside also stimulates fibroblast cells to make *more* of this extracellular matrix material, again at the level of their genes. It also dramatically enhances fibroblast cells' ability to stick to this cellular scaffolding, helping anchor these scaffolding-generating cells in place.

Enzymes that break down your tissues might be reduced with gotu kola extract. The extracellular matrix material that makes your tissues strong and supple can be broken down by certain (lysosomal) enzymes, which is a normal regenerative process, but these degrading enzymes are abnormally high in the blood of patients with vascular problems and diabetes. One study found that they are also high in people with varicose veins, but gotu kola was able to reduce their enzymes to normal.

What's In It

THE ACTIVE ingredients of gotu kola are thought to be its triterpenes and triterpene glycosides (saponins), consisting principally of asiatic acid, madecassic acid (6-hydroxy asiatic acid), asiaticosides A and B, and terminolic acid.

Gotu kola might thin your blood. One small, older study showed that gotu kola extract increased cultured cells' production of tissue plasminogen activator (tPA), a known blood-thinner. Blood thinners reduce your risk of heart attack and stroke. However, if you are already taking a blood thinner, be careful not to overdo it. People on blood-thinning medications should always consult with their doctor first before considering taking daily doses of blood-thinning herbs.

Gotu kola might slow down your brain's activity. Though most gotu kola product labels advertise its ability to do nebulously "good" things for your brain or mental state, the data on its mental effects are scant. Perhaps because someone obtained a patent for a gotu kola extract to promote "cognitive enhancement," it is being heavily marketed as such. But a patent is not an endorsement, and many consumers mistakenly assume it is some sort of mental stimulant. The "kola" in the name is reminiscent of "cola," but gotu kola contains no caffeine.

If anything, the one human clinical trial on this herb suggests it might slow your brain down. This is supported by one study, which shows that gotu kola increases gamma-aminobutyric acid (GABA) in rats' brains. This neurotransmitter is a well-known inhibitor of nerve cell signaling in the brain. So, rather than stimulate you, it might act as a sedative or antianxiety agent in theory.

Gotu kola extract is moderately antioxidant, which theoretically could shorten the duration of your healing time. In chemical assays, gotu kola was approximately as antioxidant as rosemary and sage. This may not be the sensational antioxidant power demonstrated by other antioxidant champions, like flaxseed oil, tea, grape seed, or garlic, but it may be worth a try.

Good Effects . . . and Not So Good

Gotu kola seems safe internally, but be cautious with using it if you are taking blood-thinning medication. Gotu kola has a relatively good record as a safe herb. Although one study suggests it could thin your blood, there are no reports of contraindications when taking gotu kola along with blood thinners. Nonetheless, you should be cautious with gotu kola if you are already on blood-thinning medication.

On rare occasions, gotu kola causes a rash when applied topically. A few cases of contact dermatitis have been reported when the herb was applied topically. If you have sensitive skin and you see gotu kola in an ointment or cream, go easy with applying it and note how you respond to it.

Gotu kola does not seem to perturb your DNA in any negative way, but repeated, long-term topical applications might not be the best idea. Tests for gotu kola's acting as a DNA-mutating carcinogen turned up negative. In fact, it had mild antimutagenic activity. However, gotu kola does promote the division of fibroblast cells, so it might act as a weak cell division promoter of previously formed tumor cells. A 1972 report noted that twice-weekly applications of asiaticoside from gotu kola extract caused skin tumors in mice after eighteen months.[1] Acute, short-term external usage is probably safe.

Commonly Reported Uses for Gotu Kola*

Internally

tonic, anxiety, insomnia, skin conditions, wound healing, circulatory disorders, blood vessel pathologies such as chronic venous insufficiency, venous hypertension, post-phlebitic syndrome, and varicose veins

forms available for internal use:

liquid extracts, capsules, dried leaves

commonly reported dosage:

Dosages of 60 to 120 milligrams of triterpenes or triterpene extract are commonly taken.

*These uses and dosages are from historic use and are not necessarily tested nor recommended.

Don't expect gotu kola to "stimulate" your brain. If anything, it is a sedative. Vague, unsubstantiated references for gotu kola acting as a "cognitive enhancer" have led to public misperceptions of this herb as a "smart drug" or stimulant. Also, the "kola" in the name subjectively suggests a relationship to the caffeine-containing kola nut, but there isn't one, nor does gotu kola contain caffeine. Only a few studies assessing its mental effects have been performed, and they all point to gotu kola's action as a brain-slowing sedative or calming agent.

Gotu kola may help reduce vein problems, but get a quality product. Most products have passed testing by independent labs, but not all. But don't buy the first bottle you see on the shelf. Find an extract where the label states that it is standardized to gotu kola's triterpenes, which are exclusively used in almost all of its clinical studies. Some Ayurvedic medicines have been found to be contaminated with unacceptable levels of heavy metals. Because of this, some of the more conscientious herb sellers are testing their products for contaminants and indicating on their labels that their products are guaranteed free of heavy metals.

EVIDENCE OF ACTION

There are plenty of studies demonstrating that gotu kola is good for your blood vessels. Unfortunately, what is sold commercially is not necessarily the same stuff as what was taken in these studies. Standardized extracts of gotu kola currently on the market will take a little work for you to find, yet most studies use the triterpene-containing extract of gotu kola rather than the crude, whole plant.

Around a dozen published studies have employed patients with venous hypertension or chronic venous insufficiency, caused by poorly functioning or damaged veins. Most studies have given their treatment groups between 60 to 180 milligrams of gotu kola triterpene extract daily, and all of the controlled studies have demonstrated improvements for those taking gotu kola.[2,3,4,5,6,7,8,9] These improvements are dose-dependent— that is, the highest dose tested provided the most dramatic results. A couple of studies also showed similarly positive results for gotu kola decreasing blood vessel pathology in diabetic patients.[10,11] Another couple of trials noticed gotu kola helped change atherosclerotic plaques' consistency for the better.[12,13]

One gotu kola study took volunteers on an airplane flight.[14] Prolonged immobility and dehydrating, pressurized air in airplane cabins exaggerates swelling and circulatory disturbances in certain people, which can be dangerous if it leads to a blood clot (deep vein thrombosis). The passengers who took 60 milligrams of gotu kola triterpene extract three times daily for two days before the flight, the day of the flight, and for another day after the flight had better circulation and less ankle swelling than the passengers who had no treatment. (A placebo would have been preferable in this study to no treatment at all, but the results are nonetheless encouraging.) No adverse effects of gotu kola were noted in this study.

A 1990 Italian study indirectly noted a possible improvement for those with varicose veins. People who have varicose veins were noted in this study to have higher levels of tissue-destroying lysosomal enzymes and connective tissue breakdown products (uronic acids) circulating in their blood, compared to people who do not have varicose veins. After taking 60 milligrams of gotu kola triterpene extract for three months, the levels of these disease markers dropped below baseline levels.[15]

One of gotu kola's ancient reputations is as a wound healer. Gotu kola extract did accelerate the healing of gastric ulcers in rodents in a few studies,[16, 17, 18] and it also accelerated wound repair in guinea pigs and rats,[19] indicating that it may indeed be useful for wound repair, but so far there are no human studies to back this up.

Though gotu kola's wound healing ability seems in part an effect of its stimulating effect on tissue rebuilding enzymes, its antioxidant properties may contribute to this beneficial result. Several animal and cell studies make note of gotu kola's antioxidant power, though one noticed that its ability to stimulate the synthesis of antioxidant enzymes wore off after fourteen days of application to skin wounds on rats.[20]

Though a couple of small studies suggest that gotu kola can enhance *rodents'* ability to learn,[21, 22] there are very few trials assessing gotu kola's effect on *human* mental functioning. Gotu kola actually *decreased* locomotor activity (motion) in rodents, and *decreased* the ability to quickly respond to a startling sound in both rodents and humans.[23] It had no effect on mood. This suggests that, contrary to what advertisers like to claim, gotu kola makes you less mentally alert, but the effect might be viewed as beneficial if you are looking for a sedative or antianxiety agent.

THE BOTTOM LINE

- Gotu kola's best-documented action is as a tissue-regenerating and blood vessel–strengthening agent.
- Gotu kola promotes the use of genes that instruct the manufacture of collagen and other cellular scaffolding materials. It also enhances the division of fibroblast cells, which make such materials.
- Gotu kola does not contain caffeine and is not related to the kola nut. It seems to act like a sedative, perhaps by increasing the inhibitory neurotransmitter GABA (gamma-aminobutyric acid) in the brain. Its reputation as a memory-enhancing agent is as yet unfounded.
- When buying gotu kola, be sure the label states the product is standardized to gotu kola's triterpenes and is free of heavy metal contaminants.
- Gotu kola has a good safety record but has caused a few cases of contact dermatitis.

GRAPE
Vitis vinifera, Vitis labrusca

History and Folklore

You might wonder, is grape an "herb"? It's an ambiguous designation, and not every plant gets it—there are over a quarter of a million plant species and only so much room in a health food store. According to the general public's consensus, it is an herb, for its extracts may be found in every health food store under "herbs." A large share of the growing status of grape and its extracts is owed to the public's association of red wine with health.

Grape cultivation may have originated in Egypt, and it has continued for six thousand years. Besides eating the fruits as is, they provide juice, preserves, and raisins, and some cultures use the leaves in cooking, for example, in the rice-stuffed Greek *dolmades.* But as it was in the past, most cultivated grapes are used to make wine. To the ancients who discovered fermentation, it must have seemed like magic. Yeast is everywhere, and a trace landing in any sugary drink like grape juice will eat the sugar and turn it into alcohol and carbon dioxide. Winemakers will caution, however, that wine should not be exposed to oxygen for long, lest its alcohol oxidize to acetic acid. This creates yet one more grape product: wine vinegar. The unfermented grape was used therapeutically for its sugar content to fatten up someone who needed it, a use that has rapidly dropped in popularity. The leaves and stem are tannic and were once used to stop bleeding. However, the mounting interest in grapes originated in the quest to explain the so-called French Paradox. The rate of coronary heart disease in France is relatively low, despite the typical French diet that includes lots of saturated animal fat from cream, cheese, and meat, and relatively higher cigarette smoking. Perhaps their regular, moderate wine consumption protects them, the theory goes. (That the French have far less fast food and smaller food portions than Americans doesn't hurt either.) Indeed, regular, moderate wine consumption was found to confer heart health in clinical studies; this was particularly true of red wine, which contains more theoretically therapeutic elements. Later studies showed that when controlled for confounding factors like lifestyle, it might have been the low doses of alcohol, and not any grape molecules, that provided the benefit, although high doses of alcohol are of course ruinous. Nonetheless, a massive amount of research on grapes' molecules have revealed very interesting activities, and grapes' expensive extracts sell like hotcakes off the herb shelves of health food stores.

How Scientists Think Grape Works

Grape compounds may do the opposite of the now infamous COX-2 inhibitors. Drugs companies are now ducking for cover amid the much-publicized revelation of the link between their once oft-prescribed and highly advertised anti-inflammatories, the COX-2 inhibitors (like Bextra, Vioxx, and Celebrex), to potentially life-threatening cardiovascular problems. At first COX-2 inhibitors seemed like a great idea and better than aspirin. Aspirin shuts off two similar-looking enzymes, COX-1 and COX-2, which make prostaglandins, many of which cause inflammation. But COX-1 also constantly makes stomach-protecting prostaglandins, so aspirin's turning it off can upset your stomach. The prescription COX-2 inhibitors didn't do this, so they both prevented inflammation and didn't upset your stomach—but at a cardiovascular cost. According to test tube studies, the epicatechin and catechin flavonoids in grapes—also found in other plants like tea and cocoa—do the opposite, inactivating COX-1 but leaving COX-2 alone.[1] Is it just a coincidence that they are associated with cardiovascular health?

COX-2 makes inflammatory molecules, but not everything it makes is bad. COX-2 makes *prostacyclin I2,* or *PGI2,* which dilates your blood vessels, dropping your blood pressure. Plus, PGI2 prevents platelets from clumping to form a clot. And not everything COX-1 does is good, and that's why aspirin's ability to block it confers cardiovascular rewards. Some of COX-1's prostaglandins are used to make the blood-clotting, blood vessel–constricting *thromboxane A2,* or *TXA2.* So the COX-2 inhibitors were doing exactly the wrong thing for your cardiovascular system: They were turning off an enzyme that makes blood pressure–dropping, anticlotting PGI2 and allowing another enzyme to make blood pressure–raising, clot-forming TXA2. A recent publication shows that the grape molecules catechin, epicatechin, and resorcinol selectively inhibit COX-1, and they leave COX-2 alone.

These grape molecules don't work quite like aspirin either. Part of aspirin sticks to both forms of COX irreversibly, permanently knocking them out of opera-

tion until your cells can make more. Your platelets can't make COX, however, so if you take aspirin, your body has to spend about a week making new COX-containing platelets to be able to clot blood efficiently again. The grape flavonoids may not have such a long-term effect; they don't permanently knock out your COX-1, but they inhibit it temporarily with a hit-and-run approach. Also, aspirin stops the first part of the reaction, the cyclooxygenase reaction, which makes prostaglandins. The grape flavonoids halt the peroxidase reaction, which is the second and final sequence involved in this conversion. In the test tube, epicatechin and catechin halt this second reaction at the same low concentrations found in your blood after you consume grape products, too, which is a big deal, since there has been much argument over how little of these flavonoids get absorbed into your blood and how most of them get chemically modified when they do get absorbed. Theoretically, a pool of different flavonoids in your blood could work together additively, too, boosting effective concentration.

Grape contains free-radical quenchers and scavengers. The notorious free radicals that attack our molecules are reactive, because in addition to the usual paired electrons, they have a single unpaired electron, which is usually an unstable situation for a molecule, depending on where that unpaired electron rests on the molecule. Unstable molecules in general are more harmful than stable ones; they are more likely to attack your body's own molecules. (To learn more about free radicals in general, see "Free Radicals" in appendix D, pages 382–396.) Since free radicals have all their electrons paired up except for one, they have an odd number of electrons, unlike the typical molecule, which has all of its electrons paired up in twos and thus has an even number of electrons. Stable molecules that have all their electrons paired up are far more common than the rarer free radicals. Flavonoids in grape, such as quercetin, start off with an even number of electrons, but they are able to donate one of their electrons to pair up with the unpaired one on the free radical, so it will no longer be a free radical. This "quenches" the former radical and stabilizes it. However, realize that since quercetin starts off with an even number of electrons and loses one, it ends up with an odd number of electrons. This loss of one of its electrons temporarily turns quercetin into a free radical, too, albeit usually a more stable, less damaging one (though not always; see below.) The quercetin free radical can un-radicalize itself, so to speak, by again donating its unpaired electron, quenching a second free radical. The loss of a second electron gives quercetin an even number of electrons again, making it more stable than before.

Some flavonoids quench, others scavenge. The scavenging flavonoids kidnap the single, unpaired electron from a free radical, becoming a free radical themselves in the process, but hopefully a more stable one. The concentrations needed to perform these radical tricks in an effective manner in the test tube are about ten times higher than what you find in your blood after you eat flavonoids, so there remain questions about how effective these mechanisms really are. However, it might be for the best that even consummate eaters of flavonoid-containing foods don't achieve massive plasma levels of flavonoids. If they did, they would have to worry about flavonoids themselves acting as free radicals.

Grape flavonoids could protect you from iron—or make you more vulnerable to it. Many of the flavonoids in grape and other plants are known to bind to iron, and less so to copper, a process called *chelation* (key-LAY-shun). Since flavonoids have trouble getting from your gut into your bloodstream, it's not likely the flavonoid concentrations required to capture metals in cells are much to worry about, but in your gut, flavonoids' binding these metals will decrease your absorption of them. But that could be a good thing. Iron isn't the hero it used to be. Sure, your red blood cells need it, but it is a free radical generator, and there are links between iron and heart disease and other problems. Because of this, nutritionists are now advising you shouldn't take an iron supplement unless you have a bleeding or metabolic problem that causes you to need more than what is in your normal diet.

On the other hand, the electron-donating capability of some flavonoids is a concern, because they can give iron an electron, turning *ferric iron* ($Fe3+$) into *ferrous ion* ($Fe2+$). When ferrous ion reacts with peroxide, a natural cellular waste product, it generates free radicals.

What's In It

GRAPE PRODUCTS contain polyphenols in four major classes. These are nonflavonoid stilbenes like resveratrol and viniferins; and three types of flavonoids: The red anthocyanidins, flavonols (kaempferol and quercetin), and the tannins, which are mainly proanthocyanidins (oligomeric proanthocyanidins) containing catechin, epicatechin, and epigallocatechin units stuck together. Many of the flavonoids and stilbenes can have attached sugar, which increases their water solubility but decreases our ability to absorb them. Grapes also have tangy components like tartaric, citric, malic, succinic, ascorbic, and oxalic acids, as well as the aromatic acids like coumaric acid and caffeic acid, and the fruits have a great deal of glucose.

The Dr. Jekyll/Mr. Hyde nature of flavonoids can be avoided. It's true: Although flavonoids are usually noted for their antioxidant- and free radical–neutralizing actions, on occasion they have been witnessed doing the opposite. Under certain circumstances they act as pro-oxidants and free radicals in the test tube. High dietary intakes of flavonoids *from eating plant-based foods* have not been associated with adverse effects. On the other hand, very high doses (1 gram/day) of purified, supplemental quercetin have been associated with negative effects, in the form of nausea, vomiting, tingling in the extremities, headache, sweating, and difficulty breathing. It seems safest to get your flavonoids from plants rather than supplements, and because clinical studies show that flavonoids are generally good for you, the more you get from plants, the better. It doesn't matter if a label for quercetin or some other flavonoid brags about being derived from a plant. Most flavonoids are. The fact that this sort of supplement is purified and in higher concentration than you would absorb from a plant-based food is what makes it riskier than the plant itself.

Proanthocyanidins are associated with healthy blood vessels. In the test tube, the tannins in grape, known as *proanthocyanidins* (also called *oligomeric proanthocyanidins, OPCs,* or *PCOs*), prevent blood clotting. In clinical studies they are also linked with better blood vessel function. The proanthocyanidins in pine bark extract, commonly called *pycnogenol,* are chemically quite like the proanthocyanidins in grape, and results from clinical studies on it are similar. In test tubes, both pycnogenol and OPCs facilitate the release of nitric oxide from the cells that line blood vessels, and nitric oxide relaxes your vasculature, dropping your blood pressure.

This is great news until you learn that proanthocyanidins have trouble getting into your blood. According to metabolic studies, they are hard to absorb—proanthocyanidins are both water soluble and come in medium, large, and extra large sizes. Water solubility and large size are both characteristics that make it difficult for a molecule to get through cells lining your gut out into surrounding capillaries. They also tend to stick to proteins lining your digestive tract, literally "tanning" it temporarily, which also limits their absorption. However, tests for proanthocyanidins crossing a simulated intestinal lining show the smaller proanthocyanidins could find a way through the intestinal lining into the blood.

The resveratrol from grape skins does many exciting things—in test tubes. A select group of plants—grapes, blueberries, cranberries, bilberries, mulberries, Japanese knotweed, spruce, eucalyptus, and peanuts—make resveratrol when under stress, for example, when grape skins are attacked by fungi. In grapes resveratrol comes in two forms, cis and trans (mainly trans), and may or may not have attached sugar. (Don't confuse trans resveratrol with the unhealthy "trans" fats; the chemical designation of "trans" is a very general one and in the case of resveratrol has nothing to do with healthiness or unhealthiness.) Some grape products have more resveratrol than others; it's concentrated in grape skin, and Pinot Noir is supposed to have the most among wines, for example. Consumers, inspired by the breathlessly worded media pieces generated by research on it, are now taking resveratrol in supplement form.

Yeast, worms, and fruit flies, oh my. Resveratrol is antioxidant, anti-blood-clotting, and blood vessel–relaxing—in the test tube. Its actions in animals are less clear. However, it is even thought to have anticancer activity through a number of mechanisms, inducing cell suicide of cancer cells, choking off tumors' blood supplies, hindering estrogen's cell-proliferating tendency, increasing liver detoxifying enzymes, and decreasing liver toxifying enzymes. Some researchers have even linked resveratrol to life prolongation—in yeast, worms, and fruit flies. As far as we know, the only thing that reliably prolongs the life of some experimental animals is rather depressing: caloric restriction. Many types of lab animals are now known to live much longer and healthier lives if their calorie intake is severely restricted by at least 30 percent. (A handful of courageous people have volunteered to undertake the tough task of drastically restricting their own food intake, too, as scientists watch parameters of their health. These lifetime studies are ongoing and will obviously take awhile to reach completion.) In some animals, caloric restriction stimulates a gene called *SIR2;* resveratrol's stimulation of SIR2 in yeast, worms, and fruit flies—*without* caloric restriction—mimicked this life-prolonging effect. In the test tube, resveratrol also stimulates the human form of this gene (called SIRT1 or Sirtuin1). Whether it prolongs the life of a calorically unrestrained human is another question entirely. No studies have yet tackled this question.

Unfortunately, you can't get much resveratrol inside you when you eat it. Even ridiculously small adults are much bigger than worms, and accordingly, humans also need more resveratrol to acquire comparable concentrations. The water-soluble resveratrol floating about in grape juice has attached sugar, which always makes a molecule hard to absorb, but gut bacteria can remove the sugar. The sugar-free resveratrol is much better absorbed but is not water soluble, so less of it will be in aqueous grape extracts. Even after the sugar-free resveratrol is absorbed into your blood,

it is rapidly altered in the liver to once again possess attached sugar, or sulfate. Concentrations peak at half an hour after you ingest resveratrol, but at most are ten to one thousand times less concentrated than what is commonly used in test tube experiments. This does not mean we should throw the resveratrol baby out with the bathwater. We don't know much about the activity of resveratrol's metabolites, for example. It just means that its exciting test tube studies tell us less than we'd like, and it remains an unknown.

Good Effects . . . and Not So Good

For all grape beverages and food, moderation is the key. The "French Paradox" won't work if you drink too much wine, or any other alcoholic beverage, for that matter. Excess alcohol ruins your liver, and your health along with it, and makes you vulnerable to estrogen-sensitive cancers like breast cancer. Even grape juice is not so innocent if you drink tons of it—its naturally high sugar content can turn into an unnaturally high triglyceride (fat) content in your body. If you manage only a little of either red wine or grape juice on a regular basis, however, your cardiovascular system will be grateful. Grapes and raisins make a great, healthy snack, but if you overdo them, you can get diarrhea. If you want the proanthocyanidin tannins and anthocyanidin flavonoids, go for the red grape product, since white grapes have relatively little.

There are various grape-derived supplements, too. Grapes' proanthocyanidins are a type of tannin that is called *oligomeric proanthocyanidins, OPCs,* or *PCOs,* and it is widely sold under these designations. OPCs are derived from grape seed and grape skin.

There have been no adverse effects reported for people taking this or grape seed extract, except that it is rather expensive. Large doses of tannins can, however, upset some people's stomachs.

Some people have complained of gastrointestinal upset and diarrhea, headache, and retching after taking red vine leaf, the flavonoid containing grape *leaf* extract. Resveratrol supplements so far have a good safety record, but very large doses of supplemental quercetin have caused nausea, vomiting, tingling in the extremities, headache, sweating, and difficulty breathing. If you take a lot of flavonoids in supplement form or from grape products, tea, or cocoa, they can limit your absorption of iron. It is safe and actually recommended that you get as many flavonoids as you can in the form of different plant foods.

Watch your blood thinning. If grape products do give you a blood-thinning effect, be sure that will not potentiate any blood-thinning medication you are on, and be careful if you have a bleeding disorder or are scheduled for surgery.

EVIDENCE OF ACTION

For all the hype and published articles covering grape extracts (to date there are over eleven hundred scientific publications on resveratrol alone), the number of human studies is relatively scant. While all sorts of exciting news emerged from cell studies, the oral bioavailability of the exciting components in grapes is low, perhaps explaining why results from animal and human studies are less dramatic. At least with respect to what they have measured so far in humans, nothing outstanding pops out. The results hint at antioxidant, blood-thinning, and blood vessel–dilating properties, however.

Commonly Reported Uses for Grape*

Internally
antioxidant, circulatory disorders, anti-cancer, hemorrhoids, diabetic complications, retinopathy

forms available for internal use:
juice, wine, grapes, raisins, grape seed extract, grape leaf extract, grape skin extract, resveratrol, quercetin

commonly reported dosage:
Daily doses of grape seed extract range from 40 to 300 milligrams. In clinical trials grape leaf extract was taken either at 360 or 720 milligrams per day to treat chronic venous insufficiency. A glass of red wine contains about 640 micrograms of resveratrol, and supplemental resveratrol doses range from 200 to 600 micrograms daily.

*These uses and dosages are from historic use and are not necessarily tested nor recommended.

The more exciting results so far are seen with red grape juice and red wine. Red grape juice, which is red because of its water-soluble anthocyanins, won a blood-thinning battle against orange juice and grapefruit juice.[2] Of course orange and grapefruit juice do not have these red pigments, and had, according to the study, three times less polyphenolic compounds. Subjects drank a small glass of one of the three juices a day, and after a week their blood clotting potential was challenged. While orange and grapefruit juice had no effect, grape juice drinker's blood clotting potential dipped to 77 percent of its value at to start of the study, a highly significant drop.

In case some of the former grape juice–drinking volunteers might have naughtily popped an aspirin, it's nice to know that similar significant results for lessened blood clotting were seen when a different set of subjects drank red grape juice.[3] Platelets from people drinking red grape juice also significantly decreased production of the damaging superoxide free radical. A significant rise in the blood vessel–dilating nitric oxide was observed as well, implicating a mechanism for lowering blood pressure.

This theoretical blood pressure–lowering mechanism may have manifest as an actual one in forty hypertensive Korean men.[4] Some drank red grape juice, while others drank a nongrape beverage with equal calories. The grape juice drinkers significantly reduced their blood pressure from the start of the study, and also with respect to the placebo group, although not quite significantly so.

Not all the things red grape juice does are good; when pitted against vitamin E, the juice significantly elevated plasma triglycerides—what we call "fat." This isn't peculiar when you stop to think about it: Grape juice has a lot of natural sugar, and excess sugar often turns into fat, increasing triglycerides. On the other hand, both vitamin E and red grape juice significantly improved to the same extent several antioxidant parameters that were measured, such as ability to squelch free radicals and LDL cholesterol oxidation. The grape juice drinkers even had significantly fewer oxidized proteins than the vitamin E swallowers.

Whether red wine is as powerful as red grape juice is a complicated question; specifically, it is complicated by the presence of alcohol, which has potent effects on its own. Numerous studies show that *small* amounts of wine on a regular basis (one glass per day for a woman, two for a man) offer significant protective cardiovascular rewards, but drink more than that and the health benefit plummets. Although initial studies showed that wine was more protective than other forms of alcohol, these may have been confounded. People who appreciate good wine over your basic rotgut are more likely to lead healthier lifestyles, for example, and to have better socioeconomic status. When these factors were taken into consideration in later studies, *all* forms of alcohol conferred the same benefit, but only if taken in small doses.[5, 6] The jury is still out but is leaning toward alcohol being the therapeutic constituent. One study found that although de-alcoholized red wine prevented platelets from clumping together in a test tube, a more realistic test showed that the platelets of volunteers who drank the de-alcoholized red wine were no less able to form clots than those who drank water.[7]

Be that as it may, wine contains more absorbable flavonoids than grape juice, because the fermentation process helps remove the sugars attached to the flavonoids, making them easier to absorb. So grape juice sellers who brag that their product has just as much flavonoids and resveratrol as red wine aren't telling you the whole story.

In studies of people taking grape seed extracts, allergic rhinitis sufferers taking 100 milligrams of grape seed extract twice a day weren't helped in a preliminary but well-structured (randomized, double-blind, placebo-controlled) study.[8] In another similarly designed study, a higher dose (300 mg of grape proanthocyanidin twice a day) taken for five days had no effect on serum levels of C or E, yet the volunteers taking the grape supplement may have enjoyed an increase in their antioxidant status, measured by a test called *total antioxidant capacity,* or *TAC.*[9] (However, TAC assays can be hard to interpret without more data and may be thrown off by various factors. For example, people with kidney failure may have misleadingly high TAC due to unusually high urate, which is measured as an antioxidant in the TAC assay. An increase in TAC doesn't tell you much unless you know what individual components of antioxidant status were improved.)

Grape seed did not prove itself as a short-term diet aid in a sensibly constructed (double-blind, randomized, placebo-controlled crossover) trial either.[10] Fifty-one volunteers were allowed to eat whatever they wanted for lunch and dinner for three days at a university cafe, but took either grape seed or a placebo beforehand. No significant difference in consumption was seen.

In a Japanese study, eleven women took high-proanthocyanidin grape seed extract for eleven months with the hopes of treating abnormal skin pigmentation (melasma).[11] Their skin significantly improved over the course of the study, but no control group taking a dummy medication was used, so it is hard to say whether this improvement would not have happened naturally on its own.

In treating forty patients with high cholesterol, proanthocyanidin-containing grape seed extract failed to make any dent in total or "bad" LDL cholesterol compared to a placebo or to a chromium supplement.[12] Nor was there any effect on blood pressure or homocysteine, an amino acid that is elevated in cardiovascular disease. The only positive finding was not statistically significant, but the extract showed a "trend" toward diminishing the patients' antibodies to their own oxidized LDL cholesterol. Many scientists believe fewer antibodies to oxidized LDL signifies better cardiovascular health.

Twenty-four smokers took either 75 milligrams twice daily of proanthocyanidin-containing grape seed extract for four weeks or a placebo, pausing for a "washout period," and then traded treatments, all without knowing who was taking what.[13] Smokers are renowned for having poor antioxidant status, and one of the indicators of this is increased lipid peroxidation, a sort of free radical–mediated attack of oxygen on a cell's membranes, which can cause the membranes to break down. Taking the extract significantly reduced a measure of lipid peroxidation. However, once again grape seed extract didn't budge their cholesterol and its various forms.

For studies with resveratrol alone, unfortunately most that call themselves "human" studies involve *removing* cells from humans, like blood cells, and dumping resveratrol on them in a test tube to see how the cells behave. For example, platelets removed from human subjects, treated with resveratrol, are less likely to aggregate and clot. This isn't a realistic test of resveratrol, since better-designed studies show that although we absorb the sugar-free version of resveratrol quite well, it is very rapidly turned into other things in our bodies and excreted rapidly. So it is really the action of these more mysterious resveratrol metabolites, and not resveratrol, that holds the key as to whether resveratrol offers health benefits, and isolated cell studies with resveratrol can't answer that question.

In a Danish study,[14] volunteers were placed on a very low flavonoid diet, which significantly decreased the vitamin C in their blood, perhaps because the vitamin C was being used to take over some of the antioxidant burden normally assumed by dietary flavonoids and other antioxidants found in plant foods. Then they took grape skin extract along with this diet, and another group followed the same procedure, in reverse order. Taking the extract blunted the loss of vitamin C, and some antioxidant enzymes were increased, though not all, and none were increased significantly.

Leaving no part of the grape untested, a German company offers a grape *leaf* extract, which they call "red vine extract." The leaf extract contains flavonoids, too (iso-quercitrin and sugar-bound quercetin). It is used to treat vein problems like varicose veins and chronic venous insufficiency.

According to some publications, red vine extract impressively helps blood flow, reduces leg swelling, and other symptoms.[15] The studies are at least well designed, although they may raise an issue over objectivity, since they were funded by the company selling the red vine extract.

THE BOTTOM LINE

- Flavonoids in grape act may like selective COX-1 inhibitors, thinning your blood and dropping your blood pressure in a manner similar to, but not exactly like aspirin.
- Grape flavonoids are most often seen as antioxidant and free radical–scavenging. Under certain circumstances they may do the opposite and be harmful, in theory. Thus it is not a good idea to take very large doses of purified flavonoids in supplement form. It is safe and healthy to get as much as you can from food, however.
- The proanthocyanidins, or tannins in grape are associated with better vasculature, but your ability to absorb them is very poor.
- Resveratrol from grapes does amazing things in test tube studies, which hint at anti-cancer and even life-prolonging mechanisms, but it may be metabolized too rapidly to have these effects in people.

GUARANA
Paullinia cupana, Paullinia sorbilis

HISTORY AND FOLKLORE

If you are from South America, you already know all about this herb. It is in the national drink of Brazil, and many of my Brazilian students, eyes gleaming, proclaim their devotion to it. Guarana is both a climbing, Amazonian evergreen vine and the caffeinated drink made from its seeds. Indian legend holds the plant grew from the eyes of a divine child who was killed by a serpent. Guarani Indians were the first to process the seeds, hence its name. After the seeds are shelled and roasted, they are powdered and mixed with water to form a dough. This is molded into hard cakes or bars. Amazonian Indians used these on-the-go guarana bars by grating off a piece for themselves with a hard fish bone when they needed a little extra zip. This form of guarana is likened to bitter chocolate, but astringent and dry, without the fat found in cocoa butter. Besides abating fatigue, it is considered an aphrodisiac. Traditionally it is used to treat mild digestive upset—its tannins may help in that arena—and headache, an action probably assisted by its caffeine.

Guarana seeds are also mixed with cassava and allowed to ferment to make one of Brazil's favorite drinks. Sugary, amber-colored guarana sodas are huge in South America, and most of its devotees say it's not just the caffeine but guarana's contribution of an unusual, spicy, berrylike flavor not found in other sodas. These have made their inroads into U.S. grocery shelves, marketed under the term "energy drinks" and sporting confidence-inspiring names, like "Bawls."

HOW SCIENTISTS THINK GUARANA WORKS

Guarana's main active ingredient is caffeine. Like tea, coffee, cocoa, and maté, these unrelated plants all possess differing amounts of stimulant molecules called *methylxanthines:* the classic stimulant trio of caffeine, theophylline, and theobromine. They all tend to work the same way, with different potencies and subspecialties. Caffeine is the most prominent one in guarana, and guarana has more caffeine than coffee. People who take guarana typically experience the same effects as those who drink coffee.

You may already be familiar with caffeine's most obvious effects, such as stimulation, faster heartbeat, and an exceptional urge to urinate. Caffeine also stimulates your gut's release of digestive enzymes and acid, discourages blood clots, and briefly raises your blood pressure, as if you have been climbing a flight of stairs. Regular caffeine consumers, however, do not have high blood pressure.

A lot of caffeine's other effects are signature moves of the fight-or-flight nervous system, which readies you for action, and some of these effects can be exploited therapeutically. For example, blood vessels in muscles are widened, allowing them greater access to blood sugar. At the same time, blood sugar is released from stores in the liver, and fat breakdown is stimulated, the products of which can also be used to feed cells poised for action. Caffeine tends to suppress appetite—eating is not something you need to do while fighting or fleeing—plus its stimulating effects form the rationale for its addition to diet aids.

Blood vessels in other areas are constricted, like in the brain and skin, conserving its delivery to muscles and lungs. The constriction of blood vessels in your brain by caffeine makes it useful in treating vascular headaches, and you may notice its addition to some over-the-counter analgesics and prescription migraine medicines. Caffeine opens up the respiratory system, allowing you to get more oxygen. Theophylline, one of the other methylxanthines, is better at this than caffeine, however, and is therefore used in asthma medications. How does the caffeine in guarana and other plants perform these tricks?

Caffeine is an adenosine receptor antagonist. The main effects of caffeine are attributed to its antagonism of a molecule called *adenosine.* Caffeine does other things, too, like increasing calcium in muscle cells, making them twitchy by lowering the threshold stimulus needed for them to contract. Caffeine may also stimulate histamine receptors in your gut, too, increasing digestive juices. But the main effects of caffeine are through its inhibition of a sleep-inducing molecule called adenosine.

What's In It

GUARANA CONTAINS the stimulant purine alkaloids caffeine (2–7.5 percent) and smaller amounts of theophylline and theobromine. Its tannins are proanthocyanidins (12 percent), and also contains cyanolipids such as 2,4-dihydroxy-3-butyronitrile. It also contains trace amounts of the saponin fish poison timbonine.

Adenosine is released as part of a larger molecule called *adenosine triphosphate,* or ATP, from stimulatory nerve cells, but adenosine itself doesn't stimulate. It is released at the same time as the stimulatory fight-or-flight neurotransmitter, norepinephrine, perhaps as a means to keep norepinephrine from getting out of hand. The slow, spontaneous breakdown of ATP lingering outside the nerve cell releases adenosine. This adenosine doubles back on its tracks and binds to adenosine receptors on the nerve cell that released it. Adenosine blunts the nerve cells' ability to release the stimulatory norepinephrine, so adenosine inhibits brain activity, and it makes you sleepy.

Adenosine also accumulates throughout the day as ATP is broken down during its use to fuel reactions that just would not occur on their own; reactions that require energy. So as you spend energy throughout the day, adenosine builds up, and its binding to adenosine receptors in your brain shuts down your brain's activity. Caffeine and other methylxanthines look a lot like adenosine, and also temporarily stick to adenosine receptors, blocking adenosine's access to them. This keeps you from getting sleepy.

Besides allowing the fight-or-flight stimulant norepinephrine to work unopposed by adenosine, caffeine has indirect effects that boost dopamine and serotonin, and this could explain why we get a pleasure-enhancing mood reward from consuming it. Scientists speculate that caffeine's effect on these hormones may explain why large studies have shown that habitual caffeine consumers are less likely to get Parkinson's disease or to commit suicide. Despite our puritanical impulses to portray anything that makes us feel so good as a danger, caffeine has several health benefits, although certain people should not have it. For a summary of all of caffeine's positive and negative disease risks, see "Interesting Facts," on page 182.

Commonly Reported Uses for Guarana*

Internally

stimulant, aphrodisiac, diet aid, cognitive performance, athletic performance, vascular headaches, digestive aid

forms available for internal use:

capsule, dried herb, seeds, powder, extract, syrup, tablet, tea, carbonated sodas, energy drinks

commonly reported dosage:

Either one-half to a gram of dried herb is taken, or 200 to 800 milligrams of extract once or twice daily, not to exceed 3 grams of extract.

*These uses and dosages are from historic use and are not necessarily tested nor recommended.

Guarana also contains a lot of tannin. The effects of guarana tannin are less well known. Small doses of guarana tannin are benign and can even be helpful. Guarana tannin cross-link proteins, pulling them tight, and this skin-tightening effect is what is meant by "astringent." Tannins "tan" the lining of your mouth and digestive tract in a mild way. This forms a temporary, protective barrier against gastrointestinal irritants, hence guarana's traditional use in treating indigestion. Large doses, however, can upset your stomach. Another tannin-containing South American herb, yerba maté (see page 342), is very popular and part of South American cultural traditions, just as wine drinking is among European ones. Like guarana, it has both caffeine and a high tannin content. Maté, however, has been repeatedly linked to an increased risk of certain cancers, and we aren't sure why. It certainly isn't because of its caffeine content. Early studies suggesting caffeine was a carcinogen were confounded by coffee drinkers' tendency to smoke. Caffeine has been vindicated of these charges in numerous, better-designed studies, and the American Cancer Society officially states that caffeine does not cause cancer.

Tannin, on the other hand, theoretically could cause cancer, if you have loads of it, and some have proposed this is behind maté's increased cancer risk. There have been no associations of guarana with cancer, but no one has performed epidemiological cancer-risk studies on it either. If you want to limit any of tannin's actions, have it with protein. The tannin reacts with the protein and not with you.

Good Effects . . . and Not So Good

Guarana gives you an energy boost, and can stop a vascular headache, but don't overdo it. Too much stimulation will make you jittery and bad-tempered, and any fine motor controls you require go down the drain. Like other caffeine agents, too much guarana can induce small tremors. If you do fine artwork or anything requiring careful control of your hands, don't have guarana beforehand.

Watch out for withdrawal. Like other caffeine-containing beverages, guarana is pleasure-enhancing and addictive; though this is not as sinister as it sounds. The tolerance you develop to caffeine is mild, and unlike many other additive drugs, caffeine pharmacology works differently. It isn't something that you need more and more of to continue having the same effect. You won't end up selling your house and car to fund your caffeine habit, for example. There are also health benefits to moderate regular caffeine drinking, though not everyone should have it. It you are used to guarana or other caffeinated substances, their sudden withdrawal may cause blood to flood into your brain, causing headache, and the increased number of adenosine receptors that you make while taking caffeine makes you more susceptible to adenosine's sleep-inducing effects, making you groggy.

Certain people should limit their guarana. It is not for the insomniac. Caffeine is a common culprit in causing insomnia, and guarana's caffeine content is higher than coffee's. Caffeine can cause some people to have an irregular heartbeat, and if you think you are one of these people, don't take guarana. Certainly, if you don't like how it makes you feel, don't take it! If you are not a regular consumer of caffeine, it may temporarily boost your blood pressure, though those who take it regularly don't experience this effect. Because caffeine can enter fetal circulation, pregnant women are advised to have no more than one cup of coffee per day, and since guarana has more caffeine, guarana abstinence seems wise during pregnancy. Unless you want a fussy, sleepless baby, don't nurse while taking guarana either. The caffeine in it is transported through breast milk.

Guarana is not for pets. Although the problem is more often seen with chocolate, pets should not be exposed to methylxanthines in general, because they respond differently than humans, and in some cases it can kill them.

Various forms of guarana have precautions, too. The diet and cognitive aids containing guarana typically contain many other herbs with unknown safety records, and since it's not clear how they work, avoid them. And although there are some "diet" versions, most guarana sodas and "energy drinks" are brimming with sugar. Since energy is measured in calories, "calorie drinks" is a more truthful designation than "energy drinks," especially since the energy the calories provide may not be used and will more likely get stored as fat. The sugar in them can also cause tooth decay.

The tannins in guarana are an unknown but are a concern. It is not known if their presence in the herb maté causes cancer, for example. Tannins do limit your absorption of protein, because they bind to proteins in your gut. To limit the action of tannins in your gut, some have suggested taking high-tannin-containing herbs like guarana with milk, to keep them preoccupied enough with milk proteins.

Interesting Facts

Through caffeine, nature teaches us once again that no molecule is entirely bad or entirely good.

REGULAR CAFFEINE consumption has been associated with a decreased risk of committing suicide and developing Parkinson's disease, gallstones, liver disease, and type 2 diabetes. On the other hand, it can increase urinary loss of calcium, although studies attempting to link it to osteoporosis have been inconclusive, perhaps because dietary calcium compensated for the loss in the people studied. It was once believed that caffeine stimulated breast cyst formation, but this is no longer held to be true, as no well-designed studies have found evidence to support this. Caffeine can cause some people to have an irregular heartbeat, although it is not associated with causing heart disease. It can enter fetal circulation, and its effects on fetuses are unknown but not associated with birth defects. However, a Danish study found that women consuming the highest amounts of caffeine a day were more likely to risk having a stillborn child, so pregnant women who have increased risk for miscarriage should limit caffeine intake to less than 300 milligrams a day, it or avoid it entirely.[1]

Evidence of Action

There are not many studies of the effects of guarana on humans. Its effects on cognitive performance are contradictory. One study where neither the researchers nor the elderly volunteers knew who was taking what discovered that guarana had no significant effect on volunteers taking it, compared to caffeine or placebo,[2] while another similarly constructed study suggested that guarana gave participants moderately better attention on mental tests but slightly worse accuracy in their answers.[3]

Two studies examined guarana as a weight loss agent, but unfortunately the guarana was mixed with other herbs, so it is hard to say which herb was doing what. Healthy volunteers who consumed guarana mixed with yerba maté and damiana showed significantly delayed gastric emptying compared to a placebo, theoretically helping them retain a feeling of fullness.[4] (However, in another study, mice fed solely guarana, or caffeine, showed no change in gastrointestinal transit.[5]) After forty-five days of taking this mixture, significant weight loss of around eleven pounds (5 kg) was seen, and

for those who continued on the extract for a year, the weight was not regained.

Another mixture containing guarana and the now widely banned ephedra showed a significantly greater loss of weight and fat in those taking the mixture than in those taking placebos,[6] but it should be noted that eleven of the thirty-five subjects in the active group withdrew before the study was complete, complaining of chest pain, heart palpitations, increased blood pressure, and irritability, and it is likely that a lot of these side effects were caused by ephedra, which was banned for its toxic and sometimes fatal effects on the heart. Guarana contributes caffeine, which is an appetite suppressant and stimulant, and this theoretically could have contributed to the effects in these studies. However, there is no way to tell whether guarana caused the weight loss in these studies of herbal mixtures. Caffeine also stimulates an increase in blood sugar, blood pressure, and heart rate, all of which were significantly elevated in the later studies' herb-taking volunteers as well.

Mice fed guarana also experienced a significant surge in blood sugar after an hour, from its storage form, glycogen, in the liver.[7] This significantly prevented them from experiencing a drop in blood sugar during exercise. Rats fed guarana had better endurance in swimming tests and showed no ill effects from the herb.[8]

Animal studies hint that guarana isn't harmful, and it could provide certain health benefits. A study with rabbits fed guarana showed their platelets were less likely to clot,[9] and this blood thinning is already a known effect of caffeine. Guarana also prevented chemical-induced liver cancer in mice,[10] and protected rats from indomethacin or alcohol caused stomach injury.[11] No toxic or adverse effects of guarana on behavior or organ tissues of rats or mice were seen even at high doses.[12] Additionally, an antioxidant effect was observed in the form of decreased membrane oxidation (lipid peroxidation.) This prevention of membrane oxidation is positive, since membrane oxidation causes cells and their constituents to break down prematurely.

THE BOTTOM LINE

- Guarana exhibits therapeutic actions through its high caffeine content. Caffeine works primarily by blocking a sleep-inducing molecule called adenosine.
- Because of its caffeine, guarana is a stimulant and can be effectively used to treat vascular headaches. However, it is not clear whether it boosts mental ability or works as a diet aid.
- Guarana also has tannins, which in small doses can relieve indigestion but in large doses can cause it. The high dose of tannins from another stimulant, the South American herb maté, might increase cancer risk, but no one knows whether guarana is associated with cancer.
- Although regular, moderate caffeine intake is associated with health benefits, it should not be taken in excess, as it can cause withdrawal, and certain people should not have it. People prone to irregular heartbeat and pregnant or nursing women should avoid guarana.

HAWTHORN

Crataegus laevigata, Crataegus monogyna, Crataegus oxyacantha

History and Folklore

This member of the rose family (*Rosaceae*) is a small tree or shrub that, like roses, also sports thorns and festive red berries resembling rose hips. These fruits, or "haws," were once commonly used to make jams, jellies, and alcoholic beverages. The leaves and flowers, however, are considered the more pharmacologically active parts. "Haw" is also an old term for hedge, so its common name literally means "thorny hedge." It was also once called mayflower, for its white, early blooming flowers.

Though hawthorn's early blooming flowers made it a symbol of hope, their malodorous scent once also paradoxically linked the plant with death. Some of the small amines released by these flowers are identical to those produced by rotting corpses. One old superstition warned that bringing the flowers into your house would result in the death of a loved one.

Hawthorn is found throughout the world in the temperate northern hemisphere. Both Europeans and Asians used hawthorn medicinally. It was one of the thirteen sacred trees of the ancient Celts, and though both the ancient Greek Dioscorides and the medieval father of toxicology, Paracelsus, noted its action as a heart therapeutic, this use was not popularized in Europe until the nineteenth century. Europeans more often used the leaves, flowers, and berries for kidney stones and as a diuretic. Chinese traditional medicine uses hawthorn berries, or *shan zha,* for indigestion and diarrhea. However, current Chinese traditional medicine now more often includes hawthorn's more modern and well-documented use as a heart medication.

How Scientists Think Hawthorn Works

Most medical references suggest hawthorn acts like a type of antiarrhythmic heart drug known as a PDE-3 inhibitor. "PDE-3" stands for an enzyme known as *phosphodiesterase 3*. PDE-3 normally breaks down a key signaling molecule known as *cyclic adenosine monophosphate (cAMP)*. It's customary for signaling molecules like cAMP to get broken down like this; otherwise they would keep signaling forever, and that would cause problems. However, you can slow the breakdown of cAMP by inhibiting the PDE-3 that disables it. Some heart drugs, like inamrinone ("Inocor") and milrinone ("Primacor") work by inhibiting PDE-3, and hawthorn has traditionally been placed in this category, too. By inhibiting PDE-3, you boost the concentration of cAMP. What does boosting cAMP do? Some flight or flight hormones like adrenalin (also known as *epinephrine*) also boost cAMP directly, and you know your heart beats harder when you get an "adrenalin rush" because of fear or excitement.

The actions of cAMP differ from cell type to cell type, affecting functions as diverse as fuel usage and blood sugar levels, nerve cell signaling, cell division, and the immune system. But in the heart, cAMP ultimately allows calcium that is stockpiled in closed compartments inside of heart cells to be released into the cell's main interior, increasing the active calcium concentrations inside heart cells. Increased calcium inside muscle cells causes them to contract. This includes the heart muscle, and thus if hawthorn is a PDE-3 inhibitor, hawthorn ought to help the heart pump blood more forcefully. (In the involuntary muscle cells lining blood vessels, increased cAMP has the opposite effect, relaxing the muscles, and opening the blood vessels to allow blood to flow more easily, and blood pressure drops.) The scant number of studies claiming PDE-3 inhibitory activity for hawthorn used various rodents, not people, and since PDE-3 behaves differently in different species, this is not proof that hawthorn works as a PDE-3 inhibitor in humans.

PHOSPHODIESTERASE-3 INHIBITORS are not the same as the more recently famous phosphodiesterase-5 inhibitors, such as sildenafil ("Viagra"), which are used for male erectile dysfunction. There are different types of phosphodiesterase enzymes, and they have different functions. Phosphodiestase-5 inhibitors prevent the breakdown of cyclic GMP (cGMP) by phosphodiesterase-5 in the penis, and PDE-3 inhibitors don't do this. So don't expect hawthorn to treat erectile dysfunction.

Preliminary new evidence suggests the former theory may be incorrect, and hawthorn might work like a class III antiarrhythmic drug, instead. The most recent experiments with hawthorn surprised the investigators, because although they used the same animal model that was used to determine PDE-3 inhibition above, they could not detect the type of altered heart calcium concentrations expected for a PDE-3 inhibitor.[1] Instead, they discovered hawthorn behaving like a class III antiarrhythmic drug. (The number "III" here has nothing to do with the "3" in the PDE-3 inhibitor name; it's just coincidental.) What hawthorn and class III antiarrhythmic drugs have in common is that they block the flow of potassium ions in the heart, and are therefore also known as *potassium channel blockers.*

The heart uses several different ions, including potassium ions, in order to beat. Think of the heart as being like a battery that can continually recharge itself. Each time it beats, it discharges, and these charged particles called *ions* (or *electrolytes*) are released to flow in directions that cause them to disperse (either out of heart cells or into heart cells, depending on the type of ion.) Before the next beat, your heart has to recharge, and energy is spent to push the ions back into their original positions, so they can be rereleased to create the next beat. The ions involved are calcium, sodium, and potassium ions. Other herbs and types of heart medications block sodium (type I antiarrhythmics) or calcium (type IV antiarrhythmics) flow, but hawthorn and class III antiarrhythmic drugs delay the recharging action of potassium ions. As a consequence of hawthorn's potassium channel blocking, the heart takes longer to "recharge" between beats. This delay in recharging of the heart "battery" is what all class III antiarrhythmics have in common. The delay can prevent abnormal, fast arrhythmias of the heart.

Hawthorn might widen coronary arteries, allowing more oxygenated blood to nourish the heart. Most experimenters who observe this effect on isolated animal blood vessels postulate that hawthorn does this by increasing the creation of a blood vessel–widening hormone called *nitric oxide*. One paper attributes this to hawthorns' procyanidins, which are a common type of plant tannin. Increased nitric oxide could also result from secondary effects of some of the theoretical antiarrhythmic mechanisms mentioned above.

What's In It

THE ACTIVE ingredients of hawthorn are thought to be mainly its proanthocyanidins and flavonoids. Hawthorn leaf, flower, and berry extracts contain 1-3 percent oligomeric proanthocyanidins. Its flavonoids include hyperoside, vitexinrhamnose, rutin, and vitexin. Hawthorn has around 0.6 percent triterpenes, including oleanolic acid and ursolic acid; and small amines such as choline, acetylcholine, and the malodorous trimethylamine.

Hawthorn's flavonoids and proanthocyanidins have several actions in your body. They can act as mild antidiarrheals and are antioxidant and free radical–scavenging. The larger proanthocyanidins are technically *tannins*. Tannins bond to the inside of your gut, forming a temporary, tough lining that can reduce contact with chemical irritants. Though hawthorn is not heavily promoted as a digestive aid these days, traditional Chinese medicine reported its use for diarrhea, and its tannins probably account for this use. They should be used in moderation—large amounts of tannins can irritate your gut, too. Also, regular ingestion of inordinate amounts of tannins from other herbal preparations with higher tannin content than most (see yerba maté, page 342) is postulated to increase cancer risk. Smaller amounts of tannins are found in classic herbal remedies for diarrhea and indigestion, and moderate doses of the proanthocyanidin type of tannins such as those in hawthorn are thought to be good for the cardiovascular system in general.

Unlike hawthorn's big proanthocyanidins, its smaller proanthocyanidins and flavonoids can more easily slip through your gut lining, making it into your blood stream.[2] These molecules are found in many other plants, too, and many investigations report that they are antioxidant and free radical–scavenging. This further protects your heart from chemical damage.

Good Effects . . . and Not So Good

Doctors are rethinking their use of antiarrhythmic drugs in general, and this includes those that act like hawthorn. This may lead you to rethink using hawthorn as a heart medication as well. Early on, doctors and scientists just assumed that suppressing abnormal heart rhythms with antiarrhythmic drugs would allow people to live longer. To their consternation, several long-term trials noted that many (but not all) antiarrhythmic drugs, not only did *not* prolong life, but also were associated with an increased risk of mortality! Indeed, the use of implantable devices like ICDs (Internal Cardiac Defibrillators) and pacemakers is for some heart patients associated with a better life-prolonging track record than antiarrhythmic drugs. We are also now learing that the hearts which can easily adapt to a greater range of different rhythms may fair better than ones that are maintained at a constant rhythm. There are many different types of heart problems and treatments, and what works well for one person may be hazardous for another. The uncertainty in the long-term benefits of antiarrhythmic drugs highlights why you should be under a doctor's care if you have any sort of heart problem.

Most people are not adversely affected by hawthorn, and interactions with other drugs are not documented. However, it should be used cautiously. Hawthorn has potent effects on the heart, so most experts recommend it be taken with a doctor's supervision. It should probably not be taken by pregnant women or children under twelve years of age. There are reports of hawthorn having a sedative side effect, but this action has not been clinically documented nor its mechanism outlined.

Commonly Reported Uses for Hawthorn*

Internally
    heart tonic, digestive aid, sedative
    forms available for internal use:
    capsule, dried leaves, flowers and
    berries, infusion, tablet, tincture
    commonly reported dosage:
    Three doses adding up to no more than
    5 grams of crude plant material or 1
    gram of extract daily is reportedly taken.

*These uses and dosages are from historic use and are not necessarily tested nor recommended

---

If you have heart disease and want to try hawthorn, talk to an understanding doctor first. Don't be afraid to ask. More and more doctors are becoming herb-savvy and sympathetic to those who want to try herbs. And if they do give you permission to take hawthorn, a responsible doctor ought to monitor your heart rate and blood pressure on a regular basis.

Whether or not you want to try hawthorn, you ought to be under a doctor's care if you have heart disease. Don't drop your heart medication and substitute it with hawthorn. A doctor can best decide whether any heart medications you currently take could theoretically be interfered with by hawthorn.

If you want to buy hawthorn, use a standardized preparation. Get one standardized to proanthocyanidins (also called oligomeric proanthocyanidins, OPCs, or procyanidins.) According to research, the active ingredients are reportedly the mixture of proanthocyanidins and flavonoids. Proanthocyanidins are sometimes also called *oligomeric proanthocyanidins,* or *OPCs*—these are the same thing, so don't be baffled by these similar-sounding terms. Procyanidins (without the "antho" in the middle of the name) are a particular *type* of proanthocyanidin, and these are thought to be active ingredients, too.

The antioxidant flavonoids are good to have, too, if you can find a label that standardizes to both. The product might be standardized to a particular flavonoid. (Flavonoids in hawthorn include hyperoside, vitexinrhamnose, rutin, and vitexin.) However, some hawthorn products are standardized to the flavonoid vitexin, and the vitexin from unrelated plants is thought to interfere with a thyroid enzyme (thyroid peroxidase) if consumed regularly. If you have thyroid problems, you might want to avoid taking vitexin-standardized products on a regular basis.

EVIDENCE OF ACTION

There is excellent evidence that hawthorn is a potent heart medicine. An analysis by two independent reviewers, published in the 2003 *American Journal of Medicine*,[3] scrutinized all available published and unpublished clinical trials where hawthorn was used for chronic heart failure. Of these, only eight of the most carefully constructed (the randomized, placebo-controlled, double-blinded ones) using pure hawthorn extracts met their criteria as the most reliable. The studies encompassed 632 patients with chronic heart failure, with treated individuals taking between 160 and 1,800 milligrams of hawthorn daily for three to sixteen weeks.

This analysis concluded that hawthorn significantly improved the heart's "maximum workload"that is, the hearts of volunteers taking hawthorn were better able to take on challenges such as exercise stress tests on stationary bicycles. Hawthorn also significantly improved heart patients' labored, uncomfortable breathing (dyspnea) and fatigue. A beneficial decrease in a parameter quantifying heart rate and blood pressure was also seen. Side effects were uncommon and temporary, but included mild nausea, dizziness, cardiac and gastrointestinal complaints.

THE BOTTOM LINE

- Older references and data imply hawthorn may act like antiarrhythmic drugs known as *PDE-3* (*phosphodiesterase-3*) *inhibitors.* These ultimately increase a signaling molecule known as *cAMP* (*cyclic adenosine monophosphate*), which increases calcium in heart cells, increasing the force of their contraction.
- New contradictory but preliminary data suggest hawthorn may alternatively work like a class III antiarrhythmic heart drug, slowing potassium's electrical "recharging" of your heart before each beat. This increases the heart's force of contractions, improving your heart's pumping power.
- Antiarrhythmic drugs may alleviate symptoms of heart problems, but there is concern that several types of antiarrhythmic drugs actually increase mortality. The use of hawthorn as an antiarrhythmic drug is a concern for this reason.
- Hawthorn dilates blood vessels, probably by increasing the synthesis of a hormone called *nitric oxide.* This drops blood pressure and improves blood flow.
- Hawthorn's flavonoids have protective antioxidant and free radical–scavenging action.
- Although hawthorn is not known to interact with other drugs, and side effects are rarely reported, it should be taken while under a doctor's supervision, because of its potent effects on the heart. Pregnant women and children under twelve should avoid it.

HOODIA
Hoodia gordonii

History and Folklore

Verifiable hoodia isn't readily available just yet, despite what you might glimpse on some of the Internet's shadier sites. Despite this, "hoodia" products are doing a brisk business worldwide because of sensational-sounding news stories featuring its appetite-suppressing power. Hoodia is a cactuslike plant with spiny, cucumber-like protuberances that grows in the Kalahari Desert of Southern Africa. The San Bushmen eat it to quell their hunger during long hunting forays. South African scientists noticed in the 1960s that hoodia dramatically suppressed lab rats' desire to eat—by up to 50 percent—but the studies were neglected for a while, possibly because weight loss is normally considered a sign of toxicity in animal studies, although the animals did not appear worse for the treatment. Newer unpublished studies report that hoodia banishes appetite in people in the same extraordinary way and did them no obvious harm. Consequently, interest in the rare desert plant has soared, fueled by features on *60 Minutes,* the *BBC World News,* and other prominent media. With health food shelves groaning under the weight of diet aids assigned flunking grades by the Western world's growing obese population, the dietary supplement market is primed and itching to pounce on hoodia. In some cases they have done so, however, before it has made its rounds through clinical studies, bringing out the worst in human behavior. It is a potential goldmine for whoever sells it.

IDEALLY, A patented herbal product ought to benefit any ethnic culture that discovered it, introduced its properties to the rest of the world, and did all the work of testing it in their everyday lives. Yet it often does not work out that way, and that has human rights organizations alarmed. Those who steal traditional knowledge and profit from it without compensating the robbed are dubbed "biopirates." The case of hoodia and the San Bushmen is classic.

The heart-wrenching part of the hoodia story contrasts the frenzy over this latent commercial jackpot with some of the poorest people in the world, the San Bushmen. First oppressed by Bantu tribes, the San Bushmen were subsequently repressed by European immigrants who considered them like animals and in fact treated them worse than animals. Europeans once legally hunted them for sport. Today they live out in the open, or in primitive huts, making do off the desert with bows and arrows. Many of them are addicted to drugs and alcohol. Under ideal circumstances, if hoodia does all that has been promised and is safe, and if its sales can be channeled into helping the San Bushmen, their nightmarish history could change to happily ever after. This will not happen on its own. It absolutely requires that knowledgeable consumers use their purchasing power to draw the line between what is right and wrong.

The South African Center for Scientific

and Industrial Research (CSIR) heard rumors of hoodia's appetite-squelching effect and took some into their labs. When the commercial potential for the herb dawned on them, they patented what they believed to be its active ingredient, P57, in 1997, and sold the license to a British company called Phytopharm, for half a million dollars. Phytopharm promptly sold the rights to develop the drug to Pfizer for 32 million dollars. The San, despite pronouncements of the finest intentions toward them on the parts of CSIR and Phytopharm, were not informed of all this and have not received any money. The head of Phytopharm claims this was because they were not sure the herb would live up to its promise, despite the massive amounts of money invested in it. He also says, with some embarrassment, that the company's failure to notify the San was because they could not find any, although they looked very hard for a long time. They had several years to do so.

Nonetheless, there are around one hundred thousand Bushmen, and some of them were found within a day by Action Aid, an international development agency. The San organized themselves and hired human rights lawyer Roger Chennells, who negotiated with CSIR and Phytopharm and won the argument that the San were essential to the development of the patent. The agreement is confidential, but now Phytopharm officially states that they have entered a benefit-sharing plan with an organization representing the San.

Now the company is growing plantations of the rare hoodia, because its active ingredient is too hard to synthesize on a large scale. It takes about five years for the plant to mature, and it is difficult to grow. These plantations are fenced off and guarded. The CSIR has patents relating to hoodia in all the territories where it is known to grow in the world, over which Phytopharm has exclusive license.

Hoodia is protected by conservation laws and can only be grown and collected with a permit. Hoodia is additionally protected by CITES (Convention on International Trade in Endangered Species of Wild Fauna and Flora), an international agreement that not only conserves rare plants and animals, but also ensures that indigenous people who are dependent upon them for survival maintain access to them. Thanks to all the hype, though, shady people have been caught wandering around the Kalahari digging up this rare plant, and gray-market hoodia plantations are rumored to be growing in secret locations. Any profits made from these do not benefit the San.

How Scientists Think Hoodia Works

A component in hoodia appears to fool the brain into thinking you are full, but there are unanswered questions. The dramatic appetite-banishing power of hoodia on rodents led to the hunt for the herb's active components. A molecule resembling cardiac glycosides, which are plant molecules that have effects on the heart, attracted the attention of scientists, who dubbed it P57. Druglike molecules often stick to human receptors, so they did a reasonable thing. They tested P57's affinity for a full range of receptors for neurotransmitters, bioactive neuropeptides, and ion channels. It didn't stick to any of these. It didn't even stick to the standard target of cardiac glycosides, which is called the *sodium-potassium pump* (also commonly known as the *sodium-potassium ATPase*).

Yet their attention centered on this pump in their efforts to discover how P57 worked. They found that a poison called *ouabain,* which normally subverts the action of this essential pump, was unable to work in the presence of P57, despite P57's failure to bind to ouabain receptors or for P57 to affect the pump on its own. Since the pump requires the universal energy-carrying molecule ATP, they shifted their focus to P57's effect on ATP.

They ultimately found that food-deprived, hungry lab animals had significantly less ATP in the brain's hypothalamus. Injections of P57 into their brain (an act consumers will not wish to duplicate) preserved ATP. They formed the reasonable hypothesis that ATP in the hypothalamus is a means of sensing energy levels, and when it gets low, you get hungry. Phytopharm's (the corporation that holds a patent on P57) official position so far is that when you are fed, your increased blood sugar causes nerve cells in your hypothalamus to fire, and you sense you are full. P57 is, according to them, ten thousand times as active as glucose in performing this trick, which fools your brain into thinking you are full.

What's In It

AN EXTENSIVE chemical analysis of hoodia has not been published. The alleged active ingredient is a trirhabinoside-14-hydroxy-12-tiglyoyl pregnane steroidal glycoside with a molecular weight of 1008 amu. This is termed either P57AS3 or P57.

How does P57 get to the brain, assuming it is the active ingredient? According to Phytopharm's studies, P57 is a glycoside, meaning it has attached sugar.

Sugar-bound molecules are difficult to absorb into the blood from the digestive tract, although there are some exceptions to this rule. This could mean that you have to eat a lot of hoodia to get an effect. Usually bacteria in your gut remove and eat the sugar from a glycoside. The remaining *aglycone,* or sugar-free molecule, is usually more pharmacologically active and absorbable than the glycoside, but they found the aglycone of P57 had no effect on appetite suppression or the ATP-preserving brain effects. Assuming the allegedly active P57 glycoside gets into the blood after you eat it, it still has to perform an additional trick of crossing a chemical barrier to many molecules called the *blood-brain barrier* in order to enter the brain, assuming the brain is where it exerts direct action. Phytopharm's study got around such digestive issues anyway, by injecting the compounds directly into rat brains. These questions don't mean hoodia doesn't work. It just means there remain a lot of unanswered questions about *how* it works.

Good Effects . . . And Not So Good

Don't buy hoodia just yet, for a number of very good reasons. Anything that affects the brain as dramatically as Phytopharm claims must be extensively tested in clinical trials for safety. These trials are not yet complete.

Don't give money to pirates. You are likely to end up with a very expensive caffeine pill with no hoodia in it. That's what was revealed in the analysis of one "hoodia" supplement that was marketed off an Internet site. Most Web sites that advertise and sell the purported supplements boast incorrect and oftentimes outright false claims, while also cutting and pasting more official news reports and the scant scientific literature onto their site, making them look more official than they really are. Please keep in mind that the herb is not yet approved and that research is still in its early stages.

Commonly Reported Uses for Hoodia*

Internally
appetite suppressant, aphrodisiac, digestive aid, protection from illness
forms available for internal use:
Verifiable hoodia is not currently available.
commonly reported dosage:
No typical dosage has been reported.

*These uses and dosages are from historic use and are not necessarily tested nor recommended.

Upon analysis, most of these products contain no hoodia, or only traces that are unlikely to have any effect. Despite being warned by the FDA, they close their shops and open them up elsewhere. If they using hoodia, it is unlikely the San Bushmen, who are now integral to the patent on it, are benefiting from their profits.

If and when hoodia becomes approved for safety and available, become a detective before you buy it. Go the extra distance to see who benefits from its sale. This is hard investigative work, too, because very little of the herb market is strictly regulated. It's worth it, though, because San Bushmen have suffered long enough. Please ensure that any profits from hoodia you buy end up in the hands of the San Bushmen.

EVIDENCE OF ACTION

Exhaustive searching reveals only two publicly available, officially published papers on the testing of hoodia. The first describes how both lean and genetically obese rats were fed either normal Purina rat chow, or the same plus hoodia.[1] Neither group appeared visibly

THE BOTTOM LINE

- Hoodia is a plant the San Bushmen of the Kalahari use for appetite suppression. Very preliminary evidence suggests it works dramatically, by keeping ATP concentrations in the brain's hypothalamus high.
- Hoodia's presumed active ingredient P57 is patented and currently undergoing clinical trials.
- The desperately poor San Bushmen are considered essential to hoodia's patent and legally require compensation from its use. Although human rights organizations are aware of the situation, vigilance in pursuing this end is required on the part of consumers as well.
- Most hoodia products sold over the Internet contain no hoodia or trace amounts that are unlikely to be effective. They may also be spiked with undeclared drugs like caffeine. Sales from these products are not likely to benefit the San Bushmen.
- For such a popular herb, there are almost no studies on it to date, compared to most herbs. Its safety and effectiveness are big unknowns.

worse for their treatment. Those rats that were fed hoodia ate less by more than 50 percent, and their blood glucose dipped by 15 percent within forty-eight hours, compared to those not getting the hoodia. In addition, the obese rats became almost as lean as their lean counterparts after three weeks, and both groups' fat losses were noteworthy.

The other publication noted similarly dramatic results with rats who received injections of P57 into their brains.[2] This included an additional study where thyroid hormone, used to increase rats' metabolic activity and hunger, was unable to make rats hungry if their brains were injected with P57.

Phase I clinical trials are ongoing, and while those reports of preliminary findings have been released, they have not been published. Phytopharm states that morbidly obese volunteers were split into two groups of those taking hoodia and those taking a placebo. After fifteen days, the hoodia group reduced their calorie intake by one thousand calories a day. This is almost half the number of calories that most adults consume in one day.

HORSE CHESTNUT

Aesculus hippocastanum

HISTORY AND FOLKLORE

You have probably seen this handsome, ornamental tree towering about parks and lawns. The horse chestnut shares its genus with buckeye trees, so it is also loosely called buckeye, as well as *Spanish chestnut, conkers, conquerors, fish poison,* and *seven leaves tree.* They are common in North America and Europe, and though once thought to have come from Tibet, are now considered natives of the Balkan Peninsula.

Horse chestnuts are easy to recognize, with distinctive, serrated "palmate" leaves. A palmate leaf's veins diverge from one central point, somewhat like fingers radiating from the palm of a hand. The leaves do resemble large, goofy hands, each divided into five to seven oblong leaflet "fingers," further distinguished by their conspicuous veins. The large seeds, or "conkers," are also unique. Their spiked capsules break into three parts, revealing big, shiny brown seeds that children use in a game (described below). Do not eat them. They are not very tasty, they can be toxic, and they are not actual chestnuts.

It is not clear what these trees have to do with horses either, but medieval sources suggest that Constantinople residents gave horse chestnut seeds to horses that were "broken-winded" or coughing. Others think the Welsh word *gwres,* meaning "heat" or "fever" advertised the seed's pungent taste, and this word degraded into "horse." The unprocessed seeds are poisonous to humans, but many people who survive eating them report they are mouth-puckeringly tannic.

Cows are often said to love the seeds, but prudent livestock experts advise keeping all parts of the tree away from animals. The 1911 *Encyclopedia Britannica,* however, portrays the seeds as feed for poultry, sheep, deer, and other animals: "Given to cows in moderate quantity, they have been found to enhance both the yield and flavour of milk. Deer readily eat them, and, after a preliminary steeping in lime-water, pigs also." (One assumes the seeds, not the finicky pigs, were soaked in lime water.) The old reference goes on to quote the *Edinburgh Pharmacopoeia*'s instruction to take ground horse chestnut seeds as a *sternutatory,* to encourage sneezing, assuming you are in need for such a thing. Horse chestnuts carried in your pocket are supposed to magically ward off arthritis, but fiddling with them compulsively may at least grant arthritic fingers a workout.

The seeds are in fact considered the medicinal part, and the other bits are more toxic and avoided. Indeed, fish are particularly sensitive to all parts of the tree, especially the twigs and buds, a phenomenon that Yuchi and Creek Indians used to their advantage. Horse chestnut pieces were thrown into ponds, and stunned yet edible fish would rise to the surface. Humans should use seed extracts only after special processing removes its more poisonous components.

Horse chestnut seeds have been used for centuries to treat colds, coughing, various pains, arthritis, and fever. Today their best-known uses are vascular, such as for treating varicose veins and chronic venous insufficiency, inflamed veins (phlebitis), edema, hemorrhoids, and ulcers.

How Scientists Think Horse Chestnut Works

Horse chestnut constricts your veins. This might explain how it helps treat chronic venous insufficiency (CVI) and varicose veins. The theoretically active ingredients from horse chestnut seeds are certain triterpene glycosides (saponins) that are collectively called either escin or aescin. The increased venous tone appears mediated by aescin's ability to increase one of your prostaglandins, called *prostaglandin F2-alpha,* or *PGF2a.* This molecule acts locally to cause contraction of certain involuntary muscles, like those surrounding both arteries and veins, and their constriction increases vascular "tone." Constricting the inept veins found in these conditions aids the return of blood through the heart. It also prevents vein swelling, which can lead to a varicose vein. Constricted vessels also tend to be less leaky, so constricting your veins prevents surrounding tissues from swelling with uncomfortable water retention.

Horse chestnut also keeps your blood vessels from leaking. Leaky blood vessels allow water from the blood to penetrate into surrounding tissues, and this water retention is a classic uncomfortable symptom of CVI and varicose veins. Aescin might keep blood vessels from leaking by preventing serotonin and histamine from making the blood vessels more permeable to fluid. In tissue cultures, aescin-treated blood vessels remained leak-proof even when antagonized by serotonin and histamine.

Aescin could help keep your tissues from breaking down. Aescin inhibits lysosomal enzymes, which are more active in

people with CVI and varicose veins. Lysosomal enzymes are normally stored in safe storage units (lysosomes) in cells, but when released they break large molecules into smaller ones and break down your tissues. This is normal, but it ought to be balanced with tissue construction projects. Since these enzymes break down some of the building blocks of capillaries, aescin inhibiting them theoretically helps preserve the integrity of inflamed regions around veins.

What's In It

THE THEORETICALLY active ingredients from the seed are certain triterpene glycosides (saponins) collectively called either *escin* or *aescin (diacylated tetra-* and *pentahydroxy beta-amyrins).* Flavonoids include biosides and triosides of quercetin. Its tannins are of the proanthocyanidin type.

Horse chestnut could also stop inflammatory actions that make vein pathologies worse. Inflamed blood vessels display distress signals on their inside linings. Like billboards on a highway, these signals catch the attention of immune cells that flow past them. The immune cells stick to these display signals and are alerted that something is wrong. The method works well if there is a pathogen in the area, but if not, it does more damage. The defensive immune cells start attacking randomly, causing even more damage and inflammation. Horse chestnut extracts were seen in animal studies to prevent the expression of these molecular distress calls in blood vessels, so the white blood cells did not linger in them to do any harm. Horse chestnut's quercetin flavonoids also help protect you from inflammation by reducing oxidizing agents and free radicals.

Good Effects . . . and Not So Good

Be careful what you use. Children have died after drinking unprocessed tea from the leaves and following ingestion of the seeds. Because the seed extract must be carefully processed prior to commercial use, buy products where the label states it is standardized to aescin (also called escin), and only from companies with an impeccable reputation. The product label should also clearly indicate that aesculin (also called esculin) has been removed (not to be confused with the similar-sounding active ingredient aescin). Aesculin is similar in structure to coumarin, a type of plant molecule with a tendency to prolong bleeding times. *Aesculin (esculin) can cause severe bleeding, and in isolated cases even death.* Products that contain derivatives from parts other than the seeds, such as the bark or twigs, should be avoided. Don't try to make the extract yourself.

After processing, the commercial products seem relatively safe except for mild side effects. Many large studies of humans taking horse chestnut seed extract have been performed with relatively minimal side effects reported. However, some people experience gastrointestinal distress, and taking the extract with food may be helpful in preventing this. Side effects reported include nausea, vomiting, diarrhea, dizziness, itching, headache, and weakness. Don't overload on horse chestnut, because overdoses may induce kidney failure in some people. Topical formulas are also available, and the relatively few studies on them suggest they are effective as well.

Interesting Facts

Watch horse chestnut seeds fly in a historic English battle.

IF YOU find yourself near Ashton, England, in October, you may wish to take in the excitement of the annual World Conker Championship. Organizers typically collect around three thousand conkers, or horse chestnut seeds, for the event. These are then rated for quality and only the best conkers are used. Lately, hot, dry summers have created chronic conker shortages, and shrewd collectors sensing their worth have sold choice ones on eBay for 5 to 15 British pounds per bag. Worried organizers even resort to importing them, to avoid catastrophe.

This championship, now celebrated by papers like the *London Times*, the *Guardian*, and the *Daily Telegraph*, evolved from a popular children's game. Holes are drilled through nuts deemed superior, and a string is threaded through the hole. Two opponents face each other brandishing one strung conker apiece. Each opponent takes turns dangling their weapon while the other swings their nut at it, attempting to dislodge the dangling one from its string. The owner of the intact conker wins. Serious conker swingers experiment with nut-toughening methods and apply protective finishes to them. In Australia the game is called "Bullies." "Conker" derives from "conqueror," but either term makes sense nowadays since contestants conk each other's conkers until one of them "conks out."

Certain people should not take horse chestnut. Although recommended doses of horse chestnut seed extract appear safe for most people with chronic venous insufficiency and related problems like varicose veins, it should be avoided by women who are pregnant or nursing, because it could elevate a labor-inducing chemical (prostaglandin F2), and its effect on fetuses and infants are unknown. Those with liver or kidney problems, because of their possible inability to efficiently metabolize its potentially toxic saponins, should not take it.

EVIDENCE OF ACTION

Many clinical studies assessing horse chestnut seed's efficacy in treating chronic venous insufficiency generally support its use, but they affirm that the herb should be taken as recommended and avoided by those with kidney or liver problems. In 2004 a comprehensive review of randomized controlled trials using horse chestnut seed extract for chronic venous insufficiency (CVI) concluded, "The evidence presented implies that HCSE (horse chestnut seed extract) is an efficacious and safe short-term treatment for CVI. However, several caveats exist and more rigorous RCTs [randomized controlled trials] are required to assess the efficacy of this treatment option."[1]

In one study, 240 patients with documented early stage CVI were randomly placed into groups that either took a placebo or horse chestnut seed standardized to 50 milligrams of aescin twice daily, or were treated with compression stockings and a diuretic. Swelling was measured by lower-leg volume repeatedly up to twelve weeks, and though the placebo group's leg volume increased during the trial, the compression stocking and horse chestnut groups significantly improved and achieved comparable results.[2] A similar study using 350 patients with later-stage, more severe CVI observed similar results, with both horse chestnut

and compression stockings improving leg volume with respect to the placebo, but horse chestnut did not achieve the significant decrease that compression stockings did. Also, some people who took horse chestnut seed extract complained of gastrointestinal upset.[3]

Commonly Reported Uses for Horse Chestnut*

Internally
chronic venous insufficiency, varicose veins, edema (swelling), hemorrhoids, ulcers, and inflamed veins (phlebitis)
forms available internal for use:
capsules, extracts, pills, herbal blends
commonly reported dosage
Package instructions should be followed. A dose equivalent to 10 to 140 milligrams of aescin per day, sometimes taken in divided doses, is often recommended.
Externally
chronic venous insufficiency, varicose veins, edema (swelling), and inflamed veins (phlebitis), hemorrhoids
forms available for external use:
gel, lotion, ointment
commonly reported dosage:
A 1 to 2 percent aescin is applied topically several times daily.

*These uses and dosages are from historic use and are not necessarily tested nor recommended.

Another review in 2002 included thirteen trials where subjects were randomly assigned either horse chestnut, or a placebo, as well as three observational studies totaling 10,725 patients. Overall, variables associated with

THE BOTTOM LINE

- Horse chestnut seed extract may help with vascular problems, such as chronic venous insufficiency and varicose veins.
- Aescin is a mixture of saponins, detergent-like plant molecules from horse chestnut seed extract, and considered its active ingredient. Aescin constricts blood vessels and makes them less leaky, reducing swelling. Aescin may do this by antagonizing serotonin and histamine's actions on blood vessels, or by increasing prostaglandin F2, which constricts certain blood vessels. The extract also inhibits tissue-degrading enzymes and prevents recruitment of inflammatory white blood cells to blood vessels.
- Formulas containing commercially prepared horse chestnut seed extract from reputable companies are the only form recommended, because poisons (aesculin, also known as esculin) must be reliably removed.
- People with liver or kidney problems, as well as pregnant or nursing women, should avoid horse chestnut seed preparations.
- Some people experience gastric distress after taking horse chestnut seed products.

CVI such as leg volume, edema, pain, leg heaviness, cramps, and itching were assessed. The authors noted that the three observational studies showed significant effectiveness for pain, edema, and leg fatigue or heaviness. In the thirteen other trials horse chestnut seed extract reduced leg volume by 46.4 milliliters and increased the likelihood of improvement 4.1-fold for leg pain, 1.7-fold for itching, and 1.5-fold for edema compared to the placebo, but provided insufficient evidence of an effect on leg fatigue and heaviness or calf cramps.[4]

A more recent study suggested that a topical aescin mixture decreased damaging free radicals. Aescin was combined with phospholipids, molecules that are common to all cells that comprise a cell's outer membrane. (Phospholipids are commercially available in the form of lecithin, which is usually derived from soy, page 281.) Phospholipids applied topically are moisturizing and can form cell-like bubbles called *liposomes* around drugs. Since liposomes penetrate skin more readily than many drugs, its inclusion in topical mixtures may enable a drug—or in this case, aescin—to penetrate skin more efficiently. For two weeks the phospholipid-aescin mixture was applied three times daily to the ankles of ten patients with either venous hypertension, no ulcerations or infections, dysfunctional small veins (venous microangiopathy), or varicose veins. All groups' plasma showed statistically significant decreases in free radicals.[5] This correlates with a study using donated human umbilical veins, which when subject to low oxygen levels attract inflammatory white blood cells, but aescin was able to inhibit their adhesion and release of free radicals and inflammatory mediators.[6] A molecule isolated from aescin (beta-aescin) also showed potential to reduce inflammation. Beta-aescin prevented the display of inflammatory, adhesive molecules called *ICAM-1* and *E-selectin* on cerebral arteries The protrusion of ICAM-1 and E-selectin from blood vessels into the blood is associated with inflammation. They ordinarily stick to and provoke immune cells that flow past them in the bloodstream, mediating a local immune response that can damage the arteries.[7]

The mechanism of horse chestnut appears related to its ability to improve venous tone and prevent enzymes from degrading tissue associated with inflamed veins. Aescin's ability to contract vein segments from patients with varicose veins was comparable to a reference chemical (phenylephrine), although neither agent affected the vein in the calf region.[8] The contraction of veins by aescin seems mediated by its ability to stimulate the production and release of prostaglandin F2 alpha.[9] Aescin inhibits some tissue-degrading enzymes, such as hyaluronidase, but not elastase,[10] and horse chestnut extracts inhibit the proteoglycan-destroying enzymes from cell lysosomes.[11]

KAVA KAVA
Piper methysticum

History and Folklore

Kava kava, now more often known simply as "kava," is both a plant and the lip-numbing, bitter-tasting drink that is made from the plant's roots. Kava drinking is an important social and ceremonial tradition among Pacific Islanders, not unlike wine drinking in other cultures. The roots are ground, chopped, or even chewed, and then soaked in cold water to make the communal beverage.

Piper methysticum means "intoxicating pepper," as this member of the pepper family (*Piperaceae*) is said to produce feelings ranging from contentment to exhilaration, relaxation, and sociability. Traditionally, it has been used not only as a sedative but also as an anesthetic, as well as a treatment for infections and asthma. It may actually work as an anxiolytic, or antianxiety agent.

On the downside, kava's abuse, even in its traditional form, has long been associated with health problems. The association with several rare but frightening cases of liver failure put the brakes on the sale of what was, in the 1980s, one of the world's best-selling herbs. One of these cases, as noted in the introduction, was my stepmother's teenage niece, who after drinking many cups of kava tea daily, turned a bit yellow. Her family was shocked to learn she was suffering catastrophic liver failure, and thankfully, she is now surviving very well following her liver transplant. Cases like this prompted kava's ban in several countries, and it remains subject to health advisories in the remaining countries where it is not banned.

How Scientists Think Kava Works

Like some local anesthetics, kava probably blocks sodium ion channels on your nerve cells. Kava numbs your lips and mouth, and it probably does so by acting like certain local anesthetics that are used by your dentist and doctor. One of the things that triggers a nerve cell to respond is the influx of sodium ions into the nerve cell, which occurs through special sodium channels in the nerve cell membrane. Kava molecules are termed kavalactones or kavapyrones. On cultured nerve cells, certain kavalactones behaved as though they parked inside inactive sodium channels, prolonging the channels' inactive states.[1] Other kavalactones appear to reduce the action of sodium channels indirectly.[2]

Kava probably blocks your muscle's calcium channels, too. One of the triggers for getting muscles to contract is an inflow of calcium ions into the muscle cell, which occurs through various types of calcium channels on a muscle cell membrane. There is decent evidence that a kava molecule called *kavain* blocks a calcium channel known as an *L-type channel,* causing relaxation of involuntary muscles.[3]

Kava appears to act on your brain's limbic system, perhaps by affecting GABA. When your inhibitory neurotransmitter gamma-amino butyric acid (GABA) binds to its receptors on nerve cells in your brain, those nerve cells become less responsive, and so do you. Since GABA is a brain-slowing neurotransmitter, a lot has been done to uncover how kava might affect

GABA. The answers aren't clear-cut, but here is what we know.

There are two types of GABA receptors, called *GABA-a* and *GABA-b*. Kavalactones don't stick to GABA-b, but they do weakly stick to GABA-a, particularly in the brain's limbic system, according to studies with rats.[4] The limbic system is one of the oldest parts of the brain, evolutionarily speaking, so it is involved with pretty primitive stuff, like sexual arousal, fear, aggression, emotional bonding, hunger, thirst, smell, and the formation of emotionally charged memories. Several publications have suggested that kava relaxes this primitive brain region, so the preferential binding of kavalactones to GABA receptors in this area lends credibility to this assertion.

The antianxiety, sedative drugs known as *benzodiazepines* (Valium) also work on GABA receptors, but not at the same spot on the GABA receptor as kava. So kava doesn't act *just* like benzodiazepine drugs.[5] Kava may not enhance the binding of the relaxing GABA neurotransmitter to its receptor, but it does enhance the binding of some GABA-receptor binding drugs.[6] Some data suggest kava instead increases the number of GABA binding sites, which would make the brain more sensitive to GABA.[7] The bottom line is that, based on this research, kava doesn't act just like the antianxiety benzodiazepine medications. It may instead enhance the brain's own calming mechanisms.

Kava could affect other neurotransmitters, too. Several kavalactones inhibited monoamine oxidase (MAO), which is how some antidepressants work—those that are appropriately called *MAO inhibitors*. MAO is an enzyme that breaks down several neurotransmitters, including serotonin, adrenaline, histamine, and dopamine. These neurotransmitters are either diminished or less effective in certain depressed people.

MAO inhibitors boost their concentrations. When you inhibit MAO, it no longer mops up these lingering neurotransmitters, and they are consequently elevated in your brain. This makes some depressed people feel better (although kava appears to work more as an antianxiety agent than an antidepressant).

Kava failed to act like certain popular antidepressants known as SSRIs. Kava was tested for its ability to work like the ever-popular antidepressant SSRI drugs, or selective serotonin reuptake inhibitors, known by brand names such as Prozac, Zoloft, or Paxil. SSRI drugs boost the concentration of the neurotransmitter serotonin in the brain, but not everywhere in the brain at once. SSRIs increase serotonin only in places where the brain is using it. Nerve cells that release neurotransmitters such as serotonin often soak up some of the neurotransmitter that they have just released, a phenomenon called *reuptake.* Drugs that limit reuptake thus boost the amount of released neurotransmitter, and this makes some people feel better. Kavalactones failed to inhibit serotonin reuptake, so they don't act like SSRIs.

Perhaps kava acts like norepinephrine reuptake–inhibiting drugs, instead. Individual kavalactones did, however, inhibit nerve cells' reuptake of norepinephrine, a different brain neurotransmitter that, like serotonin, can also alleviate some forms of depression when it is increased in the brain. There are drugs that do this, too, known as *norepinephrine reuptake inhibitors,* which are prescribed to treat either depression (reboxetine) or attention deficit disorder (ADD) and attention deficit hyperactivity disorder (ADHD; amoxetine). Though the norepinephrine-boosting power of individual kavalactones was weak, they may cooperate to produce more potent effect when consumed together in kava.

But wait, there's more: Kava may affect glutamate and dopamine. Kava may keep glutamate, an excitatory neurotransmitter, from escaping a nerve cell. The release of glutamate is triggered by the influx of calcium ion into certain nerves cells, and synthetic kavain prevented this calcium-ion-dependent glutamate release.[8] This theoretically could prevent nerve cells from getting excited by glutamate, thus keeping them calm.

In addition, different kavalactones had variable and even opposing effects on the concentration of dopamine in rat brains.[9] However, large doses of kava extract increased dopamine in rat brains. If it does the same in human brains, it may help explain why kava drinking is pleasurable. Dopamine not only serves fundamental roles in the brain in coordinating smooth body motions, but is also associated with pleasure and the anticipation of pleasure, and is thought to play a role in the addictive nature of certain drugs like cocaine and amphetamines.

Kava could damage your liver by altering drug-metabolizing enzymes and lowering glutathione. Most of the molecules that you consume, regardless of whether they are from herbs, drugs, or your breakfast cereal, head first to your liver. (Certain dietary fats are an exception and are more directly released into the blood). Within your liver, alterations are often performed on these molecules, by various enzymes, before the molecules can be released into the general circulation. Remarkably, this often—but not always—produces a less toxic molecule. (In rare cases it produces a *more* toxic molecule, but that is another story.) When you mess with your liver's enzymes, you change your liver's ability to respond to various toxins that your body might consume. Kava certainly alters several of your liver's so called P450

enzymes, limiting their power to process toxins.[10] This increases your liver's exposure to toxins.

Additionally, kavalactones react with glutathione.[11] Glutathione is one of the most important protective molecules made by cells, and the liver particularly relies on it, since the liver is routinely exposed to all the strange molecules we consume. Kavalactones react with glutathione, sticking to it, and this bound glutathione is rendered ineffective, no longer able to detoxify. More glutathione can be made, but this takes time, during which liver damage can occur. Kavalactones theoretically exhaust the supply of one of your liver's most protective molecules. Depleting glutathione is a classic method of initiating liver poisoning; literally hundreds of different liver poisons and disease states are known to cause harm by depleting glutathione.

GOOD EFFECTS . . . AND NOT SO GOOD

Are you so anxious that you are willing to try an effective herb that has a very small chance of killing you? It's up to you to contemplate this serious question before you try kava. The odds of kava causing your liver to fail are small, but they are not zero. Remember, there are many other treatments for anxiety besides kava. If you are truly suffering from anxiety, it makes sense to exhaust all of your safest treatment options before you turn to kava.

There are additional problems with kava besides liver poisoning. Since kava-induced liver failure is rare, your odds of avoiding catastrophic liver damage are good, but long-term or heavy use of kava is still likely to damage your liver, reducing your overall health. In traditional cultures, indulgent kava use is associated with loss of hearing, hair, appetite, and weight. On occasion, kava drinkers develop uncontrollable eye spasms (saccade or blepharospasm) and an inability to control other muscles (ataxia).

Kava is bad for your complexion. "Kava dermopathy," or "kavaism," a condition caused by habitual kava use, has been documented for ages. A late eighteenth-century, intrepid Westerner concluded after observing South Pacific natives, "After some continuance of yava [kava] drinking, the skin begins to be covered with a whitish scurf, like the leprosy, which many regard as a badge of nobility: the eyes grow red and inflamed; and the soles of the feet parched and cracked into deep chaps, as some lips in winter." Yellowish, scaly, flaky skin and eye irritation develops with chronic kava use, but this condition does reportedly disappear over time with cessation of kava intake.[12]

"Traditional" preparations can still hurt you. Don't believe persistent rumors claiming this herb does not hurt members of traditional cultures who prepare kava "properly." In 2003 a couple of South Pacific Island natives who consumed large doses of kava in their traditional style developed hepatitis. (Hepatitis just means *liver inflammation;* and it can be caused by lots of things besides hepatitis viruses, including drugs and herbs.) Subsequent to this discovery, an investigation of traditional kava users on the South Pacific island of New Caledonia revealed that heavy consumption of traditional, aqueous kava extracts was positively associated with elevated liver enzymes,[13] what dying liver cells release into the blood. A classic sign of liver damage is the presence of a surplus of liver enzymes in your blood. Based on this data it seems obvious that heavy, traditional kava use by native New Caledonians impairs their livers. Similar findings were found in Aboriginal Australians who drank traditional kava preparations regularly. Those who downed kava more often and more recently showed significantly higher levels of liver enzymes in their blood.[14] Heavy kava use among Aborigines is also reportedly linked with sudden death, though poverty and poor diet confound this data.[15]

TRADITIONAL KAVA-MAKING disgusted colonists, who consequently outlawed the procedure. On his Pacific travels in 1777, one of Captain James Cook's companions related how Pacific Islanders made this beverage:

"[Kava] is made in the most disgustful manner that can be imagined, from the juice contained in the roots of a species of pepper-tree. This root is cut small, and the pieces chewed by several people, who spit the macerated mass into a bowl, where some water [milk] of coconuts is poured upon it. They then strain it through a quantity of fibers of coconuts, squeezing the chips, till all their juices mix with the coconut-milk; and the whole liquor is decanted into another bowl. They swallow this nauseous stuff as fast as possible; and some old topers value themselves on being able to empty a great number of bowls."

The chewing of kava prior to its incorporation into the communal beverage was so revolting to colonists that this method was once made illegal, forcing Pacific Islanders to grind the roots by hand.

Some controversy exists over whether peeled roots are safer than unpeeled ones, as traditional use reportedly involves peeling the roots. Peeling roots is arduous, especially for companies that are eager to profit on sales of the herb. However, there is only *one* published study on the toxicity of root peelings, which contain more of a liver toxin (*pipermethystine*) than peeled roots,[16] but this preliminary study is based on tests with cells in petri dishes, and this is hardly the basis for concluding whether peeled roots are safe. Keep in mind that even traditional users of kava have elevated plasma levels of liver enzymes, which is a concern.

Aqueous extracts are not necessarily safer either. Some optimists protest that the more traditional water-based extractions do not cause toxicity, but that our more modern acetone or alcoholic extractions are to blame. However, this assertion rests on very little evidence. One surprising preliminary study notes that large aqueous kava extracts given to rats actually failed to damage their livers.[17] However, rats and humans have different liver enzymes, and we don't know how this study applies to humans: rats may respond differently than humans, and they did not test other types of extracts to see if those had any different effects.

Another publication made a more eyebrow-raising claim and stated that aqueous kava extracts were not toxic to humans. This startling conclusion was based on studies not with actual humans but with a single-celled *amoeba*. The conclusion is questionable since amoebae are strikingly different than humans—for example, they do not have livers. Thus the theory that water-based extracts are safe is certainly not rigorously substantiated as of yet. Even isolated kavalactones, the active principles in the herb, given to men in one clinical study gave everyone a rash, and though it relaxed

the scaly men, their conditions forced the study to be discontinued. The truth is that we do not yet know what sort of kava preparation is safest, if any.

What's In It

THE SEARCH for active ingredients in kava turned up around fifteen molecules, alternately termed kavalactones or kavapyrones, including (+)-kavain, dihydrokavain, (+)-methysticin, dihydromethysticin, and yangonin.

If you *must* try kava, take these precautions. What do you do if you are offered kava at a luau? If you want to be polite, it probably won't hurt you to drink one cup. However, don't take it if you have any known liver problems, and don't take it with any other drugs, herbs, or alcohol. Some cases of kava-associated liver failure may have involved multiple factors such as these, and kava definitely shuts down many of the liver's drug-detoxifying enzymes. It seems prudent to limit kava to small doses and extend its use to no longer than a few days. Most cases of liver failure were seen after a person had been consuming kava for two to three months. As with alcohol, avoid kava if you are pregnant or nursing.

Don't drive under the influence of kava. Even the newly popular "kava bars" in Hawaii post signs admonishing customers not to drive under the influence of kava. In 1996 a Utah driver was spotted weaving in and out of traffic. Staggering out of his car to greet the highway patrol officers who had stopped him, he showed signs of intoxication, yet his blood alcohol was zero and there was no sign of illegal drug use. He admitted

Commonly Reported Uses for Kava*

Internally

antianxiety, sedative, antidepressant, aphrodisiac, pain reliever, ant-arthritic, anesthetic

forms available for internal use:

capsules, decoction, liquid extract, powder, peeled or unpeeled roots or rhizomes, tea

commonly reported dosage:

Clinical trials for treating anxiety disorders have most commonly used kava extract standardized to 70 percent kavalactones, and 100 milligrams of this extract (containing 70 milligrams kavalactones) was taken three times daily. The daily dosage of kavalactones reported typically ranges from 50 to 250 milligrams.

*These uses and dosages are from historic use and are not necessarily tested nor recommended.

drinking sixteen cups of kava tea and was the first Utahn convicted for driving under the influence of kava. There are two similar cases in California, both involving inordinate amounts of kava (eight cups in one instance and twenty-three in the other!) and no other intoxicants.

EVIDENCE OF ACTION

There is good news and bad news about kava. Here's the good news: Kava really does appear effective in reducing anxiety. No one is clear on how it works, but it persistently reduces anxiety in both human and animal studies. The most recent meta-analysis of the best clinical trials—that is, eleven of the most scrupulously designed (randomized, double-blind, placebo-controlled) trials using kava root extracts with no other complicating herbs— found that kava significantly reduced participants' Hamilton score, a standard test of anxiety.[18] Subsequent trials constructed in the same careful manner confirm this,[19] plus they indicate it helps create a "cheerful" mood.[20]

THE BOTTOM LINE

- Kava appears to be an effective antianxiety agent; however, there is also good evidence that it is bad for your health, particularly your liver.
- The risk for kava initiating catastrophic liver failure is small, but the odds of incurring lower-grade liver damage increase with increased kava use.
- There is currently very little evidence indicating what sort of kava preparation may be safest. Evidence that traditionally prepared kava, aqueous kava extracts, or preparations made from peeled roots are safer is either completely lacking or tenuous as of yet.
- There are many mechanisms that suggest how kava may affect brain neurotransmitters, nervous conduction, and muscle contraction, yet we are not clear which of these fully explain kava's effects.
- Since kava alters your liver's metabolizing enzymes, do not take kava if you have liver problems or are taking any medications or alcohol. Do not drive under the influence of kava, and avoid kava if you are pregnant or nursing.

Now for the bad news. Alas, kava is positively linked with causing potentially fatal liver damage, and though the risk is small, this is the sort of liver damage that can ruin your whole life, if not end it. You ought to seriously consider whether taking this small but potentially fatal risk is worth reducing your anxiety. A total number of seventy-eight cases linking liver toxicity to kava use have been reported in scientific literature, including eleven cases of liver failure, with four fatalities.[21] Perhaps not all were truly or completely caused by kava, but kava alters liver enzymes in a worrisome way, thus kava-induced liver failure is theoretically quite plausible. In January 2003, concerned scientists convinced the European Union and Canada to ban it, and the U.S. FDA has published several cautionary notices concerning its use.

LAVENDER

Lavandula angustifolia, Lavandula dentata

History and Folklore

The word "lavender" comes from the Latin "lavare," to wash, and people have used lavender-scented water to cleanse themselves, as well as their clothing and linens, since ancient times. Its pleasant-smelling oil is still commonly incorporated into modern soaps.

This Mediterranean plant became popular in European perfumery, particularly in France. Lavender was valued for repelling flies and for preventing moths and other insects from attacking clothing and linens. Bees don't seem to mind it, though, which is nice, because their pollination of the plant gives us lavender-scented honey.

If you look at "aromatherapy" products today, you will find lavender inevitably classified as calming. This traditional association of lavender with rest perhaps inspired medieval ladies to sew lavender-filled pillows. You can still find lavender pillows today, sold with the intention of initiating pleasant sleep. These lavender "dream pillows" have superseded the now amusingly obsolete medieval "swooning pillows," which made the presumably recurrent landings of fainting women more luxurious.

Patches of lavender, with its purple or white flowers, make soothing silvery green clumps of foliage about your garden, and you can enjoy dried lavender inside your house, too. It may have originally entered homes as a purifying agent. The American Botanical Council published the curious statement that lavender was "used as a bactericide to disinfect hospitals and sick rooms in ancient Persia, Greece, and Rome," which makes you wonder how ancient people knew about the existence of bacteria. Nonetheless, lavender oil is mildly antiseptic, as are many other plant oils.

Along with its pleasant smell and appearance, lavender is edible. New gourmet food sensations such as lavender ice cream and lavender chocolate are enjoying increasing popularity and are easy to create by adding a couple drops of lavender oil to the ingredients. Since it does not smell or taste very minty, it may surprise you to learn that lavender is a mint and is in the mint family (*Labiaceae*). Like other mints, it's traditionally consumed as a treatment for digestive disturbances and gas. The soothing action of lavender oil on nerves is its best-documented effect, which may explain its legendary power to assist sleep and quell digestive upsets.

How Scientists Think Lavender Works

Involuntary muscles treated with lavender relax, perhaps because lavender increases cyclic adenosine monophosphate inside them. The next time you rub lavender oil on your body, consider that the odiferous molecules in lavender can cross through your skin, entering your blood to have a relaxing effect on your involuntary muscles. One British team isolated small intestines from guinea pigs, and treated them with lavender oil and various agents designed to either block or activate particular nervous reflexes. They found that lavender increases the concentration of a common cell-signaling molecule inside gut cells, called *cyclic adenosine monophosphate,* or *cAMP,* perhaps by directly enhancing its synthesis.[1]

This is one of your body's most important signaling molecules, and it has different and even opposing effects on different tissues. Yet like lavender, some medications also increase cAMP in involuntary muscles, which relaxes most involuntary muscles—the muscles that you don't have conscious control over. In your respiratory tract, this relaxation opens up airways. In your gut, it calms cramping spasms. In your blood vessels, the vessels relax, causing them to widen, which lowers your blood pressure.

These researchers reported that lavender oil calms voluntary muscles, too. Italian researchers may have uncovered another mechanism for lavender's muscle-relaxing power in mice. *Linalool,* a small molecule responsible for one of the primary fragrance "notes" in lavender oil, acts at the neuromuscular junction, which, as the name implies, is a place where a nerve cell meets a muscle. Specifically, the researchers found that linalool prevented nerve cells from releasing the neurotransmitter acetylcholine, which would otherwise contract the muscle.[2]

The linalool in lavender blocks glutamate's nerve cell-stimulating action. More recently, another research group linked linalool's sedating action to its effect on the brain's glutamate receptors by competitively blocking them.[3] Glutamate is an excitatory neurotransmitter and a necessary amino acid that we can synthesize or eat.

What's In It

THE PRIMARY constituents of lavender oil are the monoterpene linalool, also known as *linalyl alcohol* (20–38 percent) and its ester, *linalyl acetate* (25–55 percent), which may serve as an oil-soluble, time-release form of linalool, since the body's enzymes probably metabolize it to linalool. Other terpenes in the oil are cis- and trans-ocimene, 1-terpinen-4-ol, 1,8-cineole (also known as *eucalyptol,* and found in eucalyptus oil), alpha-terpineol, camphor, and lemony-smelling limonene. Like other mints, it has a decent amount of tannins (5–10 percent), too.

Glutamate can't get into your brain very well after you eat it (i.e., it can't cross the blood-brain barrier.) This is good, because an inordinate amount of glutamate in your brain excites nerve cells to the extent that they party themselves into oblivion, so to speak, and die. Unlike glutamate, lavender's fragrant molecules are not water soluble, and thus can penetrate your blood-brain barrier after you inhale them. So the aromatherapists are really on to something with their insistence that you can use fragrances to temporarily alter your brain biochemistry. In cell culture, linalool prevented glutamate from bonding to rodent brain receptors, protecting nerve cells from having these perilous little festivals. Besides protecting your brain from its own supply of glutamate, this also implies that lavender smell becalms your brain by blocking the excitatory action of glutamate.

Do You Have a Taste for Glutamate?

GLUTAMATE IS present in all foods, but is most concentrated in foods like tomatoes, mushrooms, cheese, soy sauce, Worcester sauce, and seaweed, as well as the so-called flavor-enhancer food additive monosodium glutamate (MSG). Many people relish the savory, meaty taste of glutamate. In fact, scientists have created a special name for glutamate's flavor, called *umami*. The four traditional taste bud sensations have expanded past the original quartet of sweet, salty, sour, and bitter. We now know that humans also have glutamate-sensing taste buds on our tongue, which provide the sensation of umami.

Since glutamate can't cross into our brain's circulation after we eat it, reports of people responding with a wide variety of different negative symptoms to MSG after they are aware of having eaten some are considered questionable. MSG immediately releases its attached sodium to become glutamate in water, and this also happens right after you eat it. So there really isn't any difference between eating natural glutamate and MSG, other than the load of extra sodium consumed along with MSG. This extra sodium is more likely to affect you than glutamate. Negative responses to MSG were once termed "Chinese Restaurant Syndrome," since Chinese restaurants once liberally sprinkled it on their entrees, but now most advertise they are "MSG-free" because of negative publicity surrounding its use. (Some scientists have joked the term be made more cosmopolitan in the form of "Italian Restaurant Syndrome," since Italian food naturally contains several foods that are naturally high in glutamate.) Although in rare instances certain people may be more sensitive to MSG, the effect, if there is one, is not understood, because the daily consumption of natural glutamate from food far outweighs the amount contributed to by additive MSG in the typical diet.

Lavender's linalool also enhances the action of a brain-calming neurotransmitter. A small handful of cell studies show that linalool better enables gamma-amino butyric acid, commonly known as *GABA*, to work. GABA's binding to nerve cells in the brain temporarily puts them in them a state where they are slow to respond to stimuli. Linalool appears to act indirectly, enhancing the binding of GABA to its receptors. Enhanced GABA binding produces a calmer brain.

GOOD EFFECTS . . .
AND NOT SO GOOD

Lavender is generally safe for external use. Lavender-induced dermatitis is rare but has been reported. Like tea tree oil, which contains some of the same terpenes (oily, fragrant molecules) in different concentrations, lavender oil may generally destabilize cell membranes, causing skin irritation.[4] The mild antiseptic action of lavender oil may result from a moderately toxic action of its terpenes on cells similar to that of tea tree oil. One study suggests that lavender oil might increase the skin's absorption of other drugs,[5] so you may wish to avoid applying it with skin-soluble medications.

Smelling and eating lavender in moderate amounts is reportedly safe. There is a dearth of studies for lavender's internal use, but lavender is at least not associated with deleterious effects when taken in recommended doses. The German Commission E health authority seems comfortable recommending its internal use without much apprehension, for "restlessness or insomnia and nervous stomach irritations, Roehmheld's syndrome, meteorism, and nervous intestinal discomfort." Meteorism, by the way, has nothing to do with shooting stars but refers to abdominal distension due to gas.

Evidence of Action

Although the calming effect of lavender oil is well documented in animal and test tube studies, only a smattering of small trials have investigated its effects in people. Of course, odiferous herbs are impossible to give in "blinded" placebo-controlled situations, because subjects notice the herb's smell. With that in mind, lavender oil generally elicits a positive response from people, maybe just because it smells nice. Fifteen volunteers ranked various essential oils subjectively, and most associated lavender with "happiness."[6]

Pitted against rosemary oil, lavender oil won in something like an aromatherapy competition assessing forty subjects' mathematical skills.[7] Half of the volunteers were given three minutes to inhale lavender oil aroma, and the other half breathed in rosemary, which is generally considered stimulating in aromatherapy circles. The electroencephalograms of lavender-treated people showed enhanced beta wave activity, which is associated with active thinking, attention on the outside world, and solving problems. However, beta wave stimulation can occur just with all the excitement of having your brain waves measured. In contrast, though, the rosemary inhalers showed decreased beta activity, as well as decreased alpha wave action. Alpha waves are associated with relaxed awareness. Although the rosemary group reported feeling more alert and nimble with math questions, the lavender group actually solved the math problems more accurately.

Lavender was tested for its capacity to refresh exercisers. Twenty men exercised moderately for a couple of minutes and then were divided randomly into those who breathed lavender and those who did not.

Commonly Reported Uses for Lavender*

Internally
fatigue, restlessness, nervousness, insomnia, indigestion, gas
forms available for internal use:
decoction, dried flowers, infusion, tincture, oil
commonly reported dosage:
Tea is made with 1 to 2 teaspoons (5 to 10 grams) of leaves steeped in 1 cup of boiling water for 15 minutes, and this may be drunk several times a day, particularly before bedtime. Some recommend one to four drops of lavender oil on a sugar cube, but greater amounts of the pure oil should not be ingested.

Externally
fatigue, restlessness, nervousness, insomnia, antiseptic
forms available for external use:
decoction, dried flowers, infusion, tincture, oil, soaps, cosmetic products of all kinds
commonly reported dosage:
Two to 4 drops are added to 2 to 3 cups of boiling water, and vapors are inhaled several times daily or as needed. Around 5 drops of lavender oil, or ¼ to ½ cup of dried lavender tied in a bundle or contained in cheesecloth, is added to a bath. For massage, 1 to 5 drops of lavender oil can be added to each tablespoon of massage oil.

*These uses and dosages are from historic use and are not necessarily tested nor recommended.

The lavender inhalers were said to "recover" slightly faster, as measured by dropping blood pressure, but the effect was not statistically significant.[8]

Lavender has also been assessed in some small trials for attenuating psychological disorders. There is conflicting evidence for lavender scent calming agitated psychiatric patients, with one study showing mild improvement[9] and another showing none.[10] though both trials suffer statistically from using an inadequate number of test subjects. Also, lavender was not as effective as the antidepressant imipramine in forty-five depressed patients, although people receiving both lavender and imipramine did significantly better in this preliminary study.[11]

Researchers who observed the soothing effect of a lavender oil massage on patients with advanced cancers noted that massage alone exerted the lion's share of the sedation observed. Forty-two patients were given either weekly lavender oil massages, massages with carrier oil without lavender, or no massage at all, for four weeks. All massaged patients slept better than the unrubbed ones, and the presence of lavender did not seem to make any difference.[12] There are a number of similar studies of lavender aromatherapy or lavender treatments failing to produce a statistically significant effect to improve mood, and a couple of studies also show it does not help relieve perineal discomfort following childbirth when added to mother's bathwater.[13] Nonetheless, most trials' participants report enjoying lavender's smell.

THE BOTTOM LINE

- Lavender is traditionally used for calming nerves, promoting sleep, soothing the digestive tract, and decreasing gas pains.
- Lavender relaxes certain involuntary muscles. It may do this by increasing cyclic adenosine monophosphate (cAMP) in involuntary muscles lining the digestive tract and blood vessels, thus soothing digestion and decreasing blood pressure.
- Lavender might quell voluntary muscle action by inhibiting the release of acetylcholine at the neuromuscular junction.
- Lavender may calm your brain by blocking the excitatory action of glutamate and by enhancing the calming action of gamma-amino butyric acid (GABA).
- Lavender seems generally safe for internal and external use, when used moderately.

LEMON BALM
Melissa officinalis

History and Folklore

Lemon balm is a plant in the mint family (*Labiatae*), with a strikingly refreshing, lemony, and slightly minty fragrance. It is often alternately called *melissa,* or just *balm,* and is sometimes confused with another mint family plant, bee balm (*Monarda didyma*), because lemon balm is so good at attracting bees. Both have the classic mint family's opposing leaves on a square stem, but bee balm has showy red flowers and lemon balm bears tiny white ones.

Native to the Mediterranean and western Asia, lemon balm was revered by the ancients. The Greek Dioscorides and Pliny recommended it enthusiastically for poisonings, mad dog bites, and wounds, and the eleventh-century Arabian physician Avicenna said it made the heart merry. It was often referred to for aiding menstrual problems, perhaps because of its association with women and the Greek goddess Diana.

Carmelite water, first made by seventeenth-century nuns, featured lemon balm as the prime ingredient, but over time the less expensive and harsher smelling citronella oil was substituted for it. Maud Grieve's 1900s *A Modern Herbal* indicates lemon balm's use for indigestion and fever, which are typical uses for mint family plants. *A Modern Herbal* and other historical references also often suggest it to treat "wens" (warts), blemishes, and sores, and we are now learning it may prove useful in treating cold sores.

Also intriguing are many historical admonitions to use lemon balm for failing memory.

There are several texts mentioning its use for the brain. Nicholas Culpeper writes, "It is very good to aid digestion and open obstructions of the brain," while the seventeenth-century diary of John Evelyn says, "Balm is sovereign for the brain, strengthening the memory and powerfully chasing away melancholy." The 1696 *London Dispensary* additionally instructs, "Essence of Balm, given in Canary wine, every morning will renew youth, strengthen the brain, relieve languishing nature and prevent baldness." Its use for baldness hasn't panned out, but alcoholic extracts of lemon balm may help those with Alzheimer's disease.

How Scientists Think Lemon Balm Works

Something in lemon balm sticks to your brain's acetylcholine receptors, and it might help those with Alzheimer's. Scientists screened several alcoholic extracts of various herbs, and found some, like lemon balm, stuck to acetylcholine receptors better than others.[1] (The molecules in it that are doing the sticking aren't known yet.) There are two forms of acetylcholine receptor, actually, the nicotinic and muscarinic receptors, and both are vital in nerve cell signaling. Alzheimer's patients' brains lose the nicotinic version over time. Their symptoms are linked to losing the action of acetylcholine at those sites. Providing Alzheimer's patients with drugs that boost acetylcholine activity doesn't cure them, but it does help slow their memory loss.

The above researchers screened several different herbal extracts to find which of them best adhered to nicotinic receptors. Cooking sage (*Salvia officinalis*) didn't bind either type of receptor. Sage (see page 266) was tested because it has clinically helped people with Alzheimer's, but in a different way; it seems to prevent acetylcholine from breaking down. Conversely, lemon balm doesn't seem to act like sage—it doesn't prevent acetylcholine from breaking down. Other species of sage, however, showed binding to one or the other type of receptor, depending on the species tested. Wormwood (*Artemisia absinthium*), a plant unrelated to sage or lavender but known to affect the brain, had several components that bound strongly to both types of receptor, but its toxic thujone content precludes its use.

It's noteworthy that lemon balm bound nicotinic receptors in particular, because drug companies are now testing such agents. They reveal a new mechanism by which Alzheimer's drugs could work. Most prescription Alzheimer's drugs were thought to work by preventing acetylcholine's breakdown, or at least that's what scientists assumed. The problem with this original idea is that the ability of an Alzheimer's drug to prevent acetylcholine degradation isn't very well correlated to its clinical efficacy. In addition, some of these medications seem to keep working even after patients stop taking them. It has been found that some of these drugs actually bind the acetylcholine receptor, yet at the same time they don't block the receptor or prevent acetylcholine from acting on its receptor. Instead, these Alzheimer's drugs enhance the action of acetylcholine or acetylcholine-like molecules at the receptor after they stick to the receptor. Plus, they can stimulate the production of more nicotinic receptors, the very receptors that Alzheimer's patients lose.

Lemon balm is most likely not a cure for Alzheimer's, but it helps. Drugs that work in the same manner as lemon balm seems to do not cure the disease, they just slow it down. They do not prevent the underlying cause of Alzheimer's disease, which is not completely understood. Alzheimer's disease development is associated with excess brain inflammation, and it also involves the accumulation of a brain protein (beta-amyloid) that mucks up its gears, so to speak.

Aromatherapists may be on to something. When it comes to the relaxing properties of inhaled plant fragrances such as lemon balm, a theoretical mechanism has emerged. The fragrant oils from plants contain molecules called *terpenes,* which are rapidly absorbed through the lungs and thenceforth enter the brain. This is a noteworthy feat, since the brain is protected by the blood-brain barrier, which prevents most foreign and potentially dangerous chemicals from accessing it. But oil-soluble molecules like terpenes are better at crossing it, and studies show they do so after they are inhaled.

We don't know exactly what lemon balm's terpenes do in human brains, but in cell cultures, some of them, such as citronellal, eugenol,[2] and oxidized linalool,[3] enhance the activity of a nerve cell-slowing neurotransmitter called *GABA* (*gamma-aminobutyric acid*). These and other terpenes are ubiquitous in the plant kingdom, so this theoretical mechanism is not likely confined to lemon balm. If lemon balm's terpenes are responsible for the acetylcholine receptor activation shown in cell studies, another mechanism besides enhancing GABA's action for calming pops up that involves acetylcholine. Lemon balm apparently enables acetylcholine to work more effectively, and acetylcholine is the "rest and digest" neurotransmitter. Lemon balm, according to studies, tends to make you do just that—rest and digest.

Internally, lemon balm probably relaxes gut muscles that are involved in digestion. It's not surprising, since most plants in the mint family relax gut muscles. This gut-soothing effect is usually attributed to the plant's terpenes, which are present in the fragrant oils of lemon balm and other mint plants. Both the oil and its main component, citral, were shown to relax isolated muscle preparations to the same extent, even when provoked by chemicals that normally contract them.[4] At least in peppermint, this same effect works when a related terpene, menthol, prevents calcium from rushing in to the muscle cells, which would otherwise make them twitchy.

Something in lemon balm might work against viruses. Scientists have observed that aqueous lemon balm extracts work against both types of herpes (cold sores and genital herpes). Its inclusion in some popular cold sore commercial preparations plus its success in a clinical trial for treating cold sores have encouraged some scientists to seek out a mechanism. Consistently, an assortment of water-soluble polyphenolic acids, such as caffeic acid and rosmarinic acid, have been noted as having antiviral activity in cell assays. When the lemon balm plant is stressed, the molecules oxidize and stick to each other, forming a sort of defensive tannin that is unique to plants in the mint family. Of course, different lemon balm plants have varying amounts of this putative active ingredient, depending on its growing conditions. The mechanism for its antiviral action isn't known, but publications repeatedly state that it works early in the stage of viral replication.

One way the tannin could work is by preventing viral attachment to cells. The first thing a virus has to do to infect a cell is stick to it, before it injects its genetic material into it. Since tannins cross-link proteins, the tannins could alter and protect the surface of the cell by coating it, or it could coat viruses, which are covered with a protein shell (although some viruses, like herpes viruses, are further covered with a protective fatty envelope, which would subvert the latter mechanism).

What's In It

THE VOLATILE oil is mainly (50–75 percent) geranial and neral; two cis-trans isomers which are collectively called *citral*. The oil also contains citronellal. The oil may includes-maller amounts of linalool, geraniol, geranyl acetate, methyl citronellate, trans-beta-ocimene, 1-octen-3-ol, beta-caryophyllene, and eugenol. Glycosides of these are also present. Like another putatively cholinergic herb, sage, it contains rosmarinic acid (up to 5 percent), as well as caffeic and ursolic acid. Its flavonoids include cynaroside, cosmosiin, rhamnocitrin, luteolin, apigenin, and iso-quercitrin, and their glycosides.

Other theorized actions for lemon balm's caffeic acid oxidation products involve the tannin getting inside the infected cell, which is more difficult—water-soluble molecules have trouble getting into cells without crossing though a specialized port that recognizes and admits them. Nonetheless, in test tubes these tannins from lemon balm inhibit a factor required for protein synthesis (elongation factor eEF-2, which is something a virus needs in order to make more copies of itself), so this could stop a virus from replicating. Lemon balm tannin also inhibits an inflammatory enzyme called *lipoxygenase* in test tubes, and if it does the same thing in human cells, it could provide an additional anti-inflammatory benefit.

Lemon balm could affect your thyroid gland, at least in theory. The thyroid gland helps control metabolic rate—it is the body's metabolic gas pedal. Messing with it sometimes slows you down, and you feel tired and depressed and gain weight. Sometimes antagonizing your thyroid has the opposite effect, though, and paradoxically it causes your metabolic rate to increase too much, resulting in trembling, heart palpitations, weight loss, hair loss, and ravenous hunger. Some people worry about herbs affecting the thyroid, and lemon balm is on the list. Tests show that some components in lemon balm and other plants (caffeic, rosmarinic, chlorogenic, and ellagic acids), as well as lemon balm extracts, stick to the cow's version of thyroid-stimulating hormone (TSH). This alters TSH's structure, preventing it from sticking to its receptors on human thyroid cells in cultures. Since TSH is needed to kick your thyroid into action, lemon balm could theoretically affect thyroid activity. However, people taking lemon balm aren't known to have affected thyroid function. The issue remains a theoretical unknown.

GOOD EFFECTS . . . AND NOT SO GOOD

Lemon balm has an excellent safety record. People have used lemon balm since ancient times. There are no historical records or modern case studies showing any obvious side effects from using it.

Lemon balm may affect your mood. Clinical tests imply it has soothing power. However, don't use it prior to taking timed tests. It also seems to decrease skills requiring rapid functioning.

Lemon balm might work to speed healing of cold sores. Hypothetically, the active ingredient is in the water-soluble extract. Some herbalists recommend making a tea of the herb, cooling it down, and using a cotton ball to apply it to sores.

It's too soon to know how well lemon balm will help Alzheimer's patients. First of all, regardless of the potential treatments for Alzheimer's disease, anyone with the disease should be under a doctor's continuing supervision. Although lemon balm looks promising, more studies need to be done. Also, remember that it won't be a cure for Alzheimer's, because drugs that show the same action don't cure it either, but it could slow the disease's progression. Simply put, it might not be effective for Alzheimer's. Some lemon balm extracts have no nicotinic receptor binding activity, because the concentrations of constituents in one lemon balm plant from the other are highly variable.

Don't use lemon balm every day if you have thyroid disorder. There aren't any reports, so far, of lemon balm adversely affecting a person's thyroid function. Yet test tube studies show it could, in theory. Some people with a type of thyroid disorder called Graves' disease have popularly tried lemon balm, but based on its theoretical actions, this could backfire and make someone with Graves' disease worse. If you do have any sort of thyroid disorder, including Graves' disease, you probably don't want to dose yourself with it regularly. The occasional mild exposure to it probably won't hurt you, though.

EVIDENCE OF ACTION

There are not many human studies employing lemon balm on its own, not mixed with other herbs. The studies that do assess the effects of lemon balm on humans investigate its mood and cognitive effects, its use in Alzheimer's disease, and its ability to treat herpes. Lemon balm appears more or less active in all three cases. Although all the studies below have placeboes, keep in mind that lemon balm is pretty fragrant, so unless the herb was well encased in capsules, it's likely some of the active group members knew they were getting something, especially in the topical preparations. Still, a study with a placebo group is better than a study without one.

According to three studies at the University of Northumbria,[5, 6, 7] lemon balm might make you calmer, but, as you might expect, correspondingly less alert. The authors of these studies first searched for some effect of lemon balm on nerve cell receptors in test tubes. After testing their lemon balm extract to see how well its components stuck to nicotinic and muscarinic acetylcholine receptors, they found that the affinity of the extract for the receptors was low compared to previous studies. Nevertheless, they tested various doses of this extract or placebo on twenty healthy volunteers and assessed them in a double-blinded manner. Each took one of the doses or a placebo after seven-day intervals, in different orders, so their dosing sequence would not affect the results of cognitive and mood tests they were given following the treatment. Those who took lemon balm had improved calmness, but were significantly less alert after taking the highest dose of the herb (900 mg).

Before repeating another similar study, the researchers decided to screen a number of lemon balm extracts again for an action similar to the fundamental nerve cell-signaling molecule acetylcholine, which was a reasonable thing to do, since concentrations

Commonly Reported Uses for Lemon Balm*

Internally

indigestion, agitation, fever, headache, depression, poor memory, Graves' disease, menstrual cramps

forms available for internal use:

drops, extracts, oil, fresh and dried leaf, tea, tincture

commonly reported dosage:

In aromatherapy the smell of the oil or extracts is inhaled. Dried leaves are crushed and 1 to 3 teaspoons are added to a cup of water to make a lemon balm tea.

Externally

cold sores, herpes, warts, calming lotion

forms available for external use:

drops, extracts, oil mixed in lotion, some commercial lip balms

commonly reported dosage:

For cold sores the cooled tea is applied with a cotton ball.

*These uses and dosages are from historic use and are not necessarily tested nor recommended.

of the components in lemon balm are quite variable from plant to plant and season to season. While another plant in the mint family, sage, appears to enhance acetylcholine by inhibiting the enzyme (acetylcholinesterase) that breaks it down, they found no similar acetylcholinesterase-inhibiting activity in lemon balm. However, the researchers did find a different lemon balm extract from another sample of different lemon balm plants with better binding to acetylcholine receptors than before and used it in another study with a similar setup. Again twenty healthy volunteers were used, and this time researchers found the higher the dose of extract ingested, the better the volunteers tested on calmness and recall. But it also slowed the volunteers down. The more lemon balm extract they took, the worse they did on timed memory tasks and rapid processing of visual stimuli.

The same researchers finally repeated yet one more similarly designed study with eighteen healthy volunteers, and further determined the highest dose of lemon balm extract tested (600 mg) improved mood and significantly improved volunteers' opinion of their level of calmness. Also, it significantly decreased volunteers' opinions of their degree of alertness.

A similar effect was observed using lemon balm topically.[8] This time, it was used on patients with severe dementia, assessing their agitation level and quality of life. Either a sunflower oil placebo or lemon balm extract was mixed with a base lotion and applied by caregivers to the arms and faces of seventy-one patients two times a day for four weeks. In a double-blinded manner they were tested on their degree of agitation and rated for quality of life by quantifying factors such as time spent social-izing and working on constructive projects. Both groups improved, as you might expect, because receiving human touch with or without active ingredients comforts most people. Yet those who received the lemon balm treatment showed significantly better quality of life than those who didn't, and reductions in their agitation were statistically highly significant when compared to the placebo group.

On the Alzheimer's disease front, lemon balm extracts had first popped up as a winner in a few test tube screenings of various extracts for activity at the acetylcholine receptor. Since this receptor is key to several treatments for Alzheimer's, Iranian scientists investigated further by providing large daily doses (60 drops) of lemon balm alcoholic extract to a random portion of forty-two patients with mild to moderate Alzheimer's disease.[9] The rest got placebos. At the end of the four-month study, those who took the lemon balm had significantly better cognitive function and significantly less agitation than those who took the placebo. Shahin Akhondzadeh, the principal investigator, reports that the effects were comparable to those exerted by prescription Alzheimer's drugs.

THE BOTTOM LINE

- An unidentified ingredient in some lemon balm extracts binds to nicotinic acetylcholine receptors. This may help reduce the speed of memory loss in patients with Alzheimer's disease. It is not likely to hold a cure for Alzheimer's, however.
- Lemon balm is likely calming, but hampers alertness and skills requiring rapid thinking. When it is inhaled, terpenes may enter the brain and sedate nerve cell impulses, perhaps through the inhibitory neurotransmitter GABA.
- Lemon balm aqueous extracts may work therapeutically on herpes cold sores by an unknown mechanism.
- Lemon balm is relatively safe. Because it affects TSH (thyroid-stimulating hormone) in test tube studies, it may theoretically adversely affect people with thyroid problems, but evidence for this has not yet surfaced.

Cell studies have suggested that lemon balm prevents herpes virus replication as well. Because of this, a randomized, double-blind clinical trial enlisted sixty-six people with recurrent cold sores (herpes simplex labialis) to use either placebo cream or a lemon balm—containing cream on their mouth four times daily for five days.[10] Compared to those who used the placebo, those who used the lemon balm had significantly fewer cold sores by the second day of treatment.

LICORICE
Glycyrrhiza glabra

HISTORY AND FOLKLORE

The first thing you may think of when considering licorice—or "liquorice," if you are in Europe—is that it is candy, but historically it is better known as an herb. The candy is traditionally prepared from the sweet-tasting root of the licorice plant, a member of the bean family (*Fabaceae* or *Leguminosae*). It is native to the Mideast and has been recommended by ancient healers, such as the Greek Dioscorides, who used it as a wound healer. Perhaps signifying its value, it was found at Tutankhamen's burial site. Konrad von Megenberg, one of the most prolific German writers of the fourteenth century, who wrote *Das Buch der Natur* (The Book of Nature), called licorice "bear's droppings," which remains a good name if you want to keep your friends away from your candy. Napoleon himself was reportedly addicted to licorice, which theoretically could have hampered his sex life (see below).

Commercial licorice is mainly harvested from the Mediterranean, Spain, Asia, and the former USSR. Millions of pounds are imported to the United States, not so much for candy, as you might think, but 90 percent is used in flavoring cigarettes and other tobacco products. Real licorice is far more popular in Europe. Licorice candy in the United States often has no licorice at all but is flavored with anise oil. However, real licorice candy is now being sold more often in the United States, too.

Licorice has traditionally been used for ages around the world, for congestion, sore throats and cough, digestive problems, ulcers, arthritis, and constipation. Some of these uses appear valid, but the herb contains a potent drug that produces both benefits and dangerous side effects. As such, licorice should be used with care.

HOW SCIENTISTS THINK LICORICE WORKS

Licorice temporarily shuts down some members of a family of enzymes called short-chain dehydrogenase reductases (SDRs). This does both good and bad things to you. SDR enzymes are a large family of enzymes that accomplish a wide variety of chemical transformations in the body. Some SDR enzymes that licorice hampers break down stomach-protecting molecules, and other SDR enzymes that licorice inhibits help keep blood pressure low by balancing sodium and potassium concentrations. SDR enzyme inhibition by licorice can thus protect your stomach but raise your blood pressure.

This disabling of SDRs occurs by glycyrrhizinic acid or its salt, glycyrrhizin, the molecules that give licorice root its mild sweetness. Their structures somewhat resemble human steroids, yet unlike steroids they are also attached to sugar molecules. Both licorice molecules have the ability to impersonate your own steroids, and this enables them to "competitively" inhibit your SDR enzymes, meaning that an SDR enzyme temporarily docks with these imposters instead of its customary targets, which prevents the enzyme from performing its usual task.

After you eat licorice, glycyrrhizinic acid or glycyrrhizin reaches your gut, and the bond between the steroid part and the sugars is cleaved, yielding just the sugar-free and unsweet steroid mimic, glycyrrhetinic acid. If the names of these licorice molecules all look like Welsh to you at this point, you are not alone. The thing to remember is that they are all biologically active. The sugar-free metabolite *also* inhibits short chain reductases, and it can get absorbed into your bloodstream. That's where the trouble starts. Before we go there, let's discuss the nice thing licorice does for your gut.

What's In It

LICORICE'S ACTIVE ingredient, which also makes it taste sweet, is due to about 5 to 9 percent glycyrrhizin, the acid salt of a saponin glycoside. The free, acidic version of this molecule is also active, and is called *glycyrrhizic acid.* Both are bound to two glucuronic acid sugar molecules. Licorice also possesses 1 percent flavonoids, primarily liquiritin and liquiritigenin, and related chalcones isoliquiritin, isoliquiritigenin. Isoflavonoids include formononetin, glabren, glabridin, and glabrol. Hydroxycoumarins include herniarin and umbelliferone, and sterols such as beta-sitosterol and stigmasterol. The root contains trace anethole, estagole (also present in anise and fennel oils), and eugenol (also found in cloves).

By raising your supply of gut-protecting prostaglandins, licorice increases mucous and decreases acid. You have many sorts of different prostaglandins, each of which has varied and even opposing effects, yet they have acquired negative connotations in popular health articles, because many prostaglandins promote damaging inflammation. However, not all of your prostaglandins are bad. Some of your *gut* prostaglandins decrease acid secretion and increase the production of protective mucous, which coats your stomach, shielding it from acid and protein-degrading enzymes. Stomach mucous creates a slimy barrier that literally prevents acid and digestive enzymes from digesting the stomach lining itself, which would cause sores on the lining of the stomach that are otherwise known as ulcers. Aspirin, in fact, blocks the synthesis of these gut-protecting prostaglandins, initiating the classic gastric distress associated with aspirin, sometimes causing ulcers. Licorice, on the other hand, inhibits the SDR enzymes that break these gut-protecting prostaglandins down. This allows the prostaglandins to hang around for a longer period of time, consequently enhancing the safeguarding of your stomach lining.

What helps your stomach may help your throat, too. The mucous that licorice increases protects not only your digestive tract, but may help with coughs and sore throats, too; however, that idea is more controversial. Some think it is simply the pleasant, sweet taste that encourages salivation and swallowing, which suppresses a cough reflex.

Licorice may induce uterine contractions. Licorice does not increase *all* prostaglandins. Licorice specifically hampers the SDR enzyme 15-hydroxyprostaglandin dehydrogenase. This enzyme breaks down prostaglandin F2-alpha and prostaglandin E2. Therefore, licorice raises the concentrations of these two prostaglandins by slowing their metabolic conversion to less active forms. Both prostaglandins are used medically to induce either labor or abortion, because they contract the uterus. Increasing these prostaglandins is worrisome for women who are prone to painful uterine contractions, better known as menstrual cramps, and even more troublesome for pregnant women. Increasing these specific prostaglandins by using licorice could induce premature labor; thus most reputable sources advise you should not take licorice if you are pregnant. Don't panic if you are pregnant and have innocently eaten one licorice candy. To my knowledge, cases of single doses of licorice inducing acute abortion have not been documented, but *heavy* use of licorice (500 mg per week) has been positively linked to premature delivery.[1]

Eating an inordinate amount of licorice causes a potentially dangerous syndrome called *apparent mineralocorticoid excess.* It's a common story: A person with high blood pressure innocently enjoys a lavish amount of licorice on a regular basis and winds up in the emergency room. It may surprise you to know that this scenario is quite familiar to medical professionals. In repeated tests of people taking large doses of licorice, *all* volunteers begin to show signs of apparent mineralocorticoid excess after twenty-four hours, beginning with potassium loss, sodium retention, and water retention, which is then followed by gradually climbing blood pressure. Thankfully, it takes a lot of licorice to cause these side effects, and these symptoms go away after licorice is discontinued. Prolonged consumption (weeks or months) of licorice exceeding a products' suggested serving size leads to more severe symptoms, however, such as lethargy, paralysis, and heart failure.

It's called "apparent mineralocorticoid excess," because a specific hormone known as a mineralocorticoid *appears* **to be overactive.** The most striking effects of licorice overdose—potassium loss, sodium retention, and high blood pressure—are all classically associated with a hormone called *aldosterone.* Aldosterone is in the category of hormones known as a *mineralocorticoid,* because it affects mineral balance, specifically potassium and sodium, and because it is produced by the outer core of the adrenal glands, the adrenal *cort*ex. It appears as though licorice increases aldosterone, based on the symptoms it causes; however, in people who overdose on licorice, aldosterone remains low and may even be suppressed. Since aldosterone *appears* to be in excess, the term *apparent* mineralocorticoid excess is used for the syndrome that it causes. Here is what licorice *really* does.

It isn't aldosterone that licorice increases, but cortisol, which looks like aldosterone to your kidneys. At first scientists postulated that licorice simply mimicked the hormone aldosterone, which certainly seemed reasonable, because aldosterone is a steroid, and licorice contains steroid mimics. You can still find many old herb books that say that licorice binds to aldosterone's receptor and acts like aldosterone. That theory, however reasonable, proved incorrect. Researchers in the late 1980s were puzzled by this, until a link was made with people who had apparently identical symptoms to licorice toxicity but instead possessed a rare genetic disease rendering them with a defective version of the enzyme 11-beta-dehydroxysteroid reductase type 2 (11-beta HSD2). Since this enzyme is in the family of SDR enzymes that licorice inhibits, researchers made the connection that licorice inhibits this enzyme. This theory has withstood testing in test tubes, isolated cell cultures, animals, and humans, and is now the currently accepted mechanism for licorice causing apparent mineralocorticoid excess.

In the kidney this 11-beta HSD2 normally inactivates cortisol, another steroid hormone. Cortisol (called *hydrocortisone* when used therapeutically) has a wide range of different actions, such as quelling inflammation and altering blood sugar levels. Normally cortisol's action on the kidney is blocked, however, because an SDR enzyme in the kidney turns cortisol into a less active form called *cortisone.* If left active, cortisol works on the kidney just like aldosterone, binding to aldosterone's receptor and triggering the same effects as aldosterone: potassium wasting through the urine, sodium retention, water retention, and hypertension. The problem with cortisol acting just like aldosterone in your kidney is that cortisol is several times more concentrated than aldosterone in your plasma, and if cortisol remains unchecked at your kidney, it will appear as though your kidney is flooded with aldosterone when it is actually cortisol doing all of this. Normally, the 11-beta HSD2 enzyme inactivates cortisol in the kidney, preventing it from impersonating a flood of aldosterone hormone. This explains why aldosterone appears out of control but remains low in both licorice overdose and 11-beta HSD2 deficiency; it is actually surplus cortisol acting like aldosterone.

In normal circumstances in the kidney, the SDR enzyme 11-beta HSD2 turns cortisol into the less active corti*sone,* which is not capable of binding to the aldosterone receptor and is thus not capable of acting like aldosterone. When licorice inactivates 11-beta HSD2, cortisol is no longer deactivated in your kidney, and a flood of cortisol binds to your kidney's aldosterone receptor, mimicking aldosterone.

Remember, however, that licorice also can protect the stomach lining by preventing an SDR enzyme from breaking down gut-protecting prostaglandins. It's a shame that a potentially good ulcer medication has such serious side effects, which begin when licorice's molecules enter your blood stream. If some smart chemist out there wants to synthesize a nonabsorbable form of these licorice molecules, which remain in the gut, there might be a new ulcer medication on the market.

GOOD EFFECTS . . . AND NOT SO GOOD

Licorice overdose is a thoroughly documented and common occurrence. Licorice toxicity is more common in Europe, where more licorice is consumed, and the licorice that is eaten there is *real* licorice. In the United States licorice often has the syndrome-causing ingredient, glycyrrhizin, removed, and it is called *deglycyrrhizinized* licorice. It is flavored with similar-tasting anise oil, which does not have this problem. In fact, many U.S. "licorice" products contain *no* licorice, mimicking its taste with anise oil. Demand for real licorice in the United States is growing, however, so check the label to be sure.

If you don't have a condition that precludes eating licorice, you can use it to treat ulcers, gastrointestinal upset, cough, and sore throats. Just use it cautiously. There is reasonable evidence that real licorice helps in treating these conditions. Multiple serving sizes of licorice per day for a period on the order of a week or more are usually required for licorice overdose symptoms to show up in healthy people, and the occasional dose of licorice can certainly help people who have ulcers. Be sure you have actual licorice, since many so-called licorice products don't contain any, and make sure the licorice has not been deglycyrrhizinized. Don't take too much of the product, and don't take it for too long. Most pharmaceutical references suggest limiting your treatment to less than four to six weeks, and avoid taking more than 100 grams a day. If you feel any strange symptoms coming on, like weakness, dizziness, water retention, headache, or heart palpitations, stop using it.

Commonly Reported Uses for Licorice*

Internally
   used for gastrointestinal ulcers, stomach upset, sore throat, cough, congestion, expectorant, sweetener, flavoring
   forms available for internal use:
   dried whole, chopped, or powdered root, capsule, extract, infusion, tea, powdered extract, tincture, candies, gum, lozenges, syrup, liqueurs
   commonly reported dosage:
   A typical dose of licorice is 1 to 4 grams of powdered root, or up to three cups of licorice tea, daily, taken for no longer than four weeks.

*These uses and dosages are from historic use and are not necessarily tested nor recommended.

Certain people should avoid licorice. Do not take licorice if you have high blood pressure, heart disease, low potassium (hypokalemia), kidney disease, or are pregnant. Certain hormonal disorders may be exacerbated by licorice. This includes adrenal disease, Cushing's disease, primary hyperaldosteronism (Conn's disease), secondary hyperaldosteronism, and pseudohyperaldosteronism. Since licorice may have estrogenic action, those with estrogen-sensitive conditions (breast, uterine, and ovarian cancers, endometriosis, and uterine

fibroids) may find it helpful to avoid excess licorice, too.

Licorice may not be the most romantic treat for your male partner. If you are male, recent evidence suggests licorice could have a downside for your love life. In some small studies it decreased testosterone levels of both male and female volunteers, and because of this it was suggested as a possible culprit in male sexual dysfunction.

You may be surprised at how many products contain licorice. If you take the time to read labels, you will see that many herbal teas, for example, contain licorice as a sweetening agent, even though they are not labeled "licorice" tea. One case report describes a man who drank 100 grams of licorice in an herbal tea daily for three years, and he had to be hospitalized for extremely low potassium and muscle weakness, which developed into paralysis. His symptoms retreated slowly, even after his licorice was discontinued.[2]

The literature is replete with similar cases. For example, one woman habitually chewed licorice-flavored gum and developed serious symptoms;[3] another did so after she ate five licorice sticks a day for a month.[4] Licorice is of course found in licorice candy, but it is also present in some candies that don't have "licorice" in the name. Some licorice candies sport festive titles like "Turkish Pepper" or "Fisherman's Friend," and though they contain licorice, their names do not make that obvious. Licorice is also added to many tobacco and smoking products. There is a case report of a man who chewed roughly ten bags of chewing tobacco a day and swallowed the juice. The resulting paralyzing weakness that he suffered was attributed to the licorice content of the tobacco.[5] He recovered when his chew was taken away from him. Many other tobacco products contain licorice as flavoring agent, but it is unlikely that licorice-laced tobacco will affect someone who smokes it. When burned, physiologically active licorice molecules most likely degrade. (What tobacco molecules transform into after they are burned is more of a concern for cancer doctors.) Licorice is also added to certain cough drops, lozenges, and syrups for flavoring.

An occasional small dose of licorice won't kill you, but you should limit it, especially if you have any of the conditions listed above. Overdosing on licorice takes some effort, as evidenced by the existing case reports, and the occasional bit of licorice won't kill you. However, if you have condition that could be worsened by licorice, there is no sense in aggravating it either; you should reasonably limit your licorice consumption to amounts far less than what most people would consume. Better yet, treat yourself with deglycyrrhizinized licorice, which has had most of its active ingredient removed.

EVIDENCE OF ACTION

The evidence for licorice's producing untoward and even dangerous side effects—high blood pressure and potassium loss—are far more thoroughly documented than its therapeutic actions. Nonetheless, it may promote the healing of ulcers, although because of its side effects, it should only be taken for limited time periods. Licorice was able to prevent ulcer caused by aspirin in rats,[6] and licorice increases stomach-protective mucous formation and decreases stomach acid production. Both of these actions shield the stomach from damaging acid, allowing old ulcers to heal and preventing new ulcers from forming.

Carbenoxalone, a semisynthetic derivative of glycyrrhetic acid that releases licorice's natural glycyrrhetic acid when consumed orally, has been shown to accelerate the healing of ulcers, too.[7] Unfortunately, people taking carbenoxalone also experience worrisome blood pressure elevation and potassium loss; it causes the same problems as licorice. It is sold in the United Kingdom, but is not available in the United States.

Deglycyrrhizinized licorice has also been tested as an ulcer aid. This is licorice that has had most of its offending, side effect–causing glycyrrhizin removed (sold commercially as "Caved-S"). Unfortunately, it is the glycyrrhizin and its aglycone metabolite that are responsible for the ulcer-protecting, beneficial effects. Indeed, animal studies show deglycyrrhizinized licorice had no effect on gastric prostaglandins, which are thought to mediate licorice's protective effects. Consequently, it is not a surprise that *most* deglycyrrhizinized licorice trials for ulcer have been unimpressive,[8, 9] although a few actually boast modest benefits.[10, 11] This may be due to the trace glycyrrhizin (about 3 percent remains) in the treatment; or perhaps unknown factors are at work. At any rate, deglycyrrhizinized licorice is certainly safer than licorice, but probably doesn't help ulcer sufferers either.

Licorice has been tested for other possible benefits on a limited scale. There is preliminary evidence that licorice reduces testosterone in both men[12] and women,[13] which is usually a detriment for the men, but could theoretically help certain women, such as those with polycystic ovarian syndrome. Licorice might reduce body fat, but small trials testing licorice's ability to help you lose fat are conflicting, possibly because of the weight gain that it causes through water retention.[14] Also, some preliminary studies show that licorice has action against hepatitis B and C,[15, 16] but the studies are too small to draw conclusions as of yet. Additionally, a skin preparation using licorice was able to reduce redness and itching in dermatitis.[17] More evidence is needed to evaluate licorice for these uses.

THE BOTTOM LINE

- Licorice raises blood pressure, causing you to retain sodium and lose potassium, by inactivating an enzyme that normally keeps cortisol from acting on your kidneys. In extreme cases these side effects can be dangerous and have even been fatal.
- Licorice may help those with ulcers or stomach upset, but should not be taken for extended periods of time. Licorice protects your gut by inactivating an enzyme that normally inactivates mucous-producing and acid-decreasing prostaglandins in your gut.
- Deglycyrrhizinized licorice is safer than licorice, although it may be less effective in healing ulcers.
- Don't use licorice if you are pregnant. It may cause premature delivery.
- Several medical conditions are aggravated by taking licorice, such as hypertension, heart problems, and kidney disease, and estrogen-sensitive diseases, such as certain cancers, endometriosis and uterine fibroids, hyperaldosteronism and pseudohyperaldosteronism, low potassium, and male sexual dysfunction.

MARSHMALLOW
Althaea officinalis

History and Folklore

The marshmallow candy you know was once made from the root of a plant in the mallow family (*Malvaceae*). It typically grows, as you might expect, in marshes. An old-fashioned name for marshmallow plants was "cheeses," because their tiny seeds resemble cheese wheels. It has also been nicknamed *althea, sweet weed,* and *mortification root.* The latter, unappetizing label refers to marshmallow's reputed ability to heal gangrene.

This native of Europe and western Asia has made a home in the eastern United States, although there are many related "mallows" to be found throughout North America. Marshmallow plant has pink to white flowers and resembles a smaller version of another mallow, hollyhock. Living in the western United States, I am more familiar with its ubiquitous desert-dwelling relative, globe mallow, which has lovely orange flowers. You may be more familiar with other mallow family relations, like rose of Sharon, hibiscus, cotton, and the remarkably slimy okra. Marshmallow is slimy, too, and this is what makes it so special: "The mucilage or slimie juice of the roots, is mixed very effectively with all oils, ointments, and plasiters that slacken and mitigate paine. It cureth rifts of the fundament, it comforteth, defendeth, and preserveth dangerous greene wounds from any manner of accidents that may happen there, it helpeth digestion in them, and bring old ulcers to maturation" (*Gerard's Herbal,* 1636).

I recall my first experience with the "slimie juice." After purchasing powdered marsh-mallow root, I mixed it with water, eager to discover whether historic references to its mucilaginous properties held true. Indeed, the powder transformed into a cohesive slime, which was cool and soothing to the touch, though swallowing some was an exercise I felt better left to hearsay. My own inexpensive purchase was perhaps insufficiently cleaned, as it smelled like dirt. Cleaner preparations in teas, however, have a mild sweet flavor.

What's In It

THE SLIME, or more properly, *mucilage,* in marshmallow can be obtained from either the leaves or roots, which contain 5 to 10 percent polysaccharides, specifically galacturonorhamnans, arabinans, glucans, and arabinogalactans. Beyond the mucilage, there are also flavonoids; tannins; coumarins; caffeic, chlorogenic, ferulic, and syringic phenolic acids; and sterols.

Perhaps its sweetness encouraged its incorporation into candy. Ancient Egyptians could have been the first to invent marshmallow candy, since they united the slimy root with honey. The plant consecutively impressed ancient Greeks and Arabs. It then made its way into Indian Ayurvedic tradition, where it is still recommended to soothe inflamed, irritated tissues and wounds, both inside and out. Charlemagne ordered the plant's cultivation for use as a vegetable in his garden.

The self-described "gastrophysicist" Harold McGee's utterly engrossing tome *On Food and Cooking* describes how the French *pâte de guimauve* reestablished marshmallow root as a confection. The juice of the root was beaten into a foam with eggs and sugar to became a posh dessert. By the twentieth century the plant was replaced with gums or gelatin. Our modern marshmallow foodstuffs no longer have any hint of the plant.

How Scientists Think Marshmallow Works

Marshmallow's action is all in the slime. The slime, or more properly, *mucilage,* in marshmallow can be obtained from either the leaves or roots and is composed of polysaccharides. These are large chains of smaller sugar rings linked together. Sugars of all sizes recruit water with electrostatic attractions. The polysaccharide chains are too big to dissolve in water the way small sugars like table sugar do. Instead, the chains stick to one another, forming a network of fibers holding loosely attached water molecules. A loose molecular fabric filled with water forms the slimy mucilage. This is what makes the cohesive ball of slime-exuding gel when you mix marshmallow root powder with water. It's rather like a sponge. Touch it, and the pressure will squeeze out its loosely bound water, making it feel cool and moisturizing.

The polysaccharides themselves do not interact chemically with your body; they just form a physical barrier. Marshmallow gel can be applied to aggravated skin, as well as used on irritated membranes in throats and digestive tracts. Wounds repair more rapidly when protected and moist. Healing requires that biological components move around so they can perform their construction projects, and water allows this mobility.

Good Effects . . . and Not So Good

Marshmallow is probably quite safe. No rigorous studies of the physiological effects of this plant on humans yet exist, but at

Commonly Reported Uses for Marshmallow*

Internally
cough, hoarseness, inflammation of the stomach and intestines, ulcers
forms available for internal use:
capsules, decoction, dried leaves, dried root, syrup, teas, tincture
commonly reported internal dosage:
Teas are made with cold water and then gently warmed. The tea is made with 1 to 2 teaspoons of leaves per cup of water. For the syrup, 10 grams is recommended.
Externally
irritated skin, burns, inflammation, insect bites, wounds
forms available for external use:
gargle, gel, ointment, dried leaves, dried root, paste (made from powdered leaves or root and water), tincture, cosmetic preparations
commonly reported external dosage:
Enough water is mixed with the powdered leaves or root to make a paste, which is then applied.

*These uses and dosages are from historic use and are not necessarily tested nor recommended.

least historically it is not associated with any remarkable side effects. Allergic responses to marshmallow are rare. The FDA are popularly applied to inflamed skin and wounds, and are said to immediately take away the pain of insect bites and stings. An improperly sterilized preparation could make an open wound worse, however. Marshmallow is also used as gargle or drink to soothe a sore throat. Swallowing its mucilage could theoretically line and pacify an unruly digestive tract from top to bottom.

You may already be taking marshmallow and not know it. It is used as a binding agent in some pills, and is used to flavor strawberry, cherry, and root beer beverages. It is also added to ointments and cosmetics.

EVIDENCE OF ACTION

There are no human clinical trials using marshmallow alone. There are a few uncontrolled trials where marshmallow is taken, mixed with many other herbs, but it's impossible to sort out which herb could be doing what in these studies. Some references have blindly cut and pasted citations for what they must have thought was marshmallow plant, but had they taken the time to read the abstract, they would see the study employed the *candy* marshmallows to evaluate volunteers' swallowing ability. Since the modern candy contains no marshmallow plant, these references of course have no bearing on the subject.

allows its use as a food additive and has not placed any restrictions on its use, but acknowledges it as a medical unknown. Don't swallow it along with your medications, however. Its barrier action could limit your absorption of oral medications.

Use marshmallow for irritated membranes and skin, but not open wounds. Formulations from marshmallow leaf or root

THE BOTTOM LINE

- Marshmallow root is used for sore throat, indigestion, wounds, irritated skin, insect bites, and as a moisturizer.
- Modern, commercial "marshmallows" and related candy products no longer contain the plant.
- Marshmallow's moisturizing mucilage supports its use as a physical barrier for tissues and as a moisturizing agent.
- Marshmallow has not been rigorously tested in humans, and so is classified as a medical unknown. However, centuries of its use have not been associated with harm.

MILK THISTLE

Silybum marianum

History and Folklore

Milk thistle has also been called *Marian, Mary's thistle,* and *St. Mary's,* for its folkloric connection to the Virgin Mary's milk. According to legend, Mary was nursing Jesus beside a prickly plant. Her milk spilled onto it, and thereafter, its prickly green leaves were mottled with striking white veins, which exude a white sap when you break them.

Other prickly white-sapped plants, like the unrelated yellow-flowered sow thistles, were at one time identically named, so you may run across an excess of paradoxically contrasting milk thistles in older herb books. Milk thistle is also confused with *blessed thistle,* or *holy thistle* (*Cnicus benedictus*), even in today's commercial herb products. This probably results from centuries-old literature instructing the substitution of one plant for the other. However, blessed thistle has different ingredients and properties, which have not been as thoroughly researched. Blessed thistle was used as a digestive agent, but milk thistle was historically most often recommended for the spleen and kidneys, but most often the liver. Artichoke, a relative of milk thistle, is also thought to possess liver-benefiting molecules, although they are mainly different molecules that initiate other mechanisms.

Like artichokes, milk thistle's flower heads were boiled and eaten for ages, and every other part of the plant was eaten as well. Milk thistle's young stalks were once prized as a vegetable. Its long taproots were also boiled and eaten and were compared to salsify root, which is now almost as culinarily obscure as milk thistle. The leaves, minus their spiny edges, can be steamed and eaten, though preparing them is a fiddly task. The ancient Greek physician Dioscorides recommended milk thistle to patients with liver problems, suggesting they eat its leaves "sodden with oil and salt," which probably makes any sort of greens taste fine.

Today, the medicinal focus is on the "fruits," more commonly called seeds. Like the seeds of its fellow *Asteraceae,* the dandelion, each milk thistle seed is equipped with a parachute, or *pappus.* The milk thistle pappus is removed before the seed is consumed. Milk thistle seeds have a bitter, nutty taste and are ground and sprinkled on food or roasted for a coffee substitute.

How Scientists Think Milk Thistle Works

Milk thistle protects liver cells from many poisons, but this action is mostly seen only in the petri dish. Milk thistle seeds contain a mixture of flavonolignans that are collectively called *silymarin.* Silymarin has been shown to protect liver cells against a long list of chemical insults: acetaminophen, iron, alloxan, cisplatin, vincristin, carbon tetrachloride, galactosamine, thioacetamide, praseodymium, concanavalin A, amiodarone, pyrogallol, aflatoxin, lipopolysaccharides, and mycrocystin-LR, the *Amanita* mushroom toxins amanitin and phalloidin, and something called *cold-blood frog virus* (*FV3*), and more. As impressive as all that seems, most of these protection studies with milk thistle were not on humans, but on mere, isolated liver cells or lab animals, and some of the studies were better designed than others. Nonetheless, it seems like something is going on.

What's In It

MILK THISTLE seeds contain a mixture of flavonolignans that are collectively called *silymarin*. Silymarin contains silibins A and B (collectively called *silibinin*), isosilybins A and B, silydianin, and silychristin.

Silymarin flavonoids may boost defensive enzymes. Silymarin mildly to significantly increases the antioxidant, detoxifying enzymes superoxide dismutase, glutathione S-transferase, and quinone reductase. Some papers claim this results from silymarin's ability to induce cellular synthesis of these enzymes.

These enzymes' actions are particularly important in the liver, because it's the organ most often hit by toxins. The liver most usually takes the first hit from toxins, because most molecules that are absorbed during digestion, regardless of their source, first go to the liver to be processed and are often altered there. Since the liver is continually exposed to potentially toxic molecules, the liver is particularly sensitive to chemical assaults. To cope with this, liver cells produce molecules like glutathione, which is antioxidant, and can bind to toxins, rendering them ineffective or more easily excreted. When the liver is hit with toxins, either long term or acutely, and even when simply stressed in several disease states, glutathione is typically depleted in liver cells because of

their ongoing metabolic battles. Toxins generate, either directly or indirectly, radicals and oxidants, and silymarin assists cell's defense against them.

Some researchers suggest that silymarin limits the ability of the liver's Kupffer cells to make inflammatory molecules. Kupffer cells are specialized liver cells that are actually immune cells of the *macrophage* (meaning "big eater") variety. They hang out in liver sinuses and eat or phagocytose large particles and bacteria entering the liver from the digestive tract circulation. This prevents bacteria and foreign particles from entering the rest of the circulation. Kupffer cells, acting as circulatory system bouncers, are thus helpful, but they have a dark side and pose danger to "innocent" liver cells. When "activated" by various liver assaults, Kupffer cells make free radicals, oxidants, and other nasty chemical weapons as a defense, and nearby liver cells suffer friendly fire.

A stressed liver's long-term exposure to activated Kupffer cells is thought to play a role in liver damage. In both rat and human Kupffer cells, silymarin strongly inhibits an enzyme called *5-lipoxygenase*. This enzyme makes leukotrienes, which are pro-inflammatory and damaging, so it is helpful if silymarin really prevents these leukotrienes from being made.

Silymarin apparently keeps other inflammatory mediators low, too. Another pro-inflammatory molecule that silymarin inhibits holds the daunting title "nuclear transcription factor kappa beta," or NF-kappa-B, for short. Several different cell types, when stimulated by oxidative stress, viruses, toxins, or carcinogens, produce NF-kappa-B, and it is elevated in stressed livers. NF-kappa-B triggers more inflammation, because it causes more inflammatory molecules to be synthesized. It binds to the "promoters" of genes that encode inflammatory molecules called *cytokines.* Binding to the promoters of cytokine genes causes the gene's instructions for making the cytokines to be "read" by certain enzymes and results in the synthesis of an array of different inflammatory cytokines. To keep this process in check, an inhibitory molecule called *I-kappa-B* is normally bound to NF-kappa-B, which inactivates it. In one cell assay, silymarin directly prevented this inhibitor from being degraded, which in turn prevented NF-kappa-B from being released. The more silymarin that was used, the greater inhibition of NF-kappa-B, leading to better suppression of the synthesis of inflammatory cytokines.

Commonly Reported Uses for Milk Thistle*

Internally

liver protection and healing, digestive upset

forms available for internal use:

capsule, concentrated drops, seeds, powder solution, tablet, tea bags, and tincture

commonly reported dosage:

Pills or capsules of milk thistle seed extract standardized to at least 80 percent silymarin are most often recommended. One hundred to 500 milligrams of this is taken daily, often in divided doses. A tea of milk thistle does not contain much silymarin, because it is not very water soluble.

*These uses and dosages are from historic use and are not necessarily tested nor recommended.

Milk thistle theoretically helps your liver regenerate by increasing its pro-

tein synthesis. A cell needs protein to regenerate and divide, and silymarin may increase a liver cell's number of functional protein factories, called *ribosomes.* Ribosomal RNA, or rRNA, is an ingredient that is crucial to the operation of a ribosome's protein-making machinery. Two older studies of rat livers suggest that silymarin binds an enzyme called *RNA polymerase I.* This binding encourages the enzyme to perform its usual task, which is rRNA synthesis. The newly made rRNA then incorporates into ribosomes. A few other studies show that silymarin also enhances rRNA synthesis. Ribosomes need rRNA to build proteins. Increasing the number of working ribosomes accelerates the replacement of damaged proteins, allowing liver cells to repair and proliferate.

Milk thistle's flavonoids probably act as antioxidants and free radical scavengers and stabilize cell membranes. This is not uncommon for plant flavonoids, although a few flavonoids from other plants have the opposite activity. Numerous studies show that silymarin flavonoids can lower oxidizing agents and reduce free radicals. In doing so silymarin protects cell membranes from breaking down, and some say this keeps toxins from penetrating liver cells. Radicals and oxidants break down cell membranes by causing *lipid peroxidation,* a process in which the damaging agent binds to the cell membranes' lipid constituents and they consequently fragment.

Lipid peroxidation is quantified by measuring one of the cell membrane's breakdown products, malondialdehyde. Silymarin is often noted to prevent the malondialdehyde increase ordinarily seen in toxin-treated liver cells. Because of these observations, the scientific benediction "stabilization of membrane lipids" frequently graces silymarin in research papers. Membrane stabilization stops good things from leaking out of cells and bad things from getting in.

GOOD EFFECTS . . .
AND NOT SO GOOD

Silymarin probably won't hurt you unless you are allergic to it. The reports of adverse effects from milk thistle are rare. Occasionally it causes transient digestive upset and diarrhea. If you are allergic to plants in the daisy family (*Asteraceae*), such as ragweed, you might want to approach milkweed cautiously, but cases of allergic reaction to milk thistle are uncommon.

Interesting Facts

Are you sanguine, melancholy, phlegmatic, or bilious?

ANCIENT AND medieval physicians prescribed certain plants like milk thistle to correct imbalances in the humors of the body. These were mythical substances associated with different organs. Blood was the humor associated with the liver, and it gave one a sanguine or happy personality. Black bile, or "melancholia," came from the spleen and made one sad. Yellow bile from the gallbladder gave one a "choleric" or "bilious," angry temperament, and phlegm from the stomach made one slow and cold, or "phlegmatic." These were, in turn, associated with the four seasons, as well as air, earth, fire, and water. The physician's job was to balance the humors, accomplished through vomiting-inducing agents and purgatives, but mostly through bloodletting. Plants were used, too, and milk thistle was prescribed for excess melancholy.

Keep a doctor monitoring you if you have liver problems. Liver diseases are serious. A doctor can easily keep track of your liver status indicators, such as serum liver enzymes and bilirubin, with a simple blood test, and can keep you apprised of your condition.

Read the label. Researching available products, I recently found that a major brand's "milk thistle" caplet contained barely any milk thistle but quite a lot of blessed thistle. The two are sometimes used in place of each other, although they contain completely different ingredients. Blessed thistle is not a substitute for milk thistle. Be certain to find a standardized preparation containing at least 80 percent silymarin. Some brands are reportedly better absorbed than others. Because the active ingredients are not very water soluble, a tea made with milk thistle seeds does not contain much in the way of active ingredients, so it's usually not recommended, but it's also unlikely to hurt you either.

EVIDENCE OF ACTION

Most clinical trials of milk thistle enlist people with liver problems, such as cirrhosis (scarring of the liver) or hepatitis. (Hepatitis, by the way, broadly means any sort of liver inflammation, but many incorrectly think the term is confined to infection by the hepatitis-causing viruses.) Despite exciting results from test tube and animal studies, human clinical studies are conflicting. There is no shortage of clinical trials either. Around fifty have been published since 1966 on the National Library of Medicine's database PubMed. According to a meta-analysis examining fourteen of the best-designed trials, the authors concluded, "We found no reduction in mortality, in improvements in histology at liver biopsy, or in biochemical markers of liver function among patients with chronic liver disease."[1]

However, they did say that it was safe and well tolerated.

THE BOTTOM LINE

- Milk thistle seed extract, called *silymarin,* is used for protecting and healing the liver. Despite exciting results showing it protects cells from numerous poisons in test tube studies and lab animals, human studies with it are inconclusive and conflicting.
- Milk thistle is generally very safe.
- Silymarin's components are antioxidant, free radical–scavenging, and protect against lipid peroxidation.
- Silymarin may also stimulate liver regeneration by increasing the number of functional cellular structures called *ribosomes* in liver cells. Cells need ribosomes to make protein, and increasing the number of ribosomes may speed regeneration. Silymarin may also act against inflammation caused by liver Kupffer cells and inflammatory molecules like NF-kappa-B and leukotrienes.

NETTLE
Urtica dioica

History and Folklore

You are unlikely to forget where you were and what you were doing if you have ever encountered stinging nettle. You can find this perennial weed—or it can find you—in the wastelands and fields of the United States, Canada, and Europe.

My own first encounter with nettles was unforgettable, and as a naive, enthusiastic botany apprentice I wandered out into a Pennsylvania field of what looked like some new, interesting mint plants. Nettles resemble mints, with their square stem and opposing leaves, but they are not in the mint family, and mints don't sting you. The result was agonizing. I rubbed my stung legs with the local jewelweed leaves, based on anecdotal advice I'd remembered about nettle sting remedies, and the stinging did subside. (Anecdotes such as this are never proof of efficacy; however they can be useful when scientists guardedly make note of them for future testing.) Another common weed that is supposed to combat nettle stings, according to more unsubstantiated lore, is dock.

Nettle stings are detailed throughout history and are even included in a children's fairy tale, "The Nettle Spinner." A beautiful yarn spinner is forbidden by a jealous count to marry her fiancé until she spins her wedding gown out of nettles. Her faithfulness keeps the nettles from stinging her, and as the count dies due to his wickedness, the gown becomes his funeral shroud.

Some arthritis sufferers deliberately use nettles to induce this legendary sting upon themselves for pain relief. This seemingly masochistic treatment, known as *urtication,* was recorded by ancient Romans and survives as a folk remedy for arthritis pain today. Other folk remedies include nonstinging cooked nettles or nettles' extracts used as a diuretic, fever reducer, wound healer, allergy reducer, and in the vague-sounding category of "female discomforts." It also has been used as a "tonic," an even more vague term for something that allegedly strengthens the constitution like some mysterious herbal vitamin. Nettle greens do contain vitamins comparable to amounts found in spinach, and stories survive of nutrient-starved pioneers emerging from their cabins following a hard winter to pick nettles for a spring tonic. Cooking nettle keeps it from stinging, and nettle soup is a traditional folk dish that remains popular with weed foragers today. Also, some cheese makers still continue the tradition of using nettles to curdle milk in order to make "nettle cheese." The trick is picking the main ingredient.

Why Doesn't Cooked Nettle Sting?

THE SIMPLEST explanation is that heat pressurizes the contents of the stingers to expel their inflammatory contents, which then get diluted by the rest of the cooked material. Since the inflammatory mediators are dilute, they are less potent. A nettle stinger injects a teeny, tiny area of the skin with a relatively concentrated dose of inflammatory mediators.

How Scientists Think Nettle Works

It's no mystery why nettle stings are painful. Nettle injects you with a lot of dreadful chemicals through tiny hypodermic needle-style hairs. This brew resembles insect venoms. They contain histamine—the annoying, inflammatory chemical created by allergic responses (for which many people take *anti*histamines). Nettles also have formic acid, which is found in red ant bite stings. They even possess the human neurotransmitters serotonin and acetylcholine. When these neurotransmitters hit your pain nerves, your nerves' sensitivity to pain spikes. And if as if that were not enough, nettles also contain some leukotrienes, which our human bodies can produce in certain noxious circumstances, creating allergic and asthmatic responses. Indeed, *anti*leukotriene medications are used for asthma. Since all of these ingredients are so irritating, the real mystery is why some people find nettle stings helpful for arthritis.

Treat your arthritis pain with . . . pain? It's hard to say why testimonials and one small but intriguing study imply that urtication—stinging yourself with nettles—might diminish arthritis pain. But there are similar alternative "therapies," such as using animal venoms and stings for pain. One possible explanation for why this apparent self-abuse might work is based on "gate control theory," which still holds the status of theory but remains useful in medical practice since its birth in the 1960s. What do you do when you bump your head or have an itch? Usually we rub or scratch the affected area, but when you think about it, that seems like an odd thing to do. Even animals instinctively rub or chew on body areas that

What's In It

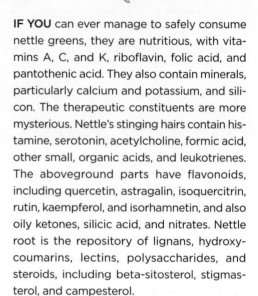

IF YOU can ever manage to safely consume nettle greens, they are nutritious, with vitamins A, C, and K, riboflavin, folic acid, and pantothenic acid. They also contain minerals, particularly calcium and potassium, and silicon. The therapeutic constituents are more mysterious. Nettle's stinging hairs contain histamine, serotonin, acetylcholine, formic acid, other small, organic acids, and leukotrienes. The aboveground parts have flavonoids, including quercetin, astragalin, isoquercitrin, rutin, kaempferol, and isorhamnetin, and also oily ketones, silicic acid, and nitrates. Nettle root is the repository of lignans, hydroxycoumarins, lectins, polysaccharides, and steroids, including beta-sitosterol, stigmasterol, and campesterol.

---

are itchy, irritated, or sore. Gate control theory tries to explain why this works.

According to the theory, before pain signals can reach the brain, they must pass a theoretical "gate" in your spinal cord, which is opened or closed by a number of factors, possibly by signals coming down from the brain itself. Additional signals to the brain, such as heat, cold, or touch, can "close the gate," preventing pain signals from reaching the brain. This is why heat, cold, massage, acupuncture, and even electrical stimulation might help reduce pain sensations. Of course, these sorts of stimuli can do other things, too, like altering blood flow to an affected part. Perhaps some signals to the brain from a nettle sting keep the brain too busy to notice other types of pain, like arthritis pain. The trick, then, would be to minimize the sting sensation while maximizing the closure of the pain gate. Since nettle stings can be horrible, this trick requires cautious consideration. Unfortunately, use of nettle stings for therapy is for now too poorly documented to advise a safe technique.

Maybe nettle stings deplete your supply of substance P. Another theory, which is better known as the explanation for why topical red pepper (see page 260) preparations reduce pain, says that nerve cells quickly "use up" a pain-signaling molecule called *substance P* when the plant-induced pain is first felt. This is followed by a period of analgesia, an inability to feel pain, because the pain nerves haven't had time to make any more substance P.

Nonstinging nettle root extracts might prevent estrogen from enlarging the prostate. Nettle is commonly used for benign prostatic hyperplasia (BPH), and the best suggestion of a mechanism lies in its ability to prevent estrogen from causing excess prostate enlargement. You hear a lot about dihydrotestosterone, a more potent, natural by-product of testosterone, as causing BPH, but the finger of guilt is moving toward this female hormone, too. Estrogen (there are actually several estrogens, plural) is normally found in men but becomes more dominant as men age. In order for the estrogen called *estradiol* to enlarge the prostate, it has to first stick to a protein called *sex hormone–binding globulin (SHBG)* while this protein is attached to a prostate cell membrane. This linkage between estradiol and SHBG on the cell membrane then directs another protein called *insulin-like growth factor* to stimulate the growth of prostate cells, causing prostate enlargement. Nettle might stop estradiol from doing this in a couple of ways.

Some aqueous lignans from nettle root can significantly bind to SHBG and prevent it from anchoring to its realm of activity, the cell membrane, at least in test tube studies. Lignans from other plants, like flaxseed (see page 123), are also exciting scientists with this SHBG binding activity, but one nettle lignan in particular (3,4-divanillyltetrahydrofuran) binds SHBG "outstandingly" well.[1] There are rumors that the same German team that reported this also subsequently noted that nettle extract prevented this estrogen from being made from testosterone, by inhibiting the aromatase enzyme that normally converts the male hormone to the female one, but this research on nettle alone is not readily available for review and does not appear to have been repeated. Pervasive rumors that nettle is an aromatase inhibitor are thus premature.

Oral nettle may affect the heart and increase urination, but how that works has yet to be determined. Rodents injected with nettle extracts urinated more than those receiving saline. The rats also and excreted more sodium. Nettle may have even damaged their kidneys at higher doses, but not at lower doses.[2] The excess sodium excretion could be caused by a number of different factors, and its mechanism has not been investigated further. Urinating more decreases your blood volume and blood pressure, which may explain why nettle is a popular antihypertensive herb in the Mediterranean. Nettle extracts contract the aorta and slow the heart's beat in isolated organ perfusion studies.[3] Since the mechanisms behind these actions remain unknown, using nettle long-term, solely as a diuretic or antihypertensive, seems to be a gamble.

GOOD EFFECTS . . . AND NOT SO GOOD

Feel the medicine working. . . . ouch! If you are thinking of stinging yourself with nettles, please be careful! Deliberately stinging oneself with nettles, or "urtication," is not to be approached lightly. This most curious use of nettles for arthritis might make you feel worse than before, so regard nettle stings as a last resort. They can really hurt. Colin Randall, a doctor who studies this treatment, had subjects rub nettle leaf on an arthritic limb for thirty seconds. On the one hand, he reassures, "It doesn't hurt as much as you would think," and implied that a long-lasting anesthetic effect made subsequent treatments less painful. However, he also suggests you should be very cautious handling these stinging objects. People who know how to gather them for nettle soup wear heavy gloves. Particularly nasty nettle stings can last longer than twelve hours.

Side effects are uncommon, but don't assume nettle is completely safe. Damaging effects are so far only noted in lab animals that are given inordinately large doses of nettle, and the occasional cup of nettle soup probably won't hurt most people. However, large doses of the herb caused uterine contractions in rabbits, so pregnant women should avoid oral nettle just to be on the safe side. Rodent studies suggest nettle might exacerbate diabetics' attempts to keep blood sugar low after meals. There are reports of gastric upset following ingestion of oral nettle, so you should stick to typically recommended dosages and follow package directions.

EVIDENCE OF ACTION

According to an old folk remedy, "urtication," or deliberately stinging yourself with stinging nettle in a controlled manner, might actually relieve arthritis pain. A highly popularized paper published in 2000 supports what had previously remained the domain of testimonials and anecdotes.[4] Colin Randall, a British doctor who headed

the study, had previously been intrigued enough by the phenomenon to publish an exploratory case report of eighteen joint pain sufferers who routinely used nettle urtication, and all but one were convinced it helped them.[5] Testimonials, however, mean very little scientifically, because there are always many people who are certain about something that turns out to be incorrect.

Commonly Reported Uses for Nettle*

Internally
allergies, diuretic, benign prostatic hyperplasia, arthritis, mineral and vitamin supplement
forms available for internal use:
root extract, powdered root, leaves and stems, juice, capsule, decoction, extract, tea
commonly reported dosage:
Either 8 to 12 grams of aboveground plant material or 2 to 3 grams of powdered root is commonly taken per day. For a diuretic, herbalists suggest 1 to 2 teaspoons of leaves and stems be steeped in 1 cup of hot water for tea.
Externally
arthritis
forms available for external use:
lotion, tea, tincture, fresh leaves (for "urtication," deliberately stinging yourself with stinging nettle in a controlled manner)

*These uses and dosages are from historic use and are not necessarily tested nor recommended.

To clarify these reports, Randall experimented with twenty-seven people who

- Nettle's stings, like ant bites and bee stings, are painful and pro-inflammatory. Inflicting inflammation upon yourself is generally not recommended. Nonetheless, some evidence suggests nettle stings might help relieve arthritis pain. Of course, the stinging plant must be handled with utmost caution.
- Nettle extracts are diuretic and could possibly slow the heart's beating. The mechanisms for these actions have not been unveiled as of yet. Nettle root extracts might help reduce symptoms of benign prostatic hyperplasia, possibly by preventing estradiol from binding to sex hormone–binding globulin.
- Nettle should be avoided by pregnant women and diabetics. High doses might be damaging to the kidneys or heart.

complained of thumb osteoarthritis and had never tried nettle. Continuing to take their painkiller medications, for thirty seconds once a day for one week the subjects also rubbed on their aching joint either stinging nettle leaf or a sham treatment of a leaf that resembled nettle but did not sting. However, there is a possible problem with this study: The two groups swapped treatments after a five-week "washout" period. Crossover studies like this are quite respectable, but the fact that one "treatment" stung and the other did not might have allowed the placebo to be detected, although the studies' authors showed wisdom in telling the volunteers not to expect relief from either leaf. Still, patients reported significantly less pain and disability when treating themselves with nettle leaf. Seventeen of the twenty-seven wanted to continue using nettle afterward.

Nettle is an old Middle Eastern standby for hypertension and heart disease, but according to one study, it might have toxic side effects.[6] Rats injected with nettle leaf extracts had lower blood pressure, probably because of the pronounced diuretic and sodium-excreting effect also observed. However, this effect persisted when a more concentrated infusion of nettle extract was halted, indicating that the extract did some

permanent damage, perhaps to the kidneys. Although the study used rats instead of people, and also used highly concentrated, injected extracts, which can behave substantially differently than the more common oral preparations, it does raise questions about nettle's safety in high doses.

The use of nonstinging nettle extracts as a diuretic has gradually evolved into several investigations of its use in benign prostatic hyperplasia, or BPH, which can restrict an affected man's ability to urinate. Unfortunately, studies of this kind mainly use mixtures of herbs, and it is impossible to sort out which herb is doing what in these trials. This leaves only one German trial employing nettle by itself, and the results are encouraging.[7] Two hundred and forty-six men with BPH took either a placebo or nettle in the form of 459 milligrams of dried root extract for one year. For those taking the nettle extract, their IPSS (International Prostate Symptom Score) decreased significantly, indicating improvement. Other good things they experienced were faster urine flow and less residual flow, though these two effects were not statistically significant. They also experienced fewer adverse effects than the placebo group.

Less encouraging are results from a study using nettle for allergies. A randomized, placebo-controlled study of freeze-dried nettle enlisted sixty-nine volunteers, and those taking nettle reported their allergic rhinitis improved only slightly but not statistically significantly better than the placebo group.[8]

Nettle may be bad for diabetics. It is important for diabetics to keep their blood sugar from spiking up after a meal. Although there are plants that help keep diabetics' blood sugar low following a meal, nettle is not one of those plants, according to a couple of rodent studies. In diabetic mice[9] and rats,[10] nettle either had no effect on blood glucose or elevated it. In nondiabetic rats, however, nettle lowered blood glucose and was postulated to reduce the intestinal absorption of glucose.

PARSLEY

Petroselinum crispum

History and Folklore

What plant terrified ancient Greeks and medieval virgins? Surely it couldn't be the meek and oft-ignored adornment to modern-day restaurant platters. Parsley has a surprisingly colorful history and contains several interesting pharmacologically active ingredients to boot.

This prototypical member of the *Umbelliferae* (or *Apiaceae*) family grows in rocky soil (hence the *petros,* Greek for "rock," in its Latin name) and is cultivated worldwide. Both the curly-leaved and flat-leaved parsley varieties are the same species, and you should expect them to have similar properties. We eat many common *Umbelliferae* (also called *Apiaceae* by many botanists) vegetables and herbs, such as carrots, parsnips, fennel, celery, cilantro, chervil, cumin, caraway, and anise, and many share common molecules and properties with parsley. *Umbelliferae* possess a classic "umbel" type flower, which, looks like curved metal spokes of an upside-down umbrella, each originating from a common point and each supporting a small flower. *Umbelliferae* are

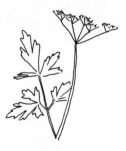

parsley umbel

easy to recognize, but please don't try eating wild ones—because the poisonous and abundant hemlock is one as well.

Unlike its cousin hemlock, parsley is relatively harmless as a green. But though the Romans enjoyed eating it, the Greeks were more hesitant to do so, using it more for medicine and occasionally feeding it to horses and warriors. The Greek ambivalence toward parsley stemmed from their association of the plant with death, for it was said to have sprung from the blood of their beloved, snakebitten Archemorus, the herald of death. Thereafter the Nemean games, created in honor of the slain prince, awarded winners with wreaths of parsley in remembrance of the fallen. Parsley decorated Greek tombs, and their expression "to need only parsley" means to be at death's door. According to the Roman historian Plutarch, an under-equipped Celtic army took advantage of the Greeks' superstition and created something like a guided herbal missile. They successfully shattered the nerves of an invading Greek army by loading hundreds of mules with the herb and sending them toward their would-be conquerors.

The association of parsley with death— and hence, evil—continued into medieval Europe. The seeds—which inhibit their own germination with chemicals called *furanocoumarins,* common to members of this plant family—were thought to be hard to grow, because they had to take several trips to the devil first (explaining the period needed for groundwater to wash away the furanocoumarins). A virgin planting the seed was said to risk impregnation by the devil, and only the man of the house could safely plant this herb on Good Friday.

Parsley has traditionally been used as a diuretic and digestive aid, for fevers, and of course, its abundance on dinner plates passively suggests its use as a breath freshener, too. Its purified oil was used "to bring on the flow of menses"—a polite, old-fashioned phrase for anything that aborts a fetus. The 1898 *King's American Dispensatory* noted these properties as well as the oil's hallucinogenic effect if taken in overdose.

How Scientists Think Parsley Works

Parsley might increase your trips to the bathroom. Something in the extract of parsley seed worked as a diuretic and mild laxative in rats. And for those of us who are not rats, folklore has long maintained that parsley is a diuretic and digestion aid. Both effects were determined to originate from the extract's hindrance of something called the *sodium-potassium pump* (also commonly known as the *sodium-potassium ATPase*).

What's In It

PARSLEY CONTAINS the volatile oils myristicin, apiole, beta-bisabolene; flavonoids such as apiin, apigenin, and luteolin; and furanocoumarins such as psoralen, 8-methoxypsoralen and 5-methoxypsoralen; and several vitamins and minerals, such as vitamins A, B, C, K, iron, potassium, and calcium.

Both human cells and rat cells both have this sodium-potassium pump; in fact, all animals have them. Human cells are constantly spending energy to pump out sodium ions and pull in potassium ions, which maintains cells' water balance. Cells also use the unequal distribution of these ions to power various processes in a mechanism similar to how batteries work. So this pump "charges the battery," so to speak, for various cellular effects, which differ from cell type to cell type. This sodium-potassium pump in kidney cells is not only interfered with by parsley, but by some types of prescription diuretics, either directly or indirectly. When this pump's action in your kidney cells is quelled, more water enters the kidneys, thus generating more urine.

Parsley's inhibition of cells' sodium-potassium pump helps explain its mild laxative effect, as well as its diuretic effect. This same type of pump works in colon cells in a more complicated way, but ultimately it pulls sodium ions through the cells that line the colon into the blood of surrounding capillaries, and water passively follows, because water is attracted to sodium ions. (This is why you retain water when you eat too much sodium; sodium readily enters the bloodstream through the gut lining, and water follows it, increasing blood volume and swelling.) This process removes water from your intestinal contents, making them more solid. Of course, if you block this process with something like parsley, the reverse happens. Your intestinal cargo becomes more watery, and in more extreme cases is transformed into diarrhea.

Parsley's laxative effect is apparently mild, however, as is its diuretic effect. This could be because the active ingredient does not strongly inhibit the sodium potassium pump, or perhaps because the active ingredient is not concentrated in parsley leaves.

Parsley's diuretic and laxative effects are more noted for parsley seed oil, and

less so for parsley leaf. Oily constituents concentrated in the seed oil (apiole and myristicin) are found in lesser amounts in the leaves, and these are tentatively attributed to these effects. Eating large amounts of parsley leaf, such as in the Mediterranean, parsley-based tabbouleh salad, may produce a mild diuretic or laxative effect. Also, plant fiber in general can act as a simple, safe, bulk-producing laxative, so eating a lot of parsley leaf may encourage a bowel movement by an additional mechanism.

Parsley herb and water-based extracts of parsley are probably quite safe, but parsley oil and seeds contain potentially dangerous stuff. Parsley oil here refers to either the oil extracted from the seed or the pure volatile oil that is distilled from the leaf. Parsley seeds contain more than ten times as much oil as the leaves per gram, so eating a lot of parsley seeds is similar to consuming the oil. (What cooks commonly call "parsley oil" is not the same, but merely parsley leaves macerated in cooking oil, and that is relatively safe.) True parsley oil contains the oily molecules myristicin and apiole, and you want to limit your intake of these.

The myristicin in parsley oil is detoxifying in small amounts, but a toxic hallucinogen in excess. Cases of myristicin overdose are better documented in people who consumed too much nutmeg, because it is also found in nutmeg and in mace.[1] In fact, this nutmeg component contributes to the pleasantly subtle, spicy smell of parsley. But ingesting more than 70 milligrams of myristicin (and parsley oil is typically 40 to 80 percent myristicin) will result in unpleasant hallucinations that are accompanied by vomiting, nausea, convulsions, and brain damage; it has been fatal. The liver is postulated to turn myristicin into some amphetamine-like chemicals, but this hasn't been proven.

On the other hand, the small amounts of myristicin in parsley greens, or nutmeg for that matter, used in normal cooking will not hurt you. In fact, it might be good for you, since in small amounts myristicin has been shown to induce the production of a detoxifying, antioxidant enzyme called *glutathione S-transferase* in mice.[2] The myristicin in parsley also inhibited tumor formation in mice by benzo[a]pyrene, the major carcinogen that is formed by broiling meats at high temperatures.[3]

In large doses, the apiole in parsley oil is also toxic. Greater than 10 grams of apiole causes anemia and kidney and liver failure, and parsley oil is 50 to 80 percent apiole. If you are female, there's another reason to avoid the apiole in pure parsley oil. Apiole can cause uterine cramps and miscarriage. *Something* in parsley oil does anyway, and recent evidence points to apiole, which causes uterine muscles to contract. If you read traditional herb books' references to parsley, you will probably come across the flowery phrase "brings on the flow of menses." It's surprising how many authors echo this phrase yet seem ignorant of its historic significance. But this is an old euphemism for an *abortifacient,* an herb used to terminate an unwanted pregnancy, and parsley oil is still used for this purpose today. Since parsley oil is toxic in large doses, its use in terminating pregnancies has led to the deaths of some women in developing countries.[4] According to physician's texts, raw or cooked parsley in amounts typically used in food should not frighten you if you are pregnant, but you should avoid pure parsley oil, as well as parsley seeds, which contain a lot of parsley oil.

Don't worry about tripping out after eating a salad bowl filled with parsley greens, or from your own homemade parsley-infused cooking oil. Parsley greens are good for you. The myristicin content is far too low, and a little myristicin isn't bad. You *should* avoid commercially prepared oils that are *distilled* from parsley, which is *pure parsley oil* and not something you normally consume anyway, as it is full of myristicin and apiole. Besides activating detoxifying mechanisms, parsley herb is loaded with vitamins and minerals, such as carotene (the precursor to vitamin A), other carotenoids like lutein, C and B vitamins, antioxidant flavonoids like apigenin, and also many minerals, particularly calcium, iron, and potassium.

Contrary to popular belief, chlorophyll in parsley will not freshen your breath. But chewing a sprig of parsley will. If you look for a cure for bad breath on the Internet, zillions of adds for parsley pills will pop up, all claiming that the chlorophyll in them is a "natural deodorant" or that it works internally in some mysterious manner to scavenge malodorous molecules. Experimentally, chlorophyll doesn't work.[5] However, chewing a sprig of parsley after a meal does stimulate salivation and abrasively cleans your mouth.

If you use parsley topically, sunlight may give you a rash. Parsley isn't normally used topically, but if you do happen to get a lot of it on your skin, topical exposure to molecules called *furanocoumarins* (in parsley and other *Umbelliferae* family plants, such as celery, parsley, fennel, and parsnips, as well as the unrelated limes, lemons, and figs) are known to give some people a rash following sun exposure.[6]

The furanocoumarins in these plants are in the category of molecules known as *psoralens,* molecules that bond with DNA when exposed to light. Furanocoumarins are flat molecules that can slide comfortably in between the rungs in the ladder of your DNA molecules, a process called *intercalation.* There they rest harmlessly until ultraviolet light triggers their bonding to DNA. Their cross-linking to DNA strands kills the cell. So psoralens from parsley in skin cells can damage skin cells if you activate the psoralens with sunlight. Psoralens, in combination with UV light, are used in medicine to treat psoriasis and vitiligo and are even being tested for killing cancer cells. But don't try it at home. This sort of therapy requires a trained specialist's supervision. Eating parsley is unlikely to cause this photosensitization reaction.[7]

Good Effects . . . and Not So Good

Avoid pure parsley oil, especially if you are pregnant. This is oil derived from distilling the root, greens, or seeds of parsley. Its volatile oil myristicin is a toxic, nauseating hallucinogen. It also contains an agent that sends the uterus into spasms, which can cause cramps that may abort a fetus. Parsley seeds have a higher oil content than its leaves, so don't munch on the seeds as a snack.

Some cooks make "parsley oil," but this is not the same thing as *pure* parsley oil. You can do this by soaking or heating a bunch of parsley in a cup of your favorite cooking oil and blending the mixture to make a vibrantly green oil. This is drizzled onto entrees for flavor and aesthetic appeal. Though the cooking oil will liberate the myristicin and uterine stimulant to some extent, these are still relatively dilute, and a couple tablespoons of this common kind of culinary parsley oil is probably more good for you than bad.

Parsley as a green, used in cooking, is nutritious, and you may expect a slight diuretic and laxative effect from them. There is nothing dangerous about eating a salad bowl full of parsley greens or making parsley tea from the leaves. Parsley is full of vitamins and minerals. Pregnant women should probably not eat loads of parsley greens every day, but should limit parsley to normal amounts used in cooking, however, to reduce risk of uterine stimulation.

If you want parsley to clean your breath, you have to chew it. There is no evidence that popping parsley pills works on bad breath, despite scads of herb sellers trying to tell you otherwise. Chewing a sprig is more work, but it is effective.

Parsley is not normally used topically, and you might get a rash if you do. The rash is triggered by ultraviolet light or sun exposure. There is no evidence that it can happen if you take parsley orally.

Evidence of Action

Though commonly encountered on dinner plates, parsley is surprisingly uncommon in human clinical trials. Nonetheless, there is moderately good experimental evidence that something in aqueous parsley seed extracts increases urine output, at least in rats.[8] Control group rats given the same volume of water were less productive. The same extract also worked as a mild laxative in rats.[9]

THE BOTTOM LINE

- Parley acts as a diuretic and mild laxative, perhaps due to its inhibition of the cellular sodium-potassium pump.
- Pure parsley oil and parsley seeds should be avoided. Overdoses of the oil can cause brain damage, hallucinations, and miscarriage.
- There is no evidence that parsley pills will treat bad breath, but chewing parsley sprigs cleans your mouth.
- Parsley greens are nutritious, antioxidant, and full of vitamins and minerals.
- Pregnant women should confine their parsley consumption to amounts no greater than what is normally used in cooking. They should also avoid the volatile oil and seeds altogether. Topical exposure to parsley increases your risk of sun damage.

PEPPERMINT
Mentha piperita

HISTORY AND FOLKLORE

Peppermint does not have as long a story as other herbs, because it was classified relatively recently in herbal history. It is the offspring of nature's random cross between spearmint (*Mentha spicata*) with water ("wild") mint (*Mentha aquatica*). Discovered in a southern English field in the seventeenth century, it quickly became vogue to cultivate. Whether or not it was used in the Middle Ages is unknown, but one of the oldest documented specimens comes from the botanical collection of John Ray, a leading taxonomist and naturalist of the seventeenth century. He claimed his "peper mint" was better than any other mint for treating stomach weakness and diarrhea.

Though peppermint was hailed for treating all sorts of indigestion Dr. William Cook's 1869 *Medical Dispensatory* noted that in certain people it doesn't work as well: "Most stomachs receive it gratefully, and it often allays vomiting; yet some persons greatly dislike it, and its stimulating qualities unfit it for use when the stomach is sensitive."

Peppermint has been traditionally hailed as a *carminative* (gas-relieving agent) and *spasmolytic* (reducing gastrointestinal spasms). It is also thought to improve the flow of bile, although this effect has not been supported by evidence. It is considered stimulating and is used to treat headache, fatigue, and stress. Its cooling and numbing action is employed in many ointments, cosmetics, and medications today. Of course, it is also enjoyed in food and now forms the basis of classic Western foods such as candies

and mint juleps, as well as Middle Eastern main dishes.

The herb quickly spread to the United States, which now grows more peppermint than any other country. Like all members of the mint family (*Lamiaceae* or *Labiatae*) it sports the classic square stem with leaves directly opposite each other on the stem.

HOW SCIENTISTS THINK PEPPERMINT WORKS

Peppermint relaxes the muscles of your digestive tract. This could either ease your indigestion or make it worse, depending on what kind of indigestion you have. Muscle cells contract if the concentration of calcium ions rises inside them. Peppermint prevents this rise, acting like something clinically known as a *calcium channel antagonist.*[1] This means that peppermint blocks calcium influx into the muscle cell, and calcium is what helps make a muscle cell twitch. As a result, peppermint relaxes the involuntary muscles surrounding your digestive tract. Normally these muscles slowly push food through in the traditional direction.

Stress, irritating food, and illness can cause digestive muscles to spasm, however. These paroxysms are cramps, and since they impede the normal traffic, gas can accumulate in painfully pressurized pockets, potentially resulting in bloating as well. Relaxing these muscles makes the cramps disappear and can allow trapped gas to be liberated both upward and downward. An after-dinner mint can do more than cleanse your palate.

What's In It

UNLIKE ITS parents, peppermint has a good deal (30–45 percent) of menthol in its oil, and menthol is its major therapeutic ingredient. (Water mint oil has menthofurane, instead, which is minty but smells sweeter than menthol. Spearmint oil has essentially no menthol but is mainly L-carvone, which structurally resembles menthol but smells and tastes distinctively different from it.)

Besides menthol, pure peppermint oil has menthone (up to 31 percent), methyl acetate (up to 10 percent), menthofurane (up to 7 percent), and tiny amounts of pulegone, pinene, and lemony smelling limonene. The intact herb has, in addition to the previous ingredients, flavonoids, phytol, tocopherols, carotenoids, betain, azulenes, choline, rosmarinic acid, and tannins.

Be careful with peppermint if you are constipated. Peppermint might worsen a ploddingly sluggish digestion. Sometimes constipation really is caused by paralyzed digestive muscles, and further stunning them with peppermint won't help. But constipation can also be caused by erratic digestive muscle spasms, creating mini traffic jams in the gut. So, depending on what is causing constipation, peppermint could either help or make things worse. Those with chronic indigestion typically suffer the same faulty digestive mechanism repeatedly. Therefore, experimenting conservatively with small sips of peppermint tea during a typical episode of indigestion once or twice is not very risky and is usually enough to determine whether peppermint is right or wrong for you in the future.

People with gastroesophageal reflux disease (GERD) should take enteric-coated or delayed-release peppermint capsules only, if they want to take peppermint. Some people just have a hard time closing their esophageal sphincter. This ring-shaped muscle sits above the stomach and seals off the throat from stomach acid. Normally it contracts when you swallow, but for people with gastroesophageal reflux disease (GERD), the esophageal sphincter stays relaxed, and these poor people burn and damage their throats with stomach acid. Obviously, further relaxing this sphincter with direct application of peppermint is disastrous for such folks, but they can still take enteric-coated or delayed-release peppermint capsules safely.

Peppermint is said to help humans produce bile, but it might actually prevent the gallbladder from releasing it. Peppermint is often said to be a *choleretic.* Other herbal choleretics, at least according to unsubstantiated lore, are artichoke, dandelion, and turmeric. Choleretics stimulate the flow of bile, a digestive detergent that emerges from the gallbladder after a greasy meal, to facilitate grease management in the digestive tract. Choleretics supposedly prevent indigestion associated with poor fat digestion. There is not much research on peppermint's action as a choleretic. There is some evidence that peppermint stimulates your ability to *make* bile,[2] but it also seems to inhibit the *release* of bile from the gallbladder, because it relaxes the gallbladder, keeping it from contracting. This isn't too surprising, since peppermint relaxes muscles, and the gallbladder requires muscular contraction to release its bile. One research paper says that peppermint oil, taken by volunteers, "completely inhibited" their gallbladders from emptying,[3] although the concentration of peppermint oil was unnaturally high in this experiment. Keep in mind that peppermint might have the *opposite* effect on bile than what is customarily stated in traditional herb books.

Peppermint numbs your pain, because the menthol in it is a local anesthetic. Sore muscles rubbed with ointment containing peppermint oil or menthol may feel better. Menthol is *nonpolar,* which means that it is oil soluble, rather than water soluble. Like other small, nonpolar molecules, it can slowly dissolve and slip through the tissues of your skin, reaching nerves and muscles underneath. It also mixes well with the oily membranes of nerve and muscle cells, impeding the traffic of ions in and out of these cells, which would otherwise cause them to be stimulated.[4] Thus menthol ultimately anesthetizes these nerves and muscles, blunting the perception of pain. Menthol and peppermint don't smell as strongly as muscle rubs that contain wintergreen oil (see page 332) either, and are therefore incorporated into "odorless" versions of these creams, although they relieve pain by a different mechanism.

Too hot? The menthol in peppermint stimulates cold-sensitive nerve endings. It's not your imagination. Peppermint and other menthol-containing mints cool you off. Herbalists like to call cooling herbs *refrigerants.* Although menthol anesthetizes most nerve cells, separate research teams at the Scripps Research Institute at La Jolla in California and at the University of California, San Francisco, independently discovered a nerve cell receptor that was stimulated by menthol instead. The receptor (called either *CMR1* or *TRPM8,* depending on which lab you talk to) normally is stimulated by temperatures ranging from 8 to 28 degrees Celsius. Menthol tickles these nerve cells that perceive cold, so you think that you are feeling cold.[5] This is analogous to red pepper's mechanism (see page 260), which stimulates

heat-sensing nerves instead. If you are feverish, experiencing a hot flash, or just plain overheated, a few drops of peppermint oil dissolved in a cup of water and splashed on the skin will instantly provide a cooling effect. A few drops go a long way, however, so don't apply more concentrated solutions of the oil directly to your skin, because the excess cold-sensing nerve stimulation can hurt.

The menthol in peppermint helps you breathe more comfortably. What congested person has not felt the welcome cool air that mentholated rubs and cough drops provide? It seems as though more air is suddenly moving through your nose. But the effect might be all in your head. Sensitive measurements of airflow show that menthol does not significantly increase the amount of air moving through the nose. But menthol does stimulate cold-sensitive nerves, making the air more noticeable. However, another study suggests that menthol at least relaxes passages in the *lungs,* thus allowing more air through lower regions. Furthermore, menthol dilates and relaxes blood vessels in sinuses, and this makes the blood vessels leak fluid, which makes your nose run. While menthol's cold sensation in the sinuses is immediate, this mechanism takes a few minutes, but it can help unplug congested sinuses.

GOOD EFFECTS . . .
AND NOT SO GOOD

Peppermint as an herb is quite safe, but be careful with the oil, or any preparations with a high menthol content. The peppermint plant—its leaves, and tea made from the leaves—is very safe, according to both historical use and scientific toxicity studies. The tea actually has a rather low menthol content. The oil, however, does not.

Interesting Facts

Mints are loved and abundant, and not all are minty either.

THE MAJORITY of our culinary herbs are mints. Obviously spearmint, peppermint, and wild mint are mints, but did you know that rosemary, sage (see page 266), savory, basil, marjoram, oregano, and thyme are, too? Most of our popular culinary herbs belong to this family, and a botanist will still call them a "mint," whether or not they taste minty. Other mints that are now less fashionable to cook with are catnip (see page 62), lemon balm (see page 213), pennyroyal, hyssop, and horehound.

Most mints look similar and are fairly easy to recognize once you know what to look for. "Square stem and opposite leaves" is the catch phrase you memorize when looking for one, because their stems have four sides (you can verify this by trying to roll the stem with your fingers) and the leaves sit in pairs, directly opposite each other, on the branch. Typically, the small flowers at the top of the stem are pink, purple, or white, with two lips fused into a tube at their base. There are actually five petals, but two are fused at the top to make the top "lip," and three are fused at the bottom to make the bottom "lip."

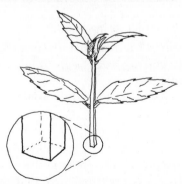

Mints have a square stem and opposite leaves

Mint can be found even as a neighborhood weed. For example, catnip commonly grows on the fringes of many suburbs. Many mints also have developed roles as decorative garden plants. There are a lot of mints, and they tend to grow like wildfire: The main problem with growing them in a garden is keeping them from annexing other plants' territories. The mint family is now officially called *Lamiaceae* (though the older term *Labiatae* is still occasionally used). There are roughly thirty-five hundred species in this family, but this is an estimate, as they can hybridize and form new varieties, as with the birth of peppermint.

If you consume the oil, you may want to dilute it or use it sparingly. No cases of overdose have been reported, but the menthol in it is estimated to be toxic when it approaches 2 grams.

Peppermint oil, applied directly to your skin even in recommended amounts, can give you a rash and irritation if you have sensitive skin. If you want to put peppermint oil on your skin, dilute a couple drops of it in a cup of water or lotion, and mix well before applying it. It should cool your skin and act as a local anesthetic.

Never put peppermint oil on the face of an infant or small child. The menthol in peppermint helps you feel like you can breathe better, but it's for adults only. Infants and children can reflexively choke and gag if they inhale peppermint oil and may even go into respiratory arrest.

Peppermint helps most types of indigestion but makes other types worse. Peppermint relaxes your internal muscles, so any sort of indigestion causes by spastic digestive muscles can be reduced with peppermint. Gas, bloating, and diarrhea usually fall into this category. It might help those who suffer from irritable bowel syndrome, too.

Sometimes constipation is caused by spastic involuntary muscles, so peppermint might help in that case. But peppermint could slow down intestinal traffic if the constipation is a result of sluggish gut muscles. Also, peppermint makes stomach acid more likely to leak through the muscular constriction that normally shuts off the stomach from your throat. Those with gastroesophageal reflux disease (GERD) should take only enteric-coated or delayed-release peppermint.

Although many sources repeat the idea that peppermint stimulates bile flow, it might actually prevent bile from being released. The data on peppermint's effect on bile is scanty so far. People with gallstones or gallbladder disease should use peppermint sparingly until they are aware of its effects.

Evidence of Action

There is no doubt that peppermint relaxes involuntary muscles, such as those lining your digestive tract; dozens of experiments bear witness to this phenomenon,[6, 7] an effect that has been observed as far back as 1920.[8] Thus peppermint has a *spasmolytic* ("spasm-cutting") effect—that is, it reduces the spasms of your involuntary digestive muscles. These sorts of spasms generate cramps, gas, and bloating. In fact, doctors have written papers recommending the best way for other doctors to apply peppermint oil to the digestive tracts of their patients who are undergoing various gastrointestinal imaging tests in order to reduce the unpleasant internal spasms that the tests induce.[9, 10, 11]

Whether or not this muscle-relaxing action makes peppermint a useful remedy for digestive complaints depends on the study. However, it can easily be reasoned that this is because not all indigestion is the same, as indigestion is not always caused by a spasmodic digestive tract. By 1990 the United States Food and Drug Administration decided that it had not been presented with data proving that peppermint acts as an effective digestive aid and banned its use in the United States as a nonprescription drug for treating indigestion. But some respected herb scientists argue that the legal language of this announcement is misleading, and it simply means the FDA was not presented with evidence of peppermint's efficacy as a digestive aid at that time.[12, 13] For example, the same FDA announcement suggests that prunes, which are famously laxative, are not effective laxatives, not because of any data reviewed, but because no prune experiments had been submitted to the FDA at the time.

More recently reviewed experiments tentatively suggest that peppermint really is useful in treating *certain* types of indigestion. Peppermint may reduce the symptoms of irritable bowl syndrome (IBS), namely diarrhea, constipation, gas, and bloating. IBS is a mysterious, difficult-to-treat ailment that usually inflicts its victims with a lifetime of chronic diarrhea alternating with constipation. A review of five carefully constructed (double-blind, randomized, placebo-controlled) trials cautiously stated that peppermint seems to help IBS, but requested that more carefully designed trials be performed to confirm this conclusion.[14] A more recent similarly designed trial of forty-two children with IBS claims that after two weeks, the children taking enteric-coated peppermint suffered less pain from IBS.[15]

However, there are two kinds of IBS. Some IBS sufferers complain that constipation is their main problem, and the others are primarily bothered by endless diarrhea. Because peppermint prolongs the time that it takes for food to travel through the intestine,[16] it seems reasonable to suggest that it

Commonly Reported Uses for Peppermint*

Internally

indigestion, gas, bloating, irritable bowel syndrome, diarrhea, constipation, cold, flu, fever, cooling agent, fatigue, tension and weariness, headache, fever, congestion

forms available for internal use:

flavoring agents for food, capsules, infusion (tea) of fresh or dried leaves, lozenges, oil, syrup, tincture

commonly reported dosage:

Teas are made with fresh or dried leaves steeped in hot water for ten minutes and then strained (it is said that after ten minutes of steeping in hot water the maximum amount of menthol and menthone are released from the leaves). The tea is taken 3 to 4 times daily. Or 3 to 6 grams of dried leaves, or 6 to 12 drops of oil, are taken daily. Capsules are available in 0.2 or 0.6 doses taken daily.

Externally

anesthetic, antiseptic, muscle aches, fatigue, tension and weariness, headache, fever, congestion, fever, cooling agent

forms available for external use:

oil, ointment, tincture, as well as oral, bath and cosmetic products

commonly reported dosage:

A few drops of oil are sometimes rubbed onto affected areas 2 to 4 times daily. This may be diluted with water or lotion if the skin is sensitive. Ointments are rubbed on the chest, back, or applied in the nose. The oil may be placed in hot water, and the steam from this can be inhaled.

*These uses and dosages are from historic use and are not necessarily tested nor recommended.

could theoretically prolong constipation. This may be true for those who suffer from IBS as well as for those who don't. Thus peppermint may be more effective for IBS associated with chronic diarrhea rather than constipation. It certainly should *not* be taken by people whose digestive problems arise from sluggish bowel activity or a condition involving intestinal paralysis called *ileus*.

Also, since peppermint relaxes the constricting muscles between the stomach and esophagus, it may enable the flow of stomach acid unpleasantly up your throat. This is the main problem in gastroesophageal reflux disease (GERD). There are no good clinical studies on this unwanted effect, but it seems a very sensible theory. People who struggle with GERD should avoid peppermint unless it is in the form of enteric-coated or delayed-release capsules.[17]

One of peppermint's most renowned attributes is its *carminative* action—that is, it is supposed to lessen gas pain. Aside from the moderately positive results observed in the studies of peppermint on people with IBS (who often complain of gas) described above, there is a dearth of research concerning peppermint's ability to treat gas alone. Theoretically, it should help by two possible mechanisms: Its antimicrobial action (because gut microbes generate excess gas) and its spasmolytic, muscle-relaxing effect (because a spasmodic gut does not evacuate gas efficiently). Peppermint did lessen the gas of pigs in one study,[18] and this was attributed not to its antimicrobial effect, but to peppermint's spasmolytic action.

Though there are frequent literary echoes of peppermint's ability to improve the flow of bile, thus aiding digestion of greasy meals, evidence for this is slim. While animal and cell studies suggest that peppermint might help your body *make* bile, it seems to inhibit your body's ability to *release* it.[19] This is probably because the release of bile requires the muscular contraction of the gallbladder, and peppermint oil prevents such muscles from contracting.

Although inhaled peppermint is often cited as "mentally stimulating," surprising results suggest it is not, but it can still help you feel better. Mental alertness tests show that peppermint does not improve various mental test scores with respect to placebo odors, such as the smell of the plain solvent that the peppermint oil was dissolved in.[20] The authors of this study conclude it seems that just smelling *anything* might wake up your brain a bit. In fact, another study suggested that the effect of inhaled peppermint on your nervous system is not stimulating but relaxing.[21] Nonetheless, most people who smell peppermint oil subjectively report its odor seems pleasant and invigorating.

Who hasn't been congested, and after inhaling the menthol from peppermint, in the form of a cough lozenge or medicated ointment, felt that they could breathe better? Some surprising studies report that inhaling menthol does not increase airflow through nasal passages.[22, 23] But it does stimulate cold receptors in the nose, making you more aware of air moving through you nose, which is pleasing if you are congested.[24] However, more recent studies have reassured us that the relief we perceive is literally not all in our heads. Menthol does open passages in the lungs by relaxing involuntary muscles around bronchioles.[25]

Like most other plant oils, the monoterpenes in peppermint oil, such as menthol, are modestly antiviral,[26] antifungal,[27] and antibacterial.[28] They can also irritate your *own* cells if peppermint oil is applied directly to your skin in its pure form.[29]

THE BOTTOM LINE

- Peppermint relaxes involuntary muscles in the digestive tract and helps some types of indigestion, but it can make other types of indigestion worse.
- Peppermint often relieves diarrhea, gas, and bloating. It may or may not relieve constipation, depending on the cause of the constipation. If you are sensitive to gastroesophageal reflux, it makes stomach acid more likely to burn your throat, unless you take an enteric-coated or delayed-release form.
- The menthol in peppermint is a skin-soluble local anesthetic, and it stimulates your cold-sensitive nerves, making you feel cool.
- Peppermint oil should not be applied to the faces of infants or small children, because they can go into respiratory arrest.
- Peppermint oil can irritate skin.

RED CLOVER

Trifolium pratense

History and Folklore

Clover was important in ancient crops, as it is today, as livestock forage and ground cover. It has an extensive symbolic history, too. For Christians, its classic, three-leaf pattern was used to represent the Holy Trinity. Clover leaves also evolved into a symbol for the clubs playing-card suit from the tarot deck's wands or rods suit. And though you can find some five-leaf clovers, four-leaf clovers are rare and considered lucky.

Depending on the color of its flowers, clover is known as either *white clover, yellow clover,* or *red clover.* White and yellow clover both belong to a different genus (*Melilotus*) than red clover, and both are sometimes called *sweet clover.* Sweet clovers are less commonly refered to in herbal literature today. Red clover as an herb is more thoroughly researched. Red clover's pink, egg-shaped blossoms are the most often used part of the herb, and country kids know they can suck the sweet nectar from them. The blooms make a mild sweet tea that was once a common beverage. It was recommended for whooping cough and bronchial distress, menstrual problems, and as an "alterative" or tonic. It was also once commonly thought to fight cancer, an issue that is still debated today.

How Scientists Think Red Clover Works

Your body turns red clover isoflavones into soy isoflavones. Red clover isoflavones are principally biochanin A and formononetin. After you eat them, biochanin A and formononetin go straight to your liver, where liver enzymes immediately transform them into genistein and daidzein. These are the same two molecules that soy isoflavones end up becoming after they are eaten.

The only difference between red clover's biochanin A and formononetin and soy's genistein and daidzein is that the red clover isoflavones both have attached to them a pattern of atoms called a *methyl,* which your body can, and apparently does, turn into soy's alternate pattern, a *hydroxyl* found on genistein and daidzein. This conversion has been proven both in people taking red clover isoflavones and in simulated liver processing of red clover isoflavones in the test tube. Red clover's formononetin becomes soy's daidzein, and red clover's biochanin A becomes soy's genistein. Soy's daidzein and genistein often start off in the soy plant with attached sugars (as daidz*in* and genist*in,* respectively), but these are promptly removed by gut bacteria prior to absorption. In other words, both pairs of isoflavones from either plant end up becoming the same two molecules in your blood.

All of these isoflavones are more or less estrogenic, and in red clover they are the presumed active ingredients. In fact, "red clover" supplements often contain nothing but the purified isoflavones from the plant. Yet both red clover and soy will end up giving you the same two molecules, genistein and daidzein. Therefore, the therapeutic effects of both soy and red clover isoflavones should be identical, theoretically. Research is confirming this, though different people may vary in their liver enzymes' ability to convert both plants' isoflavones to the same two molecules, which would cause subtle differences in the effects for some individuals.

What's In It

RED CLOVER isoflavones are principally biochanin A, formononetin, as well as daidzein, genistein, and their glycosides. Red clover possesses coumarins like coumestrol and medicagol. It also has some salicylates like methyl salicylic acid, as well as cyanogenic glycosides.

There is a second level of processing that follows the first. Whether from soy or red clover, daidzein and genistein, once they are in the blood, are further altered in the same manner. This usually makes them more water soluble, speeding their evacuation through urine. This secondary alteration is more variable than the first, from person to person— different people turn daidzein and genistein into different things. According to the study on people eating isoflavones from soy and red clover, there was less variability in people's ability to turn red clover isoflavones and soy isoflavones into the same two molecules (daidzein and genistein) as there was in their conversion of daidzein and genistein to other metabolites. The variability in these final metabolites from person to person may in part explain why the actions of either soy or red clover isoflavones in people are so inconsistent from person to person. Therefore, red clover may affect one person differently than another, and the same can also be said for soy.

Red clover isoflavones, processed or not, are partial estrogen agonists. An agonist is a drug that binds to a receptor and mimics the action of the substance that ordinarily binds to that receptor. *Partial* agonists do this, too, only weakly. This means that red clover isoflavones do some of the same things that estrogen does, only they do it less effectively. They can be so incompetent at the job, in fact, that they can end up blocking estrogen from sticking to its receptor, blocking estrogen's action, becoming antiestrogens. This is precisely what makes isoflavones so fickle in their activity and so difficult to pin down in terms of what they do. They may either act like estrogen or block the action of estrogen. (This partial estrogenic action is also true for the original, unprocessed red clover isoflavones, assuming they somehow escape the usual processing. Their structure possesses a pattern of atoms called a *methyl group* that gets in the way of their firmly docking with the estrogen receptor. This makes them even weaker estrogens than the rest of the isoflavones.) Whether any of these isoflavones work like estrogen or work against it may depend on whether your estrogen is high or low.

Theoretically, if your estrogen is low (as it generally is in men and in postmenopausal women who are not taking hormone therapy), isoflavones act as a weak estrogen replacement. They can do what estrogen does to a limited extent. They stick to estrogen's receptors in cells, stimulating the cell to make estrogen-associated proteins. These proteins are associated with the growth of sex glands and bone, among other things. Therefore, people have been interesting in trying them as hormone replacement therapy in menopausal women.

They bind a little better to estrogen B receptors than A receptors. Estrogen B receptors predominate in the bone, heart, blood vessels, and bladder, and some studies, but not all, suggest they may exert some effects there. They don't stick very well to either, however, which is what can make them antiestrogens. If your estrogen is high (as in premenopausal women), a partial estrogen agonist is more likely to sit ineptly in estrogen's receptor, blocking the activity of the more active estrogen. Since estrogen stimulates the growth of certain cancers, especially those in the sex glands, some have hoped that isoflavones might act against these cancers. Yet due to their possible estrogenic action, this could backfire. Red clover's ambivalent estrogenic behavior puts its use for cancer on the fence for now. Its possible exacerbation of cancer isn't supported by evidence and remains theoretical. However, scientists are prudently holding back on recommending it for treating or preventing cancer until this concern is better addressed with experimental data.

While the National Cancer Institute does affirm that soy products do lower the potential for several types of cancer, this is likely due to other factors in soy that are not in red clover (cholesterol-lowering sterols and substitution of soy protein for the more carcinogenic meat products). Whether *isoflavones* from either plant fight cancer or cause it remains an unanswered question for now.

One thing that red clover has that soy does not is coumarins. You have probably smelled coumarin when you mow the lawn—it imparts its sweet odor to new-mown clover hay. The coumarin and coumarin-like molecules ("coumarins") in all types of clover are famous, and in some cases they are infamous. In the 1920s farmers couldn't understand why some of their livestock sporadically died after suffering internal hemorrhaging. They used more clover-derived hay than we do today, and they more often stored it in silos. Since the weather was unusually wet, the hay tended

to rot in the silo. Mold can metabolize clover's less active coumarin-like molecules into coumarin, which is a potent blood thinner. The livestock were dying from a blood thinner.

The blood-thinning drug warfarin (researched by the Wisconsin Alumni Research Foundation, or WARF) was developed from coumarin. At first doctors were unsure of what dose was safe, so at one time it was used only in rat poison. The dose was elucidated in part from survivors either accidentally or intentionally swallowing the rat poison, and it has evolved into a common blood-thinning drug today. Both warfarin and the coumarins in clover work through their resemblance to the structure of vitamin K, the blood-clotting vitamin. They block vitamin K from working.

The action of coumarins in most red clover preparations, however, is weak, and of course absent in purified isoflavones, but you should keep it in mind if you are thinking of using the whole herb or parts of the red clover plant. Even the isoflavones resemble coumarin somewhat structurally, though less so, and they aren't known for blood-thinning activity. Just realize that red clover plant material could thin your blood, and it's probably not a good idea for your tea bag of red clover to get moldy.

One coumarin in red clover should make pregnant women think twice about taking it regularly. The coumestrol in red clover resembles diethylstilbestrol (DES), and according to some, behaves like it. DES is a particularly insidious sort of toxin, because the injury it causes stretches out over two generations, making it difficult to detect. Between 1931 and 1971 many women took this synthetic estrogen to prevent miscarriage. Its use was halted by the FDA upon discovery that it caused the daughters of these women to have an increased risk of reproductive abnormalities and a type of cancer called *clear cell adenocarcinoma*. The mothers themselves suffered an increased risk of breast cancer. Although women have stopped taking DES, DES daughters are still being discovered, because only a portion of the women taking it learned about why it was discontinued. There are far too few studies with red clover to determine if its coumestrol works the same way, but to be on the safe side, pregnant women shouldn't use red clover therapeutically on a regular basis.

Good Effects . . . and Not So Good

Red clover is probably safe, for the most part. Studies with isolated red clover isoflavones haven't turned up any obvious risks, nor have soy isoflavones, for that matter. As for the plant, the FDA includes in on its "Generally Recognized as Safe" (GRAS) list, and it is not associated with any outstanding complaints. Both forms of red clover have precautions, however.

It's not for the pregnant. Isolated isoflavones have different hormonal activities in different people, and their influence on fetal development isn't known. Besides, the coumestrol in red clover might be comparable to the birth defect–spawning drug diethylstilbestrol. The rare, limited encounter with red clover probably won't hurt a pregnant woman, but she should not use it regularly.

Watch out for bleeding. The herb, but not the isolated isoflavones, has the blood-thinning coumarin. Though red clover isn't known for its blood-thinning power, certain preparations could have more than others. For most people, a little blood thinning is good—it's better not to form dangerous

blood clots. However, if you are already on blood-thinning medication or have a bleeding disorder, be careful.

Don't treat your cancer without expert assistance. Even though isoflavones are weak as estrogens, some scientists worry about isoflavone's potential to stimulate estrogen-sensitive cancers. The issue is not resolved, because they could theoretically block estrogen, too, and fight these cancers. The National Cancer Institute is even initiating a trial for isoflavones in men with prostate cancer. Be that as it may, it's dangerous to try this on your own. If you have cancer, talk to a doctor first before trying any sort of herb, because different types of cancers can respond to the same herb in diverse ways.

Evidence of Action

If red clover's isoflavones end up becoming the same thing in your body as isolated soy isoflavones—and one test of people taking both show they do[1]—then, according to the soy studies, they don't do much. Soy's isoflavones have been much more thoroughly tested than red clover's, and they show little or no effect on hot flashes, bone loss, and cognitive ability. Blood levels of lipids like cholesterol or triglycerides aren't much budged by them either.

Just in case red clover's isoflavones *are* different somehow (and this seems biochemically unlikely), here's a summary of what human clinical trials of people taking them say.

The benefits of red clover's isoflavones are unpredictable. Studies of red clover isoflavones sometimes reveal moderate benefits in hot flashes, bone density, and blood lipids, but not always. They at least show no destructive tendencies. Most of the investigations, listed below, are well designed, with placeboes and double-blind designs, and many use the commercial products Promensil, Rimostil, or both.

Red clover's effects on mental skills are inconclusive, but this is based on limited evidence. After menopause, some people take isoflavones to prevent "senior moments"— that is, age-related dysfunction in cognitive skills. Thirty postmenopausal women took either red clover isoflavones or a placebo for six months and were then given assorted cognitive tests.[2] At first it appeared that the isoflavones caused a significant increase in visual-spatial skills but a significant *decrease* in skills related to digital recall and verbal memory. Perhaps alarmed by this, the authors reprocessed their data, applying stricter statistical restrictions, and found none of the effects to be significant.

Perhaps the most common use for red clover is in treating hot flashes. As with soy's isoflavones, most studies show red clover doesn't help.[3, 4, 5] However, one supplement with a higher concentration of biochanin A and genistein (Promensil) was better than another (Rimostil) at reducing the duration of a hot flash but not the number of hot flashes,[6] and in a different trial Promensil significantly reduced hot flashes with respect to a control group.[7]

Red clover's effects on blood lipids are variable, but at least they don't hurt. Although a couple of investigations on blood lipids reveal it exerts no change in blood lipids (cholesterol, LDL, HDL, and triglycerides),[8, 9] others showed a small but significant decrease in triglycerides.[10, 11] The effect on blood lipids could theoretically depend on who is taking the isoflavones and the type of isoflavones they are taking. Type 2 diabetics weren't able to alter their HDL or LDL cholesterol with it.[12] On the other hand, older men, but not postmenopausal

women, significantly reduced their LDL ("bad") cholesterol better when taking a supplement with more of one red clover isoflavones, biochanin, than other men who took a supplement with more of the other red clover isoflavone, formononetin.[13] HDL ("good") cholesterol was boosted significantly for postmenopausal, but not perimenopausal women.[14] Red clover isoflavones in the form of Rimostil also significantly increased HDL, but no placebo was used in this study, making the results questionable, and increasing doses of Rimostil weren't correlated with increasing benefits in HDL.[15]

Commonly Reported Uses for Red Clover*

Internally

premenstrual and menstrual problems, menopausal symptoms, hypercholesterolemia, osteoporosis, cancer, respiratory problems

forms available for internal use:

isoflavone supplements, capsule, dried flower heads, tea, infusion, extract

commonly reported dosage:

Isoflavone supplements suggest consumers take 40–160 milligrams of isoflavones daily. The flower heads are usually steeped in hot water for tea.

*These uses and dosages are from historic use and are not necessarily tested nor recommended.

The apparent effects of red clover's isoflavones on blood vessels are interesting. A couple of studies hint that they could reduce blood "resistance."[16, 17] The resistance to the flow of blood can be caused by constricted vessels, or by increased stickiness or viscosity of the blood running through them. One of these showed that this also occurred with no change in the dilation of blood vessels, suggesting the effect might be related to blood thinning. (If red clover's isoflavones aren't purified sufficiently from its coumarin-like compounds, its coumarins could theoretically thin the blood, too.) This was accompanied by significantly reduced arterial stiffness, a sign of atherosclerosis and increased risk of cardiovascular disease. The second study found that those taking the isoflavones also had a significant daytime drop in blood pressure compared to those taking a placebo.

Another measure of blood vessel integrity is protein glycation. This is a negative event that occurs with high blood sugar; therefore diabetics commonly suffer from it. It involves glucose permanently sticking to blood vessel proteins, which damages the blood vessels and can shut off the blood supply to various organs. Red clover isoflavones failed to lessen protein glycation in type 2 diabetics.[18] It appears to have no effect on blood sugar or insulin either.[19]

There is insufficient evidence yet to clarify red clover isoflavone's effect on osteo-porosis, but it doesn't seem to hurt. A couple of studies report women who took the isoflavones had significantly increased bone density, although one of these showed it only in the lower spine but not the hip,[20] while the other trial's results are highly questionable, since it had no control group.[21] The more reliable investigation also showed that although markers of bone reabsorption (breakdown) were unchanged, markers of bone formation were significantly increased.

Some people think isoflavones could prevent cancer, while others worry it might stimulate it. As with soy *isoflavones,* no link between red clover isoflavones and cancer has been established, but not enough research has been done on the subject. (Soy *protein* however, does reduce cancer risk, see page 286). In women with a type of breast density distribution associated with an increased risk of cancer, red clover isoflavones didn't change their breast density, nor did it change hormones such as estrogen, LH, or FSH.[22] Also, it didn't seem to affect endometrial proliferation in women taking it, but the study was short and had only a small number of participants.[23] Some investigators reexamined old prostate tissue biopsies of men with prostate cancer who were taking red clover isoflavones

THE BOTTOM LINE

- Most people use red clover's isoflavones, which have partial estrogen agonist activity.
- Red clover isoflavones are metabolized rapidly to become the same thing that soy isoflavones turn into in your body.
- There is insufficient evidence so far to recommend red clover isoflavones for any use, because clinical studies' results are underwhelming and highly variable.
- Red clover herb may contain blood-thinning coumarins and a theoretical birth defect–causing agent.
- Red clover is generally safe, but certain people should be careful using it, such as cancer patients and people on blood-thinning medications or with bleeding problems. Pregnant and nursing women should not use it therapeutically.

and compared them to samples from men who were not taking red clover. Although they found a benefit in a significantly increased number of apoptotic cells—that is, cancer cells that elect to "commit suicide" in a neat, helpful way—no other positive parameter of several concerning prostate cancer could be found.[24]

RED PEPPER
Capsicum annum or Capsicum frutescens

History and Folklore

Also called *capsicum, chili pepper,* and *cayenne pepper,* red pepper is a member of the *Solanaceae* family of plants and is native to South America. (Black pepper is an unrelated plant from Africa.) The ancient version of these peppers took the form of small, spicy berries. As early as BCE 7000, South American Indians started using them in cooking. Until European explorers brought this tropical plant to India, Africa, China, and Indonesia, the traditionally hot meals we now commonly associate with these countries did not include red pepper. Different cultures developed new varieties, from the mild Hungarian pepper (paprika) to the fiery South American Habanero. Botanists have recorded over ninety varieties.

People who investigate various cultural cuisines commonly wonder why the hottest countries feature the spiciest foods, while the coolest countries use blander seasonings. The habit of adding plants with violent tastes to food was very likely a means of preserving it without refrigeration. Before refrigerators were invented, using other refrigeration methods—i.e., ice and cold running streams—wasn't much of an option in the tropics. The only other convenient means of preserving food was to liberally spice it with some antibacterial herbs. The pungent oils of most spices are manufactured by plants to keep microbes from attacking the plant, so the antibacterial activity of herbal oils is widespread (but usually too nonspecific to pay much attention to). The presence of abundant red pepper and other spices dis-couraged the growth of bacteria, at the risk of discouraging the diner. There was an added but dubious "benefit": Should the spices fail to retard spoilage, they could still mask a rotten taste. Red pepper was also used to relieve indigestion and gas, to relieve sinus congestion, headache, and muscle pain. It also has a reputation of being an aphrodisiac (but don't try it for that use topically, it will probably backfire).

How Scientists Think Red Pepper Works

Even without taste buds, red pepper would still burn your mouth. Red pepper oil contains capsaicinoids, alkaloids that resemble vanillin from vanilla. They don't taste like vanilla, however. The most abundant capsaicinoid in the mixture is capsaicin (cap-SAY-sin). When you eat red pepper, you do not actually taste capsaicin with your taste buds. Like other oil-soluble, small molecules, it has the ability to penetrate tissues. It slowly moves through tissues in your mouth to trigger deeper nerves, and the classic burning sensation slowly grows. Since humans can detect one part per million, a little bit goes a long way.

Paradoxically, it relieves pain, but it isn't your usual counterirritant. This painful plant is used topically *very carefully* for pain relief, and it seems to work. At first scientists provided the classic old "counterirritant theory" to explain why: The pain caused by the herb works as a distraction from the original pain. This is sort of like hitting your thumb with a hammer so you can forget your headache, which is not the most appealing pain-relieving mechanism available. Some counterirritant action may in part explain how red pepper works. However, experimenters have unearthed a far more promising mechanism.

The capsaicin in red pepper fools your brain into sensing heat when there isn't any. Acting just like one of your own neurotransmitters, capsaicin binds to a nerve cell receptor called the *VR1 receptor* and temporarily changes the shape of the receptor. The VR1 receptor is ordinarily deformed by temperatures greater than approximately 42°C (108°F), and its change in shape opens the nerve cell's gates to charged particles called *ions*. Ions then flood into the nerve cell, producing a signal to a second nerve cell. The signal travels from nerve cell to nerve cell to reach the brain, and pain, perceived as heat, is felt. You think you are hot, but you're not. You even respond as if you are hot—for example, it makes you sweat.

Capsaicin relieves pain by depleting your nerve cells' supply of substance P, the "bad pain" neurotransmitter. Physicians classify pain as "good pain" or "bad pain." Although it may be difficult to admit that any pain could be "good," in fact, the short-term (acute) pain that you feel when you accidentally rest your fingers on a hot stove instructs you to jerk your hand away before it is burned, so it is good. "Bad pain" is long-term (chronic) pain, and is mediated by a different neurotransmitter than the one that signals good pain. Nerves that send good pain signals are fast, but nerves that send bad pain signals are slow, and they generate chronic, long-term pain.

The bad pain neurotransmitter is called *substance P* (the "P," of course, stands for pain). Just like "bad" pain, capsaicin also causes your bad pain nerves to deliver their substance P to other pain nerves leading up to the brain, and pain is felt. However, capsaicin does this so readily that the bad pain nerves lose their substance P all at once, depleting them of substance P. Initially capsaicin causes a brief sensation of pain, but since it causes such rapid dumping of the substance P supply, the nerves are no longer able to send a pain signal to the brain, because they are all out of substance P and don't have time to make any more.

CAPSAICIN BINDING to VR1 receptors initially triggers the release of the bad pain transmitter, substance P, but substance P does not bind capsaicin's VR1 receptors. As substance P travels from nerve cell to nerve cell up to the brain, it binds different receptors, called *NK1 receptors*. New therapeutics blocking NK1 receptors may also prove another method of relieving pain, since NK1 receptors are involved in sending pain messages to the brain. Incidentally, the dominant neurotransmitter signaling "good pain" is glutamate.

Whether capsaicin helps depends: are you feeling good pain or bad pain? Bad pain nerves signal slowly, because they are poorly insulated—insulation along segments of nerves in vertebrates allows the signal to jump faster from gap to gap in between each insulated segment. With less of this signal-accelerating insulation, bad pain signals build slowly but take a long time to die down. These are the same slow-signaling nerves that are active in arthritis and other types of chronic conditions, and capsaicin applied topically seems useful in dulling this pain. Fast nerves are more heavily insulated and conduct good pain, which is felt only briefly. If you burn yourself lightly on a stove and your bad pain nerves don't kick in to join the slow ones' complaint, capsaicin may not help your "good" pain get any better.

What's In It

RED PEPPER oil contains capsaicinoids, alkaloids that resemble vanillin from vanilla, oddly enough, yet an 8- to 10-carbon hydrocarbon is tacked on to the completely reduced aldehyde carbon of vanillin using an amide linkage. Most of these are capsaicin (32–38 percent) and dihydrocapsaicin (18–52 percent). The carotenoid pigments include carotene, capsanthin, alpha-carotin, and violaxanthine. Apiin and luteolin glycoside are the major flavonoids, and the mixture of steroid saponins in the seeds are collectively called *capsicidine.* The pepper also has a significant amount of vitamin C.

A new discovery reveals that your brains are spicier than you think. You don't have capsaicin in your brain, but you have similar-looking molecules called *endogenous capsaicin analogues.* You even have VR1 receptors in your brain for them to bind, but we aren't exactly sure of exactly what happens when they do. It seems they are used to signal to your brain that something is wrong in your body, and they enhance your perception of pain. For example, VR1 receptors on the heart were recently discovered, too, and the way you feel a heart attack coming on is that your own version of capsaicin binds to these receptors on your heart. They may have other physiological effects as well, like on blood pressure and respiratory airway constriction.

Capsaicin could point us toward a brand new class of pain relievers. Researchers are currently at work using this information to produce a new class of VR1 receptor blockers as painkillers. Unlike traditional painkillers that work like aspirin or morphine, they could theoretically address pain more directly and have fewer side effects. One called *capsazepine,* for example, kept rodents from feeling extreme, sensitizing pain.[1] Because capsazepine and other members of this new class of pain relievers resemble capsaicin, they are called *capsaicin analogues.* Although it will be exciting to see what drugs researchers can synthesize to relieve pain in new ways, the red pepper plant has beat them to it.

Good Effects . . . and Not So Good

It's nutritious if you can stomach it. The red color of the peppers is from carotene, the same plant pigment molecule that makes carrots orange. Carotene is used by our bodies to make vitamin A, and red peppers are also a surprisingly good source of vitamin C: One small red pepper pod contains more vitamin C than a cup of orange juice.

Red pepper can burn you twice. Capsaicin is not chemically altered by your gut after it is eaten, and any extra capsaicin you do not absorb retains its burning power all the way toward the bitter end. Thus excessive capsaicin can induce a painfully unpleasant bowel movement. Doctors have invented the term "jalapeño-proctitis" for this unpleasant phenomenon.

Here's how to remove it from your mouth and other painful places. The first step is prevention. Cooks recommend wearing rubber gloves to handle red peppers. To relieve skin irritation from red pepper, gently washing with *cold,* not hot, soapy water should be tried first. (Heat will deform the VR1 receptors even more, which is what the capsaicin is already doing.) Then, since capsaicin is oil soluble, fatty, oily things may help remove it. This is effective for burning sensations in the mouth as well. There are anecdotal reports of using milk, but relieving the burn might not work so well with skim milk, although the protein in milk may help remove capsaicin even if the milk has no fat in it. Eating buttered bread for a burning mouth is another folk remedy, but it could work in theory because of the butter. Cold beer is rumored to help as well.

Substance P makes your nose run. Capsaicin causes pain-signaling nerves to rapidly export their substance P, but substance P is more than a pain-signaling neurotransmitter. It also stimulates inflammatory processes, and if you eat enough red pepper, the consequent substance P dumping inflames your nose a bit, making it run. Some people turn this to their advantage if they are congested, and thus it is included in folkloric cold remedies.

For topical pain relief, a prepared product is probably a safer bet than doing it yourself. Such prepared products can now be found in most standard grocery stores. The FDA has approved the use of over-the-counter pain-relieving topical creams containing up to 0.075 percent capsaicin. Higher concentrations can cause unpleasant burning, worsening the pain. One medical reference tells doctors to advise their patients that they can wash off the cream with watered-down vinegar if they dislike the cream's effect.[1]

Watch where you put it. Since care must be taken not to introduce capsaicin into cuts, wounds, the eyes, or mucous membranes, some preparations come with a

Commonly Reported Uses for Red Pepper*

Internally

stimulant, poor circulation, indigestion, gas, severe or chronic pain, headache, cold symptoms such as chills, nasal congestion, inflammation, ulcers, blood clots, cholesterol reduction, cardiovascular disease, weight loss

forms available for internal use:

peppers, fresh or dried, capsules, concentrated drops, dried pepper flakes or powder, tea, tincture

commonly reported dosage:

The pepper is taken in doses of 30–120 milligrams up to three times daily. The tincture is given doses of 0.6–2 milliliters.

Externally

muscle soreness, chronic pain, back and neck pain, diabetic neuropathy, shingles, rheumatory and osteoarthritis, fibromyalgia, circulatory stimulant

forms available for external use:

creams or gels containing up to 0.075 percent capsaicin, the maximum amount allowed by the FDA

commonly reported dosage:

Three to four applications per day are recommended for maximum effectiveness. Some publications report it sometimes takes two weeks for maximum pain relief.

*These uses and dosages are from historic use and are not necessarily tested nor recommended.

ball roller, stick applicator, or patch in order to minimize this risk. Some do not, however. Anyone who accidentally transfers a little red pepper under the fingernails to a more delicate area of the body is unlikely to forget the painful result. Even after washing your hands thoroughly, a trace left on your fingers can remain for hours and be transferred to your eyeball if you change your contact lenses. The result is agony.

It could keep your feet warm. Some winter sports enthusiasts sprinkle red pepper powder in their socks, as this reportedly keeps feet toasty; in fact, red pepper powder is now being sold commercially for footwarming purposes. My mother, who suffers from poor circulation in her feet, has tried putting red pepper powder in her socks, but warns our family not to contaminate underwear drawers with socks that have been used for this purpose.

Interesting Facts

New commercial products are incorporating capscaicin.

THERE ARE some fascinating, new, products being made with capsaicin. For example, capsaicin incorporated inside veterinary sutures can prevent pets from gnawing off their stitches. And a new capsaicin-spiked paint is being tested on fiber-optic cable to prevent the cables from being chewed by rodents. The paint has even been used on boats to repel barnacles.

Capsaicin could also keep lessen the competition for your birdfeeders by creatures other than birds. In a red pepper–eating contest, even the most macho, curry-guzzling, salsa-swigging braggart would be knocked out of first place by a bird. Although mammals are affected by capsaicin, birds are not. They have a different type of VR1 receptor. The bird VR1 receptor responds to heat but is indifferent to capsaicin. Birdwatchers have observed birds nonchalantly dining on red peppers, and later these birds deposit the undigested seeds, facilitating the plant's distribution. Some inquisitive birdwatcher got the idea to lace their birdseed with capsaicin. This red pepper birdseed mix is now sold commercially. Birds happily eat the seed, while rodents avoid it. The capsaicin-eating birds reportedly suffer no adverse effects. Indeed, the trace carotenoids and vitamins in the spice are said to give them extra pep.

Evidence of Action

Well-designed clinical trials have repeatedly confirmed that topical red pepper creams are indeed quite helpful in treating a number of painful conditions, including rheumatoid arthritis,[2] osteoarthritis,[3] and neuralgias such as shingles,[4] and diabetic neuropathy.[5] It also proved effective in treating lower back pain[6] and, in a preliminary pilot study, chronic neck pain.[7] It could possibly help those with fibromyalgia, but more study is required to confirm this.[8] A few people in these studies do not tolerate the treatment, and some have especially adverse reactions to it. Others had to apply the cream several times a day for a week until they noticed positive results.

Red pepper apparently generates indigestion in some people but relieves it in others. For people who suffered ordinary chronic indigestion (without gastrointestinal reflux disease or irritable bowel syndrome), red pepper significantly reduced discomfort.[9] On the other hand, another study shows that in people who routinely had heartburn, it made their heartburn more painful.[10]

There is some controversy over eating red pepper for ulcers. It could theoretically help, and endoscopies proved capsaicin significantly protected people who did *not* have ulcers from aspirin-generated stomach injury.[11] Some have suggested it might help ulcer patients by killing the infecting *Helicobacter* bacterium frequently associated with the ulcers. Even though red pepper has bactericidal activity in the test tube, *most* herbs do, and care must be taken when extrapolating test tube studies to people. When people with *Helicobacter*-associated ulcers ate red pepper, it did not have any effect on their infections.[12] It may yet still help ulcers by other mechanisms, but more data is needed to render a conclusion.

THE BOTTOM LINE

- Red pepper contains capsaicin, which depletes nerve cells of a pain-signaling molecule called *substance P*. Red pepper creams applied topically appear successful in relieving certain types of pain.
- Red pepper creams can cause painful burning sensations if applied too liberally or when used near sensitive areas like the eyes and mucous membranes.
- Through its substance P-depleting mechanism, red pepper may help certain types of indigestion, including ulcers, but may make other kinds of indigestion worse, like heartburn. More experimental data is needed to support the effectiveness of this treatment.
- Humans make molecules similar to red pepper's capsaicin. Blocking their action may lead to the invention of a new class of pain medications.

SAGE
Salvia officinalis, Salvia lavandulafolia

History and Folklore

Today, many people regard sage as merely an essential flavoring in traditional stuffing. Appearances notwithstanding, this herb previously enjoyed a more sensational reputation. Herbalists from China, India, Europe, and North America have at one time or another recommended it for almost everything. Its genus *Salvia* stems from the Latin *salvus,* which means "health" and is related to the word *salvage.* "Why should he die, whose garden groweth sage?" a tenth-century Roman queried. A medieval exposition declared "The desire of sage is to render man immortal." And if that is not enough for you to be impressed, an old proverb instructs, "He that would live for aye, must eat sage in May."

With all these astonishing recommendations, it may be anticlimactic for you to learn that sage's principal therapeutic use today in herbal medicine is as an antiperspirant. Like so many other members of the mint family (*Labiacea*) (catnip, page 62; lavender, page 208; lemon balm, page 213; and peppermint, page 246), it is also used for digestive upset like cramps or gas. Warm sage tea has a good reputation as a soothing, astringent gargle for sore throat and canker sores and is also recommended for superfluous saliva, though that is not a widespread ailment. Sage has popped up on the radar screen of scientists lately, however, elevating its potential status beyond that of antiperspirants and drool stoppers. An association between its legendary distinction as a memory aid and its effect on the brain in treating Alzheimer's disease has gained credibility.

How Scientists Think Sage Works

Sage's tannins explain its astringent skin- and mouth-drying effects. Tannins are common plant molecules that act as a natural defense against insects and microorganisms. Tannins bind to proteins and pull them together, "tanning" a protein-containing surface such as skin. Tannins bind to several proteins at once, a phenomenon called *cross-linking,* and this makes the proteins dysfunctional. Cross-linking the proteins exposed on a plant pest renders the intruder inoperative. Tannins cause the drying, constricting sensation felt in the mouth after consuming tea, red wine, red grapes, and certain nuts. You actually "tan the hide" of your mouth with them. This is not really a flavor but a quality called *astringency.* Drinking or gargling sage tea "tans" the lining of the throat and gut, which forms a temporary, tough barrier. The barrier reduces secretions, and, in the case of the gut, reduces contact with irritants that cause diarrhea.[1] However, excess tannins can cause gastric distress. The antiperspirant activity of externally applied sage extract results from this astringent, barrier-forming action of tannins on skin, which would otherwise release sweat.

Sage could also affect one of your neurotransmitters, acetylcholine. Like other neurotransmitters, acetylcholine is released by one nerve cell and diffuses to a nearby nerve cell, thereby transmitting impulses. But should acetylcholine persist, the impulse would continue unabated, with detrimental paralytic, even deadly, consequences. Fortunately a second molecule, acetylcholin*esterase,* enters the scene to break

What Might You Expect if You *Really* Increase Your Acetylcholine?

ACETYLCHOLINE IS the neurotransmitter used by the so-called rest-and-digest parasympathetic nervous system, as opposed to the fight-or-flight sympathetic nervous system. While acetylcholine's actions vary from tissue to tissue and can be either excitatory or inhibitory, they generally produce behaviors not associated with the fight-or-flight (sympathetic) mode. That is, they tend to deal with more rest-related actions, such as digestion and dreaming.

There are far more potent acetylcholinesterase inhibitors than sage, and they boost acetylcholine to an extent that has killed people. For example, organophosphate insecticides are also acetylcholinesterase inhibitors, but they drastically increase acetylcholine to a point known by emergency care workers as a "SLUD" crisis. SLUD stands for "salivation, lachrymation (crying), urination, defecation," which are all classic acetylcholine overload symptoms. The problem with such acetylcholinesterase inhibitors such as organophosphate insecticides is that they *irreversibly* inhibit acetylcholinesterase. In this case, the amount of time cells need to make more acetylcholinesterase is too long for the patient to recover. Sage appears to be far milder that organophosphate insecticides, hampering a nerve cell's acetylcholinesterase action *reversibly*. Fortunately, sage and acetylcholinesterase-inhibiting drugs used for Alzheimer's are much milder than organophosphate insecticides in their action, and the Alzheimer's drugs do help prevent losses in memory. However, since these prescription drugs can have side effects, such as slow heartbeat, sweating, nausea, diarrhea, and vomiting, high doses of sage might in theory be expected to do the same.

down acetylcholine, preventing your acetylcholine-receptive nerve cells from firing incessantly. Sage inhibits acetylcholinesterase, and if you are into double negatives, here's the logic: it inhibits an acetylcholine destroyer, therefore it elevates acetylcholine. If acetylcholine is elevated excessively the situation can prove fatal, but for weak acetylcholinesterase inhibitors like sage, the consequent mild boost in acetylcholine may assist certain diseases where acetylcholine is in short supply.

Such an acetylcholine-boosting effect is well known in the pharmaceutical world, in the form of drugs called *acetylcholinesterase inhibitors* (*AChEIs*), also called *anticholinesterase* drugs. Acetylcholinesterase inhibitors are moderately helpful for symptomatic relief of memory loss in early Alzheimer's disease, because this disease impairs acetylcholine synthesis in particular.

Sage might be able to treat Alzheimer's disease, but will it cure it? Milder Alzheimer's disease is the leading cause of senior dementia and affects approximately 4.5 million Americans. The gradual loss of brain function associated with it has no cure, but prescription drugs afford some relief of memory loss. Since most of these drugs work by preventing the breakdown of acetylcholine, it is reasonable to expect that sage works the same way. Unfortunately, this does not address the underlying cause of Alzheimer's disease, which is not completely understood but involves inflammation and the brain's accumulation of a protein (beta-amyloid) that gums up its works, so to speak. Reduced insulin production in the brain has also recently been linked to the development of Alzheimer's disease. The prescription drugs that inhibit acetylcholinesterase do not cure Alzheimer's disease, so it's not likely that sage will either.

Sage may lead researchers toward discovering a completely new type of acetyl-

cholinesterase inhibitor. Many other plant-derived acetylcholinesterase inhibitors are known. They are too potent and too toxic for therapeutic use in Alzheimer's, but they all belong to a large class of plant molecules called *alkaloids*. Alkaloids are nitrogen-containing plant molecules that can have various profound effects on the brain and nervous system in general; some are stimulant, some are sedative, some relieve pain, others make you hallucinate, and still others act, like sage, as acetylcholinesterase inhibitors. However, the species of sage tested (*S. officinalis* and *S. lavandulafolia*) are not known to contain alkaloids, so it is surprising that sage also possesses acetyl-cholinesterase-inhibiting properties. Sage's active ingredient is thought to reside within a class of oily molecules called *monoterpenes,* instead. Many plants have different monoterpenes in their volatile oils. Monoterpenes, unlike alkaloids, are molecules that don't have nitrogen, and although some are mildly sedative, they aren't widely known for having specific effects on the brain or nervous system. Sage's isolated monoterpenes individually had weak anticholinesterase activity, but none of the monoterpenes on their own could account for the overall action of sage's oil. Therefore, these monoterpenes could act synergistically, which argues for consumption of the whole herb, which contains all the monoterpenes in the oil, rather than an isolated monoterpene.[2]

Sage could enhance your memory, maybe. Research indicates that increasing acetylcholine does aid memory slightly.[3, 4] Sage did improve the memories of healthy volunteers in one study.[5] However, images of desperate finals-week students gulping down sage, attempting to salvage (no pun intended) their grades should make you uneasy, because the most common type of sage contains a monoterpene called *thujone,* which is undeniably toxic. Famous artists

and writers once consumed thujone, and seizures, hallucinations, psychoses and suicides are associated with it.

What's In It

SAGE'S MEMORY-ENHANCING ingredient has yet to be identified, but an array of common monoterpenes are currently prime suspects, specifically: bornyl acetate, camphor, 1,8-cineole, and alpha- and beta-pinene. Other terpenes and terpenoids include ursolic acid, linalool, alpha- and beta-caryophyllene, and humulene. Like another putatively cholinergically active herb, lemon balm, it contains rosmarinic acid, and also the related chlorogenic acid. Thujone makes up 35 to 60 percent of *S. officinalis* oil, but *S. lavandulafolia* has essentially none. Its flavonoids include apigenin and luteolin glycosides, as well as various methoxylated flavonoid aglycones.

Some sage species contain thujone, a toxin with a colorful history. If thujone has acetylcholinesterase-inhibiting activity, it isn't the only monoterpene that does, because a sage species without thujone (*S. lavandulafolia*) showed acetylcholinesterase-inhibiting activity. So in theory you don't have to poison yourself with thujone in order to get the alleged memory-enhancing effect. Thujone is more commonly associated with an unrelated plant called *wormwood,* which you won't find in this book, because its toxicity overwhelms any therapeutic properties it might have. Wormwood had some acetylcholine receptor–binding properties similar to those of lemon balm (see page xx), another potential Alzheimer's herb, but again wormwood's thujone makes it too poisonous to use medicinally. To understand how sage can be toxic, it's helpful to take a look at wormwood.

Wormwood is named such because it is toxic to intestinal worms, but it is also toxic to humans and animals, so it should no longer be used as a dewormer. If you do have worms, you should immediately see a doctor, or at least a vet. Wormwood was an essential ingredient in the notorious beverage absinthe, and it made a lot of people lose their marbles. This emerald-green alcoholic drink, dubbed "the green fairy," was once very popular in the late nineteenth and early twentieth centuries, especially in France. Vincent van Gogh, Oscar Wilde, Pablo Picasso, Ernest Hemingway, Edgar Degas, Paul Gauguin, Edouard Manet, and Henri de Toulouse-Lautrec are just some of the famous people known to have enjoyed it. Its sale was outlawed in most countries after a public outcry brought attention to the resultant health epidemic from what was most likely thujone-induced brain damage. (The famously psychotic behavior of Vincent van Gogh is commonly attributed to his drinking absinthe, but then again, he also drank turpentine and ate paint, which suggests he was just mentally ill.) Since thujone is also in sage, cautions accompany the consumption of certain types of sage and sage extracts, as well.

Thujone from both sage and wormwood causes convulsions, coma, and even death if consumed in sufficient quantities. These effects are probably mediated by its ability to suppress the action of another neurotransmitter, GABA (gamma-amino butyric acid), by blocking GABA's receptor in the brain.[6] Because GABA inhibits nerve cell impulses, thujone causes nerve cells to fire uncontrollably, which helps explain thujone's psychoactive and brain-damaging reputation.[7] At one time scientists were

tempted to suggest that thujone behaved like marijuana, because thujone structurally resembles the active ingredient in marijuana, THC. However, thujone does not behave like THC in rat brains; it only very weakly interacts with the rat THC receptor and does not initiate any THC-related activity at that receptor.[8]

Although it is illegal in most countries, absinthe is making a comeback (it is still legally sold in Spain, Portugal, and the Czech Republic). And although modern absinthe has less thujone, it is not worth trying, no matter who once drank it, because it can cause permanent brain damage. Of course sage is quite legal, but its oil contains thujone as well. Thujone imparts one of the key aromas of sage. However, most cooking sage is dried, which can reduce the thujone-containing oil (by 2 to 25 percent),[9] and cooking evaporates off some of the thujone as well.[10] We can enjoy the taste of sage in our food from time to time and not risk psychosis. It may even bolster our memories. How sweetly ironic that a wise, experienced elder is still regarded as a "sage."

GOOD EFFECTS . . . AND NOT SO GOOD

Sage appears safe in externally applied applications. Sage can be used as a gargle for mouth and throat inflammations. To combat sweating, topical application may work better for you than eating it. *Internal* use of sage to combat sweating seems sketchy, because of its possible pharmacologic enhancement of acetylcholine, and acetylcholine induces sweating. *External* use of sage seems reasonable for this condition, however, because of the astringent action of its tannins on skin.

Commonly Reported Uses for Sage*

Internally

excessive perspiration, excessive salivation, indigestion, menstrual pains

forms available for internal use:

leaf infusion (tea), tincture, leaf (fresh and dried)

commonly reported dosage:

A small cup of tea made from a couple teaspoons of dried leaves is commonly recommended for the above complaints. However, this should not be taken regularly, because thujone can accumulate and cause brain damage. Cooking with sage is probably safe. Pure sage oil should never be ingested.

Externally

sore throat, excessive perspiration, excessive salivation

forms available for external use:

extracts, gargle, mouthwash, paste

commonly reported dosage:

The tea is gargled as needed for sore throat or excessive oral secretions. Pastes or aqueous extracts are applied to skin as an astringent or antiperspirant.

*These uses and dosages are from historic use and are not necessarily tested nor recommended.

Don't load up on sage if you are pregnant. Pregnant women are advised to avoid taking sage medicinally, because sage is thought by some to have estrogen-like properties. However, according to recent research, only one component in sage oil (the monoterpene geraniol) exhibited very weak binding to estrogen receptors in test tube studies.[11] Nonetheless, until studies more relevant to human beings are performed to clarify this action, it seems prudent to avoid sage if you are pregnant, just in case. Occasional pinches added to cooked foods are probably harmless.

Interesting Facts

One sage is not like the other.

SAGEBRUSH, which graces the Western deserts, resembles sage, because it also has bluish-gray leaves, and it smells somewhat similar. However, the desert plant is not related to sage. The reason it smells like sage may be that, like cooking sage, it also contains thujone. Sagebrush is more closely related to wormwood and is in the wormwood family (*Artemesia*). Another herb in the *Artemesia* family, which contains a relatively minor amount of thujone, is tarragon. Smell some tarragon and see if you think it smells slightly sagey. Opinions vary.

A hallucinogenic Mexican sage called *divining sage* (*S. divinorum*) is used ceremonially by Mazatec Indians of Oaxaca, Mexico. Unlike other species of sage, it contains molecules that interact with certain opioid receptors in the brain, and, as it is with the nerve cell–affecting molecules of cooking sage, it is again surprising that neurologically active molecules are not the nitrogen-containing alkaloids that ordinarily do such things, but are novel, non-nitrogen-bearing diterpenes.[15] Of course, an entire culture of *divinorum* users is arising worldwide, but don't play chemical games with your brain; it could cause brain damage. Researchers do hope, however, to learn enough about its active constituents to develop new therapeutics, a nobler goal than exploiting it for entertainment.

THE BOTTOM LINE

- An unidentified ingredient in sage inhibits acetylcholinesterase, an enzyme that breaks down the neurotransmitter acetylcholine. Sage could therefore boost acetylcholine.
- Increased acetylcholine may aid memory, and sage has helped decrease symptoms of early Alzheimer's disease.
- Most culinary sage species contain toxic thujone, which causes brain damage. *S. lavandulafolia,* or Spanish sage, has little or no thujone. Cooking dried sage results in a product with relatively little thujone. Thujone is probably not the acetylcholine-boosting component of sage.
- Sage oil should never be taken internally, because the thujone in it is toxic.
- Sage has a high tannin content. Tannins can dry oral secretions, soothe a sore throat, and relieve diarrhea. All tannin-containing preparations including sage should be used in moderation, because excessive amounts can cause gastric distress.

If you take sage internally on a regular basis, or large single doses of internal sage, use forms with low or no thujone. Because of its high thujone content, sage oil is toxic, causes convulsions in humans and animals, and *should not be ingested.* Frequent, long-term internal use of sage has been associated with thujone-induced mental deterioration, and large doses of sage have been associated with coma and convulsions.[12] Occasional cooking with sage-scented cooking oils and with sage itself is probably safe, since the heat of cooking evaporates off much of the thujone. Do not cook with pure sage oil, however.

Unfortunately, the most common species used for cooking contain thujone in their oils: *S. officinalis* (Dalmatian sage, harvested from the Dalmatian coast of Yugoslavia) and *S. fruticosa* (Greek sage). If you are genuinely worried about thujone, try finding the less popular *S. lavandulafolia,* or Spanish sage, which contains little to no thujone, but still demonstrates anticholinergic activity.[13] Sage's thujone content varies from season to season, being most toxic in winter, when the thujone content is the highest, and least toxic in the spring.[14] Perhaps *this* is what was meant by the old saying, "He that would live for aye, must eat sage in May." It should then be rephrased, "He that would not wish his brain to dismember, must not eat sage in December."

EVIDENCE OF ACTION

Despite much anecdotal evidence suggesting that sage aids overly sweaty people (a condition called *hyperhidrosis*), not enough research has been performed to support this claim concretely. A study as old as 1896 suggested that sage could stop perspiration, and more experiments in the early twentieth century appeared to confirm this. But in 1949, H. B. J. van Rijn failed to note any of these antiperspirant effects in small animals, although he did note that large doses of sage were toxic to them.[16] A 1998 study of thirty menopausal women treated with a combination of sage (*S. officinalis*) and alfalfa claims that 60 percent of the women stopped having night sweats, but unfortunately, there were no controls or means to sort out which herb was doing what. Although sage is approved for sweating by the German Commission E monographs, many of these monographs are outdated, and some scientists state there is no evidence as yet that it really helps this condition.[17]

S. lavandulafolia (Spanish sage) inhibits human acetylcholinesterase in the test tube, but since no specific molecule could account for the overall effect, a synergistic effect was proposed.[18] In rat brains, anticholinesterase activity of orally administered Spanish sage oil has been demonstrated as well.[19] It is noteworthy that this species does not have much or any of the toxic thujone, thus thujone is not likely responsible for inhibiting acetylcholinesterase.

More excitingly, in a placebo-controlled trial, forty-two Alzheimer's disease patients took sixty drops of sage extract (*S. officinalis*) per day over a four-month period and performed significantly better in cognitive tests than those in the control group.[20] A small, preliminary clinical trial designed to test patients' tolerance of sage noted that increased attention and fewer psychiatric symptoms were found in Alzheimer's disease patients taking sage.[21] In forty-four healthy volunteers, a double-blind, placebo-controlled study showed that Spanish sage oil improved word recall scores and significantly affected mood and cognitive skills.[22]

SAW PALMETTO

Serenoa repens, also called *Sabal serrulatum*

HISTORY AND FOLKLORE

This hardy, low-growing palm tree grows along the United States' Atlantic Coast scrub. It proved a handy, multipurpose resource used by the coasts' original occupants. The fibers of the serrated, fan-shaped palm leaves were used for making thatched huts, baskets, mattresses, straw hats, and paper. Birds also make nests from palmetto fibers. Saw palmetto's "berries," which resemble olives in size and color range, were used by the Atlantic Coast's native inhabitants as food and medicine and remain the focus of interest today. Originally claimed as a diuretic and sexual tonic, the nineteenth-century Eclectic physicians, a group of doctors who advocated the use of Native American remedies, promoted saw palmetto berries as "an old man's friend."

Imagine eating some olivelike fruits, only to find they taste like "soapy, rancid tobacco juice," which is the most common description of their flavor. They may be an acquired taste, though, because they were a staple of Atlantic Coast Native Americans, and some birds and mammals love them and seem no worse off for eating them. Though this rugged plant is not endangered, climate changes and two-legged competitors profiting off the now popular berries have wildlife watchers concerned about berry shortages.

HOW SCIENTISTS THINK SAW PALMETTO WORKS

Saw palmetto appears to hinder the formation of the more potent dihydrotestosterone from testosterone. For men, the bad thing about the hormone dihydrotestosterone is that it can stimulate excessive growth of prostate cells, leading to prostate enlargement and benign but uncomfortable symptoms. An enlarged prostate presses on both the bladder and shuts off the urine's prime escape route, the urethra, presenting a painful conflict of interest. Symptoms include increased urgency to urinate and difficulty doing so. This is known as *benign prostatic hyperplasia,* or *BPH,* and though it has no association with prostate cancer, it causes many older men grief.

For some unknown reason, the older a man gets, the more likely he is to turn testosterone into dihydrotestosterone, which is a more potent prostate stimulator. Both saw palmetto and the commonly prescribed BPH drug finasteride work by inhibiting the production of dihydrotestosterone, although they do so in different ways.

Saw palmetto allegedly inhibits both of your dihydrotestosterone-making enzymes, whereas finasteride inhibits one less than the other. The 5-alpha reductase (5AR) enzyme is responsible for converting testosterone into dihydrotestosterone, and thus this enzyme is in part culpable for causing BPH. However, the 5AR enzyme comes in two forms, or isozymes, called *5AR type I* and *5AR type II.* Both are in the human prostate, but 5AR II seems to be the major player in making dihydrotestosterone. Finasteride, a drug that is often effective in treating BPH, inhibits 5AR II, but only weakly inhibits 5AR I. Although 5AR I is not considered as offensive as 5AR II, some scientists think finasteride could work better if it inhibited both enzymes to the same extent. They are now testing new drug candidates for this dual activity, but according to test tube studies, saw palmetto already has this dual activity. This theoretically could give saw palmetto an advantage over finasteride.

Their potency is still up in the air, but it could be the berries' fatty acids that do the trick. Potency is important, because you don't want to have to take mountains of saw palmetto berries in order for it to be effective. Whether or not saw palmetto *potently* inhibits 5AR enzymes depends on what study you look at; some claim just a little bit will do the job, but others say it only weakly inhibits 5AR.[1] Although saw palmetto works as a 5AR inhibitor pretty well in test tube (*in vitro*) studies, it doesn't act as well in the real thing, the prostate. But some say it could exert an effect on the prostate by other mechanisms as well, like acting as an anti-inflammatory.

Although we aren't sure what the active ingredient or ingredients are, they are clearly oil soluble, and not found in water-based extracts. One study suggests it is the fatty acids from the berry that are the active agents, and if this is true, it is a surprise. Oil-soluble steroids are also present in the berry, and since steroids resemble our sex hormones, and have effects on them, most scientists expected saw palmetto's steroids to be its active ingredients. But according to this study, saw palmetto steroids had no effect on 5AR.[2]

One possible advantage of saw palmetto over finasteride is that it does not

seem to interfere with cancer diagnoses based on PSA. If you are a man over fifty, you should be getting your PSA, or prostate specific antigen, tested regularly to see how it changes over time. PSA is a normal substance made by the prostate to aid liquefaction of semen, but prostate damage or disease causes PSA to leak into the blood. Small amounts are normal, but increasing levels indicate prostate cancer, which can be treated if caught soon enough. A high PSA does not always signal cancer; for example, if the prostate is enlarged but benign as in BPH, more PSA may be made simply because there is more PSA-making tissue in the enlarged organ. Some drugs also interfere with PSA-based diagnostics, so it is only natural to ask whether saw palmetto also has this problem.

What's In It

THE ACTIVE ingredients of saw palmetto are thought to reside in the oil-based extract of the berries, though these have not been specifically identified. These oil-based extracts contain free fatty acids and tri-, di- and monoglycerides, mainly oleic and lauric acids (about 65 percent) and linoleic and myristic acids (about 15 percent). The oils also contain steroids such as beta-sitosterol and its esters. Saw palmetto also contains flavonoids and their glycosides, such as isoquercitrin, kaempferol, and rhoifolin.

The BPH drug finasteride (which is also used for hair loss under the name Propecia) lowers PSA, which thus lowers the chances of detecting prostate cancer. Finasteride lowers PSA by preventing the binding of a male hormone–activated complex to a portion of

DNA that instructs prostate cells to make more PSA. Saw palmetto does not do this.[3] So, theoretically, saw palmetto is less likely to interfere with diagnoses based on PSA. Even so, you should still inform your doctor if you are taking saw palmetto, because it may obscure other signs of cancer, like prostate size. Usually, however, saw palmetto doesn't reduce overall prostate size, but it has been known to shrink a portion lining the inside of the organ, the inner epitheium, a bit.

Saw palmetto could also reduce BPH symptoms with an anti-inflammatory kick. A damaged prostate sends out chemical signals recruiting white blood cells to the prostate, but the presence of these immune invaders in the prostate is not helpful. Like unruly soldiers, they contribute their own damage to the suffering prostate and are prime suspects in the development of BPH. In cell studies, saw palmetto appears to inhibit both 5-lipoxygenase[4] and COX-2,[5] which are two pro-inflammatory enzymes. 5-lipoxygenease makes white blood cell–recruiting agents called *leukotrienes,* and COX-2 creates inflammatory agents called *prostaglandins.* Increased COX-2 is even associated with a greater risk of prostate cancer. Although it's exciting that palmetto inhibits both COX-2 and lipoxygenase in the test tube, we still have not gathered data supporting these actions in actual people. If so, this anti-inflammatory activity could help reduce the problems associated with BPH.

GOOD EFFECTS . . .
AND NOT SO GOOD

If you take saw palmetto or have BPH symptoms, tell your physician. Although it seems relatively safe, and does not appear to affect PSA levels, saw palmetto might obscure other signs of prostate cancer. You should also see a doctor if you have symptoms of prostate enlargement, whether or not you take saw palmetto. These symptoms include increased frequency and need to urinate and difficultly doing so. Although BPH is not associated with prostate cancer, the symptoms are similar.

Saw palmetto tea probably won't work. Teas of the berry are sold, but though the active ingredient or ingredients are not specifically known, they are clearly in the oil from the berries. In general, teas from any herb do not possess very much of an herb's oils, simply because teas are water extracts, and oil and water do not mix. If the active ingredients in an herb are water soluble, an herbal tea will work, but this is not the case with saw palmetto. Therefore water-based extracts, such as a tea, will not give you enough active ingredient to work. Oil-based extracts of saw palmetto, on the other hand, are considered more effective.

Saw palmetto is a less expensive treatment for BPH than finasteride, but there are some concerns. Saw palmetto is an inexpensive treatment for BPH, but does cheaper equal better? One concern is that even standardized herbal products vary in ingredient levels, from batch to batch and from pill to pill, because they are not regulated. Also, while saw palmetto works for BPH, it is less likely to be effective for chronic prostatitis. Chronic prostatitis is a type of prostate inflammation that is less common than BPH, and what causes it is poorly understood, although in some cases it is caused by bacterial infection.

Why mess with your precious hormones for hair loss? Saw palmetto, on its own, *might* actually work to reduce hair loss, at least in theory, if it is similar to finasteride. And if saw palmetto *is* like finasteride, it must be taken indefinitely for maximum (potential) effect. However, consumers should generally beware of herbal hair loss remedies. These remedies are usually mixtures of many different herbs with unknown safety records, and the herbal hair loss industry and their products are poorly regulated, although some companies are now being prosecuted for fraud. Companies that sell herbal remedies usually boast of captivating "studies" substantiating their research, but they do not make these studies available for anyone to read, rendering them suspicious.

Commonly Reported Uses for Saw Palmetto*

Internally

prostate complaints, irritable bladder, sexual tonic, persistent cough, hair loss, and eczema

forms available for internal use:

dried berries, capsule, concentrated drops, decoction, fluid extract, tablet, tincture

commonly reported dosage:

Clinical studies have typically used either 160 milligrams twice daily, or 320 milligrams once daily, of an oil-based extract containing 80 to 90 percent of the volatile oil. One to 2 grams of whole berries daily are traditionally taken.

*These uses and dosages are from historic use and are not necessarily tested nor recommended.

What will saw palmetto do for women? Some claim it enhances breast growth, but there is no evidence for this. It might actually do the opposite, as some antiestrogenic and antiprolactin activity has been reported. Because its effects on a fetus or nursing infant are not clearly known, pregnant and lactating women should avoid using it.

EVIDENCE OF ACTION

Saw palmetto might act by inhibiting 5-alpha reductase, but more evidence is needed to confirm this. It at least inhibits both types of 5-alpha reductase in cell studies,[6, 7, 8] and reassuringly reduces dihydrotestosterone levels in prostate tissue biopsies from men with BPH who downed saw palmetto extract for three months, compared to those who did not.[9]

Evidence based on several small but randomized placebo-controlled trials indicates that if you have benign prostatic hyperplasia (BPH), saw palmetto may help you feel better. A 2002 review included twenty-one trials enlisting a total of 3,139 men with moderate symptoms from BPH.[10] After taking saw palmetto from four to forty-eight weeks, symptoms, such as nocturia (night urination), and various urine flow measurements significantly improved compared to those taking placeboes. This conclusion was a confirmation of the authors' older review of randomized, controlled trials.[11]

Two of the studies in the former meta-analysis found the prescription drug finasteride was similar to saw palmetto in its ability to improve symptoms of BPH, which is interesting in light of the fact that some scientists think the drug and the herb have similar mechanisms of action. But they are not identical.

For example, finasteride lowers prostate specific antigen (PSA) significantly, which can obfuscate attempts to detect prostate cancer based on PSA levels.[12] On the other hand, a randomized study of more than one thousand patients found that saw palmetto did not significantly affect PSA levels.[13] The growing use of detecting *free* PSA—that is, PSA not bound to blood proteins—may abolish such PSA-detecting concerns. Free PSA is a good sign: A higher percentage of PSA that is free PSA indicates less risk of prostate cancer. Neither finasteride nor saw palmetto appears to affect free PSA production.[14, 15]

Saw palmetto also seems unlikely to hurt you. Although formal toxicological screens remain incomplete, it is not mutagenic (does not induce cancer) nor teratogenic (does not cause birth defects) in animals,[16] does not seem likely to interfere with other medications[17] or drug-metabolizing enzymes,[18] and people taking it rarely complained of side effects any more than those taking a placebo. The most likely side effect of saw palmetto is mild indigestion, but this is uncommon and may be prevented by taking the herb along with food.

On the other hand, unlike finasteride, saw palmetto does not help with chronic prostatitis,[19] which is not the same thing as BPH. The cause of this painful condition is not well known, perhaps because it originates from several different possible sources, such as infection, inflammation, or autoimmune disease.

Saw palmetto is often compared to finasteride, which is used not only for BPH (as the drug Proscar) but also for the most common type of male hair loss, androgenic hair loss (as the drug Propecia). Because saw palmetto also appears to inhibit the production of dihydrotestosterone, which is implicated in androgenic (male hormone–influenced) hair loss, it is included in some herbal hair loss supplements, and the idea is not far-fetched. However, only one study suggests that saw palmetto extract may reduce hair loss in men with androgenic alopecia,[20] and although this was a well-designed (placebo-controlled, double-blind) study, more data is needed to confirm its results. Keep in mind most herbal hair loss supplements contain little saw palmetto and a slew of other herbs. None of these extra ingredients work to prevent hair loss, and they could cause dangerous side effects.

THE BOTTOM LINE

- Saw palmetto probably helps men with benign prostatic hyperplasia, but does not help those with chronic prostatitis. It might even prevent male androgenic hair loss, but this use is controversial. Herbal hair loss remedies have not been shown to work, and they contain multiple ingredients with unknown actions.
- Saw palmetto berries' oil-based extracts apparently inhibit both types of 5-alpha reductase enzyme, which in turn prevents testosterone from being converted into dihydrotestosterone. Dihydrotestosterone causes prostate enlargement and hair loss. Saw palmetto may also act on the prostate as an anti-inflammatory.
- Saw palmetto seems relatively safe, except in rare instances it has caused mild gastrointestinal symptoms. Its hormonal effects on pregnant or nursing women are not clearly known, so they should avoid it.

SENNA
Cassia senna, Cassia spp. (syn. *Senna alexandrina*)

History and Folklore

History's mixed feelings about senna are summed up by the medieval herbalist Nicholas Culpeper, who first writes, "It strengthens the senses, procures mirth, and is good in chronic agues." Yet he also notes that it "works violently both upwards and downwards, offending the stomach and bowels." Arabs introduced Europeans to senna's "upwards and downwards" purgative powers in the ninth or tenth century, but its use may precede written records.

Historical references to senna establish a uniform theme of delight that it helps relieve constipation and dismay at the cramps that accompany the process. Edward Lear contributed to the topic in one of his limericks:

> *There was an Old Man of Vienna,*
> *Who lived upon Tincture of Senna;*
> *When that did not agree,*
> *He took Chamomile Tea,*
> *That nasty Old Man of Vienna.*
> —Book of Nonsense, 1846

One species, *Cassia occidentalis,* is found in the eastern and southern United States and is called *coffee senna,* because its seeds can be roasted for a coffee-like drink. Drinking coffee senna can provide the same savage catharsis associated with its more renowned medicinal relations.

Senna's active ingredients, generally termed anthranoid laxatives, now enjoy widespread use in commercial over-the-counter laxatives and are found in major brands like Ex-lax. Their rise to popularity was not engendered by any recognition of new therapeutic promise, but by legal desperation. Some researchers established a questionable link between several commercial laxatives' former active ingredient, the gentler laxative phenolphthalein, and cancer in rodents. Phenolpthalein's carcinogenicity is now ironically disputed to no avail, so the commercial sennosides are probably here to stay.

What's In It

THE LAXATIVES in senna are anthraquinones including dianthrone, principally sennosides A, A1, and B, as well as sennosides C and D.

The anthranoid laxatives in the senna plant are found in several plants besides senna, such as rhubarb root, which is popular in China, the North American cascara sagrada (see page 59), the European buckthorn, or "frangula," and aloe latex (see page 19), which is used globally.

How Scientists Think Senna Works

Senna contains anthranoid laxatives, which your gut flora must act on to activate. Senna reaches the colon in about six to eight hours. In general, senna's active ingredients must first be liberated from attached sugars by intestinal bacteria in order to work.

Commonly Reported Uses for Senna*

Internally
laxative
forms available for internal use:
pill, capsule, infusion, tincture, powder, syrup, prepared tea bags, dried leaves, dried pods
commonly reported dosage:
It is best to follow package recommendations of standardized products. A tea of one-half to one teaspoon of herb per cup is sometimes recommended, made with either hot water, or the reportedly "more active" preparation that is made from soaking leaves for ten to twelve hours and then strained. Aromatic herbs like cinnamon and cloves are traditionally taken with senna to mask its nauseating taste and smell.

*These uses and dosages are from historic use and are not necessarily tested nor recommended.

They then cause a reversal in the normal flow of ions and water through the lining of the colon. Normally, water is removed through the colon to enter the blood. Senna reverses this flow, causing the colon's contents to become watery, possibly leading to diarrhea. Sennosides also stimulate an unusually vigorous version of the normal digestive process of peristalsis. During peristalsis, intestinal muscles surrounding the gut contract, propelling the gut's contents onward. Senna stimulates this activity but can do it more forcefully than is required. Excessive contraction of these gut muscles is felt as cramps. Sennosides in senna mediate this vigorous

peristalsis by stimulating the production of one of the gut's prostaglandins.

Senna could give you a polka-dotted colon, but only your gastroenterologist will know. Prolonged use of senna or other anthraquinone-containing herbs, such as rhubarb root, cascara sagrada (see page 59), buckthorn, or "frangula," or aloe latex (see page 19) or anthraquinone-containing over-the-counter stimulant laxatives commonly leads to a bizarre but probably benign pigmentation of the colon called *melanosis coli.* The colon is invaded and colonized by white blood cells that contain the half-digested remains of the colorful anthranoid pigments. It goes away when you stop using the anthraquinone-type laxatives.

Aloe latex, rhubarb root, and senna, as well as other buckthorn trees contain the same smorgasbord of chemically related molecules in varying proportions. (The mechanisms by which anthranoid laxatives like senna work are described in even greater detail in the chapter on aloe, under aloe latex—not to be confused with aloe gel; see page 17.)

GOOD EFFECTS . . . AND NOT SO GOOD

Consider the alternatives to senna and other anthraquinone laxatives. Because anthraquinone-containing herbs and medicines can cause painful cramps and their toxicity is often debated, other remedies should be considered first. If you are not worried about cramps, consider also that many references advise adding aromatic herbs such as cinnamon to senna to mask its nauseating taste and smell. There are many gentler, safer, plant-derived laxatives, such as flax seeds (see page 123), pectin, and plant fiber in general.

Some senna plants recoil from your touch.

THE "WILD sensitive plant," *Cassia nicti-tans,* is a distant relative of the remarkable "sensitive plant," *Mimosa pudica.* Both are called "sensitive" because if you touch them, the leaves that were touched rapidly fold up. The touched leaves, if left alone, perk up over a few hours, so you can repeat the process over and over. Touching these plants initiates a rapid reversal in the direction of charged ion particles in the leaves that have been touched. Water is strongly attracted to ions, and the resultant, reversible loss of water from certain cells located at the base of each leaflet causes the cells to collapse and the leaflets to droop.

Certain people should avoid senna more than others. Senna should not be taken by children, as it can give them severe rash, blisters, and diarrhea.[1] Although older references say it does not cross into breast milk, a new publication suggests it does, so nursing women who take it may risk giving their baby cramps. If you feel compelled to try it, however, use a standardized commercial formula, do not use more than the directed dose, and do not use it for a prolonged period of time.

EVIDENCE OF ACTION

That anthranoid laxatives in senna and other plants work is not in question, and senna does seem to be one of the more effective bowel evacuators of this class.[2, 3] What is debated is the toxicity of senna and other anthranoid laxatives. The anthranoid laxatives found in senna and other plants may be metabolized in the intestines to form a liver toxin, and cases of liver inflammation following anthranoid laxative use, though rare, have been reported.[4, 5, 6, 7] Chronic anthranoid laxative ingestion may be associated with cancer, but more evidence is required to substantiate these studies.[8, 9, 10]

THE BOTTOM LINE

- Senna is an aggressive laxative and can cause painful cramps and diarrhea. The active ingredients in senna are anthranoid laxatives. Their attached sugars must be removed by your intestinal flora to work.
- Anthranoid laxatives found in senna reverse the flow of ions and water in the colon by opening chloride channels, stimulating nitric oxide and prostaglandin synthesis, and initiating peristaltic gut contractions.
- Chronic anthranoid laxative abuse can produce melanosis coli, a pigmented colon, which is currently described as harmless though abnormal. Melanosis coli disappears if the anthranoid use is stopped.
- Because senna has unpleasant side effects, other methods of relieving constipation should first be considered.

SOY

Glycine max (domesticated), *Glycine soja* (wild)

HISTORY AND FOLKLORE

Many people consider soybeans, or, in the United Kingdom, *soya* beans, more of a food than an herb, except that isolated soybean extracts are taken as supplements with increasing frequency, placing soy-derived items on the shelves of every health food store. Originating from ancient China as early as BCE 1000, vegetarian disciplines of Buddhism probably helped this high-protein food spread to the rest of Asia. Soy is better than your average bean as a "compete" protein, containing all the essential amino acids. Yet it remained virtually unknown to Europe and America until its introduction in the seventeenth and eighteenth centuries, respectively. The non-Asian world ignored soy as a mere gastronomic oddity until its oil, stabilized by hydrogenation in the mid-twentieth century, exploded onto the market and into every possibly culinary application, due to food shortages resulting from World War II. Soy and soybean oil are now one of the world's largest agricultural products.

Epidemic rumors of soy isoflavones' estrogenic potential now encourage women to try it for all manner of "female complaints," such as premenstrual syndrome, menstrual problems, and menopausal symptoms. It is also used to reduce cholesterol, and traditional Chinese medicine employs it for sweating, confusion, and joint pain.

HOW SCIENTISTS THINK SOY WORKS

Soy foods lower your cholesterol and triglycerides, and there are several plausible reasons for this. The most obvious explanation is that soy foods often substitute for meat, and meat is loaded with cholesterol and saturated fat. Soy, like other plant foods, has no cholesterol and has healthier, unsaturated oils. Soybean oil possesses essential fatty acids, albeit leaning toward a preponderance of the omega-6 kind, which humans already get plenty of (and perhaps in excess, since omega-6s can be pro-inflammatory), but also has a smaller but respectable degree of the more desirable anti-inflammatory omega-3 fatty acids. Meat has relatively scant quantities of both.

Soy also is a good source of plant-derived sterols, such as beta-sitosterol. Plant-derived sterols resemble cholesterol and are thought to lower your intestinal absorption of cholesterol by mimicking the bad stuff. However they work, there is good clinical evidence that these plant-derived sterols, also called *phytosterols,* do lower your cholesterol, such that some companies now add them to foods like margarine, along with "heart healthy" claims on the label.

It's less clear that the much-touted *isoflavones* (such as genistein and daidzein) from soy help decrease cholesterol. Since they are antioxidant and free radical–scavenging, they could prevent the oxidation of LDL cholesterol that leads to atherosclerotic plaque, but this remains theoretical. Some say their estrogenic action might induce metabolism to affect lipids, but it's not clear whether isoflavones act like estrogen, or block it.

Soy isoflavones are two-faced: Sometimes they act like estrogen, and sometimes they block it. What makes isoflavones so confusing is that they are *partial estrogen agonists*. The term "agonist" means they can accomplish the same things that estrogen does, at many of estrogen's own receptors. However, the "partial" means they carry out estrogen's actions in a wimpy, weak way. For people with high estrogen levels—for example, menstruating women—isoflavones can block the estrogen receptors by sitting inside them and feebly doing what estrogen would normally do. On the other hand, in people with low estrogen—for example, men or menopausal women—these isoflavones take over the job of the absent estrogen to some extent. This may explain why some (yet not all) studies have shown soy isoflavones to aid menopausal women—they may act like a weak version of hormone replacement therapy.

What's In It

SOY CONTAINS up to 25 percent oil, and phytoestrogens known as *isoflavones,* including the inactive sugar-bound *genistin* and *daidzin* (ending in "-in"), which, after the sugars are removed by intestinal bacteria, become the active aglycones *genistein* and *daidzein* (ending in "-ein"). Soy also contains lecithin, as well as phytosterols such as beta-sitosterol, campesterol, and stigmasterol. The beans are a good source of calcium, iron, potassium, amino acids (including all the essential ones), vitamins, and fiber.

Although some studies indicate soy isoflavones may help prevent menopausal

symptoms like osteoporosis and hot flashes, most studies render a verdict of "ineffective." The isoflavones' ambiguous estrogenic behavior may explain why clinical trials using isoflavones have yielded such ambiguous results.

Soy isoflavones can mimic tyrosine, which is bad news for your thyroid hormones. The thyroid hormones (thyroxine and triiodothyronine) are made by the small, butterfly-shaped thyroid gland in the neck. They speed up metabolism, and when this system has a problem, the result is either hyperthyroidism (excess thyroid hormone) or hypothyroidism (too little thyroid hormone), and perhaps an enlarged thyroid gland, or goiter. Making thyroid hormones involves adding iodine (called *iodination*) to an amino acid called *tyrosine* in the thyroid. Then, after being stimulated by another hormone (thyroid stimulating hormone, or TSH) the iodinated hormones are released into the bloodstream to go about speeding up the metabolism. One problem with soy isoflavones is that they look somewhat like tyrosine.

The isoflavones from soy apparently resemble tyrosine to the point that they can get iodinated *instead* of tyrosine. So people who ingest a lot of soy isoflavones can theoretically make less thyroid hormone. This doesn't seem to be a problem, however, since there is enough iodine to overcome the competition for iodine that the isoflavones create. Most people probably get enough iodine. Despite the ever-present warnings of marketers attempting to sell iodine-containing supplements such as kelp, iodine deficiencies are rarely a cause of thyroid problems in developed countries (and iodine-laden supplements such as kelp can *cause* thyroid problems). Iodine deficiencies in developed countries have been virtually eliminated since its widespread addition to salt in the 1960s.

If soybean products cause gut pain, blame your colonic bacteria. Soybeans, like other beans, contain small carbohydrates that, if they reach the colon, can get enthusiastically digested by bacteria. During this feeding frenzy, these tiny microorganisms release an impressive amount of gas for their small size. Contending with these gassy bacterial waste products can be extremely painful for some people. Soy's more treacherous carbohydrates are water soluble; so one way to limit them is to drain them off with cooking water, perhaps even multiple times, if dry soybeans or other soy products are cooked in water. Some people's soybean miseries are caused by allergies. However, while the general public typically perceives soy allergies as common, experimental data show that true soy allergies are fairly scarce.

Soy lecithin allows oil and water to mix, soothes dry skin, and creates topical, drug-delivering liposomes. Lecithin belongs to a class of phosphate-containing lipids, or *phospholipids*. Lecithin is not unique to soy, but is found in most all plants and animals, because it is a constituent of an essential part of cells. It is usually the main constituent of the *cell membrane,* an outer boundary of cells that surrounds cells and keeps their contents from leaking out. However, lecithin is most often commercially obtained from soy or eggs, since it is technically easier to purify from these sources.

"Lecithin" is not one molecule, but a general term for any type of lipid with two fatty acid tails and a phosphate, all held together by a glycerol "backbone." The two fatty acid tails of a lecithin molecule could be *any* fatty acids—saturated, unsaturated, omega-3, omega-6, good, bad, or indifferent—so the term "lecithin" could mean any number of things, and lecithin varies considerably from source to source. The phosphates of lecithin molecules are usually bonded to choline, or

perhaps bonded to some other molecule (serine or ethanolamine). A portion of some lecithin molecules, choline, can be used to make the neurotransmitter acetylcholine. However, attempts to boost this neurotransmitter by dietary lecithin have not proven effective. It would be absurd to claim that anyone had a deficiency of lecithin, so claims for using it to correct its deficiency should be ignored. After eating lecithin, it may well get incorporated into cell membranes, or broken down and either metabolized for energy, or the fatty acid tails may very well get used to make fat. Soy lecithin probably isn't bad for you, but so far it isn't known to do anything remarkable as a dietary supplement either.

Lecithin is more promising when applied topically. Lecithin from any source acts like a detergent, allowing oil and water to mix. One end of the molecule (the phosphate) is charged and attracted to water, and the other end (the fatty acid tails) remains uncharged and attracted to greasier things. As such, you can add a little to your skin lotion to help keep water next to your skin. Indeed, lecithin appears effective in relieving dermatitis.

Drug designers sometimes employ lecithin to help them get drugs to penetrate the skin. Lecithin or other phospholipids are used to create microscopic bubbles called *liposomes.* Because lecithin has a detergent-like nature, when mixed with certain drugs and water it can form spheres or liposomes around the drug. The liposome can penetrate skin and carries its caged drug along with it.

GOOD EFFECTS . . .
AND NOT SO GOOD

The consensus medical opinion generally recommends soy foods and soy protein,

especially as a substitute for meat. Many soy foods, powders, and concentrates provide all the essential amino acids, making it a "complete" protein. Discarding any cooking water, if there is any, reduces common gastrointestinal symptoms of soy foods. (Soy allergies are much less common than popularly imagined, but of course if you have one, you should avoid soy entirely.) Soy foods are cholesterol-free and certainly have healthier fat, and *less* fat, than meat. There is good evidence that they lower cholesterol and reduce the risk of several cancers. Soy formula is even considered safe for infants, yet breast milk is the best option.

Commonly Reported Uses for Soy*

Internally
premenstrual and menstrual problems, menopausal symptoms, hypercholesterolemia, weight loss, sweating, aches and pains
forms available for internal use:
soy nuts, soybeans, edamame, tofu, tempeh, soy milk, soy powders, bars, meat replacements, and texturized vegetable protein (TVP), capsules, extracts, lecithin
commonly reported dosage:
For hypercholesterolemia, 20 to 50 grams per day of soy protein is taken. Menopausal symptoms have been treated with 34–76 milligrams of isoflavones in 20 to 60 grams of soy protein a day in clinical studies.

*These uses and dosages are from historic use and are not necessarily tested nor recommended.

Soy isoflavones, however, are regarded with more caution. Isolated soy isoflavones, such as genistein and daidzein, on the other hand, are more of an unknown, and because of this, scientists and doctors feel less confident recommending them than they do "whole" soy. True, soy foods contain them, but their concentrations are low enough that they shouldn't disturb your hormones unduly. It's understandable to want to try them for hormone replacement therapy, because traditional hormone replacement therapy is no longer recommended long-term, due to intolerable risks of heart disease, breast cancer, and stroke. Soy isoflavones are probably safer than traditional hormone replacement therapy, but keep in mind they are still an unknown, and it is not clear if they are truly effective in relieving menopausal symptoms.

Although soy isoflavones have not been associated with obvious health problems, remember that soy isoflavones may block estrogen if your estrogen is high, or behave like estrogen if your estrogen is low. Some worry that they may stimulate estrogen-sensitive cancers, like breast cancer.

Although soy isoflavones might slightly increase your body's demand for iodine in order to make thyroid hormones, the consensus medical opinion is that people in developed countries normally get enough iodine to avoid thyroid problems. However, those with thyroid problems should avoid taking large doses of soy isoflavones.

"Standardized to isoflavones" is ambiguous and often not true. Independent labs have found the claimed percent of isoflavones on supplement and soy food labels misrepresented in many products they tested. Confusion also arises because some companies use the weight of the inactive sugar-bound isoflavones, and others use the active, sugar-free isoflavones. So what you see may not be what you think you are getting. Like so many supplements, there is no certain way to determine whether the product contains what it claims. However, some independent testing labs, like Consumerlab, are now placing their seal of approval on products that qualify as containing what the label claims. These approval seals do not guarantee effectiveness; they merely attest the product contains what the label says.

Soybean oil is a different matter, and while it isn't bad, there are better oils out there. Canola, olive, and flaxseed oil (see page 123), and fatty fish are healthier sources of oils. Of course, all "partially hydrogenated" oils, soybean or otherwise, contain unhealthy trans fats and should be avoided completely.

Soy lecithin is not worth spending your money on, unless you want to use it for cooking or in skin lotion. Lecithin, also derived from eggs, allows oil and water to mix, and when used for this purpose in foods is called an *emulsifier*. You only need a teaspoon or so in bread, chocolate desserts, or homemade mayonnaise to keep oily molecules from separating from watery ones, but usually this insurance isn't needed. It's dreadfully sticky, so you may only want to add a tiny bit to skin lotion to help keep water molecules next to your skin.

Interesting Facts

Use your mind as a healer for hot flashes.

HERE'S A ray of hope: For some reason, the placebo effect for treating hot flashes in most studies is remarkably large. This is true not only for studies with soy but with other herbs, drugs, and supplements as well. That is, some studies do show that isoflavones help women prevent hot flashes, but place-bos help equally well. This doesn't mean hot flashes are all an illusion either. They are very real and very unpleasant. The good news is that the mind is often a more powerful healer than people tend to think, and it can be given some credit for controlling hot flashes. This leads some experts to suggest that one trick in controlling hot flashes lies in finding a way to alter states of mind through relaxation or breathing exercises—for example, training our brains to assist our bodies.

EVIDENCE OF ACTION

The best thing soy has going for it, based on human studies, is its ability to lower cholesterol and fat. Soy protein and soy foods, but not its isolated isoflavones, do this, according to several clinical trials. One review of several trials concluded that *isolated* soy isoflavones had no effect on LDL ("bad") or HDL ("good") cholesterol,[1] but another review noted that studies where volunteers consumed soy foods and protein with *higher* isoflavone levels lowered their cholesterol even more than those eating soy foods with less concentrated isoflavones.[2] It may not be the isoflavones that are lowering cholesterol, however; isoflavones may simply be more concentrated in soy products that contain chemically similar but unknown active ingredients. Soy *protein,* on the other hand, lowers the bad LDL cholesterol without affecting your good HDL cholesterol, and it can lower triglycerides, too.[3]

Soy isoflavones are most touted for relieving menopausal symptoms, like hot flashes and bone loss, which has been supported by a few animal and test tube studies, but most studies employing actual menopausal women are disappointing. They show that soy or its isoflavones have little or no effect on hot flashes, bone loss, and cognitive function.[4, 5, 6, 7]

Data on the effect of soy on cancer are all over the map: some have good news, some have bad news, and many are inconclusive. It also matters whether you are talking about soy foods or soy isoflavones. Although soy *isoflavones* inhibit cancer in many animal and test tube studies, they enhance cancer development and metastasis in other studies, placing isoflavones' cancer-halting rumors on the fence at this point. Since isoflavones can act as estrogens at some times and like antiestrogens in other instances, conflicting evidence is not surprising.

Here's a summary of current scientific thinking on soy foods and cancer: Asian women have less breast cancer than American women, and some suggest this is due to their high soy diet.[8] We can reasonably wonder whether it is the presence of soy, or the lesser amount of meat, or both, benefiting Asian women, since eating more meat *is* clearly associated with cancer, including breast cancer.[9] Also, Asians may simply be less prone to breast cancer, genetically. One study showed that Asian intestines were generally better able to remove the sugars from isoflavones than non-Asian, American intestines, a process necessary to yield active isoflavones. The genetic knack for producing sugar-free isoflavones was correlated with a lower incidence of prostate cancer in both Asian and non-Asian men.[10] According to the National Cancer Institute, groups of Americans who regularly consume soy foods are less likely to get breast, colon, endometrial, and prostate cancers than those who don't. However, they raise concern that women with estrogen-sensitive breast cancer theoretically might stimulate cancer growth with estrogenic isoflavones, particularly if their estrogen levels are low to begin with, like during menopause.

In Asia, fermented soy products (tempeh, miso, soy sauces, and natto) are generally more highly regarded for their health benefit compared to nonfermented soy products (fresh green soybeans, whole dry soybeans, soy nuts, soy sprouts, whole-fat soy flour, soymilk and soymilk products, tofu, okara and yuba), and there is a lot of commentary on this notion in the popular press. Fermentation removes the sugars from soy's isoflavones, enabling their absorption into the body. It's not clear that isoflavones are responsible for soy's benefits, however. Fermented soy products are sometimes claimed a source of the B12 that is missing in vegan diets, but data on this is inconclusive and unreliable. While fermented soy products may still have as-yet-undiscovered benefits, studies of their influence on cancer are disturbing.[11, 12] Most studies on fermented soy products indicate that consumption of large amounts of fermented soy products, such as miso, soy sauce, and tempeh, increase stomach cancer risk. For example, six case studies comprising 732 people showed that unfermented soy products prevented rectal cancer but fermented soy products did not.[13] That such products often have a high sodium content complicates the data. Also, fermented soy products also contain carcinogenic N-nitroso compounds. (N-nitroso compounds are commonly known as a byproduct of nitrites, which are used in Western cultures to preserve meats.)

Though animal and cell studies show that soy isoflavones, even diluted to the concentrations found in plasma, interfere with thyroid hormone synthesis, health authorities seem unconcerned. Women taking isoflavone supplements in randomized, controlled studies continued to maintain normal thyroid hormone levels.[14] Experts suggest that soy isoflavones won't upset thyroid function in people who have adequate dietary iodine, and iodine deficiencies in developed countries are pretty rare these days, thanks to the addition of iodine to salt. Since this phenomenon has not been extensively researched, it appears prudent that those with known thyroid dysfunction should avoid isolated soy isoflavones, but soy protein and soy foods have such low levels of isoflavones that they are probably safe.

There are some concerns that unknown hormonal actions of isoflavones affect infants who drink soy-based infant formulas. Studies of adults who were fed soy formula as infants show they suffered no ill effects, however, so it seems safe.[15] Yet some suggest even these theoretical risks reserve its use for cases where infants can't tolerate milk.

Breast milk, though inconvenient, remains the healthiest choice.

Finally, much ado was made of one study that suggested that eating more tofu, that bland champion of health foods, accelerated the mental decline of middle-aged Japanese American men.[16] This study has been widely criticized for its methodology, as it allowed volunteers to self-report previous "high" or "low" tofu consumption rather than measure their tofu intake directly. It also presents potential confounding factors—for example, poorer men ate more tofu but probably also had less healthy living environments. No similar effect pops up in other human studies or circumstances: Japanese men who regularly consume even more tofu do not suffer accelerated mental decline.

THE BOTTOM LINE

- There is good evidence that soy foods and soy protein, especially when used as a substitute for meat, can help lower your cholesterol and fat. It is uncertain that soy isoflavones aid cholesterol reduction, but soy's phytosterols clearly do.
- Evidence that soy isoflavones prevent menopausal symptoms is poor. Soy protein may reduce prostate cancer risk, but isolated isoflavones could elevate the risk of estrogen-sensitive cancers, like breast cancer. Evidence for soy reducing breast cancer is contradictory.
- There is no evidence that adults who consumed soy infant formula were adversely affected in any way. However, breast milk is healthier for infants, and soy formula should only be used if an infant has an allergy to milk or lactose intolerance.
- Soy isoflavones interfere with thyroid hormone production, but only if you are low on iodine, which is uncommon in developed countries.

ST. JOHN'S WORT

Hypericum perforatum

HISTORY AND FOLKLORE

St. John's wort is distinctive in several ways. First, its leaves appear perforated with transparent spots, which are actually oil glands. This is why the word *"perforatum"* appears in its species name. Crushing the yellow flowers or leaves with your fingers produces an odd, reddish oil that stains your fingers. Also, festive little black dots decorate the margins of the star-shaped yellow flower, which are also engaged in making chemicals. St. John's wort is in fact a curious little chemical factory, and as such it should be used with respect and caution.

Ancient Greeks employed this herb against evil spirits, and dubbed it *hypericum,* meaning "over an apparition." Christians associated it with St. John, and its blood-colored oil may explain why people so often historically tried to use it for healing wounds. The medieval Paracelsus and the nineteenth- and twentieth-century American eclectic physicians promoted its use for anxiety and depression.

HOW SCIENTISTS THINK ST. JOHN'S WORT WORKS

Some scientists believe St. John's wort acts like the popular reuptake inhibitor antidepressant drugs. It does, at least in test tube studies. Some of the most popular types of antidepressant drugs prescribed these days are various types of *reuptake inhibitors.* These come in different neurotransmitter flavors, so to speak, depending on the neuro-

transmitter that is to be boosted. Selective serotonin reuptake inhibitors, or SSRIs (Prozac or Zoloft), increase serotonin. Serotonin norepinephrine reuptake inhibitors, or SNRIs (Effexor), increase both serotonin and norepinephrine. Finally, there are norepinephrine dopamine reuptake inhibitors, or NDRIs (Wellbutrin), that increase both norepinephrine and dopamine.

Unlike these drugs, St. John's wort allegedly increases the three neurotransmitters affected in clinical depression to the same degree.[1, 2] In test tube studies, where the herb is tested on isolated tissues that differ dramatically from an actual, intact human being, St. John's wort prevents the "reuptake" of serotonin, norepinephrine, and dopamine. This increases these neurotransmitters in the following way.

Normally, a nerve cell sending a signal produces a neurotransmitter, which drifts to a receiving nerve cell. Perhaps to prevent excess neurotransmitter from loitering dangerously in between the sending and receiving nerve cells, the sending nerve cell normally mops up most of the chemical that it just let loose, a normal phenomenon called *reuptake.* Enough of the chemical signal usually gets through for the receiving nerve cell to get the message anyway. But depressed people seem to either have too little neurotransmitter or do not respond adequately to it. Reuptake inhibitors work by preventing the nerve cell that is sending its neurotransmitter from gobbling up its own chemical message. This increases the amount of neurotransmitter in between synapses, amplifying its signal. The nice thing about reuptake inhibitors is that they work only for nerve cell signals that the brain is already trying to send. Increasing all of a particular neurotransmitter in the brain by taking it orally, instead, would result in it hitting *all* receptors for that neurotransmitter rather than just the pathways the brain is trying to activate. Taking oral neurotransmitters generally does not work anyway, which brings up an important problem with St. John's wort.

What's In It

IT'S NOT clear what St. John's active ingredient or ingredients are, but there are several candidates. St. John's wort contains proanthocyanidins and other catechin tannins. Its flavonoids are primarily hyperoside, rutin, quercitrin, isoquercitrin, quercetin, and kaempferol; it also possesses biflavonoids, such as amentoflavone. Hyperforin is one of its major acylphloroglucinol derivatives. It has caffeic acid derivatives like caffeic, chlorogenic, and ferulic acids. N-alkanes, monoterpenes, and sesquiterpenes may cause its turpentine odor. Naphthodianthrones (hypericin and pseudohypericin) are anthracene derivatives; it also has sterols (beta-sitosterol); vitamins C and A; xanthones; and choline.

This reuptake-inhibiting action of St. John's wort is challenged by some studies. Hyperforin has been put forth as the reuptake-inhibiting ingredient in St. John's wort. However, hyperforin has a problem getting past something called the *blood-brain barrier*,[3] a chemical border guard that is pretty picky about what it admits into the brain. The blood-brain barrier is why a person can't just eat neurotransmitters to treat depression, as the neurotransmitters can't reach the brain. But other constituents of St. John's wort besides hyperforin could be responsible for the reuptake inhibition seen in cultures, and if they *can* slip past the brain's personal bouncer, they may work as antidepressants. And if that doesn't work, there are a dizzying number of alternate proposals for an antidepressant mechanism of St. John's wort. Here are some examples.

Amentoflavone from St. John's wort can get into your brain. Amentoflavone, a biflavone made of two flavonoids chemically bonded together, might have valium-like activity, binding to the brain's benzodiazepine receptors and actively signaling the brain to slow down. In addition, amentoflavone sticks significantly well to serotonin, dopamine, opiate, and benzodiazepine receptors. Exactly how it influences these receptors, and to what degree, has yet to be determined.

St. John's wort's miquelianin cross the blood-brain barrier, too, possibly to create a short-term stress hormone–lowering effect. This flavonoid, miquelianin, reaches the brain, and when rats eat it their ACTH (adrenal cortical tropic hormone) and corticosterone, two stress hormones, are significantly lowered.[4] However, this effect wore off after the rats ate miquelianin for eight weeks. In addition, cortisol, another stress hormone, was slightly but statistically significantly lowered in human volunteers' saliva compared to a placebo, after they were given St. John's wort for two weeks.[5]

St. John's wort even contains the hormone melatonin. You might be surprised to learn that some plants contain human hormones. Melatonin is a hormone the brain makes when it gets dark, specifically when less light hits the retinas. Melatonin conveniently makes people tired and ready to sleep, and it enhances dreaming. In plants it scavenges free radicals, but whether dietary melatonin provides humans significant protection from radicals, cancer, and disease, as some scientists now postulate, is not yet known. When melatonin is ingested from plant sources (it is also found in rice, corn, tomatoes, and bananas), it gets past the blood-brain barrier and has the same impact as the body's own melatonin.

One of the more recent human studies supports the theory that St. John's wort prevents dopamine from being turned into another neurotransmitter. This study's results challenge older ideas that St. John's wort is a norepinephrine uptake inhibitor, or that it acts like another type of antidepressant called a *monoamine oxidase inhibitor* (*MAOI*). Instead, it confirmed other studies' findings that the herb could increase dopamine. It's noteworthy that this study was performed in intact people, with a control group, rendering its conclusion more reliable than most.[6] Dopamine is a neurotransmitter that helps regulate several vital functions, such as movement, coordination, emotion, motivation, and the sense of reward. The claim that St. John's wort increases dopamine is supported by earlier studies that showed that dopamine's breakdown into other metabolites is slowed by hypericin and pseudohypericin from St. John's wort. Hypericin and pseudohypericin are two large, dyelike molecules that fall in the category of polyaromatic anthraquinone derivatives. Since they react with light, they are unstable and can make people taking St. John's wort more likely to sunburn. However, they could also be responsible for increasing dopamine in the brains of people who take St. John's wort, since they both inhibit an enzyme called *dopamine beta-hydroxylase*.[7, 8] This enzyme converts dopamine to norepinephrine. Inhibiting the

dopamine beta-hydroxylase enzyme theoretically increases dopamine, perhaps at the expense of norepinephrine.

One novel theory of depression has less to do with neurotransmitters and more to do with inflammation. St. John's wort could theoretically affect this mechanism. Maybe hyperforin doesn't need to get to the brain. One recent study shows that hyperforin inhibits the substance P–stimulated production of interleukin-6 (IL-6) in cell cultures,[9, 10] and perhaps in mice, too.[11] Substance P is a pain-signaling molecule, and the IL-6 it boosts is a protein that stimulates inflammation. Curiously, IL-6 and other inflammatory-signaling molecules appear to be elevated in depression. Perhaps mild, continuing inflammation makes people feel chronically unwell, and thus depressed. One study showed that a daily multivitamin lowered IL-6 and decreased the risk of depression. Some scientists are therefore looking for antidepressants with an anti-inflammatory kick. Whether or not this mechanism is at work in people taking St. John's wort is not yet known.

But is it safe? St. John's wort increases the liver's production of a metabolizing enzyme with the cumbersome name of cytochrome P450 3A4. (There are many different drug-metabolizing enzymes in the liver called *cytochrome P450s,* and this particular one is designated 3A4.) Many studies show that St. John's wort speeds the clearance of drugs that might very much need to remain active in the body, like oral birth control pills, or, more frighteningly, blood thinners, HIV medications, and organ transplant rejection-suppressing drugs. St. John's wort can interfere with herbal medications, too, for the same reason. The long list of medications that St. John's wort interacts with is below.

GOOD EFFECTS . . .
AND NOT SO GOOD

Weigh carefully the well-known risks with the lesser-known benefits of St. John's wort before you take it. Though St. John's wort appears quite physiologically active, ultimately it is not at all clear exactly how it affects us. The more recent studies on St. John's wort show it does not work better than placebo for treating severe depression.

There are two major concerns to consider when taking St. John's wort. First of all, even for standardized preparations of St. John's wort, the concentrations of the purported active ingredient (which is not actually known at this point) have been found to vary wildly, from zero to one hundred times what is stated on the label. If this active ingredient (usually hypericin) really *is* helpful, the effect of St. John's wort will be erratic, resulting in "on" days and "off" days, due to the natural variation in the concentrations of active ingredients from plant to plant.

The second issue is that St. John's wort can critically inactivate other herbs or medications. Can St. John's wort impregnate a woman? Yes, if she is relying on oral contraceptives. St. John's wort has caused unplanned pregnancies and breakthrough bleeding in women who are taking oral contraceptives. There are also several documented cases of St. John's wort's reducing serum levels of immune-suppressing drugs, leading to organ transplant failure. What we know so far is that John's wort decreases the circulating levels of the following medications: amitriptyline, cyclosporine, digoxin, fexofenadine, indinavir, methadone, midazolam, nevirapine, phenprocoumon, simvastatin, tacrolimus, theophylline, and warfarin. It may also affect other drugs that have not been tested yet. St. John's wort reduces the ability of the cancer drug irinotecan's active metabolite from remaining in the blood. Of course, St. John's wort probably decreases the actions of other herbs that have also been ingested, using the same rapid-clearing mechanism.

Commonly Reported Uses for St. John's Wort*

Internally
used for depression, anxiety, sedation, menstrual cramps, infections, wounds
forms available for internal use:
capsule, decoction, fluid extract, infusion, tincture, oil, sometimes standardized to hypericin
commonly reported dosage:
Usually, 2 to 4 grams of the herb are taken daily, or 0.2 to 0.1 milligrams of hypericin daily. Capsules containing 0.3 percent hypericin are reportedly taken three times a day. Historically, an infusion is made with 1 to 2 teaspoons of flowers steeped for ten minutes in 1 cup of water for ten minutes, which is then strained and drunk once or twice a day.

*These uses and dosages are from historic use and are not necessarily tested nor recommended.

It is dangerous to take St. John's wort while taking another antidepressant. A few cases of something called *serotonin syndrome* are reported for people taking both antidepressant SSRIs or selective serotonin reuptake inhibitors (e.g., sertaline and paroxetine) along with St. John's wort. Serotonin syndrome is a potentially deadly reaction to excess serotonin in the brain. This implies that something in the herb might really act as an SSRI after all, but that isn't clearly known at this point.

Photosensitization may make you want to stop taking St. John's wort. Many study volunteers dropped out of the study because sunlight burned and blistered them more readily. When hit by ultraviolet light, the hypericin in St. John's wort produces a reactive troublemaker called *singlet oxygen.* Singlet oxygen turns around and wreaks havoc on your skin. Blistering and malaise are common problems for livestock grazing upon this wild weed, too.

EVIDENCE OF ACTION

St. John's wort probably is physiologically active, but exactly *what* it does and how it does it are not clearly known. Obviously this is a concern. It significantly alters the behavior of mice. For example, it got mice moving faster when they were forced to swim, and it "significantly inhibits marble burying behavior" in mice,[12] although it isn't clear how that action translates to humans. But how does it affect people?

Though there are plenty of human clinical trials testing St. John's wort for use against depression, their results are conflicting. Such studies are difficult to begin with, because clinical depression has several different physiochemical causes, which may or may not be addressed by a particular treatment. Yet as bigger and better-designed trials are being performed, the advantage of St. John's wort over placebo is narrowing. New evidence implies that earlier claims for St. John's wort may have been blown out of proportion.

There are so many trials that we have additional studies, called *meta-analyses,* to perform statistical analysis on batches of the better-designed trials. Meta-analyses published prior to 2004 generally suggested good news for St. John's wort.[13, 14, 15, 16] It seemed more effective for treating depression than a placebo, and it appeared comparable in effectiveness to common prescription antidepressant medications. Bear in mind, however, that although some individuals are dramatically improved by prescription antidepressants, most depressed people find prescriptions to be only mildly effective.

However, the news gets more troublesome for St. John's wort promoters. Three recent, large, well-designed studies failed to demonstrate efficacy, and when these were included in one of the latest meta-analyses,[17]

THE BOTTOM LINE

- St. John's wort is physiologically active, but exactly what it does is not clearly known. Several antidepressant mechanisms have been proposed that may theoretically work, but none of these have been proven.
- Though older studies imply St. John's wort may work as an antidepressant, they were small and poorly designed. The most recent, better-designed clinical trials for St. John's wort suggest it does not reliably work as an antidepressant, with respect to placebo.
- St. John's wort significantly alters the effectiveness of other medications, including birth control pills, blood thinners, transplant rejection drugs, AIDS medications, and cancer drugs. It can also increase sensitivity to sunlight.

the authors, who previously published a paper suggesting St. John's wort was effective,[18] revised their original conclusion, saying: "St. John's wort may be less effective in the treatment of depression than previously assumed and may finally be shown to be ineffective if future trials confirm this trend." This same meta-analysis re-reviewed fifteen trials that had been previously analyzed and found the advantage of St. John's wort for treating depression was smaller than previously reported, implying an unscientific bias favoring St. John's wort on the part of the original authors.

Nonetheless, even a bit of help is understandably tempting for those who suffer from depression. Some scientists argue that St. John's wort should be considered because its side effects are less severe than those of prescription antidepressants. Yet St. John's wort does have at least one significant side effect—it decreases the potency of several other commonly used drugs by increasing the rate at which they are cleared from the body.[19] Other medications' potencies can be dangerously enhanced by St. John's wort. Though St. John's wort's ability to relieve depression is now eyed more skeptically, there is no doubt that it contains ingredients that alter the body's physiology.

TEA TREE
Melaleuca alternifolia

HISTORY AND FOLKLORE

There is more than one tree called "tea tree," but the subject of most herbalists' discussions is the *Melaleuca alternifolia,* which grows in Australia's swampy areas. Aborigines used its leaves as an antiseptic, and the explorer Captain Cook broadcast its reputation in the 1700s, increasing its popularity among Australian settlers. Australian soldiers were issued tea tree oil for sterilizing their wounds in World War II. It was even included in machine-cutting oils in ammunition factories in order to decrease the likelihood of accidental infections.

Besides its use as an antibiotic, tea tree oil seems to repel insects that find it distasteful. As a tea it is possibly distasteful to humans as well, so it's poorly named, and though the beverage has been consumed, it isn't popular. The leaves' distilled oil is a yellow, volatile oil with a pungent, nutmeg-like smell. Though relatively new on the world herb market, its inclusion in all sorts of cosmetic products in the United States is now immensely fashionable.

HOW SCIENTISTS THINK TEA TREE WORKS

Plant poisons are a dime a dozen. First of all, most herbs can kill bacteria. Herbs can kill many different types of cells, and their chemical weapons are usually in their essential oils. That's why many fragrant plant oils irritate skin cells. That herbs are antimicrobial is not news, and headlines that this or that herb killed bacteria or even cancer cells in a test tube are a bit misleading, because most cells will die if treated with enough essential oil.

One reason for this is that cells in test tubes are sensitive things, and mixing them with an extreme amount of any substance, poisonous or not, can kill them, because anything can kill you if you have too much of it, including water. That holds not just for cells but for people, too (people have indeed died from drinking too much water, but it's rare and pretty hard to do). Another reason not to be impressed by an herb killing bacteria in test tubes is that plants can't move much, compared to animals. Plants use their volatile oils to protect their tissues from pathogens, since they can't move around to perform the hygienic washing maneuvers that animals have evolved. Some plants are just better at making cell-killing oils than others, and tea tree is one of the better ones.

Tea tree oil can kill cells, all kinds of cells. Depending on the nature of the injured party, tea tree oil may be used to advantage, but it can also be irritating stuff. It is not inappropriate to consider tea tree oil potentially toxic, and that's why you should handle it appropriately and in diluted form. Most of tea tree oil's users hope for antimicrobial behavior and apply it against unwanted bacteria, fungi, or viruses. The problem with undiscerning cell-killers of higher potencies is that they also kill *people* cells, and that is at best an annoying rash and at worst a medical crisis.

Some antibiotics are more discriminating than others. Penicillins and cyclosporins interfere with the integrity of

CELL MEMBRANES KEEP CELLULAR CONTENTS FROM LEAKING OUT. A cell membrane is somewhat like a plastic bag surrounding all cells. It's the cell's "skin," so to speak; it keeps a cell's contents inside and odd things outside. The cell membrane's fabric is mainly made of molecules that are actually a lot like detergent or soap molecules and are called *phospholipids.* For the purpose of visualization, each building block may be imagined as a roughly linear object, with one small water-attracting end, connected to two long, oily "tails" that are not attracted to water. The small water-loving end is called *hydrophilic,* or *polar,* and the water-ambivalent end is *hydrophobic,* or *nonpolar.* (Hydrophobic means "water hating," but that is a misnomer; hydrophobic things are only weakly attracted to all things, including water.)

The oft-recited chemical rule "like mixes with like" means that polar is attracted to polar, and nonpolar is attracted to nonpolar (for more on *why* this rule works, see Appendix B, "Introducing the Players"). Water is polar, and organisms are mostly water.

When these cell membrane molecules are put in a glass of water, they do something remarkable: They form a microscopic film on the water's surface. It may not *look* remarkable, but it is at the molecular level. This sheet is composed of membrane molecules that are all pointing the same way. Their water-loving ends are pointing down into the water, and their water-shy ends are pointing up and out. (You can do this with lecithin, available at health food stores, because it is made of cell membrane molecules.)

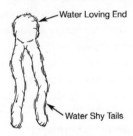

Water Loving End

Water Shy Tails

phospholipid

If you push this layer about, attempting to submerge the water-shy phospholipid tails, microscopic portions of the sheet will fold into a sandwich of two layers, with the water-shy tails inside the sandwich and the water-loving polar ends outside, in contact with the water. This double-layered sheet of material spontaneously curls into many water-filled bubbles, floating in a watery environment just like real cells. These are artificial cell membranes.

Real cell membranes have many other types of molecules embedded amid these membrane molecules, such as proteins that act like pores, channels, or receptors, and oil-anchored sugars, or *glycolipids,* that display sugars on the outside of the cell for attachment and recognition to other cells and to tissue scaffold material.

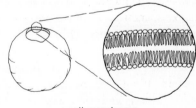

cell membrane

However, it is these phospholipid membrane molecules that give the cell membrane its essential structure. The membrane material is also essential in most cells in forming *internal* compartments, which are said to be "membrane bound." Many are internal storage units, but several have far more complicated and essential functions. This phospholipid material is thus vital to the structure of cells, and this is what tea tree oil disrupts.

bacterial cells' outermost boundaries, called *cell* walls, and neither animal nor human cells (because humans are technically animals) have cell walls. Tetracyclines and erythromycin mess with bacterial protein factories called *ribosomes,* but since these are different from human ribosomes, these antibiotics don't kill human cells. Unfortunately, both bacterial and human cells have *cell membranes,* which is what tea tree oil tangles with.

What's In It

THE OIL contains more than 100 monoterpenoids, sesquiterpenoids, and alcohols. Much of these (up to 40 percent) are terpinen-4-ol, 1,8-cineole (eucalyptol), alpha-terpineol, terpineolene, and alpha- and gamma-terpinene.

Tea tree oil works somewhat like detergent to disrupt cell membranes, although it is not a detergent. Detergents disrupt cell membranes, because they *look* like membrane molecules. Like the material making up cell membranes, they also have a water-loving end and a nonpolar, grease-loving end, and that is why detergents get grease and water to mix: They weakly stick to both and act as a molecular bridge between the two. They also will feel themselves pulled into a cell membrane by electrostatic forces, and if enough of these imposters integrate, the cell membrane will fall apart. Some detergents are better at this than others. The soaps we wash with mainly free germs from our skin and send them down the drain rather than disrupt their cell membranes. Tea tree oil constituents are not like detergents because they don't have a hydrophilic, water loving end. But

they are hydrophobic, and thus attracted to the oily portions of cell membrane molecules. They are also small enough to slip between cell membrane molecules, disrupting their attractions for one another, causing the membrane to fall apart.

Tea tree oil also compromises the integrity of cell membranes, but some membranes are easier to get to than others. All cells, including human cells, have this membranous structural material, so tea tree may have a negative impact. In fact, bacterial cell membranes are buried underneath a protective *cell wall,* so they are potentially *less* vulnerable than ours to tea tree oil. Animal cells—including human cells—do not have cell walls. True fungi also have cell walls protecting their cell membranes. Viruses don't even have a cell, much less a membrane, and for this reason, viruses are not even considered to be alive, technically speaking. Viruses simply inject their genetic material into real cells and get the cell's machinery to make more virus particles. So if we were to throw a bunch of different cells and viruses into the ring to battle tea tree oil, the most vulnerable to tea tree oil's attack, on the face of things, appears to be animal cells, including human cells.

Disrupting cell membranes can still be regarded as respectable employment for an antibiotic. Detergents do it, and we owe them our gratitude for such work. The antibacterial agent *polymyxin* does this, too. Like tea tree oil, polymyxin also disrupts cell membranes and can kill human cells by the same mechanism, so it is of limited clinical use. Because of its serious systemic toxicity, polymyxin is no longer taken internally. However, it is useful topically. Skin is made of cells that are *already* dead, along with nonliving molecular bits, so it is moderately impervious to such poisonous affronts, as long as the agent can't penetrate the skin.

Tea tree oil, likewise, should be used only topically, diluted enough to prevent its penetration into the skin.

POLYMYXIN AND tea tree oil are chemically different but work the same way.

The active ingredients of tea tree oil and polymyxin are quite different, however. Polymyxin is made in part of amino acids strung together, while the active ingredients of tea tree oil are much smaller hydrocarbon-like molecules. Yet they both integrate into cell membranes and disrupt them.

Good Effects . . . and Not So Good

Don't swallow tea tree oil, even if it's diluted. Several reports document depression, weakness, loss of coordination, and muscle tremors in people who swallowed the oil. There is even a documented case of coma. Ingestion of as little as 2.5 milliliters of oil can cause a rash and white blood cell abnormalities.

Keep it away from children and pets. There are scary case reports of inquisitive children swallowing the oil and requiring hospitalization. Pets have died from it, too. Some people are circulating the idea that it can be applied to their animal companions to use it to control their pets' fleas or skin problems. This is an especially bad idea, because pets lick themselves and are more sensitive, since they usually weigh less than we do.

Tea tree oil is for topical use only, but please be careful with it. A dilute solution of no more than 2 percent oil is recommended. It is commonly used to fight toe-

nail fungus, athlete's foot, dandruff, cold sores, acne, and oral bacteria. Tea tree oil definitely causes allergic reactions in some people, however, so you should of course discontinue using it if it gives you a rash.

You Want Me to Put It Where?

ONE TEA tree oil manufacturer went beyond the call of duty out of concern for their consumers. *New Scientist* magazine's "Feedback" section is fond of collecting and sharing such curious product labels, like the one submitted by Derek Long. His bottle of tea tree oil warned him "For external use only. Avoid skin contact."[1]

Most studies mention that tea tree oil irritates some fraction of those using it. In fact, the title of one Swedish paper is "Warning against a fashionable cure for vulvovaginitis. Tea tree oil may substitute Candida itching with allergy itching." The irritating agent in tea tree oil has consequently been a subject of some debate, and people have wondered if they can remove it from the oil to create a less irritating version of tea tree oil. Unfortunately, it is probably not just one molecule that irritates but the majority of volatile oil molecules, because they all have similar physical characteristics and are thus highly likely to work the same way. There is a lot of talk about creating a tea tree oil product that has less 1,8-cineole (also known as *eucalyptol* and present in several other plant oils, including eucalyptus oil). It is unlikely, however, that tea tree oil with low 1,8-cineole won't irritate skin. Tea tree oil contains so many molecules that are similar to 1,8-cineole that have the same activity, and removing one of these will not make tea tree oil less irritating.

Don't stick it in your ear. Preliminary reports suggest that tea tree oil could cause ear damage and impaired hearing, although this is not conclusively known.

Interesting Facts

Isoprene building blocks make terpenes: a dazzling array of fragrances and other handy plant products.

TEA TREE oil's active ingredients are its monoterpenes, but monoterpenes and related molecules are ubiquitous in the plant kingdom. If you read through most herb books, they will impress you with jargon, describing how the active ingredient is a "monoterpene" or a "sesquiterpene" or maybe a "triterpenoid," but what are they? These oily, fat-soluble molecules are collectively known as *terpenes.*

Aside from the nonsmelly and nonvolatile "vegetable oil" triglycerides that nourish embryonic plants within their nuts and seeds, much of the other types of plant oils are terpenes. Terpenes are the major component of the plant's distilled volatile or "essential" oils. They are often principal notes of the plant's odor and flavor. For example, lemony limonene is in citrus fruit oils, and citronellal is in citronella oil. Pinene is in pine oil and gives turpentine its odor, and menthol makes peppermint oil taste cool. Variations on the menthol structure give variations in different mints' tastes; for example, regular mint has no menthol but rather the similar-looking and sweeter-smelling menthofurane, and spearmint has a menthol look-alike called *L-carvone.* Camphor and eucalyptol are pungent-smelling plant terpenes in many volatile oils besides

eucalyptus, only in smaller amounts. Zingiberine helps give ginger its zip, and nerol smells like roses. These are just a few of an astounding variety of plant terpenes which provoke such strong subjective responses from our noses, taste buds, and brains.

What you may find interesting is that many herbs share the same terpenes but in different amounts. For example, nerol smells like roses and is found in roses, but it is also present in smaller amounts in orange oil and lavender oil. Eugenol is the principal terpene in clove oil, and it gives some character to cinnamon and allspice, but did you know it is also in basil and carrots? Increasing or decreasing one terpene's concentration can completely change the flavor and smell of the herb.

A great number of the active ingredients in herbs are commonly described as "monoterpenes," "sesquiterpenes," "diterpenes," or "triterpenes," but what does this mean? First, it helps to explain what a terpene really is.

Terpenes are all simply molecules made of one particular molecular building block called an *isoprene unit.* The isoprene unit is made of five carbon atoms. Isoprene units, like Tinker Toys, can join together in a number of different ways. Plants join multiple isoprene units to make an enormous number of different plant terpenes. Since all terpenes are constructed from isoprene units, and isoprene units have five carbon atoms, true terpenes have multiples of five carbons, like 10-, 15-, 20-, or 25-carbons, and so on. However, not all molecules with multiples of five carbons are terpenes! They have to be made from these isoprene units to qualify as a terpene. A trained eye can look at a molecular structure and dissect in into its precursor isoprene units, and then pronounce the molecule a terpene. If the isoprene building blocks get substantially altered during construction, it becomes a *terpenoid,* which may not have a multiple of five carbons yet was still constructed from isoprene units.

The smallest terpenes are made by joining two isoprene units to make a 10-carbon terpene called a *mono*terpene (5 + 5 = 10). It's these smallest terpenes that are light enough to fly up your nose and emit fragrance. Three isoprenes join to make a wide variety of fifteen-carbon *sesqui*terpenes (5 + 5 + 5 = 15), and "sesqui" means "one and a half," because it is one and a half of the 10-carbon monoterpenes. Four isoprenes make the 20-carbon *di*terpenes (5 + 5 + 5 + 5 = 20). *Tri*terpenes have six isoprenes, so they have thirty carbons (5 + 5 + 5 + 5 + 5 + 5 = 30), and steroids, plant sterols, stanols, and saponins are derivatives of these. Beta-carotene, from which vitamin A is derived, is a *tetra*terpene, made from eight isoprenes (5 + 5 + 5 + 5 + 5 + 5 + 5 + 5 = 40), so these have forty carbons. Vitamins A, E, and K are also derived from terpenes. The rubber plant polymerizes loads of isoprene units together to make chains out of it, and this is natural rubber.

EVIDENCE OF ACTION

Tea tree oil is possibly effective in some cases, like acne and fungal infections. It was at least as effective as benzoyl peroxide in treating acne. The study enlisted 124 volunteers with mild to moderate acne to apply either 5 percent tea tree oil or 5 percent benzoyl peroxide to their acne, and both groups experienced significant improvement. Though the tea tree oil acted more slowly, it was associated with less redness, dryness, and irritation than benzoyl peroxide.[2]

Tea tree oil also compared favorably to a 1-percent solution of the antifungal clotrimazole for treating toenail fungus. The double-blind study assessed 117 people's toe infections periodically for up to six months and observed comparable results, with absence of cultured fungus in 11 percent using the antifungal ointment and 18 percent using tea tree oil.[3]

Commonly Reported Uses for Tea Tree Oil

Externally

antiseptic: antibacterial, antifungal, and antiviral

forms available for external use:

gel, infusion, ointment, tincture, mouthwash, cosmetic preparations

commonly reported dosage:

Tea tree oil is used in concentrations ranging from 0.4 to 100 percent externally, yet most recommend not using concentrations higher than 2 percent tea tree oil.

Tea tree may kill athlete's foot fungi, too, but at concentrations that limit its usefulness. Volunteers with athlete's foot were given either 10 percent tea tree oil cream, or 1 percent of the over-the-counter antifungal tolnaftate, or a placebo. Of the tolnaftate-treated group, 85 percent enjoyed a complete cure, but tea tree oil performed no better than the placebo.[4] Higher percentages of tea tree oil were more effective yet more irritating: another study applied either 25 percent or 50 percent tea tree oil, or a placebo, on 158 patients with athlete's foot. Of those using 50 percent tea tree oil, 64 percent had no fungus after four weeks, compared to 31 percent of placebo users, but some of the tea tree oil users experienced "moderate to severe dermatitis," which ended after they stopped using the oil.[5]

Tea tree oil's success against herpes virus in test tube studies failed to carry over to any remarkable extent in people with the infection. Eighteen people with recurrent herpes labialis who had not recently undergone antiviral therapy were recruited, and half applied five times daily either a gel containing 6 percent tea tree oil or a placebo gel. They could not be "blinded" to receiving treatment because of the strong smell of tea tree oil. However, investigators were blinded as to who received which treatment and measured several parameters related to healing time after outbreaks and viral titers. Neither group showed any statistical difference, although the healing time was slightly less in the tea tree oil group.[6]

There is little doubt that tea tree oil irritates the skin of some fraction of its users. Of twenty-eight volunteers treated with a standard allergic patch test, three "tested strongly positive."[7] Thus its long-term use is not warranted, and it should be applied with caution.

THE BOTTOM LINE

- Tea tree oil is used externally as an antimicrobial agent. The oil probably works by destabilizing cell membranes and since all cells have membranes, it is nonspecific.
- Tea tree oil should never be used internally.
- Externally, tea tree oil can cause irritation and allergic responses, but in dilute solutions it may be effective against acne and certain fungal infections. Other uses have either not been supported, or there is insufficient data to rate it for other treatments.

TEA

Camellia sinensis

History and Folklore

As the world's second favorite beverage, next to water, tea has a rich history. The leaves from this evergreen bush are processed in various ways to make both black and green tea, and all the other classic tea varieties, like oolong, orange pekoe, English breakfast, Earl Grey, the newly popular white tea, and more. (The term "herbal tea" has evolved to mean any tea *not* made with *C. sinensis,* so of course this chapter won't tell you anything about them.)

Tea was probably used even in prehistory in its native region of Southeast Asia. Chinese myth holds that around BCE 2700, the Chinese emperor was a farsighted scientific sort, who requested all drinking water be boiled before it was consumed. When Shen Nung sat beneath a tree while his servant boiled drinking water, a leaf from a wild tea plant fell into the pot. Instead of tossing it, being a scholar and herbalist, the emperor experimentally drank the brew and was refreshed by the result. Another myth describes how the Buddhist monk Bodhidharam had a good long session meditating for nine years, until he accidentally fell asleep. Today, people are pleased with themselves if they can meditate for ten minutes, but the monk cut off his eyelids to keep himself from doing it again. The eyelids fell to the ground and became the tea plant, which supplied him with the means to keep awake thereafter.

Records of tea cultivation in China first appear in the fourth century, and by the eighth century its use was all the rage and was spreading to Japan. At this time Lu Yu's illustrated, three-volume *Ch'a Ching* appeared, covering the agriculture, preparation, and uses of tea. It may have inspired Buddhist priests to invent the Japanese tea ceremony.

"Tea removeth lassitude, vanquisheth heavy dreams, easeth the frame, and strengtheneth the memory. It overcometh superfluous sleep, and prevents sleepiness in general, so that without trouble whole nights may be passed into study."
—London teahouse advertisement[1]

Enough of the first samples of tea reached Europe through Venetian trading routes in the mid 1500s to rapidly hook the populace. The English and Dutch developed regular voyages overseas, and the Russians over land, to get more of it. The idea that tea was replacing the usual ale for breakfast in the 1800s had its advocates and critics, but it evolved into the customary afternoon teatime. Between 1700 and 1800, the number of pounds of tea imported to England increased a thousand-fold. The British established tea plantations in India, as did the Dutch in Indonesia. Its use remains extraordinarily high around the world today, with most of it being drunk in the form of black tea, yet Asia drinks mostly green tea.

"The drink which has come to supply the place of beer has, in general, been tea. It is notorious that tea has no useful strength in it; that it contains nothing nutritious; that it, besides being good for nothing, has badness in it, because it is well known to produce want of sleep in many cases, and in all cases, to shake and weaken the nerves. It is, in fact, a weaker kind of laudanum, which enlivens for the moment and deadens afterwards."

—William Cobbett's *Cottage Economy,* 1821

Beyond the drink itself, compounds from tea are now being added to supplements, breakfast cereal, ice cream, diet aids, health drinks, skin lotions, soap, toothpaste, mouthwash, gum, and so on. It obviously contains many interesting and potentially therapeutic compounds besides its caffeine, and we are only now beginning to learn what they do.

How Scientists Think Tea Works

Tea flavonoids and polyphenols are antioxidant in a lot of ways, but not always. A lot is made of the beneficial antioxidant nature of plant flavonoids in general. But you can't always assume they will act that way. The major flavonoids in green tea, the catechins, behave like the polyphenols in black tea: they are all antioxidant in many test tube (*in vitro*) and animal (*in vivo*) studies. Also, green tea catechins and black tea polyphenols can scavenge free radicals. Free radicals in many cases are the same thing as oxidizing agents or are generated by oxi-

dizing agents, and tea contains antioxidants, as well.

Tea protects you from iron's free radical–generating activity. The flavonoids from green and polyphenols in black tea both stick to iron, preventing iron from generating damaging free radicals, which iron tends to do (this is why iron supplements shouldn't be taken unless necessary to correct a known deficiency). If you do need to take an iron supplement, avoid having it with tea, since tea will limit your absorption of the iron.

Tea can limit the carcinogenic action of nitric oxide. Because of its free radical–scavenging ability, tea can prevent nitric oxide from causing cancer. Nitric oxide is a free radical, but it is also a necessary hormone that helps you keep your blood pressure low, among other things, and is helpful in low amounts. In inflammation, nitric oxide shoots up and can do damage because it is a free radical, a reactive molecule. In high concentrations, nitric oxide is more likely to react with an oxidizing agent called *superoxide* to stick to proteins in a reaction called *nitrosylation.* Nitrosylation can lead to cancer. That tea can stop this may explain how it reduces cancer formation in animal studies.

However, the green tea flavonoids have on occasion been witnessed doing the opposite. Their presence has been associated with the generation of damaging oxidizing agents, like peroxide, and subsequent DNA damage. This is followed by the cell's giving up and committing a noninflammatory type of cell suicide called *apoptosis.* Whether this is a direct action or an indirect influence on the cell to make oxidizing agents isn't known. You may be relieved to know that catechin's cell-killing activity has mainly been observed in cancer cells. It's been theorized as a mechanism by which the catechins could prevent cancer.

What's In It

GREEN TEA retains the plant's characteristic polyphenolic compounds (30–42 percent), which is mostly epigallocatechin-3-gallate (EGCG), with a lesser amount of epicatechin-3-gallate (ECG), epigallocatechin (EGC), and epicatechin (EC). These are collectively termed catechins. At lower levels flavonols like kaempferol, quercetin, myricitin, and their glycosides are present in both green and black teas. In the making of black tea, the catechins polymerize into larger compounds, so there are fewer catechins (3–10 percent), but most (75–85 percent) are converted to the red-brown thearubigens, some to the orange-red theaflavins (2–6 percent; theaflavin-3-gallate, theaflavin-3'-gallate and theaflavin-3,3'-digallate), and a trace to the unstable, bright red theaflavic acid. Contrary to popular belief, tea does not have tannic acid (hydrolyzable tannins), although black tea has gallic acid, which is similar. Both green and black tea have about the same amount of fluoride per cup, with tea made from the youngest leaves on the plant (in higher quality teas) having the least, and teas made from old leaves on the plant having the most. As with coffee (in the *crema*), methylxanthines complex with polyphenols, plus brewing time, grade, and size of tea leaves make the caffeine content widely variable. Black tea is often said to have twice the amount of green tea, although there are cases where green tea's caffeine content is equally high. Although tea is the source of the medicine theophylline, the theophylline and related theobromine content in tea as a beverage is negligible.

Perhaps the catechins sense something different in the environment of a cancer cell and turn on this cell-sabotaging mechanism. The green tea catechin known as *EGCG* (*epigallocatechin-3-gallate*) is especially good at this, appearing paradoxidal, since in other studies EGCG is such a great antioxidant. But antioxidant mechanisms are many, so it's quite possible that EGCG does some of these mechanisms very well while subverting others. Many free radical scavengers work by becoming a free radical themselves while they neutralize the undesirable free radical, yet usually this is fine since the scavengers tend to be less reactive as radicals and are thus less harmful. The catechins do seem better at generating free radicals if they can find any copper ions around them to stick to.

Although it's troubling to find commonly consumed plant molecules damaging DNA, we can hope this occurs more often in cancer cells than in normal ones. That neither green nor black tea is obviously carcinogenic, and that the number of animal studies showing tea's protection against cancer are strikingly numerous, should reassure you that tea is more likely to protect against cancer than cause it.

Tea components could stop both cancer formation and spread, theoretically. Both tea polyphenols and caffeine alike have been witnessed enhancing the activity of *P53,* a tumor suppressor gene. When people carry a genetic mutation in their P53, the P53 doesn't function properly and they are more likely to get certain cancers, like colon cancer. The normal functional P53 acts like an emergency brake when cancerous processes start happening in a cell. Carcinogenic DNA-damaging agents make it more active, and then it does one of two things: it freezes the precancerous cell in the middle of cell division, or it gets the cell to neatly kill itself in the helpful manner called apoptosis. So it can stop cancer at an early stage and keep a cell from becoming cancerous. Tea stimulates the activity of P53.

Another regulator of cell division that tea affects is your cell's *AP-1 protein.* AP-1 protein stimulates the production of other proteins in your cells that in turn stimulate cell growth, which is good news when this action occurs in normal cells in a wound or a regenerating liver, but bad news if AP-1 keeps cells dividing away in abnormal tumor cells. Both green tea catechins and black tea theaflavins inhibit AP-1 activity, keeping an already-formed cancer cell from turning into a tumor.

EGCG keeps blood vessels from feeding tumors, and maybe fat, too. EGCG is a potent *angiogenesis inhibitor,* that is, it prevents blood vessel cells from dividing and forming new capillaries. While new capillary formation is helpful to feed cellular construction crews in wounds, it also feeds tumors, and tumor cells even send out chemical signals telling nearby cells to deliver nutrient-laden blood to them. Angiogenesis inhibitors like the drug Avastin are now being used with promising success against certain types of cancer. There is even an intriguing new theory that angiogenesis inhibitors help prevent fat cells from getting more fat by cutting off their blood supply, but that requires more research.

EGCG's may reduce fat—at least in test tubes and obese mice. The number of human trials investigating this effect is scant but disappointing. Be that as it may, in the test tube EGCG does appear to inhibit some digestive enzymes (lipases) that in their normal home in the gut would otherwise aid dietary fat absorption. Obese mice that were fed EGCG also made less fat-constructing enzymes in their fat cells. When fed EGCG, obese mice gained less weight than they normally would. This was attributed not to reduced food intake, but the fact that "feces energy content was slightly increased by EGCG,"[2] indicating that some of their calories were going straight through them. (This is also what happens with diarrhea.) Despite the now popular custom of spiking diet aids with EGCG, these fat-reducing mechanisms remain very theoretical at this point and have not panned out in human studies so far.

Theanine could help your cells get more of the cell-protector glutathione while depriving cancer cells of it. Theanine is an amino acid unique to tea, and it resembles another more abundant one called *glutamate.* In trying to determine how tea helped mice keep their cancer under control, researchers noted that the mice were converting the theanine in tea to glutamate in their livers. Glutamate is used for a great many things, but it is also a constituent of glutathione. Glutathione is the most abundant sulfur-containing (or *thiol*) antioxidant in cells and is present in relatively high concentrations in most cells. It is a critical detoxifying agent in the liver, and it protects against cell death in all tissues.

Extra glutamate stimulates glutathione production if glutathione is low (although glutathione's other precursor, *L-cysteine,* is better at it). Low glutathione is associated with oxidative stress, deleterious health, and poor prognosis. Unfortunately, boosting glutathione in cancer patients is tricky, because glutathione is elevated in a lot of tumors, helping the tumor cell to survive. Yet the supplementation of either glutamine or theanine reduced glutathione in the tumor and boosted it in noncancerous cells.

Tea is a good source of fluoride—good news for bones and teeth. The tea plant tends to bioaccumulate fluoride from soil. While fluoride is known for helping to keep teeth healthy, it is also effective as an accepted treatment for osteoporosis. Tea also shows some hint of helping prevent bone loss, and its fluoride content is the most commonly offered explanation. (Tea doesn't have any of the assistant bone-building vitamin K, however—that's a common myth.) Some also suggest that weak estrogenic compounds in tea help build bone.

Besides its usual reanimating buzz, daily caffeine seems to prevent Parkinson's disease. No one questions that caffeine is a stimulant, and you can still have decaffeinated tea to get all the other active ingredients in tea if you don't like how caffeine makes you feel. But caffeine does have some health benefits. As it does in yerba maté and guarana products (pages 342 and 179), caffeine prevents a molecule called *adenosine* from sticking to adenosine receptors in your brain. Adenosine normally builds up during the day as a consequence of our energy output, and when it gets concentrated enough to bind to its receptors in the brain, we get sleepy. Caffeine sits inside adenosine's receptor, however, because it looks like adenosine, and this keeps adenosine from inducing sleepiness.

Scientist think this adenosine-thwarting action explains why epidemiological studies show caffeine reduces the risk of getting Parkinson's. The connection is with the neurotransmitter dopamine. When adenosine receptors are blocked, dopamine levels rise, so caffeine increases dopamine in the brain. We don't know what causes Parkinson's disease, but it starts to happen when the brain's dopamine-producing nerves cells die off. The symptoms of stiffness, tremor, writing and speech impairments are caused by the loss of dopamine signaling in the brain. Caffeine keeps dopamine levels higher, but how

this might prevent Parkinson's isn't really known, because the cause of Parkinson's isn't yet known.

Caffeine can help with some headaches and water retention. Caffeine causes blood vessels to open in some places, such as muscles and the lungs, and to constrict in others, such as the skin and brain. Vascular headaches are associated with overly dilated blood vessels in the brain. Caffeine constricts them, reducing swelling and pain; hence its inclusion in many over-the-counter headache remedies and prescription migraine medicines. Instead of popping a pill for a headache, you can try brewing yourself some caffeinated tea. Of course, caffeine's other oft-documented symptom is that it increases urination. This results from its inhibition of the antidiuretic hormone.

There is no theine. It's a marketing gimmick. Just as with yerba matés "mateine" (page 342), "theine" is just a fancy and unnecessary term for caffeine, but the caffeine in tea is no different than the caffeine from any other source. Theine, mateine, and caffeine are the same thing.

Tea tannin can reduce puffy eyes and diarrhea. Both green and black tea contain molecules that can wrap around portions of protein molecules, squeezing and shrinking them. This is the classic astringent action of tannins in tea. (However, contrary to the common myth, tea contains no tannic acid.) If you put cold, wet teabags on your closed eyelids, the water will cool and constrict blood vessels in your eyes, and the tannins will help shrink tissues a bit. If you drink the tea, tannins coat your gut's own proteins, protecting the lining of the gut from irritating agents that cause diarrhea. This effect works best only in moderate amounts. Consuming too much tannin will result in excessive tanning of the stomach lining, thus irritating your gut.

Good Effects . . .
and Not So Good

Tea drinking is safe, but don't overdo the caffeine. For millennia, billions of people have drunk tea with no outstanding adverse consequences. However, excessive caffeine from any source will cause sleeplessness, jitters, and crankiness. Some people who are sensitive may get an irregular heartbeat or digestive upset from caffeine and should try decaffeinated tea. Even in decaffeinated tea, tannin can still upset the stomach if multiple cups of a more tannic tea are taken during a short period of time. (Some teas have more tannins than others, however.)

Don't take it with iron or copper. Components in tea bind to iron, so people who take iron supplements shouldn't take tea with their iron. It's not the caffeine that does this, so decaffeinated tea will limit iron absorption, too. Most people should limit iron anyway, because of its worrisome radical-generating activity, so this is not a detriment for most, and may be a benefit. However, infants given tea absorb less iron, and this has led to anemia in some cases. Since tea flavonoids generate free radicals in the presence of copper, it seems prudent not to take tea with a copper supplement either.

Make sure you get adequate folic acid. There is conflicting evidence over whether tea, both black and green, interferes with this B vitamin's activity, causing homocysteine levels to rise. Homocysteine is an amino acid that is found in the blood. High levels of homocysteine indicate increased risk of cardiovascular disease and stroke. The effect of tea on homocysteine, if there is one, may not be significant; for example, tea is more of a cardiovascular protector than a saboteur. Since folic acid keeps homocysteine down, everyone should get adequate folic

acid in any case. Folic acid (also called *folate*) can be obtained from citrus fruits, beans, tomatoes, and leafy green vegetables such as spinach and romaine lettuce; wheat also is often fortified with it.

Tea made from old or young leaves has different components. The most expensive tea is made from the prized young buds on the plant. These have the most flavonoids, catechins, and the most caffeine. But the most expensive tea also has the least fluoride. Fluoride accumulates in the oldest leaves on the plant. Cheap tea made from these leaves has the most fluoride, so cheaper tea products are theoretically more likely to benefit osteoporosis.

Milk reduces the tannin activity. If tannin upsets your tummy, the British tradition of "cream teas" may help. Tea tannin reacts with the protein in milk instead of the protein in your gut.

Interesting Facts

How to Make Tea

ALL TEAS, other than the so-called herbal teas, are made from the leaves of *Camellia sinensis.* ("Herbal" tea is generally accepted to mean tea *not* made from *Camellia sinensis,* which is potentially confusing, since *Camellia sinensis* is technically an herb.) The freshly picked leaves of *Camellia sinensis* are full of flavonoids called *catechins.* No one drinks tea made from fresh leaves off the plant, though, because it is weak and watery. After the tea leaves are dried, they are "rolled," and the leaf gets a twist that keeps it from releasing its components too quickly when steeped. More importantly, rolling causes cellular compartments in the leaves to break open, allowing the catechins to come into contact with an enzyme called *polyphenol oxidase.* In the making of black tea, the leaf is allowed to sit after rolling, exposing the catechins to polyphenol oxidase. The enzyme oxidizes the catechins, and their products stick to each other, polymerizing to forming larger, more complex molecules that are darker in color.

This darkening process is still traditionally called *fermentation,* which is misleading because no microbes are involved. This darkening reaction by polyphenol oxidase is also responsible for the browning of fruit when cells are bruised and their contents are exposed to it. Green tea doesn't get fermented, and its catechins remain intact. Black tea does get fermented, so its catechin content is lower. Most of them polymerize into red-brown thearubigens, some to the orange-red theaflavins, and reactions between flavonoids and these products release the unstable, bright red theaflavic acid. This process creates amber-hued constituents that give black tea its distinctive color and flavor. These black tea constituents are often called *polyphenols.*

Green tea is prevented from undergoing fermentation, because it is steamed before it is rolled. Though the rolling releases the enzyme that makes the black tea molecules, the enzyme's activity has been destroyed by heat, so no fermentation can occur. This is why blanching fruits and vegetables keeps them from browning, too. Oolong tea is only briefly fermented before and after rolling, so it's something halfway between black and green, chemically. Once only a rare, pricey commodity, white tea is now becoming popular because of celebrities' publicized enjoyment of it. White tea is processed like green tea, but it is made from the choicest young buds on the plant. White tea is mainly popular because it is a new item on the market and because of media hype; whether it is more healthful than other classes of tea

hasn't been fully studied. Its properties probably mirror those of green tea more than black tea because of how it is processed. Certainly, many people relish its unique, delicate flavor.

EVIDENCE OF ACTION

If consumed regularly, both green and black tea could prevent Parkinson's disease, probably due to the caffeine content in the tea. Large-scale, epidemiological data indicate that people who drink caffeinated beverages such as tea, coffee, or cola on a regular basis are significantly less likely to get Parkinson's disease.[3, 4, 5] For women, it didn't matter how much caffeine they took, but for men, the effect was dose-dependent. A dose of 104–208 milligrams of caffeine daily was enough to do the trick.

Also, either color tea seems to improve cognitive agility. Again, it's probably the caffeine. While it's no surprise that ingestion of caffeinated tea (but not decaffeinated tea) helped improve alertness in volunteers who were given a battery of cognitive exams, it also improved their information-processing capacity, for a limited period of time.[6] It did not affect their short-term memory. A similar study found that 60 milligrams of caffeine in tea provided volunteers significant improvement in reaction time for subjects tested on pattern recognition and visual matching tests, compared to decaffeinated tea.[7]

Black tea may help women who get kidney stones. (Green tea hasn't been evaluated for this yet.) In the Nurses Health Institute study, 81,093 women were questioned on beverage use and kidney stones. After statistically controlling the data to cancel out possible confounding factors such as fluid intake and lifestyle (tea drinkers may just live healthier lifestyles, for example), they still found an 8 percent reduction in the incidence of kidney stones.[8]

Commonly Reported Uses for Tea*

Internally

beverage, stimulant, diuretic, illness, headache, osteoporosis, cancer, respiratory problems, weight loss, diarrhea, tooth decay, cardiovascular protection

forms available for internal use:

beverage, dried leaves, capsules, extracts, tablets, EGCG

commonly reported dosage:

One to 3 cups of tea are typically taken daily.

*These uses and dosages are from historic use and are not necessarily tested nor recommended.

A couple of studies hint that very long term use of either green or black tea might decrease osteoporosis. The effect was smaller for black tea in the Women's Health Initiative study,[9] than for green tea,[10] and both studies looked at people drinking tea for around ten years. However, smaller studies are inconclusive or conflicting, so the current data is insufficient to render a conclusion.

Both black and green tea have something going for them in the way of cardiovascular health and cholesterol. In the prospective Netherlands Rotterdam Study, black tea was evaluated for protecting against heart attack and hardening of the arteries. (Green tea wasn't examined.) Controlling against confounding factors like lifestyle, out of the 3,454 participants who had their arteries examined by radiography, black tea drinkers had significantly reduced atherosclerosis.[11] Also, within the 4,807 people studied, those who were black tea drinkers also had significantly fewer heart attacks.[12] A 375-milligram theaflavin-enriched green tea extract consumed daily for twelve weeks had no effect on "good" HDL cholesterol, but slightly significant reductions in "bad" LDL cholesterol in 258 hypercholesterolemic volunteers, although it should be noted that green tea naturally has no theaflavin, and black tea does.[13] However, in a large epidemiological study of 1,371 Japanese men, in which statistical manipulations helped cancel out effects due to age, weight, alcohol use, and smoking, increased green tea drinking was associated with significant decreases in total cholesterol and "bad" LDL cholesterol, and significant increases in "good" HDL cholesterol.[14] Those who drank more green tea also had significantly better blood markers of liver function.

Green tea extracts' inclusion in more and more weight loss products is causing consumers to think it helps treat obesity, but this has not been validated as of yet. The data suggesting it might be useful for losing weight are mainly based on a few test tube and animal studies. For people taking a green tea extract (AR25, Exolise) for three months, weight was decreased by 4.6 percent and waist circumference by 4.48 percent,[15] but the subjects and investigators were both aware of the treatment. A better-designed study of people who had recently lost weight on a calorie-restricted diet showed that green tea capsules (573 mg/day of catechins and 104 mg/day of caffeine) had no effect on their subsequent weight gain, with respect to placebo.[16]

In animal studies, green and black tea repeatedly showed great promise in preventing cancer. These animal studies are, for the most part, encouraging. Most animal studies have looked at skin cancer, with the tea applied topically. The rest mainly incorporate the tea into drinking water. In animals, more than eighty studies demonstrate that tea protects against cancers of the skin (23 studies), lung (14), liver (9), stomach (8), breast (7), colon (5), esophagus (4), small intestine (4), pancreas (3), oral (1), bladder (1) and prostate (1).[17] It is therefore frustrating that the human studies don't hold up as well. Although the data is still quite promising overall, with most showing pro-tection, some show it didn't do anything, and in a few cases it appeared to have even increased cancer risk. Scientists reviewing large numbers of studies have tentatively suggested that green tea appears somewhat more protective against cancer than does black tea, in both animal and human studies,[18] but that conclusion could be swayed in that more studies have been performed on green tea than on black. The question remains whether or not the animal studies are applicable to humans.

THE BOTTOM LINE

- Tea, both green and black, is made from the leaves of the *Camellia sinensis* plant. So-called herbal teas refer to any tea made from a plant other than *Camellia sinensis*.
- Besides its stimulant, caffeine, green tea catechins and black tea polyphenols are antioxidant and free radical–scavenging. Although they show promising anticancer action in animals, probably by numerous mechanisms, it's not yet clear if humans derive the same cancer-protective benefit. They do not appear to cause cancer, at least.
- Regular tea drinking seems to provide modest cardiovascular protection, and may perhaps also protect against bone loss, cavities, and kidney stones.
- Despite theorized mechanisms for tea and its extracts aiding weight loss, this has not been supported by data from the few clinical trials performed on humans.
- Epidemiological studies suggest that regular caffeine from tea or other sources prevents Parkinson's disease.
- Tea is safe as a beverage, but too much of it can cause adverse effects, primarily from excess caffeine and tannin. Tea limits iron absorption, which is only a problem if you take an iron supplement along with it.

TURMERIC

Curcuma domestica, also called *Curcuma longa*

HISTORY AND FOLKLORE

If you love Indian food, you may already know that "curry" is not one spice, but a mixture of many variable ones that almost always includes turmeric, or *haldi,* as it is called in India. Turmeric tends to stain *everything* bright yellow, and is in fact used to color American preparations of yellow mustard condiments. Turmeric has a mild, warm, bitter taste, vaguely reminiscent of its cousins ginger (see page 142) and cardamom, which all share membership in the *Zingiberaceae* family. These three spices are all native to Asia and remain traditional additions to Indian and South Asian cuisine. The Chinese term for turmeric, *jianghuang,* means "yellow ginger."

Like ginger, turmeric has been grabbing some headlines recently as an anti-inflammatory, yet it contains different active ingredients, which are based on its yellow-staining, oily pigments known as *curcumin* and chemically related *curcuminoids.* Turmeric's yellow root is powdered and is used in Indian culture as a dye, as well as a household remedy for digestive problems, sprains, swellings, wounds, arthritis, and infections. It is also commonly used in religious rituals.

HOW SCIENTISTS THINK TURMERIC WORKS

What makes turmeric yellow lowers the calcium ion concentrations inside your cells. Actually, the molecule that helps

turmeric stain everything mustard yellow, curcumin, doesn't *really* remove calcium from your cells, it just helps the cells stow calcium into internal storage units inside the cells. This may be analogous to a kid's startlingly spotless bedroom after he "cleans" it—he didn't *really* get rid of all the junk, he just stuffed it away into a closet.

Cells maintain low internal calcium concentrations by stowing calcium away inside interconnected, tube-shaped networks of internal "closets" called the *endoplasmic reticulum,* or in the case of muscle cells, the *sarcoplasmic reticulum* (the prefix "sarco-" is often tacked on to muscle-related terms in science). Pumps on the outer membranes of these cellular chambers continuously grab onto the calcium inside the cell, pulling it inside the chambers, thus keeping a cell's internal calcium concentration low. A muscle cell's normal internal calcium concentration is maintained at about a thousand times less than what it would be if this pumping action did not occur. Every now and then a calcium pump slips, however, losing its grip on some calcium, which then floats away inside the cell. Curcumin sticks to the pumps, keeping them from slipping and increasing their calcium-storing efficiency.[1] This changes a cell's behavior, since calcium is a key chemical signal, switching on and off various cellular functions. That turmeric affects several calcium-dependent cellular functions lends weight to this theoretical mechanism.

This could explain how turmeric soothes gastrointestinal cramps. Calcium provokes dramatic results inside muscle cells: Calcium makes a muscle contract. Lowering a muscle's internal calcium content prevents the muscle from contracting, and this is what curcumin does when used in moderation. Applied to all types of muscle in test tube and animal studies, small doses of curcumin are typically *spasmolytic*— that is, curcumin reduces muscle spasms.

Eating turmeric won't relax all of your muscles, however, because the curcumin inside it has a very hard time getting absorbed into your blood from your digestive tract. It's pretty much a one-way trip for curcumin after it has been ingested. Thus, the bulk of turmeric's effects will be topical if it is applied to the skin, or within the digestive tract if it is eaten. Perhaps this explains why turmeric is an age-old, Asian digestive aid. Eating a moderate amount of turmeric probably keeps gut muscles from contracting and cramping, because of the curcumin in it. However, it is possible to overdo it.

What's In It

MUCH OF the research on turmeric root has focused attention on its oily yellow pigment, curcumin, also called *diferuloylmethane*. Besides containing curcumin and related curcuminoids, turmeric's 3–5 percent volatile oil contains mainly sesquiterpenes such as its odiferous alpha- and beta-turmerone, as well as arturmerone, gamma-atlantone, and zingiberene.

High curcumin concentrations have the opposite effect. Take too much turmeric, however, and your digestive system will pay for it. This is another age-old, recognized phenomenon. The same researchers who discovered that curcumin enhances cellular calcium sequestering also found that giving a cell even more curcumin simply shuts down the cell's internal calcium pumps, and the cell's internal calcium rises. When calcium is increased inside a muscle cell, the muscle cell will contract. When gut muscles contract excessively, pain is perceived as "cramps." Thus curcumin does not always relax muscles; the more you give to a gallbladder, for example, the more this muscular organ contracts. Most people's gallbladders contract fairly well on their own, but this contraction may enhance the release of bile, which helps in the digestion of fat. On the other hand, increased gut contractions could explain why eating too much turmeric causes stomach upsets.

Turmeric is anti-inflammatory and has anticancer activity. The curcumin in turmeric is anti-inflammatory in several ways, providing reasonable explanations for how it prevents cancer from hatching and growing, as inflammation fans the flames of both processes. Curcumin acts directly as a free radical scavenger.[2] Free radicals damage tissue, exacerbating inflammation. Free radicals can also cause mutations that lead to cancer. Curcumin also stimulates cells in culture to make glutathione, a natural antioxidant and protector against toxins.

Yet there's more. Curcumin limits the body's ability to make enzyme cyclooxygenase-2 (COX-2), which would otherwise make inflammatory hormone-like subtances called *prostaglandins.* Curcumin is repeatedly found to decrease a particular prostaglandin called *PGE2,* for example, which would otherwise help initiate the classic heat, pain, redness, and swelling associated with inflammation. PGE2 is not all bad, though; in your gut it decreases stomach acid and increases protective stomach mucous. Turmeric's power to turn off PGE2 production thus explains in part how it both reduces inflammation and causes occasional gastric distress.

Curcumin also diminishes inflammatory agents like tumor necrosis factor (TNF) and NF-kappa-beta. Tumor necrosis factor isn't so much known for killing tumors as mediating some of their nastier effects, and NF-kappa-beta is similar. These in turn stimulate synthesis of other inflammatory agents, like the COX-2 enzyme, mentioned above. It's interesting to note that in test tube studies, curcumin enables cancer cells to self-destruct, something that old and damaged cells do in a neat, helpful way, yet unfortunately, cancer cells sometimes resist pulling the plug on themselves like they should. NF-kappa-beta not only promotes the manufacture of other inflammatory molecules, but also helps cancer cells resist this natural "cell suicide," in part by stopping the large influx of calcium that occurs in abnormal cells that would otherwise trigger cell suicide. That curcumin in high doses stops a cell's calcium pumps from lowering its internal calcium concentrations could explain how it sensitizes cancer cells to this natural cell death.

Scientists hope that turmeric might help those with psoriasis and cystic fibrosis because of its effect on certain calcium-binding proteins. Some proteins must bind to calcium in order to function properly, but if these proteins are causing trouble, curcumin might help, by starving them of calcium. Psoriasis, for example, is linked with excessive activity of a protein called *phosphorylase kinase,* which is linked to a calcium-binding subunit that needs to bind to calcium in order for it to work. Not only did topical curcumin reduce the phosphorylase kinase activity of people with psoriasis better than the standard medication, calcipotriol, but it also reduced symptoms of psoriasis.[3]

In cystic fibrosis, a faulty chloride channel protein can't make it to the surface of certain cells after it is made inside the cell. In places like the respiratory and digestive tract, failure to properly pump chloride results in unmanageably sticky mucous coating the cell. Affected people suffer repeated infections, chronic respiratory distress, and shortened lives. Yet for some with cystic fibrosis, even faulty channels can function to some extent, once they make it to a cell's surface. The problem is that molecular police inspect proteins on their way to the surface of the cell and banish the faulty channel protein, since it doesn't meet specifications. These molecular police are proteins, too, but they require calcium to function. Curcumin denies these inspector proteins their calcium in mouse models of cystic fibrosis, allowing the chloride channels to make it to the surface of cells, and in one study most of the treated mice appeared almost completely better.[4] However, translating this use of turmeric into a therapy for humans with cystic fibrosis has had profound ups and downs. Those with severely dysfunctional chloride channels are unlikely to be helped, and later tests in mice and cell cultures failed to confirm the exciting results of the first study.[5] Nonetheless, the U.S. Cystic Fibrosis Foundation is now investigating the use of curcumin in a human trial.

GOOD EFFECTS . . . AND NOT SO GOOD

Taking large doses of turmeric appears safe and may lower your risk of gastrointestinal cancers, but it can occasionally cause stomach upset. Centuries of using turmeric in Asia as well as a phase I clinical trial (that is, a small-scale safety test) of turmeric that investigated people taking high doses of turmeric oil have helped confirm its safety.[6] There is much discussion in scientific papers as to whether or not regular consumption of turmeric by Indians lowers their risk of cancer, and though it seems theoretically sound, the data is undoubtedly confounded by other variables, such as the prevalence of vegetarianism in India, which also helps lower the risk of cancer. Although turmeric is often recommended in India as a digestive aid, it occasionally causes stomach upset, especially if a lot of it is taken.

Commonly Reported Uses for Turmeric*

Internally

digestive aid, anti-inflammatory, antirheumatic, anticancer, stimulant

forms available for internal use:
capsules, powder, dried or fresh root, liquid extract, tincture, oil

commonly reported dosage:
Between 1 and 3 grams a day of turmeric powder is taken three times a day, or after meals. Sometimes turmeric is dissolved in warm milk.

Externally

sprains, wounds, bruises, itchy skin

forms available for external use:
capsules, powder, dried or fresh root, liquid extract, tincture, oil

commonly reported dosage:
Traditionally, turmeric oil or powder is applied to the skin, sometimes mixed with honey.

*These uses and dosages are from historic use and are not necessarily tested nor recommended.

Turmeric should be kept in the dark to preserve its activity. This goes for curry powders, too, which usually contain turmeric. The active yellow pigment in turmeric is sensitive to light and will be destroyed by it. In fact, unwanted turmeric stains can be removed by placing the stained item in direct sunlight, which may bleach the stain away.

Skip the bromelain, or use oil. Many turmeric preparations contain added bromelain, a protein-digesting enzyme isolated from pineapple. However, the curcumin in turmeric is not a protein, nor is it surrounded by protein, and breaking down proteins—which most people do very well on their own anyway—will not help with the absorption of curcumin. There is no reliable evidence that adding bromelain to turmeric will help you absorb the turmeric. For more of the oil-soluble curcumin to be pulled out of the turmeric, try consuming it with a favorite healthy oil. Since curcumin is not water soluble, don't expect to get much curcumin from turmeric tea.

People with gallbladder problems should be cautious with turmeric. Turmeric causes the gallbladder to contract, releasing its stored bile into the digestive tract, a normal process during fat digestion. This contraction can be painful for those who have gallstones in the gallbladder. Some herbalists think that regularly squeezing this organ with gallbladder-constricting herbs like turmeric helps keep it clean and stone-free, yet others worry that doing so could cause an existing stone to be pushed into the bile duct, causing impaction. If you think that you have gallstones or gallbladder disease, talk to your doctor first about using any gallbladder-contracting supplement therapeutically.

EVIDENCE OF ACTION

Turmeric is anti-inflammatory, according to numerous cell, animal, and human tests. A veterinary study that was randomized, placebo-controlled, and double-blind (both investigators and pet owners did not know what they were giving their dogs) found that arthritic dogs were significantly helped by taking turmeric extract, and the pets suffered no adverse effects from it either.[7] Curcumin from turmeric was also comparable in effectiveness to anti-inflammatory steroids in treating a serious eye inflammation called *chronic anterior uveitis,* which can lead to blindness. Unlike steroid therapy, curcumin held an advantage in producing no obvious side effects.[8] Curcumin also held its own in treating the inflammatory skin lesions of psoriasis when compared with the prescription cream calcipotriol and a placebo.[9]

Though too much turmeric can upset some sensitive people's stomachs, turmeric may still help other people with their indigestion. A study designed to examine the safety and efficacy of turmeric (a phase II clinical trial) included twenty-five endoscoped ulcer patients taking 300 milligrams of turmeric five times daily. The longer they took turmeric, the fewer of them had ulcers, and 76 percent did not have ulcers after twelve weeks. However, no placebos were used in the trial, so it is difficult to say to what extent their ulcers were diminished by turmeric. No significant changes in their blood chemistry, liver, or kidney function were seen,[10] confirming curcumin's poor ability to escape the final destination of the digestive tract.

A couple of studies also found that curcumin reliably contracts human gallbladders. Since this releases bile into the digestive tract, turmeric theoretically facilitates digestion of a fatty meal, which requires bile to solubilize the fat. A reliable (randomized, placebo-controlled) trial testing a mixture of turmeric and another herb, celandine, in those with gallbladder dysfunction found that the herbal combo provided no difference with respect to placebo for almost every symptom measured. However, "the reduction of dumpy and colicky pain" may have been faster during the first of the three weeks of the trial.[11]

THE BOTTOM LINE

- Turmeric is relatively safe and has anti-inflammatory, digestive, and anticancer properties. Turmeric could help people with psoriasis, but it is too soon to say whether it can help those with cystic fibrosis.
- Most of the effects of turmeric are topical or affect the digestive tract, since the active ingredients are not readily absorbed into the blood stream. Consuming turmeric with oil will enhance liberation of the active ingredient. It is commonly claimed that bromelain, a protein-digesting enzyme isolated from pineapple that is added to some turmeric preparations, will help you absorb it, but that is highly unlikely and disproven.
- Large doses of turmeric may upset the stomach. People with gallbladder problems should be cautious using turmeric, since turmeric contracts the gallbladder.
- Turmeric's yellow pigment, curcumin, appears to work in part by affecting a cell's ability to sequester calcium ions. It also has several anti-inflammatory and free radical–scavenging activities.

In animal studies, turmeric's curcumin prevents the development and spread of cancers of the skin and digestive tract but is less effective in treating cancers outside the digestive tract, probably because curcumin has trouble traveling from the gut into the blood. Curcumin's effect on human cancer patients is less clear, since trials have not used placebos, but instead employ increasing doses of turmeric extracts.[12, 13, 14] Such studies of colorectal cancer patients who were not responding to standard treatment indicated turmeric helped them make less of the inflammatory prostaglandin PGE2. Five of the fifteen cancer patients were deemed uncured but remained stable by radiological assessment for two to four months during turmeric treatment.

UVA URSI

Arctostaphylos uva-ursi

HISTORY AND FOLKLORE

Uva ursi means "bear's grape" in Latin, because bears are supposed to enjoy this herb. Another bear reference is the genus *Arctostaphylos,* which is Greek for "bear's bunch of berries." People are less enthusiastic than bears for their fruit. Meriwether Lewis, of the great Lewis and Clark American expedition, encountered uva ursi in Native American meals and concluded it was "a very tasteless and insippid fruit." It isn't these questionable fruits that are used by herbalists, however, but uva ursi's leaves.

The leaves' high tannin content explain its longtime use as an astringent, and several Native American tribes mixed uva ursi leaves with tobacco to create *kinnikinnik,* which they smoked. It's curious that this cousin to cranberry has been used for all manner of urinary tract complaints, as has cranberry (see page 86). For example, today uva ursi can be found in almost all herbal diuretic mixtures, although it's not clear that it is effective as such; it is probably a better urinary antiseptic. Uva ursi has similar habitats to cranberry, trailing along the ground in the colder, woodsy areas of the northern hemisphere in America, Europe, and Asia.

HOW SCIENTISTS THINK UVA URSI WORKS

Uva ursi is a source of hydroquinone, which hurts bacteria and other cells. Uva ursi leaves harbor a decent amount of arbutin. Arbutin is the same thing as a moderately toxic, antibiotic molecule called *hydroquinone,* except that arbutin possesses an attached sugar molecule, and hydroquinone does not. Unlike most sugar-bound plant molecules, arbutin can sneak through glucose-transporting receptors in the gut in order to reach the bloodstream,[1] although perhaps not very well. Gut bacteria can cut off the sugar part, too, to produce the antibiotic hydroquinone, which is better absorbed than the arbutin. (Now stop and consider that here are gut bacteria brainlessly removing a sugar from a molecule—something they do routinely—but the resultant product is an antibacterial. However, scientific literature has yet to discuss whether this affects gut flora.)

After hydroquinone and arbutin have been absorbed, the liver might then add other water-soluble bits (like sulfate or glucuronide) to some of them, something your liver often does to drug molecules. This process, called *conjugation,* makes drugs more water soluble and thus more likely to exit your body through urine. So if you have a urinary tract infection, consuming uva ursi will deliver these hydroquinone precursors, and possibly even some free hydroquinone, to the infected site.

How the modified hydroquinone molecules get turned back into hydroquinone isn't clear, but *theoretically,* an alkaline environment (otherwise known as *basic* or *high pH*) should help remove the liver's added trappings to produce the free hydroquinone. This is why herbalists usually recommend you alter your diet by eating more alkaline foods to make your urine more alkaline when you take uva ursi for urinary tract infections, to help this removal or *deconjugation* process.

What's In It

UVA URSI possesses 5-15 percent hydroquinone derivatives, mostly the glucoside arbutin, along with some methoxylated arbutin, free hydroquinone, and methoxylated hydroquinones, and these are the postulated antibiotic ingredients. The leaves have up to around 20 percent tannins, such as gallotannins, ellagic tannins, catechin, and anthocyanidins, phenolic acids, and flavonols like quercetin, kaempferol, and myricetin, and their glycosides. The triterpene ursolic acid and the flavanoid isoquercitrin theoretically provide the herb's alleged diuretic effect.

Hydroquinone is hard on cells. Therefore you may expect it to hurt unwanted bacteria and act as an antibiotic. Hydroquinone is similar in appearance, and behavior, to *phenol,* which unravels proteins, rendering proteins unable to function. Phenol may be more familiar to most people than hydroquinone: It has a sharp, sweet, "medicinal" odor; many numbing, antiseptic preparations such as medicated lip balms and sore throat sprays list phenol in their ingredients. However, because phenol is irritating to cells and removes skin layers in higher concentrations, you may want to reconsider applying it to chapped lips. In fact, what is found in some lip balms is also used in cosmetic skin "peels," and the FDA limits phenol's use in cosmetic preparations to low concentrations in order to limit its toxicity.

Hydroquinone is like this irritating phenol but has added properties of being especially good at forming those nasty free radicals, and of switching back and forth from being a good reducing agent and oxidizing agent—in other words, it is rather reactive. The more reactive a molecule is, the more likely it is to be toxic. Hydroquinone is probably one good reason why the solvent benzene causes leukemia: Benzene is transformed to hydroquinone by the liver, and this hydroquinone then damages chromosomes in bone marrow cells. This is why the wiser herbalists advise against taking uva ursi for longer than a week. Hydroquinone is an antibiotic, but due to the concerns listed above, it is also something to which exposure should be limited.

New research reveals that uva ursi contains an antibiotic's helper. Corilagin, an ellagitannin from uva ursi enabled a penicillin-type antibiotic to do its job against a bacterium that was previously resistant to that antibiotic.[2] The growing problem of antibiotic resistance, the evolving ability of bacteria to withstand antibiotic medications, greatly worries health officials, so the race is on to find a way to kill these resistant pathogens. One of these new "superbugs," methicillin-resistant *Staphylococcus aureus,* or MRSA, evades many antibiotics by making a more slippery version of a protein that the antibiotic would normally bind. These proteins, collectively called *penicillin-binding proteins,* are enzymes that help the bacterium create its cell wall, which the bacterium needs to survive. Corilagin appears to prevent these bacterial cell wall–building enzymes from forming properly. Researchers note that you get far more corilagin in a typical dose of uva ursi tea than they used in their cell cultures. Whether or not a practical, new, uva ursi–antibiotic combination can be developed to combat some forms of antibiotic resistance remains to be seen, but it's encouraging news.

Uva ursi's arbutin whitens your skin, but you should consider its toxicity. Although uva ursi is not often found in topical preparations, its constituent arbutin has been shown to prevent tanning, and it probably interferes with melanin synthesis. When arbutin has its sugar removed, you get hydroquinone, which is used in all sorts of commercial skin-"bleaching" cosmetic preparations. It isn't technically "bleaching," which implies chemical oxidation, but hydroquinone's interference with the production of the dark pigment melanin that does this. Hydroquinone resembles the amino acid tyrosine, a precursor to many things, including melanin. It's thought to work by competing with tyrosine for tyrosinase, the enzyme that turns tyrosine into melanin. Some also think it works by just *killing* melanocytes, the melanin-making cells in your skin, which is theoretically possible, given its toxicity. Although it's still allowed in low concentrations in U.S. whitening creams, hydroquinone has been banned in several European and African countries because of its toxicity. Arbutin from uva ursi is likely to behave similarly.

Good Effects . . . and Not So Good

Looking for an herbal diuretic? Consider trying something else. The diuretic action of uva ursi is not well documented and has even been questioned. Since uva ursi has potentially harmful ingredients, an alternative diuretic that is safer and more effective should be considered.

Uva ursi can be used for urinary tract infections, but for short time periods only. Hydroquinone, thought to be the active

ingredient, causes cancer and other problems, and the risk increases the longer you use it. Topical hydroquinone is banned in several countries because of these problems. One case study depicts a woman who consumed uva ursi for three years and developed retinal damage.[3] Most references suggest uva ursi should be taken no longer than one week. Of course, if you do have a urinary tract infection, you should be under a doctor's care.

Commonly Reported Uses for Uva Ursi*

Internally
urinary tract infections, diuretic, kidney stones, astringent

forms available for internal use:
tablet, capsule, fresh and dried leaf, liquid extract, tea, tincture, powdered solid extract

commonly reported dosage:
The usual dose is 1.5 to 4 grams of leaves daily for no longer than one week. Several sources suggest making an aqueous extraction by steeping the leaves in cold water overnight in order to minimize tannins, which can irritate the stomach, and this beverage is drunk up to four times a day for no longer than one week.

*These uses and dosages are from historic use and are not necessarily tested nor recommended.

Short-term adverse reactions can also occur. Uva ursi leaves have a high tannin content, and tannins can irritate the gastrointestinal tract. Tea made from the leaves should not be made with hot water; rather, the leaves should be soaked in cold water overnight. Lower temperatures reduce the amount of tannins extracted. Besides gastrointestinal upset, high doses of uva ursi have caused ringing in the ears and nausea. The hydroquinone in uva ursi can temporarily turn urine greenish-brown, and as alarming as that sounds, this effect is supposedly harmless. Pregnant or nursing women should not take uva ursi.

If you want to alkalinize your urine, here's what to do. First, it's not clear that this is necessary in order to liberate hydroquinone from its conjugates in the urine, but it's certainly chemically plausible. The easiest way to alkalinize your urine is to take a mild base, like bicarbonate. Baking soda, or sodium bicarbonate, is a source of this ion. Citrate, from potassium citrate, or calcium citrate, used in some calcium supplements, will also work. Fruits and vegetables generally alkalinize urine as well, while meat acidifies it. Some poorly informed people recommend altering the pH of *other* body fluids by diet, but this is not possible unless obvious toxic overdoses of an acid or base are taken, so it is not recommended. The rest of the body cleverly resists pH changes with its natural buffers; only the urine's pH can be affected by diet.

EVIDENCE OF ACTION

There are barely any modern human clinical trials using uva ursi, so it's difficult to say what it really does in people. Most of its actions are theorized, based on known activities of some of its components, like arbutin. Though it's most often sold as a diuretic, this effect has been disputed and even contradicted in some experiments. However, it does contain some diuretic components, like ursolic acid and isoquercitrin, and aqueous extracts increased urine production in rats.[4]

It's long been assumed that hydroquinone is liberated from arbutin after it has been consumed and that hydroquinone is the antibiotic agent in uva ursi, but this has not been strictly tested. Hydroquinone and other similar phenolic molecules are generally modestly toxic, or at least irritating to bacteria and other cells, including your *own* cells, so this seems a reasonable theory. Hydroquinone appears in the urine of people taking uva ursi, according to one study. Sixteen volunteers who took uva ursi leaf, in the form of water extracts or film-coated tablets, were found to excrete either hydroquinone or hydroquinone metabolites (hydroquinone bonded to glucuronide or sulfate) in their urine in the same amounts, regardless of what form of uva ursi they took.[5] Though herbalists advise alkalinizing the urine with diet when taking uva ursi in order to increase liberated hydroquinone, the volunteers didn't do this, so perhaps that step isn't necessary.

The liver normally processes hydroquinone by adding sugar or sulfate to it, resulting in *hydroquinone metabolites*. However, these additions require removal to liberate the antibiotic hydroquinone. One study using a commercial German preparation of uva ursi concluded that alkalinizing the urine is not necessary for hydroquinone to be released, but their theory was based on scarce evidence: only four volunteers were involved in the study, and they did not compare the effect of alkaline urine to urine with normal pH.[6] What they *did* notice was that *E. coli* bacteria are capable of converting hydroquinone metabolites to hydroquinone. Since hydroquinone is the postulated antibacterial agent in uva ursi, the fates of these antibiotic-liberating bacteria would be quite interesting to learn, but this was not mentioned in the paper. Since most urinary infections are caused by *E. coli,* hydroquinone's ability to kill these bacteria is a pertinent question. Since our cells have similar hydroquinone-liberating enzymes as the bacteria, the authors theorized we could do the same thing, with no alkalinity required, but this hasn't really been tested.

Although uva ursi isn't usually applied topically, arbutin and its metabolite hydroquinone both suppress melanin production in clinical tests.[7] That being said, it's not a good idea to use either for skin lightening, long term, because both are toxic, and increased usage increases the risk of cancer and other problems.

THE BOTTOM LINE

- Uva ursi may be useful for treating urinary tract infections, but for short periods of time only, due to toxicity concerns. Pregnant and nursing women are told to avoid it.
- Uva ursi's arbutin is a source of the toxic hydroquinone, which is thought to be its active ingredient, but this has not been strictly tested.
- It's not clear that alkalinizing the urine is required to release hydroquinone from arbutin, but it is chemically plausible.
- Although uva ursi is included in most herbal diuretics, it is not clear that it is an effective diuretic.

VALERIAN
Valeriana officinalis

HISTORY AND FOLKLORE

Valerian's tall, hollow stem bears small white, pink, or purple flowers. Its root, however, attracts more attention, even though it smells bad in a pungent, earthy sort of way. Most people say valerian root smells "like dirty socks." That people have been eating it since ancient times presumes they did so for a good reason. Traditionally it was recommended for aches, pains, epilepsy, anxiety, and sleeplessness. Allegedly your adversary could become so relaxed by valerian that they would lose the will to fight: A medieval adage advises making your potential combatant consume valerian so that they will no longer want to fight you. How one managed to get their enemy to consume valerian, however, remains unknown.

Although valerian has nothing to do with the drug Valium, the notion that valerian is relaxing has led some to mistakenly think that the drug is derived from the herb. It is not. Valerian could have some mechanisms in common with Valium, but this is not known for sure.

The word "valerian" comes from the Roman *valor,* or courage, which is what you will need to consume a valerian-based tea. A more descriptive word for valerian, used by the ancient herbalists Galen and Dioscorides, was *Fu.* Despite its obvious stench, small amounts were used in cooking as a seasoning in the Middle Ages, and a relative of valerian, *Nardostachys jatamansi,* or Indian spikenard, is a contender for having been the pungent "nard" fragrance referred to in the Bible.

HOW SCIENTISTS THINK VALERIAN WORKS

If valerian does cause relaxation, as many claim, it's not clear how it works. Several unproved but reasonable theories involve the inhibitory neurotransmitter GABA. When GABA (short for gamma-aminobutyric acid) docks with receptors on nerve cells in the brain, these cells are temporarily put into a chemical state that prevents them from responding at their normal rate. In other words, these nerve cells are slowed down. In slowing these nerve cells, GABA slows the rest of you, as well. Benzodiazepines like the antianxiety, sedative drug Valium enhance the action of GABA, and like GABA, they can help you get to sleep more quickly and may reduce anxiety. It's just a coincidence that valerian sounds like Valium, yet the herb might work in a similar fashion.

Valerian root actually contains GABA, but it probably won't do anything. Early studies on water-based extracts of valerian root showed that something in them behaved like GABA, displacing chemically tagged GABA molecules from their receptors on rat brain cells in cell cultures. However, the researchers later realized this was not some mysterious, new, GABA-like compound—it was GABA, itself![1] However, eating GABA will not relax you.

The brain cleverly protects itself from much of what you consume with a chemical obstruction called the *blood-brain barrier.* GABA is one of many things that can't cross it. So eat all the GABA you like, from valerian or any other source—it can't get into your brain. Oral GABA has not shown much effect on people.

But hold on, valerian does contain a GABA precursor that can cross the blood-brain barrier. Actually, it's a precursor to a precursor. Organisms normally make GABA from an amino acid, glutamate, which can't cross the blood-brain barrier. But glutamate can be made from glut*amine,* a related amino acid, and valerian contains a decent amount of this. Glutamine *can* cross the blood-brain barrier—it's pulled across by a special transporter:

> glutamine from valerian—> glutamine in blood—>glutamine in brain—> glutamate in brain—>GABA in brain

Glutamine looks like glutamate, except glutamine has an extra nitrogen-containing group of atoms called an *amide.* This amide can be removed and traded for a different group of atoms, transforming glutamine into glutamate, the GABA precursor, in the brain. Some scientists speculate that increasing glutamate increases GABA in the brain, but there are some problems with this theory.

Glutamine can be turned into many things—it's one of many constituents of proteins, for example. Just because you eat something does not mean it will go where you want it to go. Also, assuming glutamine increases glutamate in the brain, glutamate has an activity *opposite* to GABA and *stimulates* brain cells! So in order for this mechanism to work, the intermediate glutamate has to be converted to the relaxing GABA before it has time to excite you. Obviously this mechanism, which seems a bit of a gamble, remains theoretical.

Valerenic acid from valerian might prevent GABA from breaking down. The breakdown of molecules into smaller pieces, called *catabolism,* is a common process, especially for neurotransmitters. GABA, like all neurotransmitters, must be broken down and removed from its site of action; otherwise it would just keep acting forever. A German study using test tube–type experiments suggested that components of valerian oil—in particular, valerenic acid and its derivatives—prevented GABA's breakdown.[2] To my knowledge, the study has not been reexamined in a more rigorous fashion, yet it suggests a mechanism whereby *something* in valerian oil prolongs GABA's action in the brain. Since valerian oil ingredients are oilier than the water-soluble glutamate and GABA, they are more likely to penetrate the blood-brain barrier, because oil-soluble molecules tend to slip through into the brain more easily than water-soluble ones.

This same GABA-protecting mechanism explains the action of the prescription anti-seizure drug valproic acid, which is sold under the trade name Depakote. Valproic acid is not in valerian, but valerian contains similar-looking molecules, valeric and isovaleric acids, which are smaller and more similar to the drug than the valer*en*ic acid most often suggested as preventing GABA catabolism. Whether or not these smaller acids from valerian act like the prescription antiepileptic drug valproic acid remains to be seen, but molecules with similar shapes often behave similarly.

Yet more compounds from valerian, the valepotriates, seem sedating, but their mechanism isn't known. A small smattering of animal and test tube studies suggest that these molecules sedate rodents and inhibit involuntary (smooth) muscle contraction. Valepotriates are unstable and break down, perhaps to active ingredients. They most likely break down in the gut, having structures called *esters.* Esters are sensitive to both acid, which is in the stomach, and base, which is present in the small intestine, so the valepotriates will probably be transformed when they are eaten. Since valepotriates and their breakdown products resemble the valerenic acid structure, which is thought to prevent GABA breakdown, they could behave similarly.

Could valerian act on a completely different receptor? A newly discovered olivil lignan from valerian root (named for similar molecules previously found in olive leaves) appears to activate a different brain receptor, the adenosine receptor, in preliminary cell culture studies.[3] It may behave like adenosine, one of your normal sleep-promoting molecules. As you expend energy throughout the day, adenosine builds up in the brain and starts to stick to its receptors, making you tired. You may be more familiar with the action of a popular adenosine *antagonist* that inhibits this binding—caffeine. So valerian could have an anticaffeine action. Indeed, one study showed that a valerian-hops combination prevented caffeine-consuming volunteers from getting wired.[4]

This was a surprise, because at first glance on paper, the olivil lignan does not look like adenosine at all, yet on paper chemical structures are flat, and in nature they are most often not flat. Computer modeling of this olivil lignan in its 3-D form shows it does have some structural characteristics in common with adenosine after all.[5]

Interesting Facts

⚘

Valerian's molecules have animal magnetism . . . for some.

RATS LOVE valerian, or at least that's what people say. In fact, some claim the Pied Piper was supposed to have used valerian to drive the rats from the German town of Hamelin. Some companies even sell some valerian-stuffed toys intended to get pet rats especially excited.

The bad news for valerian-sniffing rats is that valerian attracts cats, too, or at least some of them. Some cat owners notice that their cats find valerian even more engrossing than catnip, but the effect depends on the cat, and perhaps the valerian as well, since the active ingredient or ingredients may be unstable. Since valerian's valepotriates resemble the cat-attracting molecule in catnip, nepetalactone (see page 62), it makes sense that valerian holds the same power over cats. However, rats do not love catnip and supposedly find it repulsive. All this remains hearsay: there do not seem to be any formal scientific papers quantifying valerian's appeal to either cats or rats. In my own small, uncontrolled study, my cats, Quark and Alberio, appeared intrigued by the smell of valerian but retained serious dispositions.

Good Effects . . .
and Not So Good

Valerian could relieve anxiety and insomnia, but you might have to take it for a while. Human clinical trials are inconclusive but suggest it might work better if taken over a few days. The most benefit was seen when insomniacs took 400–900 milligrams of valerian two hours before bed.[6] Topical preparations, such as oils added to a bath, don't appear to work.

Valerian is safer than many prescription sleep and antianxiety medications. It doesn't cause loss of coordination and generally seems free of side effects when not taken in excess. Of course, anything in excess, including herbs, isn't a good idea. One young woman tried to commit suicide with about 20 grams of valerian and failed, but suffered abdominal cramps, tremor, lightheadedness, and chest tightness. She felt better after a day in an emergency room having her digestive system cleansed with activated charcoal.[7]

What's In It

VALERIAN CONTAINS iridoid esters called *valepotriates,* such as isovaltrate, isovaleroxyhydroxy didrovaltrate, didrovaltrate, acevaltrate, and others. The volatile oil mainly contains isovalerenic acid and its bornyl ester, bornyl acetate, isoeugenyl valerenate, and isoeugenyl isovalerenate. The free acid sesquiterpenes valerenic acid and isovalerenic acid are also present. Pyridine alkaloids like actinidine may contribute to its cat-attracting power by behaving as feline pheromones. The root also has caffeic acid derivatives, as well as GABA (gamma-aminobutyric acid) and glutamine.

Most sources report valerian is not addictive, but there is a recent case of a possible withdrawal reaction. An older man who had taken 0.5 to 2 grams of valerian five times daily for many years became delirious and developed acute cardiac symptoms following general anesthesia. Although he had congestive heart failure and was on multiple medications, the fact that a benzodiazepine drug was able to relieve his symptoms during his hospitalization led his doctors to believe he was suffering valerian withdrawal symptoms.[8] Cases of withdrawal are probably rare, however, typically occurring only after prolonged consumption of high doses of valerian.

Avoid taking valerian with other medications, particularly alcohol, barbiturates, and benzodiazepines. Cell studies show that valerian can affect drug-metabolizing enzymes in the liver, indicating it could interfere with other medications. It actually appears to antagonize the effects of alcohol, but it should not be used by the intoxicated to speed sobriety. This could harm the liver by making it metabolize too many odd substances at once.

Although valepotriates have the notorious epoxide ring, it's not clear that they harm you. Epoxide rings are three-sided molecular triangles made of two carbons and one oxygen. Since the bonds holding the atoms in the triangle together are sixty degrees apart, they are forced to be next to one another. A bond is repelled by a nearby bond, however, since chemical bonds are made of particles that repel each other (electrons), so forcing these bonds so close together in this structure is unstable. Epoxide rings' unstable structure readily breaks open, forcing the three atoms to bond to the nearest molecule, which damages that molecule. Epoxides are associated with cancer, and though valepotriates are indeed toxic to cells in test tube studies, they probably degrade quickly after you eat them. The risk they pose to the average consumer is not clear. Although no birth defects have been associated with them, it seems wise for pregnant or nursing women to avoid valerian.

One dose of valerian is not like the next. The constituents of valerian root preparations vary widely, partly because different plants display large concentration differences of their constituents, and partly because some of the constituents are unstable and break down. So don't expect a consistent effect if you take it, over time, even from one bottle. Most herbalists recommend the freshest root products, but since the unstable constituents are likely to break down in the gut, it's hard to say whether this helps. Valerian root preparations may be standardized, but no one knows for sure what the active ingredients are—if there are any. Nonetheless, a fresh, standardized product is likely higher quality than a nonstandardized old one.

Valerian stinks. It really does. It is reminiscent of a locker room requiring sanitation. Despite what some may say, there is no correlation of smell with efficacy—since no one knows what the active ingredients are. The smelly constituents are probably small acids, like valeric and isovaleric acids.

Evidence of Action

Some human clinical trials of valerian for treating insomnia or anxiety look promising, yet others don't, and show no effect whatsoever. Although we don't know what the active ingredients in valerian really are—if there are any—what we *think* might be its active ingredients are unstable, and their concentrations deviate greatly from plant to plant. Even "standardized" preparations can vary in concentration for these ingredients within the same brand. This could certainly explain why test results have been so variable. The verdict on valerian so far is an unsatisfying "inconclusive." More evidence is needed.

In some short-term trials, where one single dose of valerian was used to treat insomnia for one night,[9] or to affect mood,[10, 11] the herb simply showed no effect compared to a placebo. Thus, optimists hope valerian might work better if taken for a longer period of time. Indeed, polysomnographic readings, which include EEG (electroen-

cephalographic) readings of brain waves, and other parameters, such as muscle activity, showed that taking one dose of valerian had no effect on sleep, yet multiple doses taken over several consecutive nights significantly improved sleep parameters with respect to placebo over time.[12] (The placebo also showed a significant effect all on its own, indicating that your mind has some power of its own in treating insomnia.)

Commonly Reported Uses for Valerian*

Internally

sedative, calmative, hypnotic, anti-seizure, antianxiety

forms available for internal use:

capsule, tablets, decoction, dried root, infusion, tincture, extract

commonly reported dosage:

For insomnia, most studies have used 400–9,000 milligrams of valerian extract around two hours before bedtime for up to four weeks. In other studies around 100 milligrams of valerian extract was given three times daily for up to thirty days.

*These uses and dosages are from historic use and are not necessarily tested nor recommended.

Also, taking valerian for four weeks may have helped some patients with their chronic anxiety. A preliminary pilot study of thirty-six patients with generalized anxiety disorder found that those who took 81.3 milligrams of valepotriates from valerian daily reduced some anxiety measures on a standard anxiety test (Hamilton Anxiety Scale) with respect to placebo. The small size of the study unfortunately prevents making dramatic pronouncements as of yet, but the data look promising.

Valerian's apparently meager action might be viewed as a plus. Although valerian had no effect when weighed against benzodiazepines (temazepam, or Restoril) and antihistamines (diphenhydramine, or Benadryl) in promoting sleep,[13] it produces fewer *unwanted* effects than these medications, too, as long as the recommended dose isn't exceeded.[14] And if you are unhappily hooked on benzodiazepines for a good night's rest, valerian may help you kick the habit, according to one study where patients tapered off their benzodiapines gradually over two weeks and took 300 milligrams of valerian extract three times daily.[15]

One review of nine randomized, placebo-controlled, double-blind clinical trials of valerian for sleep disorders found flaws in the designs of all of them, but the three designated as the best-designed trials suggest that valerian *could* be effective and that it does not cause obvious side effects when taken as recommended. However, even these trials had problems; for example, one used a combination of hops with valerian, making it impossible to sort out which herb is doing what. Because of such ambiguities in the data, the review rendered valerian's ability to promote sleep inconclusive.[16]

THE BOTTOM LINE

- Valerian root may relieve insomnia and anxiety, though human clinical trials are currently inconclusive. Taking it on consecutive nights may be more effective than taking it on one night only.
- Valerian root contains ingredients that could enhance the action of the inhibitory neurotransmitter GABA. It could also act at the adenosine receptor and have the opposite effect of caffeine.
- Although valerian appears relatively safe, avoid taking it with other medications or alcohol, and don't take it if you are pregnant or nursing.

WILD YAM

Dioscorea villosa

History and Folklore

Americans or Europeans must be adventurous to encounter "true" yams. True yams, also called *Mexican* or *wild yams,* are relatively rare as comestibles in the nontropical zones, yet are the world's third most important tropical "root" crop, after cassava and sweet potatoes. What agriculturally oblivious Americans insistently refer to as "yams" are actually sweet potatoes. For some reason, Americans call the softer, yellower varieties of sweet potatoes "yams," but these traditional Thanksgiving entrees are not related to true yams, nor are sweet potatoes even potatoes. (Sweet potatoes are in the morning glory family and are only distantly related to potatoes). So you are unlikely to obtain the allegedly medicinal wild yam from grocery stores in cold climates, despite any apparent bins labeled "yams."

Nonetheless, wild yams are one of the world's chief "root" crops, with around 25 million tons of them produced annually. As such, they have a rich history. This tropical vegetable is cultivated in Africa, Asia, and South America, and the West African *nyami,* which means "to eat," provides its name. While normally harvested for food at a respectable two to six pounds, they are among the world's largest vegetables, growing from six to nine feet long and weighing up to 150 pounds. In New Guinea and Melanesia, gigantic ceremonial yams are grown for ritual exchanges, which you can imagine make memorable gifts. A fall yam festival also employs these mammoth tubers, which are covered in beautifully constructed,

intricately woven masks, like exquisite, colossal versions of Mr. Potatohead.

Although yams are mostly tropical, the species *D. villosa* grows in the northeastern and southern United States, and since early Americans used it for colic, it was once popularly called *colic root.* There are actually more than 850 species of *Dioscorea,* with just the edible ones designated "yams." Some of the less edible species contain toxic, detergent-like molecules called *saponins,* which are used by African tribes to stun and capture fish. Various species of yams have also traditionally been used by different societies for treating arthritis, congestion, menstrual cramps, and childbirth pain. Like potatoes, yams are starchy, modified stems called *tubers* and not actual roots. They are cooked in every manner imaginable and usually mixed with more flavorful items, because they are so bland. Insoluble calcium oxalate crystals in the peel cause itching and irritation on contact, so the peel is removed.

A more historically pivotal constituent of yam is a steroid called *diosgenin.* Steroids are any molecule with a specific structure of four carbon rings fused together in a particular manner, and variations on this fundamental structure produce a wide assortment of important molecules, including sex hormones, cholesterol, and the anti-inflammatory cortisone. While many steroids are of inestimable therapeutic value worldwide, they were once prohibitively expensive. Yam supplied the world with the first affordable steroids.

In 1938 the going rate for just one gram of cortisol was one hundred dollars. Steroids were arduously obtained from cattle organs: Forty oxen were once required to get enough cortisone to treat one patient for one day, and fifty thousand cows were needed to yield twenty milligrams of progesterone! After a 1940s scientist figured out how to turn wild yams' diosgenin into human steroids, the cost of such steroids dropped dramatically. Besides saving future cows, yam provided the first affordable birth control pills. After eight chemical transformations, wild yams' diosgenin could be converted to testosterone, and after five synthetic modifications it became progesterone, a steroid that is still the main component of many birth control pills today.

None of these synthetic processes converting diosgenin to human hormones takes place in yams or the body, however. They must occur in a laboratory, and involve all the odd, unnatural manipulations that synthetic organic chemists employ to add or subtract atoms here or there to the steroid ring structure. Human hormones can't be extracted from wild yam either. Wild yam does not contain estrogen, progesterone, testosterone, cortisol, or other human hormones.

Some supplement companies have been naughty. Since supplements are currently not regulated, we are lucky that watchdog groups can occasionally afford supplement testing. Some yam-based products have been recalled because of this testing, as progesterone and other hormones (DHEA) were discovered in them. Of course, adding hormones to supplements without mentioning them on the label is illegal.

How Scientists Think Wild Yam Works

Wild yam supplements do not provide human hormones, and its constituents do not bind to estrogen or progesterone receptors. Wild yam products are often sold with the claim that they contain progesterone precursors, which are said to convert to progesterone or other hormones in the body. This is not true. Testing shows that wild yam does *not* contain human hormones, nor can the human body convert yam molecules into human hormones. It has also been suggested that the wild yam steroid diosgenin could behave like estrogen or progesterone, binding to these hormones' receptors and initiating similar responses (agonist action) or blocking the receptors (antagonist action). There are such molecules in *other* plants, like soy (see page 281) and red clover (see page 253), and they are called *phytoestrogens* or *phytoprogesterones,* depending on which receptors they bind. However, yam does not appear to contain phytoestrogens or phytoprogesterones: an extract of wild yam molecules did not readily bind to estrogen or progesterone receptors.[1]

What's In It

WILD YAM root contains the saponin dioscin, from which its algycone diosgenin is derived. It also has isoquinuclidine alkaloids, such as dioscorin, and pyrridinal alkaloids, like dioscorine.

Wild yam might act weakly against estrogen. Although yam has no apparent receptor-binding activity, it may still exert weak hormonal effects, but these are currently poorly characterized. Since steroid hormones get certain cells to make specific proteins, a good way to detect steroid hormone activity is to determine whether or not a cell makes the specific proteins that the hormone typically commands it to make.

Steroid hormones work by entering cells (they do this relatively easily), where they bind to an internal receptor. The receptor-hormone complex then travels into the nucleus of the cell, where the DNA is kept. There, information from the DNA is used to make specific proteins. So a specific hormone-related protein is the end product of the hormone's action. This is sort of like a person—let's call him Joe—(the hormone) coming into a house (the cell) and telling another friend (the receptor) to go into the kitchen (the nucleus) to use a cookbook (the DNA) to make Joe's favorite sandwich (the characteristic protein). If you find Joe's favorite sandwich, you know that Joe was around. Similarly, if you find the steroid hormone–associated protein, you know the hormone was around, or at least something that acted like it, like an herbal molecule that has hormonal activity. Specific protein-related hormones were quantified in a test tube study after cells were treated with various herbal extracts. Wild yam weakly prevented an estrogen-promoted protein from being made, so it may have mild *anti*estrogenic action.[2]

Some evidence tentatively suggests wild yam does not increase the hormone DHEA as claimed. Since chemists have used wild yam to synthesize DHEA (dehydroepiandrosterone), it is also misleadingly sold as a "natural" source of this hormone. DHEA, a human precursor to estrogen and testosterone, is of questionable therapeutic value and could even be dangerous,[3] but it has undergone the usual wave of hysteria associated with anything found to decline as we age. The fallacious logic goes like this: "_____ has been found to decline as you get older, therefore you need more _____." (Filling in the blanks with terms like "acne" quickly demonstrates a problem with this sort of reductionist logic. Of course, many supplement companies are

happy to promote items that are said to decline with age.) A very small study where yam was unfortunately mixed with other herbs showed no increase in DHEA at least.[4]

Commonly Reported Uses for Yam*

Internally

premenstrual syndrome, breast enlargement, osteoporosis, stimulant, aphrodisiac, cramps, arthritis, diverticulitis

forms available for internal use

capsule, decoction, drops, powder, tincture, dried root

commonly reported dosage

One-half teaspoon of tincture is taken twice daily, or two 500-milligram root capsules are taken twice daily.

Externally

hot flashes, breast enlargement, vaginal lubricant

forms available for internal use:

commercial creams

commonly reported doseage:

The cream is applied according to package directions.

*These uses and dosages are from historic use and are not necessarily tested nor recommended.

Wild yam might suppress your ability to make progesterone. There are some preliminary, unconfirmed reports coming out that diosgenin might even *suppress* progesterone synthesis.[5] This could be because it might block some human steroidal precursor along its way to becoming progesterone by mimicking it. So any claims that yam increases progesterone are challenged by this new data. Because the data on yam's hormonal actions are currently sketchy, using yam for any hormonal action seems unwise for now.

Wild yam might lower your cholesterol. Some plant steroids (called *plant sterols* or *phytosterols*) are now included in margarines marketed to lower cholesterol, and there is good evidence that they actually work. Yam steroids might be able to do this trick as well, but the studies on this are still scanty. The most cited study used a mixture of herbs, only seven volunteers, and the diosgenin content of the mixture taken was not assessed.[6] One proposed mechanism behind the cholesterol-lowering effect of plant steroids is lowered intestinal absorption of cholesterol, because the plant steroid assumes the place of cholesterol in particles called *micelles,* which are cholesterol-carrying units that get absorbed from the intestines.

Wild yam, eaten as a vegetable, is probably good for you. Until more is known about the pharmacology of yam molecules, it seems prudent to avoid purified yam extracts or diosgenin, which so far appear to have effects that are the *opposite* of supplement sellers' claims. However, the vegetable itself seems relatively harmless, and, like most vegetables, is probably beneficial.

GOOD EFFECTS . . .
AND NOT SO GOOD

Don't use wild yam for breast enhancement, it won't work anyway. There are all sorts of professed hormone-related effects for yam, but none are justified at present. The most common hormonal use for yam is for menopausal or premenstrual symptoms, but wilder applications abound. A quick search on the Internet for "wild yam" will blast you with advertisements of bust-increasing yam creams or pills. The companies selling yam for this purpose insist they have studies that support breast growth, but they never make these available for anyone to read. (Testimonials are usually offered, too, but these are not valid scientific data.) If they did work, it would be a wonder, with such products readily available, that women are not universally more buxom. No bust-enhancing herbs are thought to actually work anyway, and some might do harm.

Estrogen and progesterone can cause increased breast growth, but only with an unacceptable risk of increasing breast cancer significantly. Because products that increase estrogen or progesterone increase the risk of breast cancer, they should never be taken for breast-size enhancement but taken for more serious matters. Even if you neglect the risks, remember yam possibly has the *opposite* effect on estrogen and progesterone and decreases their activities.

Don't use wild yam as a contraceptive. Yam has even been sold as an oral contraceptive. Since yam does not contain progesterone or estrogen, it will not work as birth control.

Wild yams' hormonal effects are unknown, so it should not be used to influence hormones. Any uses for yam based on its alleged hormonal action are questionable, because we really don't know what it does yet, if anything. The vegetable, however, is good for you—if you can find it. Those who dwell in the tropics seem to benefit from wild yams in the diet. This is probably because, like other relatively nontoxic plants, vegetables provide antioxidants, vitamins, nutrients, and perhaps even cholesterol-lowering sterols. While there is probably nothing wrong with eating true yams as a vegetable, the main problem is in obtaining one.

Interesting Facts

Saponins are soapy and some are toxic.

DIOSGENIN IS the steroid most studied in wild yam. This steroid is also classified as a saponin. Saponins are any natural molecules that have the four-ring carbon structure mentioned above, or a related carbon structure (called a *triterpene*), plus attached sugar molecules. A curious thing happens whenever a molecule has both a water-soluble polar portion (the sugars) and a water-avoiding nonpolar portion (the carbon rings). It becomes soap. Saponins are common in plants, some saponins are poisonous, and the yam genus Diascorea has plenty of different saponins. Saponins from plants can be used as soap as well.

You know that soap removes greasy things from your hands and clothing. The way soap works is that the water-avoiding carbon portion is attracted to grease, and the water-loving portion of the molecule is attracted to water. Water and grease don't mix, but soap molecules form a molecular bridge that allows the two to mix. Our modern soaps are not saponins, but they do have a water-loving portion and a grease-attracting carbon portion.

Saponins aren't generally toxic, but some are notably so. One species of yam, Hottentot's bread (*D. elephantipes*), has a tuber that can grow up to seven hundred pounds! The yam must be cooked laboriously to remove the toxic saponin molecules. The more toxic plant saponins break down red blood cells in cold-blooded animals and do the same if injected into the blood of mammals. Saponin-laden plant pieces were used to paralyze fish by throwing these plants into ponds or streams. The stunned fish can be eaten safely. Fortunately, the wild yam that is commonly eaten contains none of the toxic saponins.

EVIDENCE OF ACTION

Wild yam does not contain molecules that bind to estrogen or progesterone receptors.[7] Nor does yam contain estrogen, progesterone, testosterone, DHEA, cortisone, or any other human hormones. After eating yam, these hormones are not seen to increase.[8] There is some preliminary evidence, however, that consuming yam might suppress progesterone synthesis.[9] Also, yam prevented an estrogen-promoted protein from being made in a cell culture,[10] so it may have antiprogesterone and antiestrogen actions. Until more is known about yam's hormonal effects, it should not be taken with the intention of affecting sex hormones.

THE BOTTOM LINE

- Wild yam or true yam is not the same vegetable as what Americans call "yams."
- Wild yam does not contain human hormones and does not increase human hormones after it is eaten.
- Wild yam might have antiprogesterone and antiestrogen actions, but more research is required to support this.
- Eating wild yams is probably beneficial and not harmful.

WINTERGREEN
Gaultheria procumbens

HISTORY AND FOLKLORE

Wintergreen is also known as *boxberry, Canada tea, checkerberry, mountain tea, partridgeberry, spiceberry,* and *teaberry.* You can find it trailing around the ground in the woodlands of eastern North America, from Newfoundland to Georgia. Although it has a minty taste, it is not in the mint family and so is not related to spearmint, peppermint, or mint. It's in the heather family (*Ericaceae*) and is actually more related to cranberry (see page 86) than mint. As the name implies, it stays green throughout the winter, with its glossy green leaves and red berries peeking out from under the snow.

Native Americans ate wintergreen's delightfully minty leaves and berries whole and also used these parts to make tea. Introduced to it by Native Americans, colonists used wintergreen tea as a substitute for black tea during the Revolution. This all-American herb later became sought after worldwide to flavor candy. Although the leaves smell minty when crushed, you will find that a tea made from them is disappointingly lacking in this flavor unless the leaves are steeped in water for a few days to develop the flavor. This process allows the plant's enzymes to release the aromatic ingredient from bound sugar molecules.

Native Americans and settlers also used wintergreen to treat rheumatism, headache, fever, sore throats, and water retention. External rubs for aches and pains were far more popular, however, probably because of the stomach upset that oral preparation

could cause. If the power to upset stomachs while relieving aches and pains sounds familiar, you are on to something. Aspirin is a great pain-relieving drug, but is notorious for upsetting stomachs. Wintergreen's minty-smelling active ingredient, methyl salicylate, looks like aspirin and behaves a lot like it, too. Unlike aspirin, however, wintergreen creams can be applied topically, circumventing the classic stomach distress that aspirin causes.

HOW SCIENTISTS THINK WINTERGREEN WORKS

Wintergreen oil contains a lot of methyl salicylate, which is a lot like aspirin. Both aspirin (which is made from salicylic acid) and methyl salicylate hamper an enzyme called *cyclooxygenase,* which biochemists call *COX.* COX creates molecules called *prostaglandins* that do a great many different things, and though some are beneficial, others are painful. Some prostaglandins cause fever, swelling, blood clotting, and involuntary muscle contractions (cramps). As if all that were not bad enough, they also enhance the perception of pain. The ability to inhibit these effects obviously makes both aspirin and wintergreen's methyl salicylate enormously useful.

Wintergreen's methyl salicylate looks like aspirin, but can do one thing aspirin can't do. Even nonchemists can see the similarities between these molecules:

Methyl Salicylate   Salicylic Acid   Aspirin

However, unlike aspirin, methyl salicylate can travel through your skin. Sometimes salicylic acid is applied to skin to remove outer layers prone to acne but like aspirin, it can't penetrate skin, either. The "methyl" in methyl salicylate is the "CH_3" shown in the box, and it is the only thing that makes the molecule different from the salicylic acid that is used to make aspirin. This group of atoms helps the molecule travel through the skin, because molecules that have more C (carbon) and H (hydrogen) atoms are more fat soluble and travel through skin much more easily. Enzymes often trim off the methyl after the molecule has traveled through the skin, creating salicylic acid. Thus methyl salicylate delivers salicylic acid through the skin, bypassing the stomach. This is good, because all of these molecules can cause stomach distress.

Methyl salicylate is an NSAID. All three of these molecules are classified as NSAIDs ("EN-seds"), which stands for non-steroidal anti-inflammatory drugs. This means they prevent inflammation and are not steroids like hydrocortisone, which is in a different class of anti-inflammatory drugs and works by a different mechanism. (Hydrocortisone works by preventing the precursor to the more inflammatory types of prostaglandins, arachidonic acid, from escaping your cells' membranes.)

Ibuprofen, acetaminophen, and naproxen are also NSAIDs, and they all have a similar structure and work by some various forms of the COX enzyme in different manners. COX is an enzyme, and like all enzymes, it speeds up the conversion of one molecule into another. COX turns a molecule called *arachidonic acid* into a prostaglandin. The enzyme is unchanged by this process, so it can repeat the process over and over again. One COX enzyme can do this repeatedly, becoming a prostaglandin factory.

What's In It

WINTERGREEN OIL is 96-98 percent methyl salicylate, as well as oenanthic alcohol (*n*-heptan-1-ol) and its esters, which contribute to the oil's odor.

Aspirin and methyl salicylate also show some differences in how they inhibit this prostaglandin factory. Aspirin permanently affixes itself to the business end of a COX enzyme, known as the "active site," where the enzyme would ordinarily bind arachidonic acid. The active site of an enzyme is the place where a substance with a complementary shape binds temporarily, and this substance's chemical transformation is accelerated. The binding of aspirin inactivates the enzyme forever, at least until cells make more, unbound COX enzymes. Methyl salicylate, on the other hand, binds *temporarily* to the same part of COX. Methyl salicylate physically, but reversibly, blocks arachidonic acid from binding to COX. This is called *competitive inhibition,* and it's a very common method by which drugs act. Methyl salicylate's metabolized by-product, salicylic acid, does the same thing and works the same way.

Not all COX enzymes are bad. The COX enzyme comes in two forms, COX-1 and COX-2, and both aspirin and methyl salicylate inhibit the activities of both, which is a mixed blessing. COX-1 is sometimes called the "good COX" and COX-2 is the "bad COX." COX-1 decreases your synthesis of stomach acid and also promotes your stomach's secretion of protective mucous, which coats your stomach, shielding it from acid. When COX-1 is blocked, the stomach lining makes less protective mucous and produces more acid, which ultimately may damage your stomach. Thus, both wintergreen and aspirin can hurt your stomach. The good news is that methyl salicylate and aspirin also inhibit the "bad" COX-2. COX-2 actually enhances nerve endings' sensitivity to pain. Why would our bodies increase pain sensitivity? This function has some value, as it ensures that you *know* that you are being damaged, so you can wake up and remove yourself from the lion's mouth, so to speak. Pain is often more limiting than informative, however. Inhibiting COX-2 really does decrease the message of pain, and assuming a lion isn't munching on you in your sleep, that's a good thing.

The Terms "Good COX" and "Bad COX" Are Old and Misleading

✧

THE DESIGNATION of COX-2 as "bad" and COX-1 as "good" is no longer thought so useful. The once popular COX-2 inhibitors inhibited "bad" COX and spared "good" COX, so they didn't upset people's stomachs. But some of the "good" COX's products create blood clots and can raise blood pressure. The "bad" COX-2 makes products that can do the opposite. This is why these drugs initiated cardiovascular problems.

Like aspirin, wintergreen thins your blood. COX-1 in blood platelets also ulti-

mately produce a blood-clotting substance called *thromboxane,* and aspirin and wintergreen inhibition of this action prevents blood clots from forming. Blood clots do stop bleeding, but sometimes people form clots when they have not been wounded in any way. Surplus clots can block an artery, causing a stroke or heart attack. This is one reason why aspirin and plant salicylates such as methyl salicylate help reduce the risk of stroke and heart attacks. And because of their blood-thinning activity, herbs like wintergreen are not recommended for people who are already taking blood thinners, to minimize risk of bleeding.

Wintergreen's salicylates can turn down your immune system's response, but that's often a good thing. COX-2 revs up your immune system's response. COX-1 is always active, but much of your COX-2 has to get "turned on." It gets activated by chemicals generated in infection or injury, and the prostaglandins it makes enhance the activity of your immune system's ability to fight infection and clear out damaged cells. However, an overly active immune system can be harmful. Lots of products boast about "enhancing the immune system," but this is like "enhancing the army," and giving an army too much power can sometimes cause problems. Stimulating the immune system excessively causes inflammation. "Heat, pain, redness, and swelling" are the four cardinal signs of inflammation, and besides being painful, this immune response can be so excessive that the process can be more damaging than helpful. Stimulated immune cells generate free radicals as weapons against bacteria, but this can result in friendly fire, damaging healthy tissues. Inflamed tissues have leaky blood vessels that allow immune cells (white blood cells) to leave the blood stream, like passengers getting off a subway. Allowing your white blood cells to exit the blood stream also allows water from the blood to follow them to their destination, putting pressure on swelling tissues, and pressure hurts. Wintergreen's methyl salicylate, unlike aspirin, can move through your skin rapidly to decrease swelling and pain.

Good Effects . . . and Not So Good

Think of wintergreen as a great way to deliver the effects of aspirin directly through the skin. Unlike aspirin, wintergreen's methyl salicylate has a minty odor and is the ingredient responsible for the aroma of certain pain-relieving muscle rubs such as Bengay. Also unlike aspirin, methyl salicylate can penetrate your skin. Sensible use of wintergreen topically works remarkably well for reducing inflammation and muscle pain, especially for those who wish to bypass the stomach upset that oral NSAIDs produce.

Topical preparations accelerate the healing of sports injuries, and in some cases could even prevent them. Since wintergreen decreases inflammation and swelling (which damage tissues), it also helps damaged tissues heal faster. Some athletes even apply wintergreen creams *before* they stress their body to keep low-grade inflammation from increasing risk to their muscles.

Don't use it with a heating pad. Keep heat away from the area of application. If it is heated, an unpleasant burning sensation could result.

The anti-inflammatory action of methyl salicylate comes with a minty odor. The "odorless" versions of these products do not contain methyl salicylate, but low concentrations of menthol instead, relieving pain by a different mechanism (see peppermint, page 246). Menthol is far less likely to be anti-inflammatory, but it does have an anesthetic and muscle-relaxing effect.

Commonly Reported Uses for Wintergreen*

Internally
rheumatism, headache, fever, aches and pains, gas
forms available for internal use:
infusion or tea (the pure oil is toxic)
commonly reported dosage:
One teaspoon of leaves steeped for five to twenty minutes in boiling water is used to make a tea. It is drunk slowly, not exceeding one cup per day.

Externally
muscle and joint soreness, swelling, inflammation, astringent, stimulant
forms available for external use:
creams, oils, or ointments containing 10 to 60 percent methyl salicylate, oral hygiene products
commonly reported dosage:
Methyl salicylate is diluted in a cream or rub in concentrations ranging between 10 and 60 percent, which is applied externally up to four times per day.

*These uses and dosages are from historic use and are not necessarily tested nor recommended.

Methyl salicylate is wintergreen's active ingredient, but it works the same regardless of its source. Some products use natural wintergreen for topical use, but most commercial products don't, because methyl salicylate is more cheaply synthesized or isolated

Interesting Facts

If you think you see sparks when chewing wintergreen candy in the dark, it's not your imagination.

METHYL SALICYLATE is a fluorescent molecule, which in part means it has electrons that are more easily energized by heat, light, or friction than others. Although of course electrons are nonliving subatomic particles, chemists anthropomorphize them. When energized, chemists say the electrons are *"excited"*—and here you can imagine the electrons dancing about the methyl salicylate molecule energetically—but they can't do this forever. Chemists also say that the electrons eventually *"relax"*—that is, they stop dancing around and let go of the energy, and this energy escapes in the form of visible light.

If you want to see this for yourself, don't use sugar-free candy, as the fluorescent effect is more obvious if the candy contains sugar. Chewing or crushing the candy causes sugar crystals to split along planes, scraping electrons off one surface onto another, thus causing one side to have excess electrons and a negative charge (because electrons are negatively charged). The other plane is deficient in electrons, so it has a positive charge. The electrons leap across the gap like mini lightning bolts, because negative is attracted to positive. Without methyl salicylate, this arcing does not produce much of a show, because the light is in the ultraviolet range, which we can't see. Methyl salicylate, however, absorbs the ultraviolet light by energizing its electrons. The electrons then relax and release the energy as blue light. Now you can impress your friends with a cool party trick: Crush wintergreen candy in a dark room with a hammer and watch the sparks fly.

from sweet birch tree oil. Sweet birch trees are not related to wintergreen, but they also make methyl salicylate. Regardless of its origin, methyl salicylate is identical to the active ingredient found in wintergreen, so look for either "wintergreen" or "methyl salicylate" on the label.

Be cautious with oral wintergreen. Some herbalists recommend a pain-relieving tea made from wintergreen leaves, which contains a relatively small dose of methyl salicylate. However, people whose stomachs are sensitive to aspirin should be careful about trying this. Methyl salicylate is more slowly absorbed from the gut than aspirin, so it has extra time to cause more pain there, too.

Never consume wintergreen oil or pure methyl salicylate. It can kill you. Methyl salicylate, or *oil* of wintergreen, is not the same thing as wintergreen tea, which has barely any oil in it. Pure wintergreen oil should *never* be taken orally, because it is much more concentrated and can cause a crisis resembling aspirin overdose, resulting in fatalities.

Keep wintergreen away from children. Oil of wintergreen is used in making candy, but inattentive cooks should be careful: Curious children attracted to the candylike odor of the oil have swallowed the oil and died. Less than one teaspoon of the oil can be fatal to a small child. Although the oil is usually far less concentrated in one piece of candy, children might sneakily eat of *lot* of wintergreen candy. Some pediatricians even warn parents against giving children any wintergreen candy.

For the same reason that they should not take aspirin, children should not use wintergreen products. There is the risk of the rare complication of Reye's syndrome with both, and this holds for both oral and topical products.

Grownups can overdo the wintergreen,

too. Children are more susceptible to methyl salicylate poisoning than adults due to their size, but overenthusiastic use of wintergreen muscle rubs by adults has resulted in symptoms similar to aspirin overdose, resulting in hospitalizations.

The same risks that apply to aspirin apply to all forms of wintergreen. Because of the increased risk of excessive bleeding, wintergreen products should not be used prior to surgery. If you have scheduled a surgery in the near future, you should stay off the salicylates, including wintergreen, for one week before the sugery. People taking blood-thinning, anticoagulant medicines may also have more bleeding problems if they use wintergreen.

EVIDENCE OF ACTION

There is no doubt that methyl salicylate from wintergreen is a superbly effective topical anti-inflammatory. It reduces fever, pain, and swelling for the same reasons that aspirin does. Unfortunately, there are currently no scientific clinical trials evaluating the use of wintergreen, the herb, for these conditions, perhaps because it's so obviously effective. Methyl salicylate is rapidly absorbed through the skin, which can deliver "a considerable amount" of salicylate to the blood.[1] Although this route bypasses stomach distress, some people are sensitive to methyl salicylate in the blood. Children, people taking anticoagulant medications, and people with bleeding disorders should avoid wintergreen. I know one person with aspirin sensitivity syndrome who became acutely nauseous after applying a commercial muscle rub that contained methyl salicylate.

In one study, mouthwashes assessed for antioxidant activity revealed that mouthwashes that contained methyl salicylate were the most antioxidant.[2] The authors of the study speculate that this antioxidant activity could aid in healing periodontal disease.

THE BOTTOM LINE

- Wintergreen contains methyl salicylate, which, like aspirin, inhibits COX, an enzyme that creates inflammation-promoting prostaglandins.
- Methyl salicylate decreases pain and inflammation when applied topically, but, like aspirin, can cause stomach distress when taken orally.
- Unlike aspirin, methyl salicylate travels easily through the skin, bypassing stomach distress.
- Pure wintergreen oil is too potent for medical use and can cause symptoms similar to aspirin overdose. Children have died from ingesting it.
- Wintergreen products should not be used by children or by people taking blood-thinning medications. It should be avoided for a week prior to surgery to minimize risk of bleeding.

WITCH HAZEL

Hamamelis virginiana

History and Folklore

The witch hazel tree is not named after the classical witch. The "witch" derives from the old English *wych,* to bend, because its branches are springy and flexible. Yet they still have a mystical association. These fork-shaped branches were classically used for "water witching," or dousing rods, a mystical method of divining where underground water or other goodies might lie.

The witch hazel isn't really a hazel, so it can't produce hazel nuts, but it does resemble hazel to the point of confusing young, unseasoned botanists. Its stringy-looking yellow flowers make popular ornamentals, especially as they bloom late into the fall, contrasting with other trees that have long lost their colorful leaves. The first word of its Latin name, *hamamelis,* is derived from a Greek phrase meaning "together with fruit." This refers to the fact that witch hazel is the only North American tree to possess last year's ripened fruit and this year's flowers, simultaneously, on the same branch.

Native Americans introduced early settlers to a tea of witch hazel branches and leaves, which they used externally for wounds, bruises, insect bites, and sore muscles, and internally for sore throats and internal bleeding. This tree is native to eastern North American forests, and the major producer of witch hazel water in the United States still makes use of Connecticut witch hazels in a renewable manner, using environmental methods which limit the loss of these trees.

How Scientists Think Witch Hazel Works

The active ingredient in witch hazel water has nothing to do with witch hazel. Witch hazel *water* (what you buy in U.S. pharmacies) is a watery solution of about 15 percent alcohol, with a trace of volatile oils. As such its main active ingredient is the added alcohol (ethanol), which isn't even from the witch hazel tree. Though witch hazel water does not have tannins, its most studied component, the ethanol added to it, is not inert either.

The ethanol in witch hazel water cools and dries your skin by stealing your body's warmth and water. Any molecule that can evaporate easily is called *volatile* and cools your skin in this manner: ethanol removes your skin's heat and then uses this energy to fly about the room, becoming a gas. This is the mechanism behind evaporative cooling. Ethanol is also attracted to water molecules and can stick to them before flying away with them. So when you put ethanol on your skin, water and ethanol fly off together like molecular lovers eloping. This is why ethanol acts as a drying agent. This drying of your skin tightens it, producing an astringent-like effect.

Witch hazel water is only weakly antibacterial. Higher ethanol concentrations kill bacteria by causing their proteins to become misshapen. Proteins are made of chains of amino acids, and these chains fold up into functional shapes, based on the amino acids' relative attraction, or lack thereof, for their surroundings. Ethanol is a strange environment for a protein to be in. The amino acids composing the protein that are most attracted to ethanol get pulled to the outside of the protein, distorting its shape. This renders the protein nonfunctional. However, ethanol can't kill dormant bacteria encased in chemically tougher spore cases.

Witch hazel *extract,* on the other hand, has astringent tannins. The tannins in witch hazel extract tie many of your skin proteins together at once, drawing them together. This is a true astringent effect. This tightening stops minor bleeding and forms a temporary, watertight skin barrier. In making skin more distasteful and less penetrable to bacteria, witch hazel extract is also briefly antibacterial. Though tannins can't penetrate your skin very far, shrinking skin structures immediately underlying your skin ultimately constrict the capillaries for a period of time. Most references report this creates an "indirect" anti-inflammatory effect. The tannins keep capillaries not only from bleeding but also from leaking fluid, which lessens inflammation's classic symptoms of swelling, redness, and heat from blood flow. Yet cell studies show that witch hazel tannins have some impressive antioxidant activities, which could *directly* reduce inflammation, too, at least in theory.

Tannins are both helpful and harmful. As with all substances, it's the dose that matters, and the application method. Though some people report that witch hazel's astringent action helps with hemorrhoids, itching, and varicose veins, tannins can be irritating, especially in excess. Witch hazel should be limited to external applications because of this. Inordinate amounts of tannins lead to mutations and cancer, and unlike other tannin-containing herbs, witch hazel extract is loaded with the stuff. This is why most responsible herbalists do not recommend that you take witch hazel extracts internally.

Good Effects . . . and Not So Good

First of all, know the difference between witch hazel water and tannic witch hazel. Witch hazel water is sometimes confusingly just called "witch hazel," especially in U.S. pharmacies. But the 15 percent alcohol (ethanol) content might tip you off (unless it is an alcoholic tincture). Witch hazel water is made from steam distilling the branches, to create an extract, and adding alcohol as a preservative. Witch hazel water does not have appreciable tannins, and its main active ingredient is the alcohol that is added. Witch hazel extracts are made by different means, such as soaking leaves and branches in water or an alcohol-water mixture, contain tannins. Look for labels that clearly describe what sort of witch hazel product you have.

What's In It

WITCH HAZEL'S leaves and bark contain highly variable quantities of tannins, including catechins, gallotannins, hamamelitannins, and oligomeric proanthocyanidins. It also has flavonoids like kaempferol, quercetin, quercitrin, and isoquercitrin, and phenolic acids (caffeic and gallic acids). Witch hazel also possesses safrole, a known carcinogen, but reportedly in quantities too scant to pose a health hazard when used externally.

Witch hazel is for external use only. This is true both for the tanninless witch hazel water and the tannin-containing witch hazel extracts. Bottles of the tanninless witch hazel water say "for external use only" and advise you to see a poison control center should you disobey this warning. They probably say this for a good reason. And though the tannin content of other witch hazel extracts is highly variable, it is high enough to alarm toxicologists. The modest amounts of tannins from other plants, however, can be beneficial. But the acute doses obtained from witch hazel may at best result in indigestion and at worse give you liver cancer. It's fine to use as an oral rinse or gargle as long as it is not swallowed.

Witch hazel tannins may help externally in some cases, but not in others. It might help with hemorrhoids, minor bleeding, and skin irritation. Some find it anesthetizes pain associated with sunburn or insect bites. On the other hand, it can irritate your skin if you are sensitive to it.

Interesting Facts

Watch out for projectiles.

WITCH HAZEL is also called *snapping hazel,* because as the seedpods dry, the black seeds fire off, loudly popping as they go, and they can shoot as far as thirty feet. Imagine the bewilderment of people who learn this botanical trivia the hard way, when they take a bouquet of the pretty fall flowers into their home. This violent manner of seed dispersal prevents the overcrowding of young seedlings. The seeds can be eaten, too. They reportedly taste like pistachio nuts and were enjoyed by Native Americans.

EVIDENCE OF ACTION

Witch hazel tannins have quite respectable anti-inflammatory and antioxidant actions.

There are a handful of test tube studies supporting this. Witch hazel tannins inhibited TNF-alpha, an inflammatory mediator, which can kill cells by fragmenting their DNA, and in one London study witch hazel tannins prevented this in the test tube.[1] Further anti-inflammatory activity by witch hazel tannins was evidenced by its ability to scavenge the damaging superoxide radical,[2] plus witch hazel tannins proved a potent inhibitor of the pro-inflammatory enzyme 5-lipoxygenase.[3]

Commonly Reported Uses for Witch Hazel*

Externally
astringent, coolant, minor cuts and skin irritations, sunburn, bruises, varicose veins, hemorrhoids, gargle, oral rinse
forms available for external use:
powdered or chopped bark and/or leaves, water extracts, decoction, tincture, witch hazel water, various cosmetic products such as cleansing pads, hemorrhoidal pads, and ointments
commonly reported dosage:
Five to 10 grams of witch hazel bark is boiled in a cup of hot water and filtered to make a decoction, or soaked in cool water and filtered to make a tannin-containing infusion.

*These uses and dosages are from historic use and are not necessarily tested nor recommended.

That being said, a human is not a test tube, and only a few studies address witch hazel's action on humans in controlled studies. Witch hazel extract plus ointment was able to reduce skin inflammation in human volunteers following ultraviolet exposure or "cellophane tape stripping" (technically, ripping tape of off some courageous volunteers' skin) compared to the ointment's carrier base, but was not as effective as hydrocortisone.[4] Similarly, though witch hazel extract improved patient's eczema, it worked no better than the cream the witch hazel was dissolved in, indicating it had little effect, and again hydrocortisone worked better.[5] A witch hazel tannin-containing ointment did at least prove comparable to hydrocortisone in relieving hemorrhoidal bleeding, soreness, itching, and burning in two controlled trials of seventy-five and ninety patients afflicted with them.[6]

There is not much in the way of studies examining externally applied witch hazel for treating vascular problems. Though a high internal dose of witch hazel (which is not recommended) improved venous tone in human volunteers, a more reasonable oral dose of 150 milligrams of oligomeric procyanidins (which can be obtained from several other plants, like cranberry, pine bark, and grape seed extract, see pages 86 and 170) achieved the same effect.[7]

THE BOTTOM LINE

- Some witch hazel products have tannins as the active ingredient, while others, commonly sold in U.S. pharmacies, have no tannins, and added alcohol is the main active ingredient.
- Witch hazel products, both the tannin-containing and tannin-less, should not be taken internally and are for external use only.
- The ethanol in tanninless witch hazel water cools your skin, dries and tightens it, and is mildly antiseptic.
- The tannins in witch hazel extracts are astringent and anti-inflammatory and can relieve some skin irritations when used in moderation.

YERBA MATÉ

Ilex paraguarensis

History and Folklore

Yerba maté, or maté for short ("MAH-tay"), is a tea made from the leaves of a type of holly. Drinking maté often surpasses consuming coffee as a daily social ritual in Latin and South American countries, as well as in the Middle East. This exotic tea is starting to catch on in Europe and the United States as well. To keep up with growing demand, South American maté farming has destroyed portions of precious rainforest.

This hot drink is commonly shared from a special gourd designated by the Quechua term *maté,* which provides the drink its name. Brazilians know the drink as *chimarrao.* Holly leaves at the bottom of the gourd are steeped in hot water, which is possibly flavored with lemon and sweetener, and filtered by drinking it through a metal straw called a *bombilla,* which has a sievelike bottom. Maté is an integral part of the lives of indigenous people of South America, especially the Guarani Indians, who use it as a stimulant, diuretic, digestive aid, and antirheumatic.

How Scientists Think Yerba Maté Works

Maté's methylxanthines give you a coffee-like buzz. Maté, like coffee, has a significant amount of caffeine. Smaller quantities of chemically similar stimulants, theophylline and theobromine, are also present. You don't need maté to get these stimulants, because you can get all three in either coffee, tea (page 301), cola, guarana (page 179), or chocolate, in varying amounts, so you are likely familiar with their effects already. Caffeine, theophylline, and theobromine are collectively known as *methylxanthines,* and despite historical suspicions, these stimulants have proven benign at moderate doses.

Maté wakes you up by antagonizing sleep-inducing adenosine. The most striking effects that caffeine and other methylxanthines create result from their blocking your adenosine-binding sites. Adenosine normally makes you drowsy, and it does other interesting things, too. Its docking ports are found on virtually every one of your cells, and methylxanthines block them. Not that every one of your cells is affected by maté— these stimulants get diluted and distributed unequally to various regions of your body after you consume them. Methylxanthines primarily affect your brain, the blood vessels of your heart and brain, and indirectly, your kidneys.

When these stimulants block adenosine receptors, adenosine can't do its job as well as it could. While adenosine is a component of DNA, it plays other, very different roles as well. It is also is a portion of the so-called energy-currency molecule, ATP (adenosine triphosphate). This molecule is broken down to provide energy for several processes in the body. As energy is expended, ATP gets broken down, adenosine levels rise, and you feel tired. Adenosine's binding receptors in the brain slow down nerve cell signaling and activity. Methylxanthines keep adenosine from doing this, so you feel more awake.

As with tea, coffee, and other caffeinated products, maté increases urination, speeds up the heart rate, constricts cerebral blood vessels, relaxes involuntary muscles, and makes the voluntary muscles twitchier. Most of these effects are again attributed to adenosine receptor antagonism. Twitchy muscles can result from the revved-up brain sending surplus impulses to the muscles, and caffeine also increases calcium ion concentrations in muscle cells, making them contract. Caffeine inhibits the release of antidiuretic hormone from the pituitary; without caffeine, the antidiuretic hormone would otherwise affect the kidneys. If you can follow the convoluted logic of how this hormone is named, maté inhibits a urination inhibitor, thus increasing urination.

Mateine does not exist. It's a marketing gimmick. Some maté promoters say maté has no caffeine, but a mysterious, beneficial substance called *mateine.* They even say it is the mirror image of caffeine. This is similar to arguments made for tea containing the mystrious "theine," or guarana containing the enigmatic "guaranine." Don't buy it. All of these molecules are the same thing as caffeine, and the alternate names are merely a marketing gimmick that confuses consumers. Some molecules have mirror-image structures that are different from themselves, like your right and left hands. Objects and molecules with mirror images that are not identical to themselves are called *chiral* (KY-ral) or *handed structures.* Certain objects (like your hands,) and some molecules are chiral, but many are not. A perfect sphere, for example, has a mirror image that is identical to itself, so it doesn't have an alternate form. Caffeine's structure makes an alternate version impossible, too. It's *achiral*—its mirror image is identical to itself.

Warning: maté may cause cancer. Enough studies have shown elevated cancer rates for those who consume maté regularly to raise a red flag. It isn't its stimulant methylx-anthines, so it's okay to drink alternate caffeinated beverages and eat chocolate without worrying about cancer. Why maté causes cancer is not yet known. Some maté lovers protest that perhaps the tea isn't guilty, but rather its temperature. Repeatedly burning your esophagus is more likely to occur with the traditional style of sipping maté through a long metal straw. Burning your throat certainly increases the odds of getting esophageal cancer, but it isn't enough to explain the elevated cancer rates, according to statistical studies. Both hot and cold maté are risky.

What's In It

NOT ALL hollies contain the same ingredients as maté (*Ilex paraguarensis*); for example, not all are stimulant. Maté's stimulants—caffeine, theophylline, and theobromine—are its most pharmacologically noticeable constituents. It also has a high tannin content and has caffeic and chlorogenic acids. Its flavonoids include kaempferol, quercetin, and rutin; it also has ursolic acid; riboflavin, pyridoxine, vitamin C, niacin, and pantothenic acid; and volatile oils.

If you must mutate your cells with maté, do it sparingly. One cell study employing the famous Ames' carcinogenicity test showed that maté extracts cause DNA mutations,[1] the first step in causing cancer. Mutations don't *necessarily* cause cancer, but they aren't something you want either. Usually not just one, but a handful of DNA mutations per cell are required to cause cancer, and your body fixes these mutations daily. Yet the more you expose yourself to any mutagen, the greater number of mutations slip by not getting fixed, and the more you risk cancer. Some experts suggest that maté's carcinogenicity stems from its remarkably high tannin content, and others describe evidence of damaging oxidizing agents in the drink, which can outweigh the tea's more beneficial antioxidant activity. It is best to consume maté in small amounts, and not habitually.

Good Effects . . . and Not So Good

Maté may cause cancer. Sampling maté is risky. While one maté drink may not be fatal, repeatedly drinking the stuff, or drinking a lot at one time, is not recommended. Hot maté is riskier, but cold maté has proven dangerous, too. If it is the tannins that are responsible for cancer—and we are not sure that they are—you can limit their actions by having the tea with protein, like milk. Then the tannins will react with the protein, and less with you.

You don't have to risk cancer for methylxanthines' therapeutic actions. These stimulants can be obtained from non-carcinogenic sources, like coffee, tea, chocolate, and cola. Some people with vascular headaches find that these stimulants help their headaches vanish. Methylxanthines squeeze your brain's blood vessels. Wide, dilated vessels leak fluid, causing local swelling, pressure, and pain. Constricting these vessels reverses the swelling. This is why some headache medicines contain caffeine. Also, methylxanthines, particularly theophylline, relax involuntary muscles in your respiratory system, easing airflow, allowing you to breathe more easily. Some people with asthma and respiratory problems take theophylline. While maté's stimulants are not harmful, something else in maté causes cancer, so a coffee, tea, or chocolate habit is healthier than a maté one.

Commonly Reported Uses for Maté*

Internally
stimulant, diuretic, antiarthritic, appetite suppressant, weight loss, "thermogenic"
forms available for internal use:
smoked or fermented leaves, tea
commonly reported dosage:
One teaspoon of maté per cup of hot water is steeped for a short period of time to make maté tea. Maté-drinking cultures typically drink up to three cups per day.

*These uses and dosages are from historic use and are not necessarily tested nor recommended.

Methylxanthines can be overdone. While not harmful, these stimulants can be taken to excess, making you irritable, insomniac, nauseous, and jittery. Although continued, moderate use of methylxanthines is not associated with harm, temporary withdrawal symptoms—headache, irritability, and fatigue—do occur if you stop using them.

Methylxanthines aren't for everyone. Caffeine can cause some people to have an irregular heartbeat, so don't have maté if you think are one of these people. If you are not a regular consumer of caffeine, it may boost your blood pressure, though those who take it regularly don't experience this effect. People who don't normally consume caffeine but have heart disease, high blood pressure, or are taking an MAO inhibitor should avoid methylxanthines, because they can elevate blood pressure. Caffeine's effect on a fetus is not known and is assumed to be safe at moderate amounts. Since caffeine can enter fetal circulation, pregnant women are advised to limit their caffeine intake from maté and other caffeinated sources. Babies will become fussy if their mother drinks too much caffeine, because the caffeine in it is transported through breast milk. The caffeine in maté is less of a concern for pregnant women than other ingredients with unknown activities, so they should either avoid maté or have only moderate amounts on occasion. Methylxanthine-containing items are never for pets either, because pets respond more profoundly to them and can die.

Interesting Facts

Nuclear waste tea, anyone?

ENVIRONMENTAL RESEARCHERS used a Geiger counter to scan fifty food products in stores in Argentina. Imagine their surprise when they discovered some Buenos Aires stores selling radioactive maté. Radioactive cesium in the tea was traced to fertilizer imported from the infamously contaminated Chernobyl nuclear power plant accident area in Russia.[2] This undesirable extra zip is not responsible for maté's overall carcinogenicity, but this one-time incident illustrates your need to know where your herbs come from, since herbs are largely unregulated. You might want to discover which herb sellers allow their products to be tested for unwanted heavy metals like cesium.

EVIDENCE OF ACTION

Here is bad news for habitual maté drinkers. Studies show that South Americans who have a maté habit risk a variety of different cancers. Oral,[3] esophageal,[4] oropharyngeal,[5] lung,[6] kidney,[7] bladder,[8] and head and neck[9]

cancers are all increased with increased consumption of maté.

One should keep in mind that such epidemiological cancer studies must undergo the sometimes-valid criticism that they are "confounded" by obfuscating factors. For example, perhaps maté drinkers also tend to smoke. Tobacco use undeniably increases cancer risk, and one study also investigated whether simply burning the esophagus with hot liquid might have been the culprit rather than maté itself. However, when these additional risks were statistically removed from the equation, the cancer risk remained. The data probably indicates a valid connection rather than a "confounded" one.

Other than its cancer risk, there are barely any clinical studies of how maté affects people. Its more obvious, immediate effects stem from its high caffeine content. Caffeine is not considered a carcinogen, and is not implicated in maté's ability to increase cancer risk. Maté's caffeine acts in the usual way—it increases energy and wakefulness, relieves some vascular headaches, increases urination, increases heart rate, and in high doses makes people jittery and anxious. One optimistic Swiss study suggested that maté is "theromogenic,"[10] increasing your metabolic activity. Dieters hope thermogenic herbs enhance weight loss. This was not attributed to maté's caffeine content. Yet maté did not cause weight loss, when combined with guarana and damiana, when volunteers took this mixture for a year.[11]

Maté has ingredients that are antioxidant, which is good, but it also has prooxidant agents, which is bad. Cell studies show that maté certainly does good things, like scavenging free radicals and preventing the oxidation of "bad" LDL cholesterol, which leads to atherosclerotic plaque deposits. This is not uncommon for plant extracts: There are other plants that are not associated with increased cancer risk that can do the same thing for you. In contrast to these antioxidant properties, the mutagenic activity of maté is associated with the extract's oxidizing potential.

THE BOTTOM LINE

- Because use of both hot and cold maté increases cancer risk, you should not make a habit of drinking it, nor should you drink a lot of it at once.
- Maté's stimulant methylxanthines are the same as those in coffee, tea, cola, guarana, and chocolate: caffeine, theophylline, and theobromine. These stimulants are not carcinogenic. In moderate doses they are benign, even if you take them for a long period of time. Maté's carcinogenic factors lie in other, as-yet-unidentified ingredients.
- Maté's stimulant methylxanthines increase brain activity, increase heart rate, act as a diuretic, constrict your brain's blood vessels, and can make you jumpy, mainly by blocking adenosine receptors. While generally proven safe, they can be habit-forming, and withdrawal symptoms, though temporary, can be unpleasant.
- People who have heart disease or high blood pressure, or who are taking an MAO inhibitor should avoid methylxanthines if they are not used to them, because they can elevate blood pressure. Methylxanthines can be fatal to pets, so they should not be exposed to maté.

YOHIMBE

Pausinystalia yohimbe or *Corynanthe yohimbe*

HISTORY AND FOLKLORE

The bark of this West African tree is considered to be an aphrodisiac and, as such, sells like hotcakes. Unfortunately, it may not work all that well and actually has notable side effects, like causing fear, which is contraindicated in romantic encounters.

These days yohimbe is sold in products with names like "Mega Yohimbe 9000," featuring pictures of happy, attractive men wearing knowing smirks. Product names sport dauntingly masculine-sounding prefixes such as "Super-," "Ultra-," and "Power-," often followed by an equally intimidating four digit number like 9000 or 1500, yet typically no one knows what that number means.

Before all of this commercial fuss, the bark of this tall, evergreen tree was used in traditional western African cultures as a sexual stimulant, especially for men, and as a stimulant in general. Although it is in the coffee family (*Rubiaceae*), it does not contain caffeine. However, like other members of the coffee family, it contains bitter alkaloids, which affect the central nervous system. Its isolated alkaloid yohimbine is an FDA-approved drug of questionable effectiveness and safety. The action of the yohimbe herb has not been rigorously evaluated; most of the effects of the herb are derived from studies on its constituent, yohimbine.

HOW SCIENTISTS THINK YOHIMBE WORKS

The yohimbine in yohimbe bark has different effects on your fight-or-flight nervous system. One of the alkaloids in yohimbe bark is called *yohimbine,* an FDA-approved drug (sometimes known by the outmoded names *quebrachin, aphrodin, corynine, yohimvetol,* and *hydroergotocin*). Yohimbine can have different effects on your fight-or-flight nervous system. This is the part of your nervous system that creates a surge of adrenalin when you are nervous or excited. Also called the *sympathetic nervous system,* its actions are mediated by different nerve cell receptors, designated *alpha* and *beta.* To complicate matters, alpha- and beta-receptors often have opposite actions. Alpha-receptors generally constrict blood vessels, and beta receptors relax them, but in different regions of the body.

Alpha-receptor activation typically constricts involuntary (smooth) muscles surrounding blood vessels in your gastrointestinal tract and skin, which is why your stomach feels odd and you get pale when you are scared. Beta-receptor activation generally relaxes blood vessels in your muscles, giving your muscles more fuel to run with, and it also makes your heart pump harder, which of course also happens when you are nervous.

In the peripheral nervous system, yohimbine stimulates the fight-or-flight nervous system. The perepheral nervous system includes nerve cells outside the brain and spinal cord. When yohimbine stimulates these nerve's fight-or-flight response, you become jumpy, your blood pressure rises, and your heart pounds. Yohimbine sticks to alpha-receptors, in particular, alpha-2 receptors, competitively blocking their activation. Normally, blocking *ordinary* alpha-receptors will prevent vasoconstriction and relax your blood vessels, allowing the blood to flow more easily. This lowers blood pressure, and indeed, "alpha blockers" are antihypertensive medications that are used to treat high blood pressure. But yohimbine *raises* blood pressure. What's going on?

Not all alpha-receptors are the same. Most, called *alpha-1 receptors,* are on *post*synaptic ends of nerve cells (downstream of a nervous impulse), and these do constrict blood vessels. Some of the alpha-2 receptors that yohimbine blocks are in this position, too. But most alpha-2 receptors are located on *pre*synaptic ends of nerve cells (upstream of the nervous impulse), and they inhibit the activation of the *other,* downstream alpha-receptors. So if you can follow this complicated bit of negative logic, yohimbine inhibits a sympathetic nervous system inhibitor and therefore stimulates the sympathetic nervous system. Since alpha-2 receptor stimulation on presynaptic ends of nerve cells prevents the release of norepinephrine, yohimbine inhibits this and *causes norepinephrine to be released.* Norepinephrine (called *noradrenalin* in the United Kingdom) is a primary mediator of your fight-or-flight response.

Yohimbine works differently in the penis, however. Since norepinephrine constricts blood vessels in the penis, too, it prevents erections, which require blood vessel dilation. Norepinephrine is thus notorious at ruining erotic arousal and dampening erections, so it would seem that yohimbine would make the worst sort of aphrodisiac. However, the alpha-2 receptors mentioned

above, which increase norepinephrine when blocked (called *alpha-2 adrenergic receptors*) are in short supply in the penis, so this isn't much of a concern. *Different* alpha-2 receptors (called *nonadrenergic, noncholinergic,* or *NANC alpha-2 receptors*) present in the penis are inhibited by yohimbine. NANC alpha-2 receptors ordinarily prevent nitric oxide from being released. Nitric oxide dilates blood vessels, generating an erection when this occurs in the penis. Again, if you can follow the reverse logic, yohimbine inhibits NANC alpha-2 receptor inhibition of nitric oxide release. In other words, it prevents NANC nerve cells from being so stingy with nitric oxide, and their consequent release of nitric oxide theoretically enables erection. Yohimbine may also help an erection by blocking some alpha-1 receptors of the sympathetic nervous system in the penis, which cause vasoconstriction and would otherwise disable an erection.[1]

In your central (brain and spinal cord) nervous system, yohimbine may have dual effects on your fight-or-flight nervous system. Yohimbine readily enters the brain, and parts of the sympathetic nervous system get stimulated: increased heart rate, blood pressure, and nervousness result.[2] Ordinarily, signals from the sympathetic nervous system from the brain or spinal cord prevent erection. However, yohimbine may shut this other part of the sympathetic nervous system off. Some researchers propose that yohimbine's inhibition of both the fight-or-flight-mediating alpha-1 and the less common, similar-acting postsynaptic alpha-2 receptors in the brain inhibits this sympathetic dampening to nerves cells controlling an erection.

Interesting Facts

Yohimbine could scare your phobias away.

HOW MANY old dramas have we watched where the protagonist recovers from a life-long fear by being exposed to it under safer, more relaxing circumstances? These dramas may be half right and half wrong.

It's true that exposing yourself to your worst nightmare can help you recover from it. Phobia researchers at the University of Boston successfully ease patients' irrational fears by introducing them for a short period of time to a simulation representing what they most dread, and they gradually increase the patient's exposure as their terror wanes. However, exposure therapy requires multiple sessions, and people tend to drop out, because it takes too long and becomes expensive. Since the therapy works, researchers are eager to find a way to speed up their patients' response. They tried giving their patients calming medications during exposure therapy, which certainly seemed reasonable. But according to new research, they may do better to give their already

trembling patients anxiety-*enhancing* medications, like yohimbine.

Researchers at the University of California found to their surprise that rats conditioned to associate a particular sound with an electric shock recovered from their fear of that sound faster when given the anxiety-producing medication yohimbine, along with exposure therapy, rather than propanonol, an anxiety-reducing drug. This was the opposite of what they had expected. Yohimbine is well known to stimulate the fight-or-flight nervous system. It even triggers anxiety attacks. Researchers don't understand how enhancing anxiety accelerates the success of exposure therapy for phobias. Despite the apparent extra touch of sadism required, however, they are pleased. Anything that allows patients to get through the therapy faster is a bonus, they say, and they plan to test yohimbine in people undergoing exposure therapy for phobias.[3]

Good Effects . . . and Not So Good

The active ingredient in yohimbe bark is yohimbine, and it does not work for everyone. It can work to treat male impotence, and possibly even low sexual desire in women, too, but clinical trials show it does not work reliably well, or for everyone. Men with nonorganic sexual dysfunction seem to be aided more. The German Commission E health authority doesn't approve it, because it has not proven reliably effective and can have serious adverse reactions. The FDA ruled yohimbine both ineffective and unsafe, as well, and since yohimbe contains yohimbine, some states have accordingly banned health outlets from selling it in this nonprescription form.

Since yohimbine is a powerful drug, if you decide to take yohimbe or its constituent yohimbine, you should be under a doctor's guidance. The primary side effects of yohimbine are well known: high blood pressure and anxiety. Although yohimbine may lower blood pressure and increase blood flow in the genitals, it more reliably *raises* blood pressure in the rest of your body. Conversely, large doses can cause blood pressure to plummet dangerously. Don't take yohimbe if you have either high or low blood pressure. People with anxiety, depression, liver or kidney disease, angina, or heart disease should avoid yohimbe as well.

The list of side effects is long. Even standard doses of yohimbe and yohimbine can produce severe anxiety, insomnia, racing heart, mania, gastric upset, dizziness, headache, and vomiting. Larger doses have caused paralysis, respiratory failure, severe low blood pressure, heart failure, and death.

Yohimbe and yohimbine can interact with foods and drink. Avoid taking yohimbe or yohimbine with tyramine-containing foods, as seriously low blood pressure can result. Foods that contain lots of tyramine include aged cheeses like blue cheese, beer, red wines, chocolate, and preserved or canned meats. Some foods enhance yohimbine's ability to raise your blood pressure, too, like coffee, tea, chocolate, colas, and fava beans.

Yohimbe and yohimbine interfere with several medications, too. Sympathomimetics, a category of drugs that are taken either as decongestants (pseudophedrine, or Sudaphed), asthma medications, or appetite suppressants, exacerbate yohimbine's side effects. Also, do not take yohimbe or yohimbine if you are on "alpha blockers" or any antihypertensive drug. It antagonizes the activities of the antihypertensive drugs clonidine (Catapres)

and guanabenz (Wytensin). Since yohimbine inhibits monoamine oxidase (MAO), you should not take yohimbe if you are already on a monoamine oxidase inhibitor (MAOI) drug, which are often taken as antidepressants. Taking yohimbe with tricyclic antidepressants can play havoc with your blood pressure, too. This herb can also interfere with phenothiazines, which are often taken as antidepressants or pain relievers.

Commonly Reported Uses for Yohimbe*

Internally

aphrodisiac, stimulant

forms available for internal use:

yohimbe bark, capsule, drops, decoction, tablet, tea, tincture, yohimbine tablets, yohimbine hydrochloride tablets

commonly reported dosage:

Yohimbe or yohimbine should be taken only while under a doctor's supervision. For sexual dysfunction, daily doses of 15 to 30 milligrams of yohimbine have been used in clinical studies. This corresponds to 250–500 milligrams of yohimbe bark.

*These uses and dosages are from historic use and are not necessarily tested nor recommended.

But do all herbal products containing yohimbe bark possess adequate yohimbine for the herb to behave like the drug? If you still insist on trying this herb, getting a product standardized to yohimbine seems in order, and though most of those tested by independent labs check out all right, not all do, so it is best to seek the highest quality brands. Also, none of the

THE BOTTOM LINE

- Yohimbe contains yohimbine, which affects the fight-or-flight nervous system in complicated ways. It may help in treating impotence, but its side effects and lack of proven effectiveness make it a risky herb to take.
- Yohimbe or yohimbine should only be taken under a doctor's supervision. There are numerous side effects—in particular, high or low blood pressure and anxiety.
- Yohimbe and yohimbine can both interfere with several medications, such as decongestants (pseudophedrine or Sudaphed), other sympathomimetics, asthma medications, appetite suppressants, antihypertensive drugs such as alpha blockers, clonidine (Catapres), and guanabenz (Wytensin), and antidepressants such as monoamine oxidase inhibitor (MAOI) drugs, tricyclic antidepressants, and phenothiazines.
- Certain foods taken along with yohimbe or yohimbine may increase the risk of side effects, such as aged cheeses like blue cheese, beer, red wines, chocolate, preserved or canned meats, caffeinated products, and fava beans.
- Several medical conditions preclude taking yohimbine or yohimbe, such as heart disease, liver or kidney disease, anxiety disorders, and high or low blood pressure.

combination herbs for treating impotence passed muster for containing what they claimed when tested by independent parties, so you should avoid all combination products completely. Yohimbe has enough side effects; don't complicate them further with unknown ingredients.

EVIDENCE OF ACTION

There are barely any studies of the *herb* yohimbe in people, let alone in animals. On the other hand, there are a couple thousand scientific reports mentioning its most publicized constituent, yohimb*ine,* which is an approved prescription drug (Yocon) in the United States. Just because a drug is FDA approved, however, does not guarantee it works and is free of side effects, and yohimbine is no exception. In the words of one of my pharmacology textbooks, "It currently has no therapeutic uses."[4]

Although yohimbine, the drug, was once prescribed extensively to treat male sexual dysfunction, it was never proven to work all that well for people. It does make rats more libidinous, however. That it never showed stunning success for treating human impotence may lie in part because the causes of human sexual dysfunction are numerous and complicated.

When given to men with impotence from varied causes, yohimbine showed no significant difference from a placebo in one reliably constructed (randomized, double-blind, placebo-controlled crossover) trial. In fact, the placebo worked slightly better, demonstrating that for certain conditions the brain is a valuable therapeutic tool.[5] Yohimbine may work better for treating nonorganic, or psychologically derived impotence. In a couple of carefully designed (randomized, double-blind, placebo-controlled) trials, it appeared significantly better than placebo for treating psychologically-derived impotence,[6] and rated equivalent to sex or relationship therapy.[7]

Yohimbine also worked well in combination with the amino acid arginine in treating postmenopausal women with low libidoes,[8] and in men with impotence,[9] but the positive results may stem more from the arginine than the yohimbine; yohimbine alone gave no benefit for nine women in another randomized controlled trial.[10]

Since yohimbine antagonizes serotonin, some hope it could be useful to prevent the decrease in libido occasionally caused by SSRI (selective serotonin reuptake inhibitor) antidepressant medications. Some clinical trials suggest it may help the so-called sexual side effects of these antidepressants,[11, 12] yet it did not help sexually dysfunctional women taking these kinds of antidepressants in one study.[13]

Interest in using yohimbine as a drug for sexual dysfunction has been lost amid the uproarious success of sildenafil (Viagra). Why is yohimbine still an approved drug? It's used to cause anxiety. Really. Clinicians often use it in their research studies to simulate physiological conditions of anxiety. It also reliably causes high blood pressure. These are obviously unwanted side effects if you want to use it to treat sexual dysfunction.

Some more optimistic herbalists suggest that yohimbe bark could work better than its isolated yohimbine, presumably because of unknown active ingredients. Yohimbe bark does contain other indole alkaloids similar to yohimbine, but their actions are not known, and there are no rigorous clinical trials using the herb, yohimbe bark.

Appendixes

APPENDIX A
WHAT DOES IT MEAN TO BE NATURAL?

Ridding Ourselves of Our Molecular Bigotry May Help Us to Become One with Nature.

We should judge molecules by their behavior, not their origin. Studies show that molecules from red clover and those from soy end up becoming the same thing in your body. Yet some consumers still worry that the molecules they turn into are different because of their origin. People also fret about whether synthetic vitamins coming out of a lab are different from those that are isolated from plants. Ideally we don't judge people based on their origin, who raised them, or what country they came from. Ideally, we judge them by their behavior. Why is it so hard for us to do the same for molecules?

On a gut-response level, natural molecules are assumed to be more virtuous than synthetic ones, but a quick glance at some toxic mushrooms, snake venoms, and a multitude of plants that are not in this book will help convince you this is not true. The truth is, whether a molecule is from a plant, a lab bench, or a rock, it can't be judged until we know how it behaves, so we must be more open-minded. Like people, some good ones can act badly under certain circumstances. A molecule's source won't tell us what it does, so we have to be ready for anything.

There used to be a doctrine called *vitalism,* which held that natural (organic) molecules couldn't be made by man, because they contained some mystic essence or "vital force" that we could not duplicate. In 1828 German chemist Friedrich Wohler used inorganic ammonium cyanate crystals (basically a rock) to make urea, which is something that organisms make prolifically (it's in urine). Although this disproved vitalism, the notion that synthetically derived molecules are identical to natural ones is still difficult for people to trust.

Modern chemists can make a copy of a naturally occurring molecule, with the exact same structure, in a laboratory. We know the exact, unambiguous structure of the desired molecule and can duplicate it unerringly. And according to every imaginable test, both *in vitro* and *in vivo,* the synthetic version behaves in precisely the same way as a naturally occurring molecule, and this has been verified innumerable times over since Wohler's discovery in 1828. The synthetic molecule has no "memory" of where it came from and truly is the same molecule as its naturally occurring counterpart.

Since this is true, why are we so inclined to trust natural molecules over synthetic ones? Food labelers know this, brandishing the term "natural" on a multitude of products, even though "natural" has no legal meaning. Some have suggested we're soft on natural molecules because we have philosophically isolated ourselves from nature. Especially in Christian cultures, ever since the fall of Adam and Eve, humans have been considered inherently sinful, so anything we make in a lab gets the same sinful taint. Our subconsciously collective decision to separate ourselves from nature not only confuses our understanding of herbal therapeutics but also provides us with a rationale for destroying nature. The historical abuse of various groups of people has usually been associated with pseudo-scientific rationalizations that these people were in an "animal" class, separate from humans. This unconscious mental separation of "human" and "nature" has invaded our language and thought. I have even had students ask if humans are really animals. According to scientific taxonomy, there are four other choices: bacteria, plants, pond organisms, and fungi. What do you think?

Most people want to feel part of nature, but of course we already are—we just don't know it! We just have far more elaborate "nests." The molecules we make are no less natural than the molecules other animals make. Some of the most feared industrial toxins made by man are also made by plants, and humans have cleverly learned how to make many of the same beneficial molecules that plants make, too. So the next time you ask yourself which is better, natural or synthetic, remember that it is not the origin of the molecule that matters but how it behaves in your body, because natural and synthetic are really the same. Perhaps if enough people discuss this issue, we can start looking at nature's molecules in a whole new way and realize we are part of nature. We might treat each other and our natural world more kindly if we did.

APPENDIX B
INTRODUCING THE PLAYERS:
Cells, Molecules, and Other Very Small Things

Herbs are Made of Chemicals—
Be More Concerned about a
Chemical's Action on Your Body
than Its Origin

Supplement vendors often give you their fishy assurance that "It's herbal, so it has no chemicals in it, and it can't hurt you." Alas, this is simply not true. All matter, anything that can be weighed on a scale and occupies space, is made of chemicals, even the air we breathe. Plants are completely made of chemicals. If plants were not made of chemicals, they would be empty vacuums, made of nothingness, without much therapeutic usefulness. Animals are made of chemicals. Humans are made of chemicals. Everything is made of chemicals. Even the so-called vacuum of outer space is not a perfect vacuum; it has chemicals drifting around in it, although they are spaced quite far apart.

There are all sorts of chemicals in living things, but most of the important ones in living creatures are of a kind called *molecules,* so you will more often see the term "molecule," rather than "chemical," in this book. (If you want to know more about molecules and other sorts of chemicals, see "Chemistry 101" at the end of this section.) Society has developed a curious bias against the word "chemical," because there are some truly horrible ones. But you should know that most are not that bad. Although the term "chemical" has acquired negative connotations for many, it is just a general term for *what all things are made of.*

The term "chemical" may conjure up images of foul-smelling vats of synthetic sludge that will cause genetic mutations. Let's not be so prejudiced. Before you criticize a chemical, you first ought to see what it does. Our historic tendency is to evaluate chemicals based on their source, whether they are "natural," "synthetic," "plant," "animal," "mineral," or whatever. This classification system is useful, but it can be deceptive. We have evolved the wisdom to judge people by their behavior rather than their origin. Why not do the same for chemicals? Where chemicals come from is less important than what they do to you, what they do to other creatures, and what they do to our environment.

THE BOTTOM LINE

PLANTS ARE completely made of chemicals. Where chemicals come from is less important than what they do to you. A molecule is a particular type of chemical. Most of the chemicals that we are interested in, in organisms, are molecules, so you will more often see the more specific term "molecule," instead of "chemical," in this book.

Herbs Affect You through
Molecules Called *Secondary*
Metabolites

Plants contain a tremendous variety of tiny chemicals called molecules. All living things have molecules and need them to live, but plants make more molecules than they need for their own survival. Molecules that plants make for basic living functions are classified as *primary metabolites,* and these are fairly similar from plant to plant. But plants spend valuable energy making extra molecules called *secondary metabolites,* too. These vary more from plant to plant. You are actually pretty familiar with some secondary metabolites whether you know it or not. You can smell and taste the different secondary metabolites in peppermint and cinnamon, distinguishing one herb from the other. It is these secondary metabolites that make herbs so interesting. Eating some secondary metabolites can change your whole day.

Some secondary metabolites can cure headaches, calm nerves, moisturize our skin, give us energy, sedate us, kill bacteria, and banish indigestion. But others can cause rashes. Others induce vomiting. Some of them can even cause fatalities. Why should such passive organisms go to the trouble of creating extra molecules that so actively affect us?

Plants can't run away. They can't perform karate on voracious predators either. They have to synthesize their own chemical weapons to prevent being eaten. Alas, this means that some plant molecules are toxic. Some *are* toxic to humans, but fortunately more are mainly poisonous to bugs and microorganisms, the most common plant predators. Also, plants use less toxic, more colorful or flavorful secondary metabolites to attract pollinators. Some secondary metabolites accidentally have powerful effects on the body. These powerful herbal molecules, and all molecules in general, are actually chemicals. Chemicals in drugs affect us, and plant chemicals work in our bodies by similar mechanisms.

Other secondary metabolites protect plants from sun damage, otherwise known as *radiation,* and harmful things called *rad-*

icals and *oxidizing agents* (see Free Radicals, page 385, and Oxygen and other Oxidizing Agents, page 388.) You can usurp these herbs' protective molecules to defend *yourself* against harmful things like radiation, bacteria, bugs, and oxidizing agents, using these molecules for your own advantage.

THE BOTTOM LINE

PLANTS MAKE extra molecules called secondary metabolites, which they don't need for basic living functions, to protect against pests, chemical and radiation damage, and to attract pollinators. Secondary metabolites can accidentally affect us by the very same mechanisms that modern drugs exert their actions on us.

CELLS ARE THE BASIC UNIT OF LIFE, AND THEIR BEHAVIOR DEPENDS ON THE ACTIONS OF THE CHEMICALS THAT COMPOSE THEM

You can think of the word "chemical" to mean "what all things are made of," but despite their abundance, chemicals remain mysterious. They are mysterious only because you can't see them individually. When huge numbers of them stick together in a clump, you *can* see the clump—for example, as a grain of sand, or a crystal of salt or sugar. But chemicals are simply very small, inanimate objects. They are not alive.

However, trillions upon trillions upon trillions of chemicals can organize themselves in complicated ways to create a vastly larger structure, called a *cell,* which *is* alive and is considered the basic unit of life. All living things are made of cells. Imagine a cell to be a tiny container full of all the machinery that it needs to reproduce, obtain and use energy and nutrients, and expel wastes. Cells come in all sorts of shapes and sizes. Plant cells tend to be more angular and boxy, while animal cells are more varied in shape and are more rounded, for example. While we can't see chemicals with our eyes, we can easily see cells using a microscope. A modern criterion for life is to be cellular— to be made of cells.

Some organisms like bacteria, pond organisms, and yeast are made of just one or a few cells, while others like plants, fungi, and animals are multicellular collections of specialized cells. It may surprise you to learn that despite lots of loose talk about "killing viruses," viruses are not officially considered to be alive, because they do not have anything like a cell. Viruses are made of a much smaller number of chemicals and must exploit a cell's internal machinery to make copies of themselves. Whether you want to call them alive or not depends on the cell-requiring technicality. In any case, these odd, intracellular parasites on occasion can be permanently disabled, if not "killed." Both viruses and officially living things are made of inanimate chemicals; therefore they will behave in a manner determined by the behavior their constituent chemicals. So, to really understand how cells behave and how herbs affect them, you must understand how the chemicals that compose them behave.

THE BOTTOM LINE

CHEMICALS ARE not alive, but many chemicals can constitute a cell, which is alive. Cells are the basic unit of life. The behavior of a cell depends on the behavior of the chemicals it is made of. The behavior of an herb depends on how its chemicals affect your cells' chemicals.

HERBAL CHEMICALS ARE DRIVEN AROUND BY A SIMPLE FORCE

The behavior of chemicals is understandable, operating by basic laws of cause and effect. A chemical from an herb is a real object, the cause, which goes on various journeys. Where it ends up in the body, and what it does there, is the effect that interests us. If there is a gap in the journey that can't be accounted for, you may be less certain about how an herbal chemical works. I will try to avoid any gaps in our journeys, if possible, but I will also try to be clear where they occur.

Also, you have to be sure that the chemical's journey logically accounts for its effect. You would not expect that changing a car's spark plug would refill its windshield fluid. Similarly, you will find the actions of plant molecules should ideally be related to their effects on your body in obvious ways.

You also can't assume that an herbal chemical will do what you think is best. There is a common assumption that molecules in our bodies are somehow compelled to do whatever is best for our survival, but this optimistic fancy is wrong. This impression is a simple result of the fact that chemicals often do end up supporting the well-being of the organism they occupy. But chemicals do not *try* to do anything.

This fact makes it even more remarkable that these inanimate objects so often (but not always) end up doing what is best for the body anyway. It's enough to give you goose bumps, even though you can reason that nature has sorted out and saved the processes that work, while the processes that fail are discarded by a cell's inability to reproduce and pass them on, and we call this evolution. Nonetheless, if you need inspiration, remind yourself of this remarkable tendency of your molecules—these small, inanimate objects—to promote your health.

Despite the fact that our constituent chemicals usually end up doing things that promote well-being, these *chemicals do not care about our health*. Chemicals are not under any compulsion to maintain your health, any more than your car, which is a very large inanimate object, spontaneously drives itself to the store because it wants to do so, or because you think it would be for the best if it did. Chemicals are nevertheless driven around by a real force.

The force that moves chemicals is not like the one we are most familiar with in our everyday experience. It is not gravity. Although we are all intimately acquainted with gravity, gravity is actually a relatively weak force, compared to the force that acts on chemicals. Earth's gravitational energy will not wrench our heads off if we lean over too far. Thus there is a force *stronger* than gravity attracting the chemicals in our heads to the chemicals in our necks. Gravity has far less of an effect on individual chemicals than it does on large collections of chemicals such as a whole person. This is because more massive objects feel greater gravitational pulls. Individual chemicals have far less mass than we do, so gravity does not have a great effect on chemicals. Chemicals are dominated by a law called the *electrostatic force*. This law works by simple rules that you can learn.

THE BOTTOM LINE

OVER THE millennia, chemical journeys that support life have been perpetuated in reproducing cells, and chemical journeys that were fatal have been discarded by a cell's inability to reproduce and pass them on. Therefore, the chemicals of a cell often end up supporting the life of the cell. But chem-icals will not necessarily do what we might think is best. They do not act in order to support life. They are dominated by a force called the *electrostatic law.*

The Electrostatic Force Causes Herbal Chemicals to Affect You

The force that influences most chemical behavior is called the electrostatic force and results from a property of matter called *charge*. Now, the funny thing about charge is that many scientists probably couldn't tell you exactly *what* charge is. Nonetheless, we know a great deal about what it *does,* and we know that it is a property of certain bits of matter.

Charge comes in only two flavors, which scientists call positive and negative. We do know that two different, or "opposite," charges (positive and negative) attract and will move toward each other, and like charges (positive and positive, or negative and negative) repel and will move away from each other.

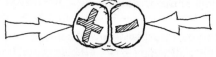

opposite charges attract

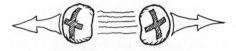

like charges repel

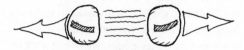

like charges repel

The electrostatic force causes opposite charges to attract and like charges to repel. This simple force is the main reason herbs affect us.

Having a bad hair day? Your hairs have probably all acquired the same sort of charge, and they stand up in the air because they repel each other. Anything with no charge is called *neutral*. If you are politically neutral, you do not get pulled to the right or the left, and a neutral chemical isn't terribly attracted to one thing or the other either.

The basis of *most* chemical behavior, and most of your herbal phenomena—because you and herbs are made of chemicals—is the electrostatic force. Because of the electrostatic force, our lifeless molecules attract and assemble to create our cells. Some of us may find this inspiring, as philosophers have asked the perhaps unanswerable question: If the electrostatic force behaved in a slightly different way, would life even be possible?

Magnets are attracted or repelled by each other by a consequence of this force. What child playing with magnets has not been awed that these forces do not require physical contact? Even though there is space between the magnets, you can feel a push or pull. The chemicals in our bodies, like magnets, feel a similar push and pull, too. Although we are made of chemicals, these chemicals are mostly empty space. We are mostly empty space. The reason we can't walk through walls, which are also mostly empty space, is the strength of this force. This "action at a distance" force is what keeps the different parts of a chemical together and also attracts one chemical to another. It holds our heads onto our necks. It drives herbal chemicals around our bodies. The electrostatic force pushes herbal chemicals upon the body's own chemicals, influencing a change in them.

In multicellular organisms, cells become highly specialized for different tasks, creating tissues. We have our own animal tissues, such as blood, skin, nerve, and muscle, but herbs also have their own tissues: dermal, ground, and vascular. Several different tissues also organize, forming specialized organs, such as animal hearts, livers, and brains, or herbal leaves and roots. All these tissues and organs are assembled by and obey the electrostatic force.

THE BOTTOM LINE

THE ELECTROSTATIC law says that opposite charges attract, and like charges repel. This force creates chemicals and also assembles these lifeless chemicals into living cells. The electrostatic force also determines much of the behavior of chemicals, including those from herbs.

Herbal Chemicals Are Polar or Nonpolar, Based on Whether or Not They Have Localized Charges.

It turns out that all chemicals can roughly be divided into two categories, based on whether or not they have localized charges on them or not. Curiously, whether the charges are positive or negative is not as important as whether they have some charge or no charge. How an herbal chemical behaves in your body actually depends a lot on which type it is.

Nonpolar chemicals are neutral.

Chemicals that have no charge are the chemical slugs and are not very attracted to much of anything around them. Air molecules are like this; they don't stick to one another, so they bounce off of each other, and they bounce off of our bodies, too. They form a gas that you can easily walk through, with the air chemicals bouncing out of your way as you go. Chemicals that have no charges are called *nonpolar.*

Nonpolar chemicals don't repulse each other; they just aren't terribly attracted to other chemicals around them. To be honest, they *are* made of tinier, randomly moving positive and negative charges, but the charges are so evenly mixed everywhere, at any given time, that in no place is the charge predominantly one flavor or the other. If you could imagine one charge to be black and the other white, they would be so smoothly distributed that a whole nonpolar chemical would appear gray, and not black or white. So overall, nonpolar chemicals appear to have no charge and are neutral—they don't get involved much. More precisely, they do have tiny, mobile charges, but the positive and negative charges are so symmetrically distributed that they even out to zero everywhere.

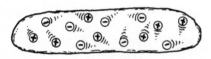

nonpolar molecule

Many molecules from herbs are nonpolar. A nonpolar molecule behaves as if it had no charge, overall. Its small, randomly moving charges are distributed evenly around it.

Nonpolar chemicals derived from living things are called *lipids* or *oils.* Herbs have lots of nonpolar chemicals. Most herbal flavors and smells come from small, nonpolar chemicals. They don't stick to each other very well in the plant, so they depart the herb, fly up your nose, and you perceive a smell. Some take their time lazily drifting through your tongue, and after a few seconds, you notice the burn of red pepper, or the cool anesthetic effect of menthol from mint.

Larger nonpolar chemicals from herbs have more surface area to stick to one another, which they feebly do, using the tiny, randomly moving charges that compose them. The oppositely charged bits of one herbal chemical align against the oppositely charged parts of another. Because they cling to each other weakly, they can slip and slide over one another in a liquid or clump up together in a soft solid.

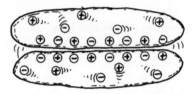

two nonpolar molecules sticking

Nonpolar molecules can stick to each other weakly. The bigger they are, the more area they have to stick together. Flavor and smell molecules from herbs are often nonpolar. Fats, waxes, and oils from herbs are always nonpolar. They often associate with other nonpolar molecules in your body.

Big bumper stickers are harder to unstick from your car than smaller ones, not because the glue is different, but because there is just more of them to unstick. Likewise, the bigger the nonpolar chemical, the more likely it will stick to another of its own kind and form a denser material. The larger nonpolar herbal chemicals are what we call fats, oils, and waxes. Even nonpolar solids are not very hard, though. You can stick your finger right through wax, because the nonpolar chemicals inside it can be separated from each other pretty easily. Nonpolar molecules don't stick to anything very well, including each other.

Polar chemicals have fixed charges.

The other type of chemical we find in herbs are the polar ones. If you find yourself in a polarized political discussion, you are aware of two persistent, opposing points of view. Similarly, a polar chemical has a permanent positive region and a permanent negative region. The charges are stuck in their places on the chemical, so they can't move around and even themselves out as they do in nonpolar chemicals.

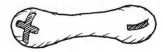

polar molecule

Several herb molecules are polar. A polar molecule has a permanently positive area and a permanently negative area.

Polar chemicals are strongly attracted to other polar chemicals, because their opposite charges attract. You might wonder why they don't repel each other with like charges instead. They might, but eventually they will bump back into each other and stick together.

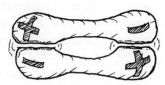

polar molecules sticking

Polar molecules stick strongly to each other. Sugars and amino acids from herbs are polar, plus herbs have many other polar molecules as well. They tend to associate with your body's polar molecules, including water.

Many chemicals from herbs are polar. Sugars, for example, are quite polar and stick so well to each other that they form hard little rocklike crystals when you get a whole bunch of them together in a pure lump. Water sticks well enough to itself that it forms a liquid and doesn't fly apart the way molecules in a gas do.

OF COURSE TEMPERATURE CAN CHANGE WHETHER A SUBSTANCE IS A SOLID, LIQUID, OR GAS. Water is too small—that is, it has too little surface area—however, to make a solid, or ice, at room temperature. But if you keep it from moving around so much, it will slow down enough so it has time to stick to itself and freeze. That is what cooling does—it slows down molecules' motions. The best definition of temperature is that it relates to the average speed of molecules. No matter what they are, the faster they go—that is, the hotter they are, the more likely they are to bounce off of each other and exist as a gas.

The water is so cohesive that it rounds up into spherical droplets, unlike nonpolar oils, which flatten out. Water also mixes well with different polar chemicals, like sugar. It does not find nonpolar chemicals like oil terribly attractive, because nonpolar chemicals have no localized charges for water to cling to.

ACTUALLY, MOST molecules are polar not because of charges but because of *partial* charges. Partial charges are less powerful than whole-number charges, like +1 or –1. These charges are fractional, like +1/4 or –1/4 or so, but we don't bother to measure their exact value. They are less than 1 but greater than –1, and can be either "partially negative" or "partially positive." It is their permanent location on one part of a molecule that makes the molecule more like a magnet, and less like the sluglike nonpolar molecule.

You may have heard that water and oil repel each other, but this isn't exactly true. They just are not very attracted to each other. Water is much more attracted to other polar things, like other water molecules. So it sticks to its own kind, and the oil is excluded from this interaction. Oil going into water is sort of like a person who goes to a party and no one talks to them. It isn't that no one likes them. It's just that everyone at the party likes everyone else better.

Like mixes with like. One of the most important chemical rules governing herbal molecules—and every other molecule, for that matter—is the rule of "like mixes with like." Polar molecules mix and stick to other polar ones fairly strongly. Nonpolar molecules mix and stick to nonpolar ones, although more feebly. Nonpolar and polar chemicals don't mix, and tend to separate.

You will see other names for polar and nonpolar in herbal literature. "Hydrophilic" means "water loving," so it refers to polar chemicals. "Hydrophobic" means "water fearing" and is synonymous with nonpolar. Sometimes you will see "lipophilic," or "fat loving," to refer to nonpolar chemicals as well.

It is actually quite important whether herbal molecules are watery or oily, polar or nonpolar. Polar molecules will interact with polar things in your body, and in some cases are more likely to depart your body through urine, which is mostly water. Nonpolar molecules will be more likely to *enter* your cells, which are surrounded by a nonpolar barrier that they can mingle with and penetrate. They can also reside along with your fat and hang out in your body for a longer period of time. But often your body modifies nonpolar herbal molecules, turning them into polar ones, so you can excrete them more easily.

Also, you should pay attention to whether a successful clinical trial of an herb

used a water-based herbal extract or an oil-based extract, because they contain different active ingredients. Teas or "decoctions" are water-based and contain more polar herbal molecules. A water-based extract will not provide you with much vitamin E, which is nonpolar, but it could have vitamin C, which is polar, for example. Similarly, a tea of saw palmetto berries is not likely to provide the berries' oily active ingredients, but a tea of chamomile is likely to contain the water-soluble flavonoid glycosides that can become sedative, anti-inflammatory agents in the gut.

Tinctures or elixirs are alcoholic extracts and contain either polar or nonpolar molecules, depending on the type of alcohol used. For what most people call "alcohol"—that is, the kind found in alcoholic beverages (ethanol)—extracts contain more nonpolar ingredients than you will find in a water-based extract but will still contain some polar molecules, too. Some natural products companies take an alcohol extract and distill it, which concentrates the nonpolar herbal molecules into an oil. This contains mostly nonpolar herbal chemicals. Another way to pull out nonpolar molecules is to soak the plant in an oil. The principle of "like mixes with like" will cause nonpolar molecules to enter the oil.

So nonpolar molecules dissolve in oil, but polar ones usually can dissolve in water. Even some polar molecules have trouble dissolving in water, however, if they happen to be very large. Plant fiber is like this. It's very much like paper (and in some cases it is). The fiber molecules are attracted to water molecules because both are polar, but the water is too small to surround the giant fiber molecule, so it can't separate the fiber from other fiber molecules, which it needs to do to dissolve. The fiber molecule just grabs onto some nearby water molecules, sticking to them and swelling to form a pulp. These sorts of very big molecules from plants will just go right through you on a one-way trip. Clinical trials where they were injected won't apply to you if you eat it. Pulpy, goo-like fiber from plants such as aloe or marsh-mallow can be useful, though, either topically or to soothe an inflamed gut.

THE BOTTOM LINE

A NONPOLAR chemical has no permanently charged regions and appears uncharged overall. A polar chemical has a permanent positive region and a permanent negative region. The rule of "like mixes with like" means that polar mixes strongly with polar, nonpolar mixes more weakly with nonpolar, and polar and nonpolar do not blend well; they separate like water and oil. An herbal chemical will act differently in your body, depending on whether it is polar or nonpolar. Size also matters, too.

CHEMISTRY 101: IF YOU REALLY WANT TO KNOW . . . MORE DETAILS ABOUT DIFFERENT KINDS OF HERBAL CHEMICALS

Atom

Atoms are made of three smaller particles—protons, neutrons, and electrons.

Protons, Neutrons, and Electrons

WHILE PROTONS and neutrons constitute the bulk of an atom, electrons are often pictured as whizzing around this blob of protons and neutrons, like planets orbiting around the sun. The number of protons alone gives an atom its name: Whether it is hydrogen, oxygen, carbon, or whatever. Anything with one proton, even an isolated proton, is called *hydrogen,* anything with six protons is *carbon,* and anything with eight protons is *oxygen,* for example.

Atoms are classified as being either metals or nonmetals, and most of them are metals. There are approximately 116 different types of atoms known, but fortunately only a small handful of these, mostly nonmetals, regularly occur in molecules in organisms, which makes herbal medicine a lot less complicated. While electrons each bear a negative charge, each proton is positive, and they occur in matching sets in atoms, in equal numbers, because atoms have no charge overall, by definition. Neutrons are also uncharged and occur in varying numbers in all atoms, increasing their weight.

What Kinds of Atoms Are In Herbs?

THE ATOMS you see most often in plants (and in all organisms) are carbon, hydrogen, oxygen, nitrogen, sulfur, and phosphorus, and there are others that are less common, too. They are more often stuck to (bonded with) other types of atoms, rather than isolated in their pure form. *Isolated atoms are not commonly active ingredients in herbs. They are more commonly bonded to other atoms.*

Element

The terms "atom" and "element" are sometimes used interchangeably. An atom is singular, while an element is plural and refers to a whole bunch of atoms *all of one kind.* These atoms may or may not be bonded together. If they bond together, they will make either an elemental molecule or what you would recognize as a shiny metal, depending on whether it is made of nonmetallic atoms or metallic ones.

What Kinds of Elements Are In Herbs?

ELEMENTS ISOLATED into their pure form are found scattered around in herbs but are not as common as other chemicals. With the exception of simple gases like molecular oxygen (O_2) and nitrogen (N_2), it is more common to find atoms of one kind bonded to atoms of a different kind in organisms. *Elements are not commonly the active ingredients in herbs.*

Compound

This is just a general term for anything with two or more *different* types of atoms or ions bonded together in some way. Thus, it is the not an element, which is made of atoms of all one type. Molecules that have different types of atoms in them are considered to be compounds. Some molecules, however, are not compounds, but elements, because they are made of the same type of atom bonded together. All ionic compounds are compounds, because they require a positively charged ion and a negatively charged ion, and these are of different types of ions.

What Kinds of Compounds Are In Herbs?

MOST OF the active herb ingredients in this book fall under the category of compounds and are molecules, since they are made of different atoms bonded together into a unit. *Molecular compounds are often the active ingredients in herbs. Ionic compounds are not.*

Molecule

A molecule is a bunch of atoms stuck together into a unit. The atoms in molecules are almost always nonmetal atoms. The atoms can be the same or different types; thus, molecules can be either elements or compounds. The smallest molecules have only two atoms, like the oxygen we breathe, which is two oxygen atoms bonded together. Since this molecule is made of only one kind of atom, it is technically also an element. The hydrochloric acid molecules making our stomach acid are also made of only two atoms, hydrogen and chlorine, bonded together, which makes them both a molecule and a compound. Water has three atoms—two hydrogens and an oxygen. Some DNA molecules can have more than a billion atoms joined together.

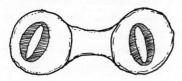

O₂ molecule

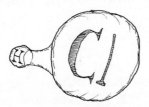

HCl molecule

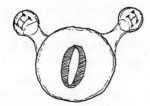

H₂O molecule

Molecules are the most common chemical making up organisms. They are usually the active ingredients of herbs. A molecule is two or more atoms joined to make a larger object. The oxygen you breathe is a molecule made of two oxygen atoms. Your stomach acid is a molecule made of one hydrogen atom and one chlorine atom. Water is a molecular compound of two hydrogens and one oxygen.

Molecular Bonds

MOLECULES ARE, by definition, held together by a particular type of bond called a *covalent bond,* represented by a straight line connecting the atoms in chemical drawings. This type of bond is quite strong, so it is hard to break apart one molecule into its individual atoms. When a molecule's bonds break, it changes into a different chemical or chemicals, and that is called a *reaction.* A diamond is tough because it is actually one giant molecule—a bunch of carbon atoms all bonded together.

A covalent bond is strong but is actually made of only two electrons. Sometimes electrons are shared between two atoms, because these negative particles are attracted to the positive protons of both atoms at once, and this sharing creates the bonds between atoms that hold a molecule intact. Each covalent bond is made of two electrons. You might fantasize these two particles swishing back and forth between both atoms so quickly that they blur, forming the straight line used in conventional chemical drawings to represent bonds.

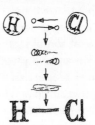

Each bond that hold atoms together in molecules is actually made of two electrons shared by both atoms simultaneously. You might imagine the two electrons zipping back and forth so fast they make the straight line used in conventional drawings of molecules.

Almost all the important molecules in life contain carbon, and carbon-containing molecules are called *organic molecules*. Many organic molecules are just made of carbons and hydrogens and are called *hydrocarbons*. When a molecule is mostly carbon and hydrogen atoms, it will be nonpolar, because carbons and hydrogens tend to share charges evenly over the molecule. The presence of more electron-greedy atoms like oxygen or nitrogen bonded to the more electron-generous carbons and hydrogens make a molecule more likely to be polar, with isolated negative regions on the electron-greedy atoms, and isolated positive regions on the electron-generous ones.

Sometimes a molecule has an unequal number of protons and electrons, which gives it a total charge. It is then called an *ion,* or a *molecular ion*. While a molecule does not have to be an ion in order to be polar, all molecular ions act like polar molecules.

What Kinds of Molecules Are In Herbs?

THERE ARE a great many different classes of molecules found in herbs. They may either have no charge (be neutral) or be charged, and if they are charged they could also be classified as an ion. Molecules are further classified by what sort of atoms are in them, how these atoms are arranged, and the molecule's physical properties. For example, lipids are mostly carbon and hydrogen and do not dissolve in water. Sugars have lots of OHs (*oxygen-bonded to hydrogen*) attached to their carbons, and alcohols have at least one OH bonded to a carbon. By recognizing common patterns of bonding like this, molecules are easily classified into a great many classes. This is convenient, because molecules in the same class tend to behave similarly.

Molecules that are strongly attracted to one another clump up and form a solid in an organism. Others are more attracted to water and are dissolved, floating around in watery fluids in organisms. Molecules that are not strongly attracted to water incorporate into oily parts of an organism, like the fat in fat cells, seeds, nuts, or cell membranes. *Molecules are the most common chemicals in organisms, so they are the most commonly found chemical in herbs. Molecules are usually the active ingredients of herbs.*

Ion

Ions have charges. An ion always has a charge, so you will always find a charge written next to its chemical representation. It is either an atom or a molecule with an unequal number of positive protons and negative electrons, resulting in a total positive or negative charge. Thus, there are negative ions (which have more electrons than protons) and positive ions (which have more protons than electrons). Negative ions are sometimes called *anions* (AN-eye-on), and positive ions are sometimes called *cations* (CAT-eye-on). Metal atoms like to lose electrons, so they often form positively charged ions. Nonmetal ions, if they don't bond to form molecules, sometimes gain extra electrons, which turns them into negative ions.

For example, sodium *atoms* are rare in nature, because they are unstable. They tend to immediately lose an electron, forming a positively charged sodium *ion*. It is positive because it still carries a positive proton that no longer has a matching electron to cancel its charge. When people refer to "sodium" in their diet, they mean sodium *ion*. Sodium *atoms* explode easily and are poisonous. But you need sodium *ion* for life. So it really matters whether something has a charge, whether it is an ion or not. You do not ever have to worry about eating sodium atoms. They are too unstable for you to find them, unless you purchase them from a chemical company.

What Kinds of Ions Are In Herbs?

MANY DIFFERENT ions are required for life, so *you will find lots of ions in all organisms, including herbs. The active ingredients of many herbs are ions.* Because ions of one type have the same charge, they repel each other, so you won't find ions of one kind all in one place. You always find ions floating in watery environments, like blood, and the insides of cells. Water molecules separate ions from one another, because water is polar and is attracted to charges of all kinds. *The ions you will most often find in herbs are sodium ions, potassium ions, chloride ions, calcium ions, magnesium ions, iron ions, sulfate ions, phosphate ions, carbonate ions, ascorbate ions, and oxalate ions, and there are many, many others.*

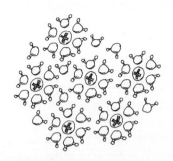

Ions are things with charges; they are either molecules or atoms that have lost or gained electrons. They are abundant in organisms and often the active ingredients in herbs. You will usually find ions surrounded by water. This is because water has both positive and negative regions—it is polar, and is attracted to ion's charges.

Ionic compound

An ionic compound is a solid crystal made of countless numbers of positive and negative ions, attracted to each other through the attraction of opposite charges. Ionic compounds are all solids, so they all look like rocks or crystals (but not all rocks or crystals are ionic compounds). A crystal of table salt, or sodium chloride, is made of zillions of positively charged sodium ions (Na+) and negatively charged chloride (Cl−) ions, attracted and held together into a lump.

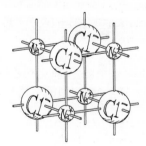

NaCl crystal

Ionic compounds are solids made of huge numbers of positive ions and negative ions. They are not that common in organisms, because water in organisms often breaks the ions apart and they dissolve into isolated ions. However, some are resistant to breakage by water, and they can form gritty or irritating crystals in herbs.

Ionic Bonds

THE BOND holding ionic compounds together, called an *ionic bond,* is usually not as strong as a covalent bond, which holds molecules together. So an individual molecule, while much, much smaller than an ionic compound crystal, is generally tougher to break apart. Ionic bonds, however, are still strong; that is why all ionic compounds are solids. However, many ionic compounds, like table salt, fall apart and dissolve when you place them in water. This is because many ions are even more attracted to water than they are to ions of the opposite charge. Ionic compounds are separated into individual ions by water molecules, and organisms are mostly water. When they dissolve in water, they disappear, because you can't see individual ions with your eyes, they are too small.

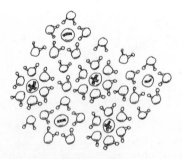

Most ionic compounds get broken apart by the water in organisms. They break apart into individual ions separated by attracted water molecules. The ions are too small to see, so the solid ionic crystal disappears. This is why ions are more common in herbs than ionic compounds.

Some ionic compounds are tougher and do not dissolve in water, so they are more permanent. The ions in lime deposits (calcium oxiop) on your sink aren't as attracted to water as they are to themselves. They will not run down your drain along with water, as they are an insoluble ionic compound—they don't dissolve in water.

What Kinds of Ionic Compounds Are In Herbs?

IONIC COMPOUNDS are not generally as common in organisms as molecules. This is because organisms are mostly water, and many ionic compounds fall apart in water; they dissolve into individual ions. Ionic compounds are not as common in your body as molecules, but they do make up some solid materials, such as bones and kidney stones. But most of the other solids in your body, like hair and fingernails and skin, are mostly made of molecules clumped together tightly. *Ionic compounds are also not as common in herbs as other types of chemicals. They are not often active ingredients in herbs.*

Insoluble ionic compounds can give herbs a gritty or even irritating texture when you touch or eat them. Some plants have needle-shaped calcium oxalate crystals. In *Dieffenbachia,* or "dumb cane," these crystals can even paralyze your vocal cords, making you temporarily unable to speak.

APPENDIX C
NONFATAL ATTRACTIONS:
Herbal Interactions with Receptors and Enzymes

Every cell in our bodies is awash in a constant stream of chemical signals. Some of these chemicals are homemade by your own body, and others are foreign, such as chemicals from an herb. Yet each of your cells only responds to some chemicals and ignores the rest. How does each cell pick which chemicals to respond to?

Chemicals from herbs often mediate effects on your cells by temporarily fitting into either *receptors* or *enzymes*. Like a key fitting into a lock, particular herbal chemicals can fit only into particular receptors or enzymes. They do this using the attractive version of the electrostatic force.

Receptors and enzymes are types of proteins. (To learn more about proteins in general, see Chemistry 101: If You Really Want to Know . . . More Details about Proteins, page 378.) These proteins have specific shapes, with pocketlike indentations that are analogous to a keyhole. When an herbal chemical fits into the keyhole, so to speak, these proteins in turn have an effect on your cells and on your body.

Receptors and enzymes both accept certain chemicals like locks accepting keys, but receptors function differently from enzymes. Receptors are like on/off switches for various actions in a cell. Each cell has an assortment of switches with different jobs. When a receptor switch encounters a chemical "key" that binds to it, the receptor inhibits or activates certain functions in the cell.

Enzymes, on the other hand, are found everywhere in your body, both associated with your cells and existing outside of them. Enzymes transform other chemicals. Our enzymes help us transform one molecule into a different one. When an herbal chemical binds to an enzyme, the herbal chemical may be transformed into a different one, too. Sometimes an herbal molecule prevents one of your enzymes from performing its usual transformation on another molecule.

The Bottom Line

Some herbal chemicals are attracted by the electrostatic force to particular receptors or enzymes and temporarily fit into them like a key fits into a lock. If an herbal chemical binds to a cell's receptor, it inhibits or activates functions in the cell. If an herbal chemical binds to an enzyme, it might get changed by the enzyme or affect the enzyme's ability to alter a different chemical.

HERBAL CHEMICALS CAN BIND TO YOUR CELL'S RECEPTORS, ACTING AS AGONISTS OR ANTAGONISTS

Receptors act as on or off switches for various jobs in a cell.

Receptors are proteins associated with cells, and different cells have different sorts of receptors. They function like on or off switches for various cellular actions. For example, insulin receptors turn on the ability to import the sugar glucose into your cells, when it binds to insulin. Other receptors turn on or off your cells' programs to grow and divide. Herbal chemicals often interact with your receptors, which in turn may have dramatic effects on your cells. For example, some herb-receptor interactions protect your cells from cancer. Others can kill the cell.

Many receptors sit right on the surface of the cell, so an herbal chemical encounters the receptor when it approaches the cell. External receptors are given the really obvious term *cell surface receptor.* Other receptors are inside the cell, so an herbal chemical has to penetrate the cell to interact with it, which can be extra difficult. These receptors are called *intracellular receptors.* Each of your cells has both cell surface receptors and intracellular receptors.

But how does an herbal molecule actually get these cellular switches to work? It might help to imagine a receptor protein as a three-dimensional lock, into which various chemical keys may or may not fit. Chemical keys that fit a receptor are called *ligands.* These keys fit into specialized pockets called *receptor sites,* where, based on the pocket's size, shape, and location of charged regions inside of it, a specific chemical will be electrostatically attracted to it and temporarily fit inside it. Receptors are picky about what fits inside their pockets. Not only is a physical fit required, as with actual keys, but charges within the receptor site must line up with opposite charges on the ligand. The discrimination of the receptor for binding only particular chemicals is called its *specificity.* Some receptors are more picky, or specific, than others.

When the proper fit is attained, the receptor protein changes its shape slightly in order to maximize electrostatic attractions. The receptor's deformation, in turn, nudges some *other* molecules into creating a biochemical effect. The effects are usually not permanent—the electrostatic attractions of the ligand-key for the receptor's active site are usually weak enough for the ligand to drift off on its own after a while. Sometimes

the cell even takes in the ligand and "eats" it—breaking it down into other chemicals.

Herbs that activate receptors are agonists.

Chemical keys that successfully get a receptor to respond to them are called *agonists.* Partial agonists initiate weak responses, while full agonists produce more pronounced effects on a cell. Partial agonists are found in many herbs. For example, soy, and red clover contain partial agonists for estrogen receptors, and they can block the more potent effects of this hormone by their temporary occupation of estrogen's binding site. If you are a woman suffering from menopausal symptoms, you are probably aware of the recent Women's Health Initiative studies that linked conventional hormone replacement therapy for menopausal women to heart disease, stroke, and some types of cancer. Shaken by these unexpected findings, scientists are seriously searching for safer, alternative estrogen receptor agonists, including ones from these herbs.

Full agonists are also found in many herbs. A striking example is that of the Mexican "divining" sage, *Salvia divinorum,* which has chemicals that cling to opium receptors in your brain. Fortunately, ordinary sage used in cooking does not have these chemicals, because they make you hallucinate.

Herbs that block receptors' activity are antagonists.

Have you ever inserted a key into a lock, only to have it fit but not turn in the lock? Some chemicals do the equivalent of this: Although they bind to a receptor, they can't get it to work. They also physically block the "right key," preventing the natural ligand from doing its job. This is a competitive *antagonist,* a chemical imposter obstructing the natural ligand. Noncompetitive antagonists also inhibit receptor functioning, but do so in a more roundabout way, without competing with the natural ligand for its binding site. Herbal receptor antagonists are extremely common.

You might even consume herbal receptor antagonists daily if you drink tea or coffee or eat chocolate. These plant-derived goodies contain chemicals that inhibit the adenosine receptor. Adenosine makes you sleepy. As you spend energy throughout the day, adenosine builds up in your body. Adenosine is a leftover piece of a larger chemical (adenosine triphosphate) that is degraded to give you energy. The more energy you spend, the more adenosine builds up in your brain. The binding of adenosine to its receptors in your brain causes your brain to slow down, making you groggy.

Early in human history, we stumbled across plants that contain adenosine look-alikes and treasured them. We now routinely use them to undermine this elegant connection between energy expenditure and tiredness. Coffee, tea, and chocolate are the most popular sources for adenosine impersonators, called *methylxanthines*. You are probably more familiar with the most renowned methylxanthine, caffeine, but *theophylline* and *theobromine* also occur in varying amounts in coffee, tea, and chocolate, and they work the same way. Methylxanthines are found in many other plants, too, like the South American herbs maté and guarana. Because methylxanthines resemble adenosine, they park inside your brains' adenosine's receptors, preventing adenosine from binding. When adenosine can't bind, it can't make you sleepy.

The effect of an herbal agonist or antagonist can be good or bad, depending on what function it affects and how much it affects it.

Is it *bad* to play with your receptors? Sometimes it helps. It really depends on which receptor and how much it is affected. The hallucinogenic divining sage doesn't seem like the brightest idea, especially if you are driving or working in a factory with lots of sharp blades whirling around. However, other plants that interact with the opium receptor in a more refined manner could act as useful pain relievers. The adenosine receptor antagonists from coffee, chocolate, and tea appear fairly harmless for humans (but not for pets; see the text box Your Pet Has Different Receptors and Enzymes, page 377). Our perhaps puritanical need to vilify such alluring substances has continuously been thwarted by years of research on these beloved comestibles. These studies show that although their methylxanthines can make you jittery and sleepless at worst, they are relatively benign and might even do good things, like decrease your risk of Parkinson's disease. Coffee, tea, and chocolate also contain beneficial plant antioxidants, so perhaps less guilt is required when you consume them. Overall, you should judge an herbal ligand by the receptor switch that it affects and how much it affects it.

THE BOTTOM LINE

AN HERBAL chemical can temporarily bind to a cell's receptor, which initiates or halts an activity in the cell. Chemicals that act on receptors are *agonists:* effective ones are *full agonists,* and weaker ones are *partial agonists.* Chemicals that block a receptor's action are *antagonists.* Whether the effect is beneficial or not depends on what receptor is being affected and how much it is being affected.

―――――――――――――

Herbal Chemicals Affect Your Enzymes, Too

Enzymes are like little machines that transform other chemicals.

Enzymes are proteins that can be found everywhere in your body, both inside cells and existing outside of them. Most enzyme names end in "-ase," by the way, so if you see a name ending in "-ase," you can bet it's an enzyme. Enzymes transform other chemicals but remain unchanged themselves. Thus, they are like tiny chemical-processing machines. A drill does not change when it drills a hole in something, so it can be used repeatedly. Likewise, the same enzyme can transform many chemicals of one type into chemicals of another type, one at a time, like a machine on an assembly line. And like machines on assembly lines, different enzymes have different tasks, each carrying out various chemical transformations. Sometimes herbal chemicals are worked on by these tiny machines and changed into something new. In other cases, herbal chemicals affect the machine's function, so to speak, either hampering or enhancing their ability to transform other chemicals.

But how do your enzymes work? Like receptors, enzymes have similar pockets, called *active sites,* which electrostatically attract chemicals with the right fit, again like a key fitting into a lock. While a *receptor's* keyhole accepts a *ligand,* an enzyme's keyhole accept its *substrate.* A substrate is a chemical that a particular enzyme works on, and it is common for herbal chemicals to become substrates for

an enzyme. But they won't be substrates for just any enzyme. Each enzyme only works on certain chemical substrates. Like receptors, enzymes are picky about what fits into their active sites. Just as some keyholes accept more than one type of key, some enzymes are more picky, or *specific,* than others.

A substrate clinging to an enzyme's active site may feel its parts tugged one way or the other because of electrostatic forces, and this can break pieces off the substrate, turning it into something new. For example, the enzymes of gut bacteria commonly cleave sugar molecules off of herbal molecules, so the bacteria can consume the sugar, and the leftover piece of the herbal molecule typically gets absorbed into the blood, where it could act as a drug.

Sometimes an enzyme introduces its substrates to other chemicals that it is also hanging on to, and the two newly introduced chemicals bond together, again forming something new. For instance, herbal molecules that pass through the liver often are introduced to sulfate, or to a sugar called *glucuronate,* by liver enzymes, and the herbal molecule and the sulfate or glucuronate are then bonded together. This creates a larger molecule called an herbal *conjugate,* which is more water soluble and more easily excreted through the urine.

Enzymes both break down large chemicals into smaller ones and join smaller ones to make bigger ones. Sometimes they just rearrange the parts on one chemical, unhooking parts and rejoining them in different ways to make a new, rearranged thing. For example, one plant enzyme (*lycopene beta-cyclase*) can take the red tomato pigment lycopene, a chain-shaped molecule, and loop the chain around to form a couple of rings, creating the orange carrot pigment beta-carotene, without adding or subtracting any parts from lycopene.

Enzymes are responsible for most of your body's alteration of chemicals.

Many people think of enzymes as simply things that aid digestion, breaking large food chemicals into smaller, more digestible ones. But you should not underestimate all that enzymes do in your body. Enzymes do a whole lot more than help you digest your dinner. They carry out most of your body's chemical transformations.

Some enzyme-affecting herbs make headaches and fevers go away. Others prevent blood clots. A few herbs act like the popular prescription statin drugs, hindering an enzyme that makes cholesterol. Some inhibit bacterial enzymes from chewing their way into your tissues. Others stimulate liver cells' enzymes to make protein and regenerate. And a few herbs, in excess, can inhibit nerve cell-associated enzymes to paralyze your muscles and kill you. Ultimately, herbs that influence enzymes can do a whole lot more than modulate your digestion.

Some herbal chemicals must first get changed by your enzymes in order to work.

Herbal chemicals frequently get altered by enzymes, and this alters their functions. Sometimes an herbal chemical requires an enzyme to turn them into a working product. For example, many herbs contain *glycosides,* chemicals that have sugars bonded to them (and their names sometimes end in "-oside," but not always). Some glycosides just don't work unless your gut's bacterial enzymes (*glycosidases*) remove their sugar appendages to release the effective, sugar-free chemical. For example, sennosides are glycosides from the herb senna and are now quite popular in over-the-counter laxatives. But sennosides don't work as laxatives as well as their sugar-free versions, so you have to count on your intestinal enzymes to chop off the sugar to activate them.

Other herbal chemicals are disabled by your enzymes.

Other herbal chemicals suffer disablement after enzymatic tinkering. The active ingredients from papaya and pineapple aid digestion, because they are actually enzymes that help break down your food. However, they don't last long, as they are quickly broken down into less useful forms by your own digestive enzymes.

Herbal chemicals often work by inhibiting the action of one of your enzymes.

Herbs frequently work by hindering enzymes. Herbal chemicals can do this by sitting inside an enzyme's active site, but they remain unaffected by enzyme's business end. Like a wrench inside the machine, the chemical blocks the enzyme from working on its substrate. This type of interaction is called *competitive inhibition.* On the other hand, sometimes an herb will bind *outside* an enzyme's active site, and though it doesn't block the business end, it can still hamper the enzyme. For example, it is difficult to operate a drill while wearing big, clunky gloves, even though there's nothing blocking the drill bit. This type of interaction is called *noncompetitive inhibition.* Sometimes herbal molecules affect an enzyme in a roundabout way without even touching it. They get another molecule to do the job. In some cases, an herbal molecule can even make an enzyme more active.

Some of the Best-Known Herb-Enzyme Interactions Are COX Inhibition

MANY HERBS possess chemicals that inhibit the *cyclooxygenase* enzyme, called *COX,* for short. There are different versions of the COX enzyme, and different herbs vary by which kind of COX enzyme they affect. But inhibiting COX enzymes is just what aspirin does, so you can expect these herbs act like aspirin. In fact, you can thank herbal medicine for aspirin.

As early as the fifth century BC, the Greek Hippocrates asked his patients to chew willow bark to reduce their pain and fever. It might have had some success, because willow bark remains popular in herbal medicine to this day. Willow bark was the original source for salicylic acid, which in the late 1800s was synthetically modified to become aspirin, *acetyl*salicylic acid, which is less irritating than the herbal chemical. Your body actually converts some aspirin back into the original herbal chemical, salicylic acid, using an enzyme (esterase enzymes). Both aspirin and the herbal salicylic acid inhibit COX.

That aspirin was made from willow bark may explain why willow is the most touted producer of aspirin-like chemicals that are collectively called *salicylates.* The other most commonly noted salicylate-containing herbs are birch bark and wintergreen. But salicylates are abundant in the plant kingdom. Most herbs, including these, have salicylate concentrations too low to represent a regular aspirin pill, unless you drink an inordinate amount of their tea. On the other hand, these herbs' oils, such as wintergreen oil—

its distinctive skin-soluble ingredient provides the characteristic minty smell of some pain-relieving muscle rubs—have salicylate concentrations that are so high that if you drank it, you would experience a crisis very similar to aspirin overdose. But hindering the COX enzyme in a more limited way seems beneficial, and both aspirin and herbal salicylates do it.

Not all forms of the COX enzyme are bad, but some COX enzymes (COX-2 enzymes) are better at creating pain-enhancing, inflammatory chemicals. Herbs that block COX hamper their creation, preventing pain and inflammation. Other versions of the COX enzyme (COX-1 enzymes) make more beneficial prostaglandins, which protect your stomach from its own acid. Not surprisingly, like aspirin, these herbs can upset your stomach.

If you can stomach them, COX inhibitors seem to be a good deal, because they apparently hinder the production of inflammatory chemicals that might ultimately lead to cancer. Also, COX enzymes can create chemicals that make your blood clot, which is good if you are bleeding but bad if the clot lodges in your heart or brain's blood vessels, creating a heart attack or stroke. Trace amounts of salicylates found in plants may, in part, explain why consuming lots of fruits and vegetables protects you from stroke, cancer, and heart disease, as does aspirin. Some health writers are even effusively calling plant salicylates "vitamin S," which sounds a tad exalted but gets our collective mothers' point across: Eating more fruits and vegetables is good for you.

Some herbal chemicals *induce* some of your enzymes, causing you to make more of those enzymes.

Some herbal chemicals cause more of one of your enzymes to be made, and that enzyme is then said to have been *induced* by the herbal chemical. If you have more machines that do a particular job, that job will be done more often. And if you induce an enzyme, you make more of it, and you can be sure that enzyme's job will be accomplished more frequently.

St. John's wort, an herb used for depression, induces production of a liver enzyme that prematurely degrades hormonal contraceptives. It is not yet clear if St. John's wort relieves depression, but it does upgrade production of this enzyme. Women who take birth control should be aware that St. John's wort could subvert their contraceptive efforts.

More favorably, many herbs induce the manufacture of detoxifying enzymes—that is, enzymes that have a knack for converting bad-for-you molecules into more benign ones. Ellagic acid, found in high concentrations in strawberries, grape skins, and grape seeds, causes more production of the detoxifying enzyme *glutathione S-transferase.* Some of garlic's stinkier components induce this enzyme, too, as well as other toxin-disarming enzymes, *glutathione peroxidase* and *quinone reductase.* All of these enzymes are immediately recognized by biochemists for their power to disable damaging and carcinogenic molecules.

A lot of plants induce our helpful enzymes, which is yet another good reason to eat fruits and vegetables. But how do plants do this? In some cases, plants' trace amounts of toxic secondary metabolites induce our cells' defensive enzymes. So, while it may be paradoxical, we should thank plants for containing small amounts of toxins, because these toxins stimulate production of our detoxifying enzymes.

THE BOTTOM LINE

ENZYMES ARE proteins that, like little machines, change one chemical into a different one, and they remain unchanged themselves. Each type of enzyme performs a different sort of chemical transformation. Like a lock accepting a key, an enzyme only accepts certain things to work on, which are called its *substrates.* Some herbal chemicals must get changed by our enzymes in order to work. Other herbal chemicals are inactivated by our enzymes. Many herbal chemicals work by inhibiting one of our enzymes. Herbal chemicals often induce one of our enzymes. This means that the production of that enzyme is enhanced and that enzyme will be more active.

Your Pet Has Different Receptors and Enzymes

PEOPLE WITH pets may have noticed that more and more vets are advertising that they can provide alternative, herbal treatments for animals. If you love your pet, you should be aware that animals have different enzymes and receptors than humans do, so they will respond differently to herbal medicine. A helpful, harmless herb for a person might do real damage to an animal. Not all herbs for pets are bad, but you can't assume that something that is good for you is good for your pet. If you have a dog, for example, be sure that the herb you are interested in giving him was tested in dogs, and that its effect is well-known in dogs rather than in some other species. Ask your vet if she is aware of such studies on your species of pet. Some vets are really up-to-date on this subject, but others are just "going with the flow," so you might want a second opinion.

Herbal treatments traditionally used by humans are now enthusiastically recommended for our animal companions without much forethought. Several "natural" pet food lines even include herbs. But animal receptors and enzymes are not always shaped like ours, and they do not respond in the same way to the same herbs. Sometimes one animal species possesses a receptor that another species lacks. For example, you can only look upon your catnip-intoxicated cat with amusement, and perhaps envy, because you do not have the receptor that binds catnip's active ingredient. Disparities in our receptors and enzymes means that animal research will always provide us with an inexact estimate of how a chemical behaves in humans.

Garlic's inclusion in several lines of pet food has recently sparked a lot of unresolved debate. Garlic's best-documented effect on humans is its blood-thinning effect, because it inhibits an enzyme that causes your blood platelets to stick together in a clot. But garlic and the related onion do strange things to cats' and dogs' blood cells if the animal eats enough of these plants. It causes a type of anemia that can even kill the animal. The pet food companies claim their garlic ingredient is present in such small amounts that it does no harm and still provides benefits. This could be true, but the point is debatable, so some people buy garlic-free versions of pet food.

Chocolate, coffee, and tea are plants that block your adenosine receptor, preventing adenosine from making you sleepy. Blocking the adenosine receptor in this way is relatively harmless to humans, but it can be toxic for cats, dogs, rodents, and even birds. While the theobromine in these plants makes humans feel pleasantly awake, it can cause vomiting, seizures, coma, and death in animals. Unless valid research indicates that an herb is safe for your species of pet, you should be wary of gambling your pet's health on it.

THE BOTTOM LINE

HERBAL MEDICINE for pets has exploded in popularity, but pets have different receptors and enzymes than we do, so they will respond differently to the same herbs. If you really want to give your pet herbs, talk to a vet who is well versed in studies of that herb in your species of pet.

CHEMISTRY 101: IF YOU REALLY WANT TO KNOW . . . MORE DETAILS ABOUT PROTEINS

Proteins are chains of amino acids folded up into a functional shape.

Proteins are molecules that are made of chains of smaller molecules called *amino acids,* bonded and strung together like beads on a string. Since twenty different amino acids are used to make proteins, you can imagine the resultant *polypeptide* string as a strand of hundreds of beads strung together, with twenty different types of "beads" strung in a specific sequence that is unique to each protein. This strand folds into a particular shape required for the proteins' function.

A Gene Holds the Instructions For Making a Particular Protein

EACH GENE carries information of what the amino acid sequence is for one protein. The information on how to make a particular protein passively rests in a different structure in a cell, called a *gene.* A multitude of different genes, each with instructions on how to make different proteins, lie in strips as part of a larger molecule, DNA. The purpose of a specific gene is to give information about what the sequence of amino acids is for a protein, so different genes determine which "beads" get strung together in which order to make a certain protein. If you were to point randomly to a strip of DNA that harbored a gene, you would be pointing to the cell's instructions for making one particular protein. Each gene has instructions for how to make a different protein. Different cells "read" different gene instructions, and that is why you have different cell types—they make different proteins. The cell reads the gene's instructions using enzymes that zip along the DNA strip, making the equivalent of photocopies of the information in the form of RNA molecules, which are carried off to another part of the cell for the protein's construction to commence. So if you have a genetic disorder, you have a gene with faulty instructions on how to make one of your proteins. The disease is caused by the dysfunction of the incorrectly constructed protein that the faulty gene codes for. (This is a bit oversimplified—for example, many genes cooperate to make products that may get paired down, but eventually unite to become the final protein product—but the general theme is true.) Some herbal molecules can influence this protein-making process by influencing the enzymes that read various genes. This can result in either increased or decreased construction of particular proteins.

The amino acids' attractions for each other cause the protein to fold up into the shape required for its activity.

However, even with the correct sequence of amino acids, a polypeptide string is not technically a protein and will not function properly in your body unless it has the right *shape.* The beads, or amino acids, have different degrees of electrostatic attraction for each other, depending whether they are polar amino acids or nonpolar ones. If you had a necklace with sticky beads, the necklace would fold up into a clump. For proteins, the shape of this clump is not random. A polypeptide chain has to fold up into its characteristic shape in order to be a functioning protein. The locations of the beads on the string and their varying degrees of stickiness for each other help the string fold up into the correct shape.

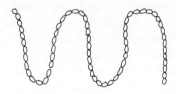

polypeptide chain

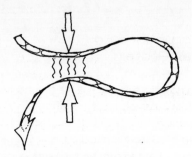

The chain folds because of differing attractions in it.

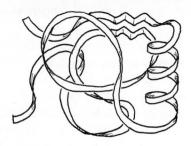

A polypeptide chain made of a chain of amino acids folds up into a protein with a specific shape because of the varying attractions of different amino acids for each other. The protein must have the right shape to function.

Proteins do many different things.

Proteins have many diverse functions. Some proteins are, like bricks and mortar, just structural building materials. These proteins don't do much except create walls and channels and other cellular architecture. For example, collagen proteins are tough fibers, and like "rebar" in concrete, they give your tissues strength. Elastin proteins are spongy proteins with flexible chains, and like little rubber bands, they give your tissues the ability to spring back into place.

Other proteins use energy to move. Actin and myosin are protein filaments in muscle cells that slide along one another, causing your muscles to contract. Some proteins tote other chemicals around, like hemoglobin in red blood cells, which transports oxygen through your blood.

Still other proteins, called *antibodies,* protect you from microscopic strangers and oddballs, like bacteria, viruses, and cancer cells. A fancier term for antibody is *immunoglobulin,* but they are the same thing. These proteins have probing ends that ideally electrostatically bind to strange and potentially dangerous things, and less ideally, they can attack your body in cases of friendly fire known as *autoimmune diseases.*

Enzymes are proteins that modify other chemicals. They are unchanged themselves during this process, so you can view them as tiny factories designed to electrostatically bind certain ingredients, which they turn into something new. You may be most familiar with digestive enzymes, which break down large food chemicals into smaller, more digestible ones in your digestive tract, but these are only a small subset of your enzymes. All cells contain enzymes, too, and enzymes do a lot more than just digest food. Enzymes perform almost all of the chemical transformations taking place in your body.

Receptor proteins also electrostatically bind chemicals, but unlike enzymes, they do not usually change the chemicals they bind. A receptor accepts a chemical like a lock accepts a key, and this binding is like a switch that turns various functions in a cell on or off.

Herbs have proteins, and herbs affect your own proteins, too.

Herbs certainly have proteins, but your digestive tract is not kind to proteins and rips them up into isolated amino acids. Thus, you should not expect an herbal protein to have an effect beyond your digestive tract should you eat it. Herbal chemicals can, on the other hand, affect your own proteins dramatically.

THE BOTTOM LINE

A PROTEIN is made of a strand of smaller molecules called *amino acids.* The strand folds up into a characteristic shape necessary for protein to work. Some proteins are just building materials, and others create movement or move other things around. Some disable disease-causing organisms. Enzymes are reusable proteins that change other chemicals. Receptors proteins are like on or off switches for various functions in cells. Herbal proteins are broken into amino acids if they go through your digestive tract. On the other hand, herbs can influence your own proteins.

APPENDIX D
PREVENTIVE MEDICINE: PROTECT AGAINST *WHAT?*
Carcinogens, Free Radicals, Oxidizing Agents, and Inflammation

It helps to understand how your enemies work. You hear the popular health media endlessly discussing benefits of herbal "antioxidants," which protect against oxygen-derived toxins, and "free radical scavengers," which neutralize other harmful types of toxins. In order to best understand how these interesting herbal molecules work, you must first understand the enemy. Doing so better enables you to live a preventive lifestyle, a way of living your life that minimizes the opportunity for health problems to arise.

Obviously it is less painful and costly for you to prevent cancer than to heal it. Thanks to various popular holistic health gurus in the 1970s and '80s, disease prevention has finally caught on in mainstream medicine, too. The only problem with preventive medicine is that it is difficult to tell if it is working on an individual basis. You might get a hint from reading large clinical trial data that coffee drinkers get Parkinson's disease less often, for example, and smokers certainly get more lung cancer. Thanks to increasing focus on preventive medicine, there are more and more large, long-term clinical studies testing herbs for their protective effects, and their details are outlined in Evidence of Action sections at the end of each herb chapter. The mechanisms of protection are also discussed in detail in each herb chapter's How Scientists Think It Works.

For just one person, all you can do is try something based on quality data and hope

it's working. If you are lucky you might feel better or have a problem resolved, but there is still no way to know if the two events were related. That you can't tell whether or not it's working is no reason not to try it, though!

After suggesting to a friend concerned about prostate cancer that he eat more plant pigments, I joked, "Now be sure to tell me when you *don't* get prostate cancer." Although it is troublesome to detect what is going on with a sample size of one person, practicing preventive medicine gives you the satisfaction of general good health and the knowledge that you are doing everything you can for yourself. A good way to get started is to understand the workings of major health enemies—carcinogens, free radicals, oxidizing agents, and inflammation. In addition to these natural enemies, we can unknowingly be our own worst enemy, fooling ourselves with misinformation. Thus understanding how to discern quality information in the health world is also part of preventive medicine.

Carcinogens

Cancer requires two events: initiation and then promotion. A chemical that causes either initiation or promotion can act as a carcinogen, a molecule that can cause cancer. Some herbal molecules can prevent cancer by thwarting either mechanism, but there are plant molecules that cause cancer, too.

Initiation damages a cell's genes, resulting in a dysfunctional protein. Initiation involves changes in the genes of a normal cell, and these sorts of accidents happen all the time, every day, and are almost always repaired by enzymes, which can detect these changes. Most genetic changes, called *mutations,* do not produce cancer. Mutations either have no effect or end up killing the cell, which is really no big deal and is usually for the best. Cells die all the time, and it is often good that they do. It is when cells do not die and instead reproduce uncontrollably that they form a clump of mutant cancer cells, called a *tumor.*

A gene carries coded instructions that passively tell the cell how to make a specific protein, designating which unique sequence of smaller building-block molecules, called *amino acids,* should be strung together, to form the protein. It's sort of like a blueprint in a book in a library, and the library is DNA, a molecule with massive collections of different genes in it. A gene's instructions may or may not get "read" by the cell, but when it does, copies of the instructions—sort of like a photocopy of the blueprint in molecular forms—leave the DNA to make themselves available to protein-making machinery in the cell. A particular protein is made with the help of the genes' instructions, which remain in place in the DNA to be read again and again.

The instructions for making a protein simply outline the proper sequence of amino acid building blocks that ought to be strung together into a chain, which becomes the protein. It's like instructions for making a necklace with twenty possible different beads, because there are about twenty different amino acids that can be linked into chains to make proteins. Because different types of amino acids tend to interact with each other in different ways, using electrostatic forces, the types of amino acids used and their sequence determine how this chain folds up to become an active, three-dimensional protein.

Most gene mutations are harmless. The trouble tends to arise if the gene codes for a protein involved in cell division or growth. If a gene carrying the blueprint for a protein concerned with cell growth or division is mutated, an unsuitable amino acid might be substituted for the right one, or some may be omitted, and then problems can arise with the protein's structure and function. Cancer can occur when the error resides in a protein concerned with cell growth or division. There are many such proteins. Some turn on cell reproduction, and some turn it off.

A mutated gene that does cause cancer is called an *oncogene.* Actually there is good evidence that it typically takes as many as five or six separate DNA mutations in one cell to create a cancer cell. While cancer can occur at any age, many forms of cancer are age-related, since it takes time for these errors to accumulate. Some people have a genetic predisposition to cancer, because they have inherited one oncogene already.

Natural and synthetic molecules alike can cause initiation events. Carcinogens that alter genes are sometimes called *mutagens* or *genotoxins.* Some carcinogens are synthetic, but there are also plenty from nature, including herbs, as well. Some work by sticking irreversibly to DNA, the molecule that contains genes, causing errors to be made when the gene is copied, or "read," to make a protein. Also, high-energy light particles, photons, can act like minuscule bullets, barreling through a cell and damaging a strand of DNA. Ultraviolet light from the sun—or any other source for that matter, including tanning booths, despite what their proprietors tell you—causes skin cancer, because it barrages your cells with high-energy photons.

In some cancers, a protein that normally turns on cell division might be faulty if its gene blueprint gets mutated, remaining stuck in the "on" position, so to speak. In other cases, a mutation might code for an incompetent growth-halting protein, which is unable to turn cell division off. Not only are there different types of cancer, based on what type of cell is growing awry, such as breast, colon, or lung, there are also different *mechanisms* that can cause one type of cell to divide continuously, so there are several different types of breast cancer, for example. This is why claims to "cure cancer"—that is, *all* cancers—reek of shadiness. That a potential cure for *some* forms of cancer exists is far more persuasive.

Initiation does not mean you will get cancer. It's just step one. Either unrestrained growth-promoting proteins or impotent growth-stopping proteins can lead to cancer, but they also might not. Initiation alone does not create cancer. Your body's DNA-repairing enzymes, like shrewd car buyers, recognize genes that are lemons and repair them. Sometimes they initiate processes that cause the cell to destruct in the neat, helpful manner termed *apoptosis.* It is rare for a mutation to go unrepaired. Your immune cells not only incapacitate foreign enemy cells but these domestic traitors as well, and this happens every day.

Doctors do not like to alarm people unnecessarily, so they do not tell you that you probably have all sorts of mutant cells, and so do I. Most people do. It is most likely, though, that these cells will never develop into actual "cancer." If a cancer cell can escape attack from our immune systems, it still requires promotion to become a tumor.

Step 2 is promotion. Some herbs and synthetic molecules stimulate this, too.

After initiation takes place, the mutant gene may sit unused and unrepaired in the cancer cell—for years, even—until an event stimulates the cell to divide. The progeny cells inherit its oncogenes and continue their own inappropriate divisions. This can be stimulated by outside factors, too. This is promotion. Some carcinogens cause initiation and mutate your DNA. Others cause promotion, stimulating the mutated cells to divide. Sex hormones like estrogen stimulate cell division; so taking estrogen increases the risk of breast cancer. Some herb molecules, too, stimulate cell division and can act as promoters. Herbs that act like estrogen worry doctors, because there is a chance they could do this, too.

Promoters are not immediately considered to be carcinogens; in tests it typically requires long term, repeated, high doses for a promoter to cause cancer, probably because it first requires the presence of an initiated cell. Not all cell-growth stimulators are necessarily bad, depending on how they are used; some accelerate wound repair, for example. Allantoin, found in comfrey, stimulates cell growth, and it its pure form is commonly used topically in skin preparations. Comfrey also contains DNA-damaging molecules called *pyrrolizidine alkaloids,* which can act as initiators, so along with the cell-division promoter allantoin, it is not surprising that when taken internally, comfrey causes liver cancer.

Step 3, metastasis, may or may not occur. But again, this can be provoked by either herbs or by synthetic molecules. There is a possible third stage in cancer, metastasis, where a cancer cell breaks free from the primary tumor and travels to another site, where it divides to create another colony of cancer cells, another tumor. *Benign* cancer cells do not do this; their tumors can be removed cleanly. Those cancer cells brandishing enzymes that are needed to chew through adjacent tissue can enter blood vessels and spread, and are *malignant*. Metastases make cancer especially difficult to treat.

Don't panic. There are many herbs, synthetic molecules, and other treatments that can stop all these events, too. Poisons that kill rapidly growing cells are the classic chemotherapy drugs used to target cancer cells. They often work by fouling up some mechanism of cell division, like the duplication of DNA prior to division. Some of these poisons have been isolated from plants. *Vincristine* and *vinblastine,* from the toxic periwinkle plant, bind to a cell protein called *tubulin,* preventing the tubulin from assembling intro structures required to organize chromosomes prior to cell division. In expert hands, these plant-derived poisons are carefully used to treat some leukemias, Hodgkin's and non-Hodgkin's lymphoma. They should never be used without expertise, because after all, they are poisons.

Radiation also kills rapidly growing cells, penetrating cells like sub-microscopic buckshot that attacks DNA with high-energy light particles. Unfortunately, chemotherapy and radiation both kill innocent, rapidly growing cells, like gut, hair, skin, and blood cells, creating nasty side effects like nausea, hair loss, and weakened immunity. If the side effects can be endured, these therapies can work to bring about remission of the cancer. New chemotherapeutics, like those that prevent tumors from recruiting their own blood supply, or ones that program our immune systems to attack the cancer, are emerging as exciting alternatives to traditional chemotherapy and radiation.

Many herb molecules prevent cancer by neutralizing genotoxins, and initiation is apprehended. Others can slow cell growth, preventing existing tumors from getting any bigger. Some herbs provoke the immune system into killing cancer cells. Toxins in small amounts in some plants stimulate the production of DNA repair and other anti-cancer enzymes. Anti-inflammatory herbs may help, because inflammation is a process known to weaken tissues and facilitate the spread of metastases. Because cancer is a complicated, multistep process, some herb molecules that affect these steps can cause cancer, but other herb molecules have the potential to prevent and cure cancer.

Free Radicals

Free radicals are chemicals with an unpaired electron. That electrons are negatively charged, and thus repel each other, yet tend to pair up in twos is a peculiar aspect of nature.

But first, what is an electron? Electrons are one of three ingredients that compose atoms. (The others are protons and neutrons. For a more complete description of atoms, see page 365.)

Electrons tend to appear in twos on a molecule. They either comprise a bond or exist as "nonbonding" electron pairs. Atoms are the building blocks of molecules. Sometimes two electrons are shared between two atoms, being attracted to the positive protons of both atoms at once, and this sharing creates the bonds between atoms that hold a molecule intact. Even though the like-charged positive protons of both atoms' nuclei repel, they are tied together by the two electrons like two dogs fighting over a bone. Every bond is made of two electrons, so we see that electrons form pairs in bonds.

Other electrons are not involved in this sharing and are called *nonbonding electrons,* which simply hang out on particular atoms

WHY WOULD ELECTRONS PAIR ANYWAY, IF THEY REPEL EACH OTHER? I have confounded this discussion by telling you that electrons are negative, but risked it because it is such a fundamentally important property of electrons. Negative does repel negative, according to the electrostatic law. Although electrons repel each other, they can "pair," which really means they share the same energy level. Energy levels are allotted rather strictly to particles that are small, compared to things that are large. In order to share the same energy level, electrons do have to physically get closer to each other, and this does increase the repulsion they feel for each other. If this repulsion is less than the attraction that both electrons feel for the protons in a nearby atom, however, they will pair and will be more stable in doing so. Yes, two electrons that repel each other are sometimes more stable when they pair up. Nature is indeed weird—and it gets weirder.

The explanation for this pairing lies in viewing electrons as being waves rather than particles. It turns out that *all* particles, not just electrons, can be described as waves. So all the particles in your body are also waves. We can represent this situation more abstractly with math. (If you are frustrated in trying to picture matter as being made of waves, don't feel bad. Most scientists don't try to visualize this situation. While such abstractions may not be very satisfying, we know that the math, on paper, works.) Equations called *wavefunctions* are used to represent particles, and since these equations predict nature's behavior quite well, we believe they are true. A wave is something that oscillates, alternates, or, well, *waves,* over a period of time. You can wave you hand up and down over time, and that is a wave. If you increase the speed, you are increasing the energy of your wave. The wavefunction of a particle allows you to predict where the particle is most likely to be found around an atom, assuming it has a particular energy. If you do not have a lot of energy, you are more likely to be in bed, for example. If an electron has less energy, it is more likely to be in its "ground state," closer to the nucleus of the atom. Higher energy electrons are more likely to be in outer regions of the atom. (They have to spend more energy remaining away from the attractive positive nucleus. Their location is like expensive real estate, and sometimes the outermost electrons get fed up, so to speak, and leave, or get shared with another atom, forming a bond.)

Waves have different energies. The smaller a particle, the more its wave energies become restricted to specific values, while other energies simply are, oddly, mathematically "forbidden." This causes very small particles to behave in ways that seem bizarre to us. For example, when they change from one mathematically permitted energy level to another, they are first in one place and then instantaneously reappear in another place, an event called a *quantum leap.* The only reason this seems strange to us is because we are so massive that the energy levels accessible to us are so close in value that we perceive no gaps between them.

This constraint upon very small particles to particular energy levels also limits them to particular regions in space. The restriction of properties associated with an electron's wave is what forces two electrons to pair up around an atom. This may not be entirely satisfactory to you, but it is the best I can do without getting into hairier quantum mechanics. Sometimes, it is unstable for a single electron to go unpaired, and any chemical possessing an unpaired electron is called a *free radical.*

in the molecule. These, too, occur in pairs, so are sometimes called *nonbonding pairs* or *lone pairs.* So, although electrons really repel each other, we still find them engaged in this remarkable pairing behavior. When a single electron occurs, it cannot pair, and this creates a free radical.

A free radical can be an atom, a molecule, or an ion, but along with its normal paired electrons, it must also have a single, unpaired electron. A free radical could be either an individual atom, the building block of molecules, or it could be a molecule, which is simply a bunch of atoms held together by bonds. It could also be an *ion,* which is either an atom or molecule with excess or missing electrons; so, unlike atoms, ions always have a charge of some sort. Atoms, molecules, or ions can have unpaired electrons, and when they do they are called *free radicals,* or just *radicals.* The adjective "free" is unnecessary but has become habitual, perhaps because it adds drama. The unpaired electron is sometimes represented in chemical drawings as a single, isolated dot on a chemical. For example, molecular oxygen, which is two oxygen atoms bonded together (O_2), can gain an extra electron to become the noxious free radical called *superoxide* (O_2-). (The added negative sign indicates it gained one unit of negative charge.)

One free radical that is unstable can damage many of your molecules in chain reactions. The bottom line of all this is that free radicals are chemicals with unpaired, single electrons, and many are unstable. The unstable ones are those that you want to watch out for. What is so bad about being unstable? You are more likely to worry about an unstable neighbor than a stable one. Unstable chemicals are scary, too. The stable chemicals really don't do much, like sub-microscopic couch potatoes,

they are long-lived, and we say they are "low energy." It is the high-energy, unstable molecules that are short-lived and do damage in the process of their becoming stable. You can be assured that they *will* become more stable, because everything in nature tends to attain the lowest energy state possible. It's one of nature's rules.

Here is how free radicals cause damage: A free radical can become more stable by kidnapping an electron from another nearby chemical and pairing the stolen electron with its unpaired one. The chemical victim of this kidnapping is now lacking one electron, so *it* becomes a free radical, in turn. It then may steal another electron, creating yet another free radical, and so on. This is called a *free radical chain reaction.* All of these victimized chemicals get altered, and when chemicals get altered, they do not function properly. So a free radical chain reaction damages many molecules. Free radicals in your body can damage DNA or proteins, possibly initiating cancer. Free radicals, in general, accelerate aging and disease.

One way to stop the chain reaction is for two free radicals to unite, and their unpaired electrons become a bond between two parts of a new molecule. (Remember that a bond is made out of two electrons shared between two atoms.) This is called *chain termination.* It is unlikely that unstable free radicals will join, because such free radicals are short-lived, which decreases the probability that they will run into one another. Unlike most reactions, which typically involve one or two molecules, a chain reaction can alter thousands of molecules, depending on the reaction. Any time one biological molecule is altered it may not function properly, and thus just one free radical can wreck many molecules. Free radicals created from chlorofluorocarbons in the upper atmosphere destroy ozone in this sort of runaway chain reaction; so one free radical can do a lot of damage. However, some free radicals are fairly stable and less harmful than others.

The more stable free radicals are helpful. For example, sulfur atoms in molecules can maintain an unpaired electron better than other atoms, so they tend to form more stable radicals. Sulfur can use its unpaired electron to "scavenge" the unpaired electron of a more damaging free radical. Also, sulfur can donate a hydrogen atom with an unpaired electron to a free radical to "quench" the free radical, and in this process sulfur becomes a free radical, but a more stable one. The unpaired electron of a sulfur radical can also simply join the unstable, damaging radical's electron, to form a stable bond, because bonds are made of two, paired electrons. All living cells synthesize sulfur-containing molecules that neutralize free radicals. Some plants, like garlic, contain many interesting sulfur-containing molecules that eliminate the more damaging free radicals. Other, non-sulfur-based herbal molecules do the same thing—flavonoids are famous for it.

Can you eat a lot of free radical scavengers and live longer? There could be a problem with having too many free radical scavengers around, as well as too many antioxidants. Since the free radical scavengers themselves often become radicals (although more stable ones) while quenching the unstable ones, having too many of them around could theoretically hurt. Mother Nature continuously teaches us that an inordinate amount of any one thing can hurt, because she maintains life through the balance of opposing forces, just as we struggle to maintain political stability through opposing parties. But this principle can help your wallet, at least, since it frustrates supplement sellers' attempts to sell you large amounts of expensive products. Although

taking large doses of *supplements* hasn't produced too many remarkable clinical outcomes, taking more in the form of fruits and vegetables does. Not only will eating more fruits and vegetables please your mother, but also less cancer and disease is seen in general for those who do, and this is attributed to the radical-scavenging activities of plant molecules in general.

It makes sense that many plants contain armories of free radical–neutralizing molecules, because plants must withstand solar radiation, being solar-powered organisms. Radiation, the sub-microscopic bullets of light particles from the sun, can knock electrons off of atoms, unpairing them. So sunlight and other forms of radiation create free radicals. Smoke from cigarettes or any other burning items contains free radicals. Inflammation, where the immune system causes damage, generates free radicals, too. Another generator of free radicals that both plants and animals protect themselves against is oxygen. The oxygen we need to stay alive is, unfortunately, a free radical.

OXYGEN AND OTHER OXIDIZING AGENTS

You need oxygen, but it hurts you, too. Most school kids learn that blood delivers oxygen from the lungs to the rest of the body and that oxygen is required for life. Most people don't know *why* it is needed but mistakenly believe that oxygen is somehow intrinsically good. Indeed, many health fads capitalize on this misconception by trying to sell you oxygen as if you could not breathe it already. Because wares designed to increase oxygen are peddled as health aids, we receive the idea that oxygen does something nebulously *good*. As a matter of fact, oxygen is very toxic and corrosive, and you

QUESTIONABLE FOLKS HAVE CASHED IN ON OUR OXYGEN ADULATION. You can shell out a lot of money for "oxygenated water," which is great if you are a fish. All water exposed to air is oxygenated anyway; otherwise, fish could not breathe in it. Oxygen from the air dissolves down into water naturally. The oxygen you obtain from breathing is significantly in excess of what you could possibly derive, if any, from drinking even superoxygenated water. Assuming you could absorb the oxygen dissolved in super-oxygenated water through your digestive tract, which is iffy, you would have to drink an extraordinary amount of this expensive water to match the amount of oxygen you get from one breath.

Many claims for oxygenated water and special waters violate so many fundamental laws of chemistry they make you dizzy. Several of the companies making these claims have been fined by the FTC yet continue selling oxygenated water, boasting supportive clinical trials, which they never release for anyone to actually read. One company, for example, claims to have even *shrunk* the water molecules in their product to make room for more oxygen! No scientist has ever shrunk a molecule. All water molecules are identical and have the same size. If you change a molecule, the process is called a *reaction,* and it is not the same molecule anymore. Unless you have gills, do not give oxygenated water a second glance.

Magnet sellers argue that their magnets attract the iron in the blood and thus bring oxygen-bearing blood to the magnetized body area. But there are many different forms of iron. The iron in blood is actually of a sort that is never capable of being attracted to a magnet, so this claim is utterly false. Magnetic iron requires that many iron atoms be crammed together into a clump, and also requires that each iron atom in the clump has unpaired electrons all spinning in the same direction, which cooperatively create a magnetic field. A hemoglobin molecule has four distantly spaced iron atoms (or more properly, *ions,* because each is missing two electrons and thus has a positive charge). They are so far apart that they cannot create a magnetic field. If you happened to be bleeding from a cut and were near a magnet, your blood would not be attracted to the magnet.

"Oxygen bars" are so-called health establishments where you can pay to stick tubes up your nose and have oxygen piped through, often accompanied by your favorite scent. Unless you are a whale or a dolphin, mammals such as ourselves do not store oxygen well, so there are no positive long-term benefits; breathing pure oxygen beforehand can't prevent you from getting suffocated later, and it could even do real damage, such as cell death and tissue injury.

Pressurized oxygen therapy is a successful, accepted medical treatment for extreme cases of necrotic, gangrenous tissue, or crush injuries, where oxygen has been cut off from cells. Supplying the oxygen to the previously deprived cells can accelerate tissue healing. It is also used for anaerobic bacterial infections, which thrive in low oxygen concentrations. Even in these cases, medical personnel must be specially trained to deliver the least amount of oxygen that has a therapeutic effect, because too much oxygen causes injury.

would do well to think twice about buying anything claiming to increase oxygen. Just think about how it rusts and corrodes metal. Most "oxygen-boosting" products do not actually increase your oxygen, thank goodness. They merely deplete your cash.

There is a very real risk of harming tissues by subjecting them to too much oxygen. Excess oxygen shuts down critical cell reactions, causing cell death and tissue injury. Oxygen overdose oxidizes, or "rusts," the iron in blood, such that the iron is no longer of a form capable of carrying oxygen. The iron capable of carrying oxygen has two missing electrons and is called *iron II ion,* or *ferrous ion.* Excess oxygen removes one more electron from iron, resulting in *iron III ion,* or *ferric ion.* Ferric ion can't carry oxygen and produces anoxia, or oxygen deprivation. Premature infants who are given oxygen risk permanent blindness. Scuba divers who dive excessively deep, or who use a high oxygen-percent mixture called *Nitrox,* must worry about "oxygen toxicity," which entails nausea, dizziness, vision problems, seizures, and the dreaded "pulmonary edema," where fluid accumulates in the lungs.

The oxygen that we require for life is unfortunately a biradical—that is, it has two unpaired electrons—and thus it is a free radical and does all the bad things that free radicals do. (You might think that the two unpaired electrons on oxygen ought to simply pair up, resolving the problem, but the reason why this can't occur involves the mathematically allowed and forbidden energies of electrons.) Not only is oxygen a free radical, but oxygen is also very good at generating *other* free radicals and free radical generators. Hydrogen peroxide (the active ingredient in peroxide bleach), superoxide, and hydroxyl radical are the customary oxygen-generated saboteurs, called *reactive oxygen species, ROS,* or just *oxidizing agents.*

Since we continually inhale oxygen to stay alive (and I will explain why, shortly), we are constantly generating these toxic oxygen by-products in addition to subjecting ourselves to damage done by oxygen itself. Fortunately we also have enzymes, such as catalase and superoxide dismutase, which perpetually convert oxidizing agents into relatively harmless molecules, such as water. The cells of healthy people also constantly produce a good number of molecules, which chemists call *reducing agents.* They inactivate oxidizing agents and repair the damage that is done by them. The more common term for reducing agent is *antioxidant.*

Everybody knows that we need oxygen, yet so few know why. We need oxygen to accept electrons in an energy-generating event called "the electron transport chain." In this process, electrons are shuttled from one protein to another in a cellular structure known as a *mitochondrion.* High school biology students dutifully learn and regurgitate the phrase "the powerhouse of the cell" in reference to mitochondria. This electron transfer flows easily because of the proteins' relative abilities to successively accept them. As a mill uses a river's current to grind flour, the electron flow is used to construct an energy-carrying molecule called *adenosine triphosphate,* or *ATP,* for short. ATP is needed for all sorts of cellular processes that require energy to run. The old phrase "the energy currency molecule" is what the same high school students apply to ATP. The problem with the electron transport chain is that all of these flowing electrons have to end up somewhere, and that is where oxygen comes into the picture. The very last acceptor of electrons is oxygen. Without somewhere for the electrons to ultimately go, the electron transport chain backs up and stops, so oxygen is required for this energy-generating process. Most of the oxygen you breathe is used to remove electrons from their conveyor belt along the electron transport chain, so more electrons can enter the flow, and the flow continues. The continuous flow of electrons is required to make the essential molecule ATP.

Too much oxygen causes this process to backfire. Ideally, when combined with electrons and hydrogen in this process, the oxygen usually becomes water, which is relatively harmless, and that is the end of the oxygen. Occasionally, however, oxygen does not pick up enough electrons, and it then becomes either the superoxide radical or hydrogen peroxide, and both of these, like hardened sub-microscopic vandals, damage nearby molecules in the mitochondrion. Their formation is more likely to occur when there are too many oxygen molecules competing for electrons.

So oxygen is both good and bad. We can't survive without it, but like a criminal whose fingerprints keep turning up at crime scenes, oxygen is a prime suspect for accelerating aging and disease. Unless you have a lung disease like emphysema, or are climbing Mount Everest, you have enough oxygen.

Oxygen also oxidizes other molecules, which damages them if the oxidizing occurs randomly. We hear of things "getting oxidized," and we know it relates to the aging of a material, but what is really happening? Oxygen readily changes other molecules, and in doing so is said to "oxidize" them. For the oxidation we are interested in, we need to focus on organic, or carbon-containing, molecules. Organic molecules are required for life and are present in all organisms. A more precise definition says that oxidation is the loss of electrons. Oxygen tends to be greedy with electrons on atoms that are less greedy, and that includes most atoms on organic molecules. When oxy-

gen attaches to a less greedy atom, it pulls electrons away from that atom. Since oxygen tends to pull the electrons in a bond toward itself, attaching it to a carbon causes the carbon to "lose" some electron density through the bond to oxygen. If the carbon in a molecule makes more bonds to oxygen atoms, we say it "got oxidized." The most oxidized, electron-depleted form of carbon is carbon dioxide. Hydrogen is more electron-generous and likely to push electrons in its bonds toward carbon, so a molecule can also get oxidized when the carbons in it lose bonds to hydrogen.

Antioxidants are reducing agents. The reverse process bears a little discussion, because it is a process that antioxidants mediate. The reverse of oxidation is called *reduction,* so reduction is the gain of electrons. This sounds backward, because usually reduction means the loss of something, as in weight reduction. But electrons are negatively charged, so this reduction refers to the drop in numerical charge that occurs when electrons are gained. When the carbon in a molecule loses bonds to electron-greedy oxygen, or gains bonds to electron-generous hydrogen, we say the molecule got reduced, because the carbon in it gained more electron density in losing a bond to an electron-greedy atom (O) or gaining a bond to an electron-generous one (H). Molecules that enable this are termed reducing agents, but in medicine they are dubbed antioxidants. They are good because they prevent oxidation. But what is so bad about getting oxidized?

The oxidation of your molecules is beneficial—if it occurs in a controlled manner. We actually benefit from oxidizing our own molecules, but in a very controlled sort of way, in order to generate energy. Another term for combining with oxygen is combustion, or burning. When we burn fuels, the fuel molecules combine with oxygen. When the fuels contain carbon, the ultimate product is carbon dioxide, where carbon is as oxidized as it can possibly get. Our bodies also burn organic molecules and produce carbon dioxide as a waste product. This is controlled carefully in multistep processes, with most steps governed by an enzyme. As with burning things, oxidizing molecules always releases energy, and that energy can either be lost as heat or it can be channeled into more useful forms. When we "burn carbohydrates," or any other carbon-containing molecules for that matter, we are using up the molecule's potential to generate energy, and that energy is stored in some other form, like ATP. This process involves successive additions of oxygen and removals of hydrogen from the nutrient. Since oxidation is the loss of electrons, oxidizing food removes electrons from the food molecules, and these electrons are then used for the electron transport chain, which, as I described above, generates energy.

Highly reduced molecules have carbons with the least oxygens attached and the most hydrogens attached. Since the molecule starts off with a lot of potential places to add oxygen, it requires the most steps to become oxidized and will provide the most energy. Fats and oils fall into this category, as well as fuels like gasoline, propane, butane, and methane, which are known as *hydrocarbons*. The more oxygen a molecule has attached, the more oxidized or "burned" it is already, and the less energy it can provide. This is not bad in itself; we require both highly reduced molecules, like fats and oils, as well as partially oxidized molecules, like carbohydrates, for energy.

Uncontrolled oxidation is oxidative stress. When oxidation runs amok and is not governed by enzymes, it can cripple essential molecules. Scientists are exten-

sively researching this *oxidative stress.* Uncontrolled molecular oxidation is accelerated by all sorts of disease processes, aging, and both short- and long-term exposure to a large number of toxins. Oxidation of molecules alters them, and when you indiscriminately alter molecules, they do not function properly. Oxidative stress, in turn, exacerbates aging and disease processes, creating a vicious circle. Organisms combat oxidative stress by producing numerous antioxidants, and some of these antioxidants are vitamins, but many are not.

For example, one of the most ubiquitous nonvitamin antioxidants is glutathione. Glutathione's depletion is clearly associated with aging, toxins, and disease, and boosting cells' production of it often proves to be beneficial. Glutathione is helpfully elevated by some herbs, like the sulfurous ones in garlic, and unhelpfully depleted by others, like kava. It is even being sold in health food stores as a supplement. When consumed orally, glutathione is broken down and is no longer glutathione. However, some of glutathione's broken-down constituents and related synthetic molecules (cysteine and N-acetyl cysteine) often increase glutathione production in situations where glutathione is already depleted.

The association of other cellular antioxidants and oxidant-destroying enzymes is very often associated with positive outcome in countless numbers of studies. Bear in mind that some studies do fail to link antioxidants with positive outcome. There are also cases where an antioxidant can turn into a damaging oxidizing agent or *pro-oxidant,* under certain circumstances, so you can't assume they are always universally helpful. However, fewer studies actually show a negative outcome. A popular theory for how regular exercise maintains good health involves oxygen. Exercise subjects cells to mild oxidative stress, which stimulates antioxidant defense systems. The suggestion that dosing oneself with antioxidants could slow down the aging process *seems* logical, at least, but just because something seems logical does not make it true!

Will antioxidant supplements help us live longer? As you may imagine, the exciting prospect of slowing aging has scientists vigorously pursuing this topic. Supplement sellers won't like this, but this is what the studies show: Although the theory certainly seems sound, it has yet to be proven that consuming antioxidant *supplements* prolongs the lives of actual people. What *is* clear is that consuming more plants, which contain lots of antioxidants, enhances your health. So it seems you are better off following the famous motherly request of eating your fruits and vegetables rather than trying to get them in a pill. Fortunately, some herbs fall under this antioxidant category, and you can either eat them or drink their molecules in a tea.

The only studies that clearly demonstrate life prolongation due to diet involve calorie restriction in lab animals. Animals that lived longer were given far less food. What is interesting about these studies is that some show this dietary restriction decreases the production of oxidizing agents, perhaps because there are fewer molecules around to get oxidized. While you can't "reverse" aging, you can lower the risk of certain age-related diseases by maintaining the antioxidant status of your body. Some of the plants discussed in this book may help you do that.

INFLAMMATION

Your immune system is a double-edged sword. Many herb peddlers brag about their herbs' "immune enhancing" potential, but your immune system is not necessarily something you want to enhance. A country needs a military to defend itself, but giving the military unlimited power may not be in the people's best interest. Like oxygen, the immune system is both good and bad. It destroys disease-bearing microbes and heals injured tissues, but it can also spiral out of control, causing damage on its own. It shouldn't surprise you that many herbs, labeled *immunomodulators* or *immunostimulants,* stimulate the immune system. Pollen comes from plants and stimulates the immune systems of people who are allergic to it. You have to ask yourself if you really want to be stimulated in this manner.

The immune system guards against many devastating illnesses, but pollen is not one of these. Pollen is simply "a stranger in these here parts" in the body, and in some people it gets needlessly attacked, and allergic fallout causes pointless tissue damage. An acute, short-term inflammatory response can be life threatening: a bee sting can kill by initiating anaphylactic shock. Chronic, long-term deterioration of tissues by inflammation also occurs, as in arthritis. Cases of friendly fire, where the immune system attacks the body itself, produce autoimmune diseases. Many common diseases fall into this category, such as type 1 diabetes, lupus, myasthenia gravis, thyroid diseases, Crohn's disease, multiple sclerosis, rheumatoid arthritis, psoriasis, and many more. Indiscriminately "enhancing the immune system" of anyone with one of these disorders is likely to make them worse. There are even controversial theories that less-understood diseases, like schizophrenia or obsessive-compulsive disorder, get initiated by an infection, during which the person's immune system attacked the wrong thing, like a part of their brain.

Your cells can die cleanly with apoptosis, or messily, generating inflammation.

The type of damage done by inflammation involves a messy sort of cell death. In order to describe this, it helps to understand the "good" kind of normal cell death, which is called either *programmed cell death, cell suicide,* or *apoptosis* (ay-pap-TOE-sis). Programmed cell death occurs in the womb. Cells in the webbing between incipient fetal digits are programmed to die, thus separating fingers and toes. In all life stages, cells divide a limited number of times, otherwise a tumor results. After a cell divides a certain number of times, apoptosis is triggered.

Chromosomes, the gene-bearing aggregates of DNA molecules and protein, must get duplicated prior to a cell's division so that each daughter cell gets a complete set of chromosomes. Cell division fritters away at structures called *telomeres,* which sit at the ends of chromosomes. So aged populations of cells, which have divided a lot, have diminished telomeres. Once the telomere has worn down, the cell breaks itself down and neatly packages its constituents for recycling by other cells.

Cell apoptosis, once enacted, cleanly breaks down a cell's molecules, which are actually packaged in membranous material, and nearby cells use the contents of these packages. (That cells manage best by recycling their contents suggests the wisdom of recycling: Cells have survived for a few billion years on this planet, so perhaps they make good role models.) The cell line continues though the activity of the enzyme telomerase, which adds telomeres back to a portion of the daughter cells. The result of cell suicide does not attract the immune system's attention, and no inflammation occurs.

The messy type of cell death attracts the immune system's attention. When cell *necrosis* occurs, however, any number of different stresses can critically diminish a cell's energy supply. A cell needs energy to maintain the integrity of its outer boundary, called the *cell membrane.* For a cell to function properly, a continuous flow of ions (a type of charged particles) must be pumped across this membrane, which takes energy. This flow is needed because it creates a net negative charge inside of cells, which a cell uses, much like a battery, to its own ends. When energy drops to critically low levels, the electrostatic force pulls ions in the opposite direction in which the cell is pumping them, pressure rises inside the cell, and the cell explodes. The contents of the cell leak messily into the surroundings, which attracts the attention of the immune system. This initiates the process of inflammation.

After a cell detonates in this untidy way, a variety of white blood cells are drawn toward its discharged innards. They travel through blood vessels and start rolling and sticking to the vessel walls in the vicinity of the ruptured cell. This is because blood vessels get altered by cellular debris, becoming sticky to white blood cells. These detained white blood cells then squeeze through the spaces between the cells that compose the blood vessel, and out into the surrounding tissue. There, they can literally eat up the remains of the dead cell in a process called *phagocytosis.* A network of protein fibers forms around the dead cell to wall it off. This traffic of white blood cells plus water from the blood flowing into the area causes swelling. The vessel is signaled to widen, or dilate, which allows more blood to flow to the area, and the area becomes warm and red. The warmth accelerates healing chemical reactions taking place in the area.

Heat, pain, redness, and swelling are the four signs of inflammation, but you might not see these. Scratch your skin gently, and you will see a red line result: This is mild inflammation. Many diseases states are associated with some sort of inflammation.

"Heat, pain, redness, and swelling" are the four cardinal signs of inflammation. "Calor, dolor, rugor, and turgor" is the phrase classically memorized by medical students, perhaps because the Latin is more impressive, and it rhymes better. But many inflammatory processes are subclinical—that is, they aren't easily noticed—because they are low grade. Nonetheless, they do damage.

Besides being painful, an immune response can be more damaging than helpful. Free radicals fired off by responsive white blood cells kill bacteria, but expose healthy tissues to friendly fire. Swelling puts pressure on tissues, mechanically damaging nearby cells. Chronic inflammation apparently ages blood vessels, causing them to harden and narrow. Inflammation causes blood clots to form, which is good if you are bleeding, but bad when they cause a stroke or a heart attack.

Inflammation is not just a result of disease; it's a cause of disease. This idea is relatively new in medicine, and ever since it's dawned on us, scientists are continually uncovering evidence to support it. We find inflammation associated with so many bad things, from pimples to pancreatic cancer, but traditionally had never thought of it as being a *cause* of disease. We used to think of inflammation as being a secondary consequence of disease and injury, but more and more, new research is turning this old idea on its head. Heart disease used to be thought of as merely some sort of plumbing problem. Cholesterol-based plaques in arterial walls were thought to restrict the blood flow to the heart, causing heart disease. Also, dislodged plaque can lodge in a narrow vessel, causing a heart attack. It is now known, however, that inflammation is what causes the plaque to build up in the first place, and it is also inflammation that causes the plaque to dislodge.

It seems that sometimes inflammation does not just fizzle out, but instead persists, causing new damage. Chris Buckley and Mike Salmon, rheumatologists at the University of Birmingham in the United Kingdom, study why inflammation occasionally fails to shut itself off. They have found that immune cells sometimes continue to hang out in the site of injury, sending chemical signals to each other, and then, according to Buckley, "The conversation starts to get dangerous." White blood cells that persist around an inflamed joint, for example, produce chemicals that cause the joint to resemble a hyperactive lymph node, recruiting white blood cells to camp out there, continuing the inflammation that wears away joint cartilage. Some scientists are even cautiously proposing that inflammation is a key element in aging, and that decreasing inflammation might slow age-related deterioration.

It really gets ugly when the immune system's shut-off mechanisms fail. Normally, the white blood cells that respond to a necrotized cell's chemical call are eventually signaled to neatly kill themselves after their job is done, through apoptosis, and inflammation dies down. This process, called *resolution,* is in part triggered by *resolvins,* discovered by Harvard Medical School's Charles Serhan, who commented, "That was completely unexpected." Resolvins are made from omega-3 fatty acids.

Omega-3 fatty acids have received a lot of press lately, because among several other good things they are anti-inflammatory. Omega-3 fatty acids, like vitamins, are not made by humans, and we must eat them to stay alive. They are found in algae, fish oil (because fish eat the algae), and several plants, such as flax seeds and purslane, and eating them is associated with all sorts of health benefits. Curiously, organic dairy products and organically raised livestock have more omega-3 fatty acids than conventional kinds. That omega-3 fatty acids are used to make signals that shut off inflammation helps explain in part its anti-inflammatory action.

Anti-inflammatories do the opposite of stimulating the immune system, and they seem to prevent disease, too. Like omega-3 fatty acids, aspirin is also anti-inflammatory and reduces the risk of many diseases. This may be a clue that inflammation itself is a culprit in these diseases. Here is a list of some of the things that you may be less likely to get if you regularly take aspirin (take a big breath): breast cancer, colorectal cancer, pancreatic cancer, stomach cancer, stroke, heart disease, heart attack, Parkinson's disease, Alzheimer's disease, staph infections, and macular degeneration. A lot of people can safely take aspirin, but some cannot stomach it. Plants are full of aspirin-like molecules, called *salicylates,* and they are anti-inflammatory, too. Some of aspirin's benefits are more striking than others, and in some cases aspirin's appear more pronounced for men than for women, perhaps because women might normally eat more plant-based salicylates than men. Since plant salicylates are common and anti-inflammatory, it should therefore not surprise us to occasionally encounter an herb with significant therapeutic salicylates.

Balance and awareness of your body's immune/anti-inflammatory state are key. More people could benefit from lowering their immune status and increasing their anti-inflammatory status than the other way around. This may stem from the modern pro-inflammatory diet, which appears to increase the risk of common contemporary diseases like diabetes and cardiovascular disease. But anti-inflammatories can be overdone, too. Use of anti-inflammatory herbs can relieve all sorts of conditions, like arthritis, ulcers, and allergies, yet they should be approached carefully if you are prone to infection or taking blood-thinning medications like aspirin already. Anti-inflammatory herbs can even cause bleeding problems if consumed prior to surgery, for the same reasons that aspirin can. It is always best to let your doctor know everything that your are taking, including herbs, especially prior to surgery.

Herbs can be used either to enhance or suppress the immune system's response. Use of an "immune-enhancing" product might theoretically shorten a cold, but it could also exacerbate an autoimmune disease or allergy. (Actually, most of the classic immune-enhancing herbs, like echinacea, don't seem to work to fight or prevent illness, according to clinical studies. Echinacea seems better able to give people rashes.) Consider whether the immune-stimulatory effect is truly needed; if used for a cold, remember that most people do not die from colds, they usually eventually recover, and this phenomenon perhaps explains why so many cold remedies are thought to have "worked." Many herbs have the opposite effect, decreasing the immune response, and are anti-inflammatory. Because an inflammatory response is a multistep process, different herbs accomplish this by several means, which you can explore in more detail in the herb chapters. If you wish to take an anti-inflammatory herb, carefully examine the herb whose anti-inflammatory mechanism best meets your own, unique needs.

APPENDIX E
HOW TO AVOID GETTING CONNED BY PEOPLE, INCLUDING YOURSELF

Science is a way of trying not to fool yourself.
The first principle is that you must not fool yourself,
and you are the easiest person to fool.
—RICHARD FEYNMAN

You could consider this section part of preventive medicine. Not only do you have to watch out for free radicals, oxidizing agents, cancer, and inflammation, you also have to watch out for errors in judgment, which can be just as harmful.

Assume nothing. This not only goes for people trying to sell you things, but also for well-meaning professionals who confidently tell you what they believe the truth is. This includes the material in this book. At the risk of losing your confidence, I'll confess I am constantly making flight corrections in my thinking based on new, incoming data. You can't hang on to any preconceptions to be a good scientist. It requires a great deal of humility and the willingness to constantly reexamine your preconceptions. It's hard work to distrust everything you hear and read and think. The payback comes when data presented repeatedly backs up a story (otherwise known as a hypothesis), and then you feel excited that this story really could be true! It's exhilarating to feel like you are on to something, to feel like you are approaching real truth. Paradoxically, we can't ever trust that we get there. We actually do not prove anything in science. We just gain more and more support for various hypotheses, and some theories we have to toss out because what we observe doesn't back them up. It's an endless journey where we get closer and closer to the truth. People who say that this or that scientific theory can't be true because scientists disagree over it don't understand the nature of science. Science is not dogmatic and never "proves" anything. We do believe that constant questioning and reexamination of even the most agreed-upon theories brings us closer to the truth, and that some theories are definitely closer to the truth than others. These are decided upon not by consensus, but by evidence and reproducible experiments.

Science has no values or morals, but people do, and they vary from person to person. Science can't tell you what is right and wrong, or how you should live your life. Some people say, "Science tells us we should take vitamins." Or become vegetarian. Or do any number of things. But science only gives us information. It doesn't say what we ought to *do* with the information. For example, science does not say whether or not you *ought* to smoke. It merely says that if you do, there is excellent evidence you will die earlier, possibly from lung cancer. It's up to you to decide if you want that. Most people want to live longer, healthier lives, because that is a highly popular value. Since more subtle values vary widely from person to person, different people use the information from science in various ways, and then they look at each other and get annoyed. When someone advises doing this or that because "science says so," the purpose of science is misunderstood. Science is merely a tool that allows us to give more credence to some theories than others.

You Don't Have to Be a Scientist to Determine Whether Information on Herbs Is Reliable.

There are simple ways to look at herb sellers' information and scientific data to determine whether or not it looks suspicious. Here are some classic red flags to watch out for. These flags don't necessarily mean the information is bad, but it does mean you need to be extra careful.

But I saw it on TV.

Consider the source. The best source of herbal data is, unfortunately, very boring and technically troublesome to read. It appears in scientific abstracts in reputable journals. But even this is no guarantee. Some journals are trustworthier than others. Sometimes the research appearing in these journals was funded—and it can be in a very roundabout way—by herb companies trying to give their product more credibility. Even with the best of intentions this can taint researchers' interpretation of the data. This is why double-blinded studies are far better than "unblinded" ones.

Is the study well-designed?

In double-blind studies, neither the investigators nor the study volunteers know who is taking what. Ideally, there ought to be a placebo, too, and some group of volunteers must swallow something with no known pharmacological action, because just the act of taking *something* will often make people feel better. That's the placebo effect. Having a placebo group "controls" for this effect. In studies of women with hot flashes, for example, a placebo group is essential. Of course hot flashes are horribly real, but they are something that the mind is better able to assume power over and fix than, say,

a broken leg. In studies of women with hot flashes taking herbal medicines, they typically do outstandingly well—in the placebo group! That they do just as well with the herb means the herb probably doesn't exert any pharmacological action. But the patients' brains did. Part of judging the source requires that you look at how the study was designed.

Is it significant?

Herbs causing an increase or decrease in this or that effect doesn't mean very much. If you lose a pound, it doesn't mean as much as losing ten pounds. Statistical methods have evolved to help estimate whether an effect is truly caused by the agent being tested, because it could be due to chance. Look for "significant" effects. The term means the effect is less likely caused by chance, but it still could be. If you want to weed through abstracts yourself, look for a *probability value,* or *P value,* of less than 0.05. You will see something like "p<0.05" in the text, which means the parameter measured was statistically significant, and the smaller the P value is, the less likely the effect is due to chance. It's no guarantee, but it's an agreed-upon standard that helps you estimate which effects you should pay attention to and which you should ignore.

In the "Evidence of Action" sections for each herb in this book, you will find summaries of some of the best clinical trial data so far on these herbs. A mind-boggling number of the hard-to-read abstracts are available for everyone to read on the National Library of Medicine's PubMed Web site (http://www.ncbi.nlm.nih.gov).

Look at the type of advertisements featured alongside articles on herbs. Eventually results from these trials, both good, well-designed ones and poorly designed ones, filter down to the more popular news media. The more a magazine features ads for herbs and supplements, the more likely they will enthuse about how wonderful herbs are, to an almost hysterical pitch. They aren't necessarily wrong about some things, but what they say should be taken with a big grain of salt.

It kills cancer cells, in a test tube . . . and every other kind of cell, too.

This is what you call *poison*. It's great if an herb can kill cancer cells, bacterial cells, and disable viruses, and many do. But the herb ought to be kind to your own cells, too. Be sure the herb does that as well. Studies performed on animals or isolated cells are not guaranteed to relate to humans. Studies of herbs on humans are more persuasive.

But they know so many big words.

Using heady terms from quantum mechanics like "quantum" to sell just about everything has recently become popular, but it doesn't mean that the person has any idea what they are talking about, because quantum mechanics has nothing to do with herbs. But it does sound very impressive. (A quantum, by the way, is not as impressive as marketers make it sound, but most marketers using the term have no idea what it means, anyway. A quantum is a small unit of energy or material that comes in fixed sizes.) If the source of herbal information uses jargon that seems out of place, be suspicious. Some companies make up new jargon.

These herbs were used for millennia by ancient, exotic people who are now all dead.

Often a romantic picture is presented of some ancient, exotic race benefiting from use of a particular herb. It assumes people in the past knew better than we do now. They surely did know a lot more about many things, like how to live off the land using their own hands, so there is a grain of truth in this. They also didn't know a lot of things we know today, and many medieval "cures," like rubbing open wounds with feces, and killing the cats that hunted their plague-infested rats, have been discarded. It helps to investigate herbs that folkloric use supports, but the herbs must be tested using modern methods, too. That people used an herb in the past is no guarantee that it works or is safe.

It's just the latest thing.

Some people are moved by images of the past, others by new technology. Like information from the past, new technology can be extremely helpful. New technology often brings with it a wave of scams. Over the past century, people have tried using soft drinks, electricity, radiation, and magnetism therapeutically because of the promise surrounding anything "new." Soft drinks don't hurt unless they are filled with sugar, and magnets don't do anything as far as we can tell, but the enthusiastic, indiscriminate application of radiation by people thrilled by science's discovery of it was a bad idea. Just because it's new doesn't make it better.

Your body is full of toxins.

A centuries-old idea that undefined toxins cause health problems has resulted in attacks of the body from above and below with laxatives and enemas, which frequently cause more harm than good. "Cleansing the blood" was a turn-of-the-century euphemism for curing syphilis, yet this phrase persists in many modern herb books. The concept of a "healing crisis," where you feel worse before you can feel better due to "released toxins," is part of this common mythology. Your body is generally great at neutralizing toxins, and it's an excellent idea to expose yourself to less of them. Give your body some credit, and trust that it can manage what toxins you do encounter without harsh purgatives.

It's all-natural, so it can't hurt you.

A quick glance at poisonous mushrooms, hemlock, and venomous snakes should convince you this is not true. We have 100 percent natural tsunamis, too. Nature can kill us, and "natural" has no legal meaning on a label.

It's a conspiracy.

Disreputable claims are accompanied by claims of conspiracy and persecution committed by the "medical establishment." Some herbal companies have even suggested that they are being persecuted because doctors secretly don't want to cure disease, so they can make more money off all the sick people. Some have even likened themselves to famous persecuted figures in history, saying, "They didn't believe Galileo either." It's pretty hard to stomach—so don't swallow it.

Your rights are being taken away from you by the government, because they want us to disclose how much mercury is contaminating our herb.

Many of the better herb sellers test their products, cooperating with independent testing groups like Consumerlab, to get a seal of approval. (Go to http://www.consumerlab .com to check on who's been naughty and who's been nice.) But those who would rather not may try to scare you into thinking that your government is trying to stop you from taking herbs. Relax. The government will not stop you from taking herbs. They aren't going to raid your garden's mint patch. It's just that some herb sellers know they have been guilty of letting products slip by that are contaminated with heavy

metals and pesticides, and they'd rather not deal with correcting the problem. Sometimes they have even been caught "spiking" herbs with drugs undeclared on the label, like wild yam with progesterone, and hoodia with caffeine. Companies who don't want their herbs tested should be regarded with suspicion.

It cured my aunt's arthritis.

Anecdotes and testimonials make wonderful, inspiring stories, and many are true. But they do not prove anything one way or another. Products that sport countless testimonials, and no clinical trials, are questionable.

This product was tested in clinical trials.

It looks impressive in an advertisement, but they don't say the results of the trials. You will find this for some products selling homeopathic arnica, for example. If you read the results from the trials on PubMed, you will see they all have very sad outcomes, even with one experiment showing that the placebo group did better than those taking the arnica! Some products are also "approved by the FDA," but this does not mean the FDA tested them, and it does not mean they are safe or effective.

It cures every kind of cancer.

If it sounds too good to be true, it probably isn't true. Some herb sellers make eyebrow-raising claims for curing every disease and living forever. One unintentionally funny advertisement for a kombucha mushroom product blindly declares the herb was "used by ancient Manchurians as a cure for immortality." However, just because a claim is extraordinary doesn't mean it *isn't* true either. We are now finding extraordinary cures in medicine, for example. Yet the more astonishing the claim, the more you should stand back and weigh the evidence. As Carl Sagan put it, "Extraordinary claims require extraordinary evidence."

Other data? What *other* data?

Scientists and nonscientists alike fall victim to selecting data that supports their claim and ignoring evidence that does not. This is called *data selection,* and it happens to the best of us with the finest of intentions. We just have to guard against it. Here's a classic case of data selection: Although many people claim that more crime, violence, or births occur on a full moon, statistics repeatedly show that this is not true. People *notice* when the moon is full and make a mental note of a correlation, yet forget the instances when they do not see a full moon. Another instance of "milking the data" has recently created a multitude of glossy advertisements suggesting that dairy products help people lose weight. Low fat dairy products probably *are* healthy for most people and these claims that diary products enhance weight loss may even be true. However, the theory requires more research and currently has very little evidence to support it, since a couple of well-designed experiments that you don't hear about contradict it. What makes these ads disturbing is that one person with a patent on the claim is profiting from them, and his claim is based on some very small, poorly designed experiments which he funded. When examining nutritional claims in advertisements, don't look at how often the advertisement is publicized. Look at *all* the data.

APPENDIX F
WARNING LABELS FOR CERTAIN HERBS

All herbs can cause side effects. But some side effects (like death) are more severe than others (an upset stomach). Below is a list of herbs that can produce *more severe* side effects than others. This is by no means a complete list, but includes those herbs that are either currently popular around the world, or have been popular in the past, and are still favored as folk remedies in some cultures. Some of these are far more benign than others, and small or infrequent use probably won't cause harm, yet others on this list should be outright avoided because they are so deadly. Also, the *form* of the plant taken—whether it is a root, fruit, leaf, or oil—matters as well. For example, most volatile, aromatic essential oils from plants are toxic if consumed orally (not to be confused with the un-aromatic "vegetable" or cooking oils).

As the father of human toxicology, Paracelsus noted: all things are toxic if you take enough of them, but some things are more toxic than others. The dose makes the medicine, and the dose makes the poison.

If you think you or someone you know has been poisoned by an herbal remedy or plant, contact your local poison control center immediately. Modern analytical methods can often "fingerprint" trace amounts of characteristic plant chemicals in blood samples from people who have been poisoned by them.

Aconite (monkshood, wolfsbane)

(Aconitum napellus)

Potential Problems: Aconite is typically used in Chinese medicine in small quantities with other herbs; however, all species of this plant are dangerous. Larger amounts of aconite causes vomiting, weakness, numbness, heart dysrhythmia, acidosis, cardiac toxicity, and death.

Mechanism of Toxicity: Aconitine, mesoconitine, and hypaconitine are fast-acting, poisonous alkaloids from the plant that activate your cell's sodium channels, producing widespread effects on the nervous system and heart.

Aloe Latex
(also called aloe juice; do not confuse with the relatively benign aloe gel, which is also confusingly called "juice" when sold as a beverage)

(Aloe spp.)

Potential Problems: The bitter yellow latex causes cramps and diarrhea, and high doses are associated with kidney irritation and failure, and heart arrhythmias. Long-term use may paralyze intestinal muscle, leading to dependency.

Mechanism of Toxicity: Long-term use causes electrolyte depletion such as potassium loss.

Angelica

(Angelica archangelica)

Potential Problems: Large oral doses of angelica can be poisonous. Both internal and external use is linked to photosensitization, burns, and possible carcinogenicity.

Mechanism of Toxicity: The psoralens in angelica become reactive when exposed to ultraviolet light, and in animal studies the plant causes cancer even if the animals are not exposed to light.

Aristolochia
(birthwort, red river snake root, mu tong)

(Aristolochia spp.)

Potential Problems: Aristolochia is an ingredient in several Chinese herbal mixtures, yet its ingestion is associated with epidemics of kidney failure. In Belgium a rapid outbreak of progressive kidney dysfunction in at least one hundred patients was linked to their use of a mixture of Chinese herbs containing aristolochia species mistakenly labeled *Stephania tetrandra*. Similar cases in at least five other countries in Europe and Asia have created the term "Chinese herb nephropathy." Contamination of flour with aristolochia seeds in Croatia caused an outbreak of kidney disorders.

Mechanism of Toxicity: Aristolochic acid is toxic to the kidney and is carcinogenic.

Arnica

(Arnica montana)

Potential Problems: Ingestion of *A. montana*–containing products has induced severe stomach upset, nervousness, racing heart, miscarriage, muscular paralysis, and death. Fortunately, its common inclusion in *homeopathic* remedies requires it to be diluted to the point of its practical nonexistence in such remedies.

Mechanism of Toxicity: There are several possible mechanisms reported. These include initiation of a severe allergic response, mucosal irritation, uterine stimulation, heart stimulation, and platelet dysfunction.

Bayberry

(Myrica cerifera, Myrica spp.)

Potential Problems: Once popular in scented candles, but when taken orally, bayberry has caused gastrointestinal irritation, vomiting, and liver damage. Rats injected with extracts of bayberry developed a significant number of malignancies.

Mechanism of Toxicity: The root bark may contain a carcinogen. It has a high tannin content, which can theoretically become carcinogenic with repeated exposure. Its myricadiol reportedly alters sodium and potassium metabolism, perhaps through mineralocorticoid hormone interference.

Belladonna (deadly nightshade)

(Atropa belladonna)

Potential Problems: Adults have poisoned themselves by confusing the attractive glossy black berries with bilberries, and children are commonly poisoned by this plant as well. Dry mouth, rapid heartbeat, enlarged pupils, hallucinations, coma, and death can occur.

Mechanism of Toxicity: Belladonna contains the tropane alkaloids L-hyoscyamine, L-scopolamine, and atropine (dl-hyoscyamine). These block the action of the neurotransmitter acetylcholine by competing for muscarinic acetylcholine receptors.

Bitter Almond
(do not confuse with sweet almond, Prunus amygdalus dulcis)

(Prunus dulcis var. amara)

Potential Problems: Sweet and bitter almonds almost always grow on separate almond trees. Culinary bitter almond oil normally has the hydrogen cyanide (HCN) removed. Children may theoretically be killed after eating just a few bitter almonds, however. Respiratory depression and death is documented for an adult who consumed the volatile oil of bitter almond.

Mechanism of Toxicity: Amygdalin in the kernel is enzymatically hydrolyzed to produce toxic hydrocyanic acid (HCN, prussic acid). Benzaldehyde (commonly used in artificial almond flavoring) from the cyanide-free oil can cause central nervous system depression and consequent respiratory failure.

Bitter Orange

(Citrus aurantium)

Potential Problems: Since ephedra has been restricted due to problems with its toxicity, some herbal diet aids are replacing ephedra with bitter orange, which has similar activity. Oral use of bitter orange is now associated with several dozen cases of serious cardiovascular crises, such as spiking blood pressure, heart palpitations, and heart attack, even in people with no previous history of heart disease.

Mechanism of Toxicity: Bitter orange's constituent synephrine (and possibly other similar-looking isomers like meta-synephrine) is a sympathetic nervous system agonist that works through alpha-adrenergic receptors like phenylephrine.

Bittersweet
(bitter nightshade, common nightshade)

(Solanum dulcamara)

Potential Problems: This plant is a common weed in suburbs, and children are attracted to its translucent red berries that arise from striking purple and yellow star-shaped flowers. Symptoms are similar to solanine poisoning from green potatoes, yet far more intense: scratchy throat, headache, dizziness, dilated pupils, vomiting, diarrhea, respiratory depression, convulsions, and death may occur.

Mechanism of Toxicity: Solanine, and to a lesser extent its aglycone solanidine, are potent inhibitors of the acetylcholine-degrading enzyme acetylcholinesterase, thus they allow acetylcholine to persist to an extent that may be toxic.

Boldo

(Peumus boldus)

Potential Problems: Boldo is approved for use in food in small amounts and in alcoholic beverages if restricted to amounts less than 0.0002 percent. Convulsions may occur if large amounts of boldo are consumed. There is one case of a man using an herbal combination for years, and after the manufacturer changed the formula to include boldo, he developed liver toxicity, which abated when he stopped using the product.

Mechanism of Toxicity: The oil contains the endoperoxide ascaridole, which is toxic to some parasitic worms, but has unfortunately caused some human fatalities as well, as it paralyzes involuntary muscles.

BLUE COHOSH
(do not confuse with black cohosh)

(Caulophyllum thalictroides)

Potential Problems: Some people have confused this plant with the unrelated, therapeutic black cohosh. Severe complications such as renal failure, heart attack, shock, seizures, stroke, anemia, and respiratory distress frequently occur when people take this herb.

Mechanism of Toxicity: Blue cohosh restricts the supply of oxygen to the heart by constricting coronary arteries. Several alkaloids and N-methylcytosine may initiate birth defect formation.

BONESET
(feverwort, Indian sage, thoroughwort)

(Eupatorium perfoliatum)

Potential Problems: Vomiting and diarrhea, as well as severe allergic responses, can occur after large amounts are eaten.

Mechanism of Toxicity: Boneset contains pyrrolizidine alkaloids known to cause liver cancer and liver poisoning.

BORAGE

(Borago officinalis)

Potential Problems: Borage seed oil, purified of its trace amounts of toxic pyrrolizidine alkaloids, is probably quite safe. The leaves have a higher pyrrolizidine alkaloid content, however, and are sometimes added to salads, drinks, and cooking. Theoretically, heavy use of the leaves over a long time can lead to liver cancer.

Mechanism of Toxicity: Pyrrolizidine alkaloids are known to cause liver cancer and liver poisoning.

BROOM
(Scotch broom, hogweed, Irish broom)

(Cytisus scoparius, Sarothamnus scoparius)

Potential Problems: Many unrelated plants are confusingly called "broom," because their dried branches were once useful for sweeping floors. Don't confuse this plant with so-called butcher's broom (*Ruscus aculeatus*), which generally appears safe and possibly even effective for vein problems like chronic venous insufficiency. *Scotch* broom, on the other hand, can slow the heart dangerously. Moldy Scotch broom flowers were once recommended in place of marijuana for smoking, despite no evidence of any intoxicating effect. Moldy broom possesses the occasionally pathogenic fungus *Aspergillus*.

Mechanism of Toxicity: Sparteine, an alkaloid in the plant, slows the heart to a potentially dangerous extent should too much herb be consumed. Smoking moldy Scotch broom has initiated pulmonary aspergillosis.

BUCHU

(Agathosma betulina, Agathosma crenulata)

Potential Problems: The oil is used commercially to impart fruity scents and flavors to various products, but it is restricted to less than 0.002 percent in foods. Miscarriage, kidney problems, and stomach irritation are reported following oral consumption.

Mechanism of Toxicity: Buchu oil contains the known liver poison pulegone. Pulegone is metabolized to a reactive epoxide molecule in the liver, which damages liver cells.

BUCKTHORN
(European buckthorn, alder buckthorn, frangula)
(Rhamnus cathartica, Rhamnus frangula)

Potential Problems: Long-term use is associated with heart arrhythmias and muscle weakness. Intestinal paralysis can lead to laxative dependency.

Mechanism of Toxicity: Long-term use leads to electrolyte disturbances such as severe loss of potassium.

CALAMUS (sweet flag)
(Acorus calamus)

Potential Problems: In the past, people candied the roots and used them for food. Some wild plant enthusiasts still recommend them. They should probably not be eaten regularly, however, because lab animals fed low amounts of calamus over time developed severe organ abnormalities and several types of cancer.

Mechanism of Toxicity: Calamus contains beta-asarone, a known carcinogen.

CASCARA (sacred bark)
(Rhamnus purshiana)

Potential Problems: Fresh bark causes nausea and vomiting. Orally, aged cascara causes cramps and diarrhea, and long-term use is associated with heart arrhythmias and muscle weakness. Long-term use may paralyze intestinal muscle, leading to dependency.

Mechanism of Toxicity: Long-term use leads to electrolyte disturbances, such as

severe loss of potassium. There is also concern over potential liver toxicity.

CELANDINE
(Greater celandine, *Bai Qu Cai*)
(Chelidonium majus)

Potential Problems: Celandine is moderately popular and sold as a digestive remedy; however, at least ten cases of liver inflammation involving five different brands from Germany are documented. Stomach pain, bloody urine, dizziness, and lethargy may also occur.

Mechanism of Toxicity: The exact cause of liver damage isn't known, but the plant contains some isoquinoline alkaloids, including berberine, which can be toxic in sufficient quantities.

CHAULMOOGRA
(gynocardia oil, hydnocarp)
(Hydnocarpus kurzii)

Potential Problems: The oil is sold on the Internet without much information to accompany it. The oil is used topically for skin problems, but kidney failure, visual disorders, and paralysis may occur if it is taken orally.

Mechanism of Toxicity: The seeds from which the oil is obtained contain cyanide-generating glycosides and are extremely toxic.

CHAPARRAL (creosote bush)
(Larrea tridentate, Larrea divaricata)

Potential Problems: Numerous cases of acute liver damage are linked with taking chaparral internally, including several requiring liver transplants. Liver biopsies of affected individuals show initial use is associated with fatty liver, and more prolonged use can result in liver scarring that is then followed by sudden, severe liver failure.

Mechanism of Toxicity: The exact mechanism of toxicity remains unknown, but its constituent NDGA (nordihydroguaiaretic acid) is commonly used experimentally for inducing kidney disease in rats. In its purified form, NDGA causes liver toxicity in rodents as well.

CLEMATIS
(devil's darning needle, old man's beard, traveler's joy, virgin's bower)

(Clematis virginiana, Clematis spp.)

Potential Problems: Prolonged skin contact causes blisters and burns. Internally, severe gastrointestinal irritation and injury can occur.

Mechanism of Toxicity: The ranunculin glycoside in the freshly cut plant is enzymatically changed into a severely irritating and toxic chemical called *protoanemonin*. This rapidly degrades into the nontoxic anemonin. Drying the herb destroys a portion of the precursor to the toxic protoanemonin.

CLUB MOSS
(Stag's horn, Lycopodium; do not confuse with Chinese club moss, Huperzia serrata)

(Lycopodium clavatum)

Potential Problems: One case of severe poisoning has been reported in Switzerland. In China, seven cases of liver toxicity are reported with use of an herbal combination of club moss and Chinese club moss. Club moss spores were once used to dust some condoms and surgical gloves, and workers in factories exposed to it had increased risk of developing asthma. Spores entering surgical wounds formed granulomas; therefore the spores are no longer accepted by the FDA for use in surgical gloves and have been replaced by cornstarch.

Mechanism of Toxicity: Club moss contains toxic alkaloids, including lycopodine, dihydrolycopodine, and traces of nicotine. It does not contain huperzine A, which is obtained from the related Chinese club moss. Huperzine A may be useful in treating Alzheimer's disease, yet has only been tested in one clinical trial to date. Both contain alkaloids with unknown safety. Purified huperzine A is also associated with side effects related to other mechanisms (acetylcholinesterase inhibition) but is likely less toxic if taken in low doses for short periods under a doctor's guidance.

COCCULUS
(levant berry, cocculus indicus)

(Anamirta cocculus)

Potential Problems: In India the leaves are used as snuff to treat malaria; it also is used to kill fish, birds, and dogs. It is diluted considerably for use in homeopathic remedies.

Mechanism of Toxicity: The picrotoxin in the herb, even in two or three kernels, can be deadly. It works by noncompetitively antagonizing GABA (gamma-amino butyric acid) A receptors, which when not antagonized help relax brain activity.

COLTSFOOT

(Tussilago farfara)

Potential Problems: A young child developed veno-occlusive disease (narrowing of liver blood vessels) and severe liver damage after his parents attempted to "assist his development" with coltsfoot tea. Several studies show coltsfoot causes cancer in rodents.

Mechanism of Toxicity: All parts of the plant have toxic pyrrolizidine alkaloids; although a tea made from the leaves may have less; it should not be taken regularly or by children and is probably best avoided entirely. The agent that causes liver cancer is probably senkirkine.

COMFREY

(Symphytum officinale)

Potential Problems: Several cases of liver cancer and veno-occlusive disorders have been documented with people taking comfrey internally on a regular basis. Theoretically, it can also be absorbed if applied to open wounds or abraded skin.

Mechanism of Toxicity: The pyrrolizidine alkaloids are genotoxic and mutate DNA, creating potential cancer cells. The allantoin in the plant stimulates cell division (mitosis), enhancing these cancer cells' likelihood of dividing into more cancer cells.

COUNTRY MALLOW (heart leaf)

(Sida cordifolia)

Potential Problems: Herbs containing ephedrine cause several side effects, the more serious including elevated blood pressure,

asphyxia, heart arrhythmias, heart attack, and sudden death.

Mechanism of Toxicity: In short, ephedrine can resemble adrenalin in its actions and produce symptoms similar to adrenalin overload. More precisely, ephedrine stimulates the sympathetic nervous system somewhat through agonist action at alpha- and beta- adrenergic receptors but primarily acts by displacing norepinephrine from storage vesicles in presynaptic neurons. The displaced norepinephrine is released into the neuronal synapse where it activates adrenergic receptors.

DONG QUAI

(Angelica sinensis)

Potential Problems: Psoralens in the plant have caused photosensitization and dermatitis.

Mechanism of Toxicity: Dong quai contains several carcinogens, including safrole, yet there is currently insufficient data concerning elevated cancer risk with large doses or with long-term use. Caution is warranted.

EPAZOTE (Jesuit tea, Mexican tea)

(Chenopodium spp.)

Potential Problems: The traditional use of epazote leaves as seasoning in Mexican cooking is probably quite safe and not associated with any side effects. The oil from the plant and its seeds, however, is more problematic. *Chenopodium oil,* as it is called, is used to kill intestinal worms traditionally, but it also can cause convulsions, paralysis, and death.

Mechanism of Toxicity: The ascaridole

not only paralyzes intestinal worms but also paralyzes the involuntary muscles of those who take it, and in excess this effect is fatal.

EPHEDRA (ma huang)

(Ephedra sinica, Ephedra spp.)

Potential Problems: Ephedra is now banned in the United States due to extensive reports of people using the herb suffering disabling and life-threatening events such as seizures, heart attack, psychosis, cerebrovascular damage, and stroke. Herbs containing ephedrine cause several side effects, the more serious including elevated blood pressure, asphyxia, heart arrhythmias, heart attack, and sudden death.

Mechanism of Toxicity: Ephedrine resembles adrenalin in its actions and produces symptoms similar to adrenalin overload. Technically, ephedrine stimulates the sympathetic nervous system somewhat through agonist action at alpha- and beta-adrenergic receptors but primarily acts by displacing norepinephrine from storage vesicles in presynaptic neurons. The displaced norepinephrine is released into the neuronal synapse where it activates adrenergic receptors.

EPIMEDIUM (horny goat weed)

(Epimedium grandiflorum)

Potential Problems: Large doses or long-term use may cause dizziness, vomiting, thirst, respiratory arrest, and spasms.

Mechanism of Toxicity: The mechanism responsible for the adverse effects isn't clear, yet it is thought to possibly block calcium channels, hinder catecholamine release, and have possible androgenic hormonal effects.

FIDDLEHEADS
(fern fiddleheads, ostrich fern, gardenhead fern)

(Matteuccia struthiopteris, Osmunda struthiopteris)

Potential Problems: Fern fiddleheads are a classic, old wilderness culinary treat and regarded as a delicacy. However, the CDC (Centers for Disease Control) has linked fiddleheads to outbreaks of severe food poisoning. It can cause nausea, vomiting, diarrhea, and abdominal cramping.

Mechanism of Toxicity: The toxins responsible for this syndrome have not been identified. The CDC recommends thoroughly boiling the fiddleheads for ten minutes before eating them, since the toxins are apparently disabled by cooking.

FO TI
(shen min, Chinese knotweed, ho shou wu)

(Polygonum multiflorum)

Potential Problems: Oral consumption of fo ti can cause cramps, diarrhea, and vomiting, and may be linked to reported cases of liver inflammation.

Mechanism of Toxicity: The anthraquinone laxatives in the plant are converted to highly reactive anthrones in the digestive tract, which may cause liver injury after they are absorbed.

FOXGLOVE (digitalis)

(Digitalis purpurea, Digitalis spp.)

Potential Problems: People once used the plant for "dropsy," or water retention, associated with heart failure. The plant is too potent and too dangerous to use, however, so its constituents are now used as prescriptions. Foxglove overdose causes blurred vision, vomiting, muscle weakness, convulsions, heart dysrhythmia, heat attack, and death.

Mechanism of Toxicity: Foxglove is the original source of the powerful heart medications digoxin and digitoxin. They are potent inhibitors of cellular sodium and potassium ion transport, indirectly causing increases in calcium in heart muscle, causing it to contract more forcefully. They also stimulate the sympathetic nervous system.

GELSEMIUM
(yellow jasmine, false jasmine)

(Gelsemium sempervirens, Gelsemium spp.)

Potential Problems: Commonly used in homeopathic remedies that fortunately dilute it to the point of its nonexistence in such remedies. Orally, gelsemium causes double vision, eyelid drooping, dizziness, seizures, trouble breathing, rapid heartbeat, and death.

Mechanism of Toxicity: All parts of the plant contain toxic gelsamine alkaloids that are postulated to act against GABA (gamma-aminobutyric acid) in the brain.

GERMANDER (wall germander)

(Teucrium chamaedrys)

Potential Problems: Germander was once a popular herb in Europe and the Mediterranean, but multiple cases of liver inflammation and death led to its ban in France and its restriction for use in other countries.

Mechanism of Toxicity: The diterpene teucrin A causes liver poisoning.

GINKGO SEEDS
(Ginkgo biloba)

Potential Problems: The leaf extract, purified of toxic ginkgotoxins, is normally used, and that is probably safe. Seeds are traditionally eaten, too, but must be boiled first to reduce the toxin to tolerable levels. If *fresh* seeds are eaten, vomiting, seizures, shock, and loss of consciousness can occur.

Mechanism of Toxicity: The fresh seeds contain the nerve poison 4-O-methylpyridoxine, which antagonizes the action of vitamin B6 (pyridoxine), which is required for amino acid metabolism, as well as carbohydrate and lipid metabolism and a wide variety of other physiological processes.

GOLDENSEAL
(Hydrastis canadensis)

Potential Problems: Goldenseal was once a very popular herb, but several fatalities have occurred in infants when used by pregnant women or nursing mothers. Prolonged use can cause hallucinations and severe digestive problems, and overdose has resulted in seizures, heart damage, and death.

Mechanism of Toxicity: The berberine alkaloid may be responsible for the herb's antiseptic action against urinary tract infections and diarrhea, yet is fatal if too much is taken. Berberine blocks potassium channels in the heart and stimulates cells' transport of sodium and calcium ions. In animal studies, berberine stimulates the vagal nerve, the cranial nerve that is essential for speech, swallowing, and the essential functions of many parts of the body and depresses heart function.

Gold Thread (huang lian)

(Coptis trifolia, Coptis spp.)

Potential Problems: Gold thread was once more popular in Western herbalism and is still commonly used in Chinese medicines. Oral use, however, can cause vomiting, breathing problems, and kidney damage.

Mechanism of Toxicity: As with goldenseal, goldthread's berberine content makes consuming it risky.

Graviola

(cherimoya, guanabana, soursop, sour sop, custard apple, Brazilian paw paw)

(Annona muricata)

Potential Problems: Cherimoya, or graviola fruit, is very popular in South America, and all parts of the plant are marketed as antibiotic and anticancer herbs. However, epidemiological studies of populations in the west French Indies show an association between regular, lifetime consumption of the plant and movement disorders resembling Parkinson's disease. Drinking tea from the leaves can cause optic nerve damage. It may be that such neurological damage from cherimoya is uncommon, or it may take years of cherimoya consumption to acquire it, but caution is warranted.

Mechanism of Toxicity: Graviola contains alkaloids that kill dopamine-secreting and GABA-secreting nerve cells in the brain. It is likely that this can in theory create a syndrome resembling Parkinson's disease.

Horse Chestnut

(Aesculus hippocastanum)

Potential Problems: Horse chestnut must have its aesculin ("esculin") removed before it is used therapeutically. Any raw parts of the plant are toxic and cause gastrointestinal distress, internal bleeding, and possible kidney damage. Don't confuse the toxic aesculin with the more therapeutic constituents aescin (escin).

Mechanism of Toxicity: For raw, unprocessed forms of horse chestnut, the high tannin content upsets the digestive tract. Its toxic aesculin resembles the blood thinner coumarin, in possessing potent anti-clottting action that may cause excessive bleeding.

Horsetail

(Equisetum arvense)

Potential Problems: Horsetail is commonly included in diuretic herbal mixtures and sold as a silica (i.e., sand) supplement for hair and nails, even though there is currently no convincing evidence that eating sand or silica helps skin, hair, or nails, which are of course made of protein, not sand. Horsetail has poisoned children and causes symptoms similar to nicotine poisoning, and it also commonly poisons grazing livestock.

Mechanism of Toxicity: The inorganic silica content can be toxic to children and livestock. The plant has trace amounts of nicotine, and children eating the plant exhibit symptoms similar to nicotine toxicity. The herb contains an agent that degrades the vitamin thiamine, causing thiamine deficiency.

INDIAN SNAKEROOT
(rauwolfia)

(rauvolfia serpentina)

Potential Problems: This plant is a source of the prescription drug reserpine, and despite warnings of its potential toxic effects it is still being sold over a few Internet sites. Small oral amounts of the herb are known to cause cramps, diarrhea, vomiting fatigue, sexual dysfunction, depression, Parkinson's-like symptoms, and convulsions.

Mechanism of Toxicity: The plant contains more than fifty potentially active alkaloids, including reserpine, which have potent effects on the heart, blood pressure, brain, and nerves.

JABORANDI

(Pilocarpus microphyllus)

Potential Problems: This plant is a source of the prescription drug pilocarpine, which is used to dilate the pupil. It fortunately is now far less popular as an herbal remedy. Ingestion of 5 to 10 grams of leaf causes slow heartbeat, respiratory distress, collapse, heart attack, convulsions, vomiting, and sweating.

Mechanism of Toxicity: Pilocarpine is a potent parasympathetic nervous system stimulant.

JAMAICAN DOGWOOD
(fish poison tree)

(Piscidia piscipula)

Potential Problems: Tinctures of bark extract are sold as herbal remedies over the Internet with very little information to accompany them. Oral consumption of bark

extracts is associated with numbness, tremors, salivation, and sweating.

Mechanism of Toxicity: The bark is a source of rotenone, which is now used as a pesticide yet appears to increase the risk of Parkinson's disease, perhaps because of it's ability to destroy mitochondrial functioning in the brain. Rotenone is carcinogenic in some experimental studies.

JUNIPER

(Juniperis communis)

Potential Problems: Juniper increases urine output but should be used with caution. If taken in excessive amounts or for a long period of time, kidney pain, kidney damage, and convulsions can occur. The oil also irritates the skin. (Much of the diuretic action of gin, which is flavored with juniper, is due to alcohol rather than to the added juniper, although juniper enhances the effect. An overdose of gin is more likely to cause toxicity through alcohol poisoning than by juniper.)

Mechanism of Toxicity: The oil's terpinen-4-ol increases kidney filtration rate but does this by irritating kidney tissues, and it can damage them.

JOE PYE WEED
(queen of the meadow, purple boneset, gravel root)

(Eupatorium purpureum)

Potential Problems: Joe Pye is a classic old herb that is still sold and used extensively, mainly for urinary tract problems and arthritis. However, it may cause vascular blockage in the liver known as *veno-occlusive disease.*

Mechanism of Toxicity: The root and

aboveground parts contain toxic pyrrolizidine alkaloids known to cause veno-occlusive disease.

KAVA (kava kava)

(Piper methysticum)

Potential Problems: For centuries, "kava dermatopathy"—dry, scaly, yellow skin—has been a historically documented side effect of long-term kava use. Liver damage is commonly observed in the form of liver enzymes leaking into the blood, as well as jaundice and acute liver failure.

Mechanism of Toxicity: Kava alters the pattern of drug-metabolizing liver enzymes such that subsequent exposure to a liver toxin may render someone more vulnerable to the toxin. Kava also depletes the liver's supply of the protective antitoxin glutathione, again, making someone more vulnerable to the damage caused by chance ingestion of a liver toxin.

KELP (bladderwrack, laminaria)

(various genera: Laminaria spp., Fucus spp.)

Potential Problems: The occasional kelp, or "sea vegetables," commonly used in Asian cooking is probably fine. However, kelp is offered therapeutically to people with thyroid dysfunction, but this could easily make such people worse. Thyroid dysfunction is common but *rarely* is it caused by lack of iodine anymore, thanks to the iodination of salt in the 1960s. Thyroid dysfunction is by far more often a consequence of an autoimmune disease (in women) and aging (in men). Only very culturally isolated communities that do not consume seafood or sea products remain at risk of critically low iodine, like some isolated rural, elderly communities in the Appalachian mountains. People who take regular doses of kelp and do not have thyroid dysfunction risk creating a thyroid problem.

Mechanism of Toxicity: The iodine in a kelp supplement can be more than 1,000 micrograms, and ingesting less than this (150 micrograms) daily is enough to cause hypothyroidism, hyperthyroidism, and to exacerbate preexisting thyroid disease.

KHAT (qat, Arabian tea, Abyssinian tea)

(Catha edulis)

Potential Problems: The stems are chewed in Arabian countries and East Africa for their stimulant, euphoric effect. Khat is considered addicting by the World Health Organization (WHO). Occasional psychotic events occur, but this is rare compared to other forms of amphetamine abuse. Users tend to have chronically higher blood pressure, and although women may have increased libido, men gradually become impotent on the herb. The herb is a common source of liver parasites known as *liver flukes.* The addictive effects of khat are blamed for fueling civil conflict and economic strife in Somalia.

Mechanism of Toxicity: Khat contains the amphetamine-like stimulants cathine and cathinone. Even imported khat leaves can harbor parasitic liver fluke eggs.

KHELLA (toothpick plant, ammi)

(Ammi visnaga)

Potential Problems: Khella is an ancient Egyptian plant once used to treat urinary parasites and renal congestion, and the accidental discovery of a potent heart medication was made from it. It is still being sold with little information on dietary and bodybuilding Internet sites. Khella can cause liver damage when taken over a long period of time.

Mechanism of Toxicity: Khellin, visnadin, and visnagin in the plant block cells' calcium channels, widening arteries and slowing and weakening the heart's beat.

LABRADOR TEA
(continental tea, St. James tea, marsh tea)

(Rhododendron groenlandicum, Ledum groenlandicum, Rhododendron tomentosum)

Potential Problems: Lots of people still drink this once popular tea made from labrador tea leaves with no ill effects. In large doses, however, the plant has caused delirium, paralysis, and death. Marsh tea is a different species but has similar precautions.

Mechanism of Toxicity: The sesquiterpene ledol can cause gastrointestinal spasms, central nervous system excitability, and paralysis. The diterpene *grayanotoxin* (also called *adromedotoxin* or *rhodotoxin*) in labrador tea is also known as a honey contaminant from bees that have pollinated rhododendrons. The grayanotoxin binds to sodium channels on cells, keeping nerve cells and muscles in an excitation-prone state where they are unable to relax. These constituents are probably too dilute in one cup of tea to do much harm.

LICORICE
(liquorice)

(Glycyrrhiza glabra)

Potential Problems: Regular consumption of *large* amounts of real licorice over a time (a few weeks or more) commonly causes a syndrome called *apparent mineralocorticoid excess,* with high blood pressure and potassium loss that can be disabling and dangerous. Much of the licorice sold in the United States is not real licorice but anise flavoring and does not have this problem. However, real licorice is becoming more popular in the United States, so an increasing number of licorice-related hospital visits are documented.

Mechanism of Toxicity: Glycyrrhizin and glycyrrhetinic acid disable the enzyme 11-beta-hydroxysteroid dehydrogenase, enabling cortisol to act on the kidneys in a far more potent manner. This results in sodium retention and potassium wasting through urine.

LIFE ROOT
(senecio herb, alpine ragwort, squaw weed)

(Senecio nemorensis)

Potential Problems: Although most herbal information sources now report this herb is potentially dangerous, a few herbalists encourage making tinctures of it for regular use and "regulating the hormones." The only thing it reliably does, however, is damage the liver. At worst, it can cause cancer, and at best it causes low-grade liver dysfunction if taken regularly.

Mechanism of Toxicity: Pyrrolizidine alkaloids in the plant react with your liver cells after you eat the plant, damaging them and possibly initiating liver cancer.

LOBELIA
(bladderpod, gagroot, Indian tobacco, pukeweed, vomit wort)
(Lobelia inflata)

Potential Problems: This herb is sometimes used in herbal antismoking products. So far it has not proved effective in mediating smoking cessation in people, however. Some of its common names give you an idea of what larger oral doses can do to you. It causes vomiting, and overdose may cause convulsions, rapid heartbeat, and death.

Mechanism of Toxicity: The alkaloid lobeline from the plant interacts with nicotinic receptors, as does nicotine, yet elicits different responses from them, which may be excitatory or inhibitory under different circumstances. Lobeline has complicated effects on the nervous system, yet does not appear addictive, at least not in studies with mice.

MALE FERN
(Dryopteris filix-mas)

Potential Problems: This herb was once recommended for expelling intestinal worms and fortunately is not recommended anymore, since it is so potentially deadly and has poisoned many people and livestock. Scattered references to its former folkloric use persist, however, which could mislead someone into taking it. Symptoms are headache, tremors, convulsions, coma, blindness, heart and respiratory failure, and death.

Mechanism of Toxicity: The phloroglucinol (benzenetriol) derived from the active ingredients generates free radicals and DNA breakage, and could be in part responsible for the plant's toxicity.

MANDRAKE
(for American mandrake, see mayapple)
(Mandragora officinarum, Mandragora autumnalis)

Potential Problems: This is a classic old plant richly associated with magical tradition, most likely because its forked root resembles a man. The herb does demand respect, for all parts of it are toxic. Several dozen recent poisonings are reported in the medical literature, with symptoms of blurred vision, dizziness, headache, vomiting, abdominal pain, rapid heart rate, hallucinations, and delirium.

Mechanism of Toxicity: Mandrake contains a high concentration of atropine, hyoscyamine, and scopolamine, which oppose the action of the neurotransmitter acetylcholine by competing for its receptor.

MATÉ
(yerba maté, Paraguay tea)
(Ilex paraguariensis)

Potential Problems: Maté is a popular caffeinated beverage in South America, and although its caffeine is not much of a problem, some other constituent, possibly its tannins, may cause esophageal and gastrointestinal cancers.

Mechanism of Toxicity: Why maté appears associated with an increased risk of cancer is not known. Scientists suspect either the high concentration of tannins, or the possibility of burning the esophagus through the traditional metal bombilla straw, or both. Other caffeinated beverages are not associated with increased risk of cancer.

Mayapple
(American mandrake)

(Podophyllum peltatum)

Potential Problems: Some people take mayapple as a mandrake substitute, yet this has resulted in hospitalizations. Side effects include loss of reflexes, coma, lactic acidosis (a buildup of lactic acid in the body), and death.

Mechanism of Toxicity: Mayapple is a source of podophyllotoxin, which stops cells from dividing (antimitotic) and is the aglycone of etoposide. Podophyllotoxin proved too toxic for use in cancer therapy. It is available diluted as a prescription for careful external use in removing warts. Internal use is potentially deadly.

Mountain Ash
(rowan)

(Sorbus aucuparia)

Potential Problems: Mountain ash berries are sometimes used to make preserves. The fresh berries can cause gastric distress, kidney irritation, kidney damage, and xanthomas (benign fatty lumps under the skin.)

Mechanism of Toxicity: The parasorbic acid in the fresh berries can irritate kidneys and skin. This compound degrades to some extent when the berries are cooked or dried, so this process makes them more palatable.

Neem

(Azadirachta indica)

Potential Problems: Neem is intensely popular and included in many cosmetic products; it is also used as an organic alternative to synthetic pesticides. However, it should be kept away from children and infants. The oil can be intensely irritating, and in children Reye's syndrome–like symptoms and death have occurred within a few hours of neem oil ingestion. Symptoms include drowsiness, seizures, diarrhea, vomiting, and coma. The EPA limits its use for nonfood crops.

Mechanism of Toxicity: The toxic constituent affecting children and infants is not known, but speculations have centered on a specific monounsaturated free fatty acid in the oil. This is not the same as the insecticidal azadirachtin component, so "azadirachtin-free" oils are still unsafe for kids.

Nutmeg and Mace

(Myristica fragrans)

Potential Problems: Both come from the same tropical tree (nutmeg is the seed, and mace comes from the red outer covering of the seed), and both are safe when used in cooking. You have to intentionally eat an inordinate amount (about 9 teaspoons) before vomiting, nausea, seizures, hallucinations, and even death can occur. Some people try to abuse it to induce hallucinations.

Mechanism of Toxicity: The toxic effect appears mediated by an effect against the neurotransmitter acetylcholine. Myristicin and elemicin are thought to become amphetamine-like compounds following their metabolism, but this has not been proven. The spices contain safrole, which in large doses causes cancer.

Nux Vomica

(Strychnos nux-vomica)

Potential Problems: This plant is commonly included in homeopathic remedies, but fortunately homeopathy requires the plant be diluted to the point of its nonexistence in such remedies. Should someone try to take even a small amount of the actual plant, however, seizures and death are likely.

Mechanism of Toxicity: The plant is a source of the poison strychnine. It is a competitive antagonist of the inhibitory neurotransmitter glycine.

Oak Moss

(Evernia prunastri)

Potential Problems: Oak moss and oak moss oil are commonly sold as a fragrance and for magical ritual use over the Internet. It is sometimes recommended as an "intestinal tonic." Long-term ingestion of thujone-containing herbs can cause brain damage, however.

Mechanism of Toxicity: Oak moss contains thujone, which probably inhibits the neurotransmitter GABA in the brain, causing nerve cells to be uninhibited and fire randomly. (Thujone probably does not act like the THC from marijuana as was once thought.)

Oleander

(Nerium oleander, Nerium spp.)

Potential Problems: Although most sources warn that this plant is potentially deadly, there are still plenty of references describing its therapeutic use, which could mislead someone into trying it on their own. It has caused several fatal poisonings, with heart failure and a wide array of side effects preceding death.

Mechanism of Toxicity: All parts of oleander contain cardiac glycosides that increase the force of contraction of the heart and critically slow its beat. They bind to sodium- and potassium-pumping channels on cell membranes, increasing sodium concentration in cells and indirectly increasing calcium concentration in them, too, interfering with the heart's normal rhythm.

Oregon Grape
(barberry, mountain grape)

(Mahonia repens, Mahonia aquifolium, Berberis repens, Berberis sonnei)

Potential Problems: No adverse effects have been documented with people using Oregon grape; however, it has only newly resurged in popularity for a wide number of uses.

Mechanism of Toxicity: Theoretically, the plant's berberine content raises a concern. In low doses berberine stimulates the heart and respiratory system, but in higher doses it depresses these systems. More than 500 milligrams of berberine causes lethargy, trouble breathing, and death.

Parsley Seed Oil

(Petroselinum cripsum)

Potential Problems: Parsley herb is probably quite safe, even in large amounts. However, pure parsley oil (not to be confused with culinary vegetable oils infused with parsley) should be limited to low doses. The pure oil is usually derived from the seed, and it has a higher apiole and myristicin content than the herb. In very *large* doses apiole (10 grams apiole) and myristicin both cause side effects. Both can cause liver and kidney dysfunction, and myristicin causes hallucinations, deafness, and paralysis if inordinate amounts are taken.

Mechanism of Toxicity: The precise mechanisms aren't known. Apiole and myristicin have structures similar to safrole, a known carcinogen and liver toxin.

PAU D'ARCO

(Tabebuia impetiginosa, Tabebuia spp.)

Potential Problems: Pau d'arco is commonly sold for use in treating infections, illness, and cancer. However, serious side effects are seen with higher doses of this plant, including nausea, vomiting, diarrhea, bleeding, and anemia. The lapachol in the plant interferes with embryonic development in animal studies.

Mechanism of Toxicity: The napthoquinone lapachol from the plant is associated with its side effects. Lapachol has many different pharmacological effects and can cause excess bleeding by increasing bleeding time by extending the time required to clot blood.

PENNYROYAL

(Mentha pulegium)

Potential Problems: Pennyroyal was once a highly popular and commonly used mint family herb, but its pulegone content has since been linked to toxicity and even death. It is no longer recommended.

Mechanism of Toxicity: Pulegone is metabolized in the liver to menthofuran, which may react in the liver and damage liver cells. It can also cause neurological and

bronchial tissue damage.

PERIWINKLE

(Vinca minor, vinca spp.)

Potential Problems: The periwinkle has historically been used to treat a wide variety of disorders, like diabetes. However, side effects not unlike cancer chemotherapy (hair loss, gastrointestinal upset, nausea) occur, and the plant can also cause kidney, liver, and nerve damage. Periwinkle and its constituents are too dangerous to use therapeutically without a medical doctor's expertise.

Mechanism of Toxicity: Periwinkle contains a large number of potentially active alkaloids, including vincristine and vincamine, which bind to tubulin proteins in cells, preventing them from dividing. These alkaloids are now made synthetically for use in cancer chemotherapy.

PHEASANT'S EYE
(Adonidis herba, herba Adonidis, herb of Spring Adonis)

(Adonis vernalis)

Potential Problems: This herb is popular in Eastern Europe and as such is becoming endangered and is classified as a vulnerable species. Because of its action on the heart, it can cause heart arrhythmias and cardiac toxicity.

Mechanism of Toxicity: Pheasant's eye contains cardiac glycosides that appear similar in function to the heart drug digoxin.

PIPSISSEWA
(love in winter, prince's pine, ground holly, bitter wintergreen)

(Chimaphila umbelata)

Potential Problems: Like uva ursi, this plant is used as a urinary antiseptic. And also like uva ursi, long-term oral use may cause hydroquinone toxicity, with symptoms of ringing in the ear, vomiting, difficulty breathing, convulsions, and collapse.

Mechanism of Toxicity: Hydroquinone is antiseptic by denaturing proteins and is hard on cells in general. It may cause cancer if taken long term.

PLEURISY ROOT

(Asclepias tuberosa)

Potential Problems: Native Americans used pleurisy root for respiratory problems, and it remains relatively popular with some herbalists today, although animal studies show it has no effect on respiratory problems. At high doses it can cause heart beat irregularities; side effects are similar to those seen with overdoses of the heart medication digitalis.

Mechanism of Toxicity: The plant's digitalis-like cardiac glycosides can produce heart arrhythmias and toxicity at higher doses.

POKEWEED
(pokeberry, pokeroot, ink berry, poke, polk)

(Phytolacca americana)

Potential Problems: The greens from this Eastern American plant were once popular as an inexpensive vegetable favored by poorer county folk for use in "poke sallet."

The berries were also used for their red ink-like juice, once used to enhance the color of red wine, yet now it is realized to be dangerous. Even one berry can poison a child, and ten berries can poison an adult. The berries have been fatal, although all parts of the plant can cause poisoning. The Herb Trade Association now advises that pokeweed should not be used in foods or beverages.

Mechanism of Toxicity: Lectins from the plant cause red blood cells to clump together (agglutinate) and can cause white blood cells to develop abnormally. A family that poisoned themselves with pokeweed salad experienced cardiac symptoms hinting at extreme excitement of the vagus cranial nerve that accompanies gastrointestinal colic.

PRECATORY BEAN
(jequirity bean, rosary pea)

(Abrus precatorius)

Potential Problems: The plant was once tentatively used for wounds, respiratory problems, as a pain reliever, and ophthalmic treatment, but is now regarded as prohibitively deadly. After a few days of stomach agony, fatalities have occurred.

Mechanism of Toxicity: Abrin in this plant is a potent inhibitor of protein synthesis, and plant extracts agglutinate (clump together) red blood cells.

PULSATILLA
(Easterflower, crowfoot, windflower, meadow anemone, pasque flower)

(Pulsatilla vulgaris, Anemone pulsatilla)

Potential Problems: The plant is recommended for so-called female complaints. However, the fresh aboveground parts that are used are severely irritating and cause dermatitis, and orally they can cause gastrointestinal, kidney, and urinary tract irritation.

Mechanism of Toxicity: The ranunculin in the plant hydrolyzes to become the toxic protoanemonin, which nonspecifically reacts with cellular components and damages them. It is unstable and quickly degrades to the nontoxic anemonin.

QUEEN'S DELIGHT
(queen's root, yawroot, cockup hat, marcory, silver root, silver leaf, pavil)

(Stillingia sylvatica)

Potential Problems: The plant is still recommended for "blood purification," liver and respiratory problems, digestive problems, and as a laxative. However, it can cause nausea, vomiting, diarrhea, aches and pains, skin eruptions, depression, fatigue, and sweating.

Mechanism of Toxicity: The diterpenes in the latex are highly irritating to mucous membranes. They could theoretically potentiate the activity of dormant viruses, or cause cancer.

RHUBARB ROOT
(rheum, rhei, rhei radix, rhein, da huang)

(Rheum officinale, Rheum spp.)

Potential Problems: The cooked *stalk,* occasionally used as food, is probably quite safe for adults, despite people's fears over its oxalic acid content. Limit children's exposure to it, however; one child who ate fresh leaves from the plant was once poisoned. People with calcium oxalate kidney stones should probably avoid rhubarb, too. The *root,* on the other hand, is not normally

eaten as food, but is dried and used as the source of a laxative around the world, especially in Asia. The laxative derived from the root causes cramps and diarrhea, and long-term use is associated with heart arrhythmias and muscle weakness. Long-term use may also paralyze intestinal muscle, leading to dependency.

Mechanism of Toxicity: In very large amounts oxalic acid binds to calcium, lowering available calcium, and forming kidney stones. Anthraquinone laxatives from the root when used long term cause dehydration and serious electrolyte imbalances, such as loss of potassium. Trace anthraquinone laxatives may be present in the stem, which is used for food.

RUE
(common rue, garden rue, German rue, herb-of-grace)

(Ruta graveolens)

Potential Problems: The dried herb is still popular in some cultures as a spice in cooking and is probably quite safe when used as a seasoning. Very large amounts of *fresh* herb or oral consumption of rue oil can cause severe kidney and liver damage, depression, sleep disorders, gastrointestinal irritation, and vomiting. Topically, reactive psoralens from the plant bind to DNA when activated by sunlight, and can cause photosensitivity.

Mechanism of Toxicity: The mechanism of toxicity is not precisely known but appears associated with the oil, which is present in greater quantities in the fresh plant than in the dried herb.

Rusty-Leaved Rhododendron
(rosebay, rust-red rhododendron, snow rose)

(Rhododendron ferrugineum)

Potential Problems: This herb is used for age-related aches and pains, arthritis, and gout. However, the whole plant is considered poisonous, and vomiting, nausea, sweating, blurred vision, seizure, heart rhythm disturbances, heart attack, and respiratory arrest can occur.

Mechanism of Toxicity: Grayanotoxin hinders nerve cell conduction by closing sodium channels on cell membranes. This plant also contains arbutin, the source of hydroquinone; so long-term use will increase risk of hydroquinone toxicity, increasing cancer risk.

Saffron (autumn crocus, crocus)

(Crocus sativus)

Potential Problems: It's probably difficult to overdose on this expensive spice, because it is bitter tasting, but reportedly 12 to 20 grams of it (which is quite a lot!) can be fatal. More than 1.5 grams a day may cause side effects like yellow skin, vomiting, dizziness, internal bleeding, numbness, and uremia.

Mechanism of Toxicity: The mechanism of toxicity isn't known.

Sage

(Salvia officinalis)

Potential Problems: Sage is quite safe when used as a seasoning in cooking. Long-term, regular consumption of large amounts of thujone-containing sage species, especially fresh sage, or consuming sage oil can cause severe brain and nerve damage. Pure sage oil should never be taken internally.

Mechanism of Toxicity: Thujone is present in several species of sage (*Salvia lavandulafolia* is an exception.) Thujone is thought to disrupt the brain's signaling by hindering the activity of the inhibitory neurotransmitter GABA. Cooking, heating, or drying sage decreases its thujone content.

Sassafras

(Sassafras officinale, Sassafras spp.)

Potential Problems: Despite it's lack of any obvious therapeutic properties, sassafras was once quite popular as a tea and medicine. Its oil was used to disguise the taste of opium medicines given to children, and was used to flavor carbonated beverages in the early 1900s. However, it is now realized to cause cancer, and 5 milliliters of ingested oil can be fatal in adults. Even safrole-free sassafras, which is approved in limited amounts for food in the United States, has caused tumors in lab animals.

Mechanism of Toxicity: According to the herbalist Varro Tyler, "No one really knows just how harmful it is to human beings, but it has been estimated that one cup of strong sassafras tea could contain as much as 200 mg of safrole, more than four times the minimal amount believed hazardous to humans if consumed on a regular basis." Safrole is a well-known carcinogen, and it damages DNA. Both safrole and it's metabolite, L-hydroxysafrole, cause nerve damage as well.

SAVIN TOPS
(savin oil, savine, sabina)

(Juniperus sabina)

Potential Problems: Topically savin tops are used to treat warts, although the herb is severely irritating to skin. It is also sometimes abused in order to terminate a pregnancy. However, internal use can be fatal.

Mechanism of Toxicity: Savin tops contain a number of potentially toxic ingredients, such as thujone (see sage), podophyllotoxin (see mayapple), and hydroxycoumarins, which act as blood thinners.

SCOPOLIA
(Russian belladonna, scopola, belladonna scopola)

(Scopolia carniolica)

Potential Problems: Scopolia is too dangerous for use. Even the use of its constituent scopolamine requires medical supervision. Dry mouth, rapid heartbeat, enlarged pupils, hallucinations, coma, and death can occur. Some rare species are harvested for medicinal use in Eastern Europe, although they are endangered.

Mechanism of Toxicity: Scopolia contains the tropane alkaloids L-hyoscyamine, L-scopolamine, and atropine (dl-hyoscyamine). These block the action of the neurotransmitter acetylcholine by competing for muscarinic acetylcholine receptors. Since acetylcholine is a mediator of the "rest and digest" (parasympathetic) nervous system, blocking its action to excess causes some toxic symptoms of overexcitation.

SENNA
(sennosides, Alexandrian senna, Indian senna)

(Senna alexandrina, Cassia senna)

Potential Problems: The constituents of senna are commonly used in over-the-counter laxatives. These cause cramps and diarrhea, and long-term use is associated with heart arrhythmias and muscle weakness. Long-term use may also paralyze intestinal muscle, leading to dependency.

Mechanism of Toxicity: Anthraquinone laxatives from called *sennosides,* when used long term, cause dehydration and serious electrolyte imbalances, such as loss of potassium.

SORREL
(sour dock, sorrel dock)

(Rumex acetosa)

Potential Problems: Though the sorrel plant has a lot of oxalic acid, when used orally in food amounts the greens are probably safe for most. Limit children's exposure to it, however; one child eating another oxalic acid–containing plant (fresh rhubarb leaves) was once poisoned, although it is not clear if oxalic acid was responsible. People with calcium oxalate kidney stones should probably avoid sorrel.

Mechanism of Toxicity: In very large amounts oxalic acid binds to calcium, lowering available calcium, and precipitates as kidney stones.

SQUILL
(scilla, urginea, Urginea Maritima Baker, sea onion, sea squill, Indian squill, and white squill)

(Urginea indica, Scilla indica, Drimia indica, Urginea maritima)

Potential Problems: The use of this plant for heart and respiratory problems, for water retention, and as an expectorant is gradually diminishing where it was once popular (Europe and the Mideast). Overdose irritates the digestive system, disturbs the heart's rhythm, and can be fatal.

Mechanism of Toxicity: Squill contains cardiac glycosides with effects similar to an overdose of the heart medication digoxin.

ST. JOHN'S WORT

(Hypericum perforatom)

Potential Problems: St. John's wort is used for depression although results from clinical studies are highly variable for this use. St. John's wort increases sun-sensitivity and the likelihood of sunburn. However, the biggest concern with St. John's wort remains its ability to interfere with a large number of other medications, either potentiating their activity to a dangerous extent (as with SSRI antidepressants) or reducing their effective concentrations so that they are no longer effective (like oral birth control, cancer drugs, HIV-AIDS medications, and many, many more. You should assume that St. John's wort is likely to interfere with any other medication that you are taking.

Mechanism of Toxicity: St. John's wort can dramatically alter the activities of drug-metabolizing enzymes in the liver known as *P450 enzymes.*

STROPHANTHUS (kombe)

(Strophanthus gratus)

Potential Problems: Strophanthus seeds were once used for heart problems but are no longer recommended because of the plant's potential toxicity.

Mechanism of Toxicity: The seeds contain cardiac glycosides with activity similar to the heart medication digoxin, which in excess causes overdose. The seeds contain ouabain, the source of the poison in poison arrows traditionally used by indigenous Africans. Ouabain blocks the essential action of the sodium-potassium ATPase pump, which cells require for water balance, ion balance, and many other functions.

TANSY
(bitter buttons, buttons)

(Tanacetum vulgare, Tanacetum spp. Chrysanthenum vulgare)

Potential Problems: Tansy was once a popular bitter-tasting seasoning added to cooking, and was used for a wide variety of ailments. It is still a common garden decoration. Long-term, regular consumption of large amounts of thujone-containing herbs like tansy is known to cause severe brain and nerve damage. Its thujone content is variable, which may explain why it has not always been toxic. However, fatalities have occurred after consuming tansy tea or powdered tansy.

Mechanism of Toxicity: Thujone is variably present in the oil, ranging from 0 to 95 percent. Thujone is thought to disrupt the brain's signaling by hindering the activity of the inhibitory neurotransmitter GABA.

TEA TREE OIL
(melaleuca)

(Melaleuca alternifolia)

Potential Problems: Tea tree oil has become a popular antiseptic and fragrant component of cosmetic products. On skin it can be extremely irritating, especially if concentrated. It may cause damage to hearing if used in the ears. It should never be used internally, as this has resulted in hospitalizations and coma, and children and pets are particularly sensitive to the oil.

Mechanism of Toxicity: The oil contains terpenes that nonspecifically disrupt cell membranes, killing the cell. This is the mechanism for both the antibiotic and skin-irritating action.

TONKA BEAN

(Dipteryx oderata, Coumarouna odorata)

Potential Problems: Tonka bean is used to impart a vanilla-like flavoring to foods and beverages, but this is illegal in the United States. It is also suggested for use treating cramps and cough, and as an aphrodisiac. However, large amounts can paralyze the heart, while smaller amounts may cause nausea, vomiting, or dizziness.

Mechanism of Toxicity: The beans' vanilla scent is due to coumarin, a blood thinner, which can be toxic in overdose.

UVA URSI

(Arctostaphylos uva-ursi)

Potential Problems: Uva ursi is used in diuretics and as a urinary antiseptic, but long-term use increases cancer risk and skin and eye problems.

Mechanism of Toxicity: Hydroquinone is antiseptic by denaturing proteins and is hard on cells in general. It may cause cancer if taken long term.

WAHOO
(spindle bark, spindle tree, arrow wood, bitter ash, burning bush, Indian arrow)

(Euonymus atropurpurea)

Potential Problems: The root bark is used as a laxative, as a diuretic, and to stimulate bile. The bark and berries are considered poisonous, and eating the seeds or berries has proved fatal in some instances.

Mechanism of Toxicity: The poison causing fatalities has not been identified, but wahoo contains caffeine and steroid-like molecules called *cardenolides* that affect the heart. Cardenolides are also toxic components in milkweed.

WHITE COHOSH
(baneberry, doll's eyes, necklace weed)

(Actaea pachypoda, Actaea alba)

Potential Problems: White cohosh was once used for "women's problems" like black cohosh is today, but avoid confusing the two. White cohosh is poisonous. It may cause gastrointestinal upset, vomiting, and circulatory failure.

Mechanism of Toxicity: The plant is a source of the severely irritating and toxic chemical called *protoanemonin*.

WILD LETTUCE
(lettuce opium, bitter lettuce)

(Lactuca virosa)

Potential Problems: This plant is not used like other lettuces, but as a sedative. According to animal studies, its debatably sedative components could be the unstable molecules lactucin and lactucopricin. It apparently does not contain hyoscyamine or morphine as was formerly suggested. In very large amounts it has caused stupor, depressed breathing, and even death.

Mechanism of Toxicity: The mechanism of toxicity is not known.

WINTERGREEN
(box berry, checker cherry, partridge berry, spice berry, tea berry)

(Gaultheria procumbens)

Potential Problems: This herb has many of the same precautions as those for aspirin. For adults, the wintergreen leaf is probably safe in limited amounts or in tea, although the methyl salicylate is likely to upset the stomach even more than aspirin. Children should be kept away from wintergreen products, because they may cause Reye syndrome, and children are more vulnerable to salicylates. Wintergreen oil, which is used to flavor candy, has killed curious children who accidentally drank it when the cook's back was turned. Even very liberal topical use of wintergreen oil can cause symptoms akin to aspirin overdose in children and adults.

Mechanism of Toxicity: Methyl salicylate in oil of wintergreen works similarly to aspirin and therefore also causes "aspirin" overdose if too much is taken.

WOOD SORREL
(oxalis, shamrock plant, sourgrass, sour trefoil, hearts)

(Oxalis spp.)

Potential Problems: I enjoyed munching on this as a kid growing up in Southern California and called it sourgrass. It is occasionally used as an exotic salad additive and for digestive problems. The plant has a lot of oxalic acid, but when used in limited quantities in food the greens are probably safe for most. Limit children's exposure to it, however; one child ate fresh rhubarb (see above entry for rhubarb), which also possess a lot of oxalic acid, and was once poisoned, although it is not clear if oxalic acid was responsible. People with calcium oxalate kidney stones should probably avoid wood sorrel.

Mechanism of Toxicity: In very large amounts oxalic acid binds to calcium, lowering available calcium, and forms kidney stones.

WORMWOOD
(artemesia, absinthe, green ginger, green fairy)

(Artemesia absinthum)

Potential Problems: Wormwood was once used against intestinal worms and is still used as a flavoring and fragrance, yet must be thujone-free prior to use in the United States for flavoring food or beverages. Wormwood is one of the principal ingredients in the alcoholic beverage absinthe, which famously caused epidemic brain damage in the late nineteenth century. Long-term or acute thujone exposure from this or other thujone-containing plants is known to cause brain damage.

Mechanism of Toxicity: Wormwood oil contains 3–12 percent thujone, considered a narcotic poison. It probably inhibits the neurotransmitter GABA in the brain, causing nerve cells to be uninhibited and fire randomly. (As noted with oak moss, thujone probably does not act like the THC from marijuana as was once thought.)

YOHIMBE
(johimbe, yohimbine)

(Pausinystalia yohimbe)

Potential Problems: Yohimbe has become a popular herb for male sexual dysfunction, but in excess it causes heart problems, severe low blood pressure, and even death. Smaller amounts can engender a state of fear or anxiety.

Mechanism of Toxicity: Yohimbine alkaloid stimulates the sympathetic nervous system.

NOTES

References for Aloe

1. D. P. West, and Y. F. Zhu, "Evaluation of aloe vera gel gloves in the treatment of dry skin associated with occupational exposure," *Am J Infect Control* 2003 Feb; 31(1): 40–42.
2. M. R. Poor, J. E. Hall, and A. S. Poor, "Reduction in the incidence of alveolar osteitis in patients treated with the SaliCept patch, containing Acemannan hydrogel," *J Oral Maxillofac Surg* 2002 Apr; 60(4): 374–79; discussion 379.
3. D. L. Olsen, W. Raub Jr., C. Bradley, M. Johnson, J. L. Macias, V. Love, and A. Markoe, "The effect of aloe vera gel/mild soap versus mild soap alone in preventing skin reactions in patients undergoing radiation therapy," *Oncol Nurs Forum* 2001 Apr; 28(3): 543–47.
4. S. Heggie, G. P. Bryant, L. Tripcony, J. Keller, P. Rose, M. Glendenning, and J. Heath, "A Phase III study on the efficacy of topical aloe vera gel on irradiated breast tissue," *Cancer Nurs* 2002 Dec; 25(6): 442–51.
5. M. S. Williams, M. Burk, C. L. Loprinzi, M. Hill, P. J. Schomberg, K. Nearhood, J. R. O'Fallon, J. A. Laurie, T. G. Shanahan, R. L. Moore, R. E. Urias, R. R. Kuske, R. E. Engel, and W. D. Eggleston, "Phase III double-blind evaluation of an aloe vera gel as a prophylactic agent for radiation-induced skin toxicity," *Int J Radiat Oncol Biol Phys* 1996 Sep 1; 36(2): 345–49.
6. D. R. Thomas, P. S. Goode, K. LaMaster, and T. Tennyson, "Acemannan hydrogel dressing versus saline dressing for pressure ulcers. A randomized, controlled trial," *Adv Wound Care* 1998 Oct; 11(6): 273–76.
7. J. M. Schmidt, and J. S. Greenspoon, "Aloe vera dermal wound gel is associated with a delay in wound healing," *Obstet Gyneco* 1991 Jul; 78(1): 115–17.
8. T. A. Syed, S. A. Ahmad, A. H. Holt, S. A. Ahmad, S. H. Ahmad, and M. Afzal, "Management of psoriasis with Aloe vera extract in a hydrophilic cream: a placebo-controlled, double-blind study," *Trop Med Int Health* 1996 Aug; 1(4): 505–09.
9. J. J. Blitz, J. W. Smith, and J. R. Gerard, "Aloe vera gel in peptic ulcer therapy: preliminary report," *J Am Osteopath Assoc* 1963 Apr; 62:731–35.
10. L. Langmead, R. M. Feakins, S. Goldthorpe, H. Holt, E. Tsironi, A. De Silva, D. P. Jewell, and D. S. Rampton, "Randomized, double-blind, placebo-controlled trial of oral aloe vera gel for active ulcerative colitis," *Aliment Pharmacol Ther* 2004 Apr 1; 19(7): 739–47.

References for Arnica

1. C. Ciganda, and A. Laborde, "Herbal infusions used for induced abortion," *J Toxicol Clin Toxicol* 2003; 41(3): 235–39.
2. Martin Gardner, *On the Wild Side* (Buffalo, NY: Prometheus Books, 1992), 31–40.
3. G. S. Kaziro, "Metronidazole (Flagyl) and Arnica Montana in the prevention of post-surgical complications, a comparative placebo-controlled clinical trial," *Br J Oral Maxillofac Surg* 1984 Feb; 22(1): 42–49.

4. E. Ernst, and M. H. Pittler, "Efficacy of homeopathic arnica: a systematic review of placebo-controlled clinical trials," *Arch Surg* 1998 Nov; 133(11): 1187–90. Review.
5. A. J. Vickers, P. Fisher, C. Smith, S. E. Wyllie, and R. Rees, "Homeopathic Arnica 30x is ineffective for muscle soreness after long-distance running: a randomized, double-blind, placebo-controlled trial," *Clin J Pain* 1998 Sep; 14(3): 227–31.
6. O. Hart, M. A. Mullee, G. Lewith, and J. Miller, "Double-blind, placebo-controlled, randomized clinical trial of homoeopathic arnica C30 for pain and infection after total abdominal hysterectomy," *J R Soc Med* 1997 Feb; 90(2): 73–78.
7. L. Baillargeon, J. Drouin, L. Desjardins, D. Leroux, and D. Audet, "The effects of Arnica Montana on blood coagulation. Randomized controlled trial," *Can Fam Physician* 1993 Nov; 39:2362–67.
8. D. Tveiten, S. Bruseth, C. F. Borchgrevink, and K. Lohne, "Effect of Arnica D 30 during hard physical exertion. A double-blind randomized trial during the Oslo Marathon 1990," *Tidsskr Nor Laegeforen* 1991 Dec 10; 111(30): 3630–31.
9. M. Kucera, O. Horacek, J. Kalal, P. Kolar, P. Korbelar, and Z. Polesna, "Synergetic analgesic effect of the combination of arnica and hydroxyethyl salicylate in ethanolic solution following cutaneous application by transcutaneous electrostimulation," *Arzneimittelforschung* 2003; 53(12): 850–56.
10. O. Knuesel, M. Weber, and A. Suter, "Arnica montana gel in osteoarthritis of the knee: an open, multicenter clinical trial," *Adv Ther* 2002 Sep–Oct; 19(5): 209–18.
11. D. Alonso, M. C. Lazarus, and L. Baumann, "Effects of topical arnica gel on post–laser treatment bruises," *Dermatol Surg* 2002 Aug; 28(8): 686–88.
12. S. L. Jeffrey, and H. J. Belcher, "Use of Arnica to relieve pain after carpal-tunnel release surgery," *Altern Ther Health Med* 2002 Mar–Apr; 8(2): 66–68.

References for Artichoke

1. W. Englisch, C. Beckers, M. Unkauf, M. Ruepp, and V. Zinserling, "Efficacy of Artichoke dry extract in patients with hyperlipoproteinemia," *Arzneimittelforschung* 2000 Mar; 50(3): 260–65.
2. H. Heckers, K. Dittmar, F. W. Schmahl, and K. Huth, "Inefficiency of cynarin as therapeutic regimen in familial type II hyperlipoproteinaemia," *Atherosclerosis* 1977 Feb; 26(2): 249–53.
3. M. Montini, P. Levoni, A. Ongaro, and G. Pagani, "Controlled application of cynarin in the treatment of hyperlipemic syndrome. Observations in 60 cases," *Arzneimittelforschung* 1975 Aug; 25(8): 1311–14.
4. R. Gebhardt, "Inhibition of cholesterol biosynthesis in primary cultured rat hepatocytes by artichoke (*Cynara scolymus L.*) extracts," *J Pharmacol Exp Ther* 1998 Sep; 286(3): 1122–28.
5. G. Holtmann, B. Adam, S. Haag, W. Collet, E.

Grunewald, and T. Windeck, "Efficacy of artichoke leaf extract in the treatment of patients with functional dyspepsia: a six-week placebo-controlled, double-blind, multicentre trial," *Aliment Pharmacol Ther* 2003 Dec; 18(11–12): 1099–105.

6. G. Marakis, A. F. Walker, R. W. Middleton, J. C. Booth, J. Wright, and D. J. Pike, "Artichoke leaf extract reduces mild dyspepsia in an open study," *Phytomedicine* 2002 Dec; 9(8): 694–99.

7. A. F. Walker, and G. Marakis, "Cynara scolymus: Artichoke leaf extract relieves the symptoms of Irritable Bowel Syndrome," *Phytotherapy Research* 15, 58 2001.

8. E. Speroni, R. Cervellati, P. Govoni, S. Guizzardi, C. Renzulli, and M. C. Guerra, "Efficacy of different Cynara scolymus preparations on liver complaints," *J Ethnopharmacol* 2003 Jun; 86(2–3): 203–11.

9. R. Gebhardt, "Prevention of taurolithocholate-induced hepatic bile canalicular distortions by HPLC-characterized extracts of artichoke (*Cynara scolymus*) leaves," *Planta Med* 2002 Sep; 68(9): 776–79.

10. T. Saenz Rodriguez, D. Garcia Gimenez, and R. de la Puerta Vazquez, "Choleretic activity and biliary elimination of lipids and bile acids induced by an artichoke leaf extract in rats," *Phytomedicine* 2002 Dec; 9(8): 687–93.

11. A. Betancor-Fernandez, A. Perez-Galvez, H. Sies, and W. Stahl, "Screening pharmaceutical preparations containing extracts of turmeric rhizome, artichoke leaf, devil's claw root, and garlic or salmon oil for antioxidant capacity," *J Pharm Pharmacol* 2003 Jul; 55(7): 981–86.

12. J. E. Brown, and C. A. Rice-Evans, "Luteolin-rich artichoke extract protects low-density lipoprotein from oxidation in vitro," *Free Radic Res* 1998 Sep; 29(3): 247–55.

13. A. Jimenez-Escrig, L. O. Dragsted, B. Daneshvar, R. Pulido, and F. Saura-Calixto, "In vitro antioxidant activities of edible artichoke (*Cynara scolymus L.*) and effect on biomarkers of antioxidants in rats," *J Agric Food Chem* 2003 Aug 27; 51(18): 5540–45.

14. R. Gebhardt, "Antioxidative and protective properties of extracts from leaves of the artichoke (*Cynara scolymus L.*) against hydroperoxide-induced oxidative stress in cultured rat hepatocytes," *Toxicol Appl Pharmacol* 1997 Jun; 144(2): 279–86.

References for Astragalus

1. J. Xue, Y. Xu, Z. Zhang, G. Shen, and G. Zeng, "The effect of astragapolysaccharide on the lymphocyte proliferation and airway inflammation in sensitized mice," *J Tongji Med Univ* 1999; 19(1): 20–22, 30.

2. X. S. Weng, "Treatment of leucopenia with pure Astragalus preparation—an analysis of 115 leucopenic cases," *Zhongguo Zhong Xi Yi Jie He Za Zhi* 1995 Aug; 15(8): 462–64.

3. Z. Q. Huang, N. P. Qin, and W. Ye, "Effect of Astragalus membranaceus on T-lymphocyte subsets in patients with viral myocarditis," *Zhongguo Zhong Xi Yi Jie He Za Zhi* 1995 Jun; 15(6): 328–30.

4. Z. Y. Lei, H. Qin, and J. Z. Liao, "Action of Astragalus membranaceus on left ventricular function of angina pectoris," *Zhongguo Zhong Xi Yi Jie He Za Zhi* 1994 Apr; 14(4): 199–202, 195.

5. H. M. Luo, R. H. Dai, and Y. Li, "Nuclear cardiology study on effective ingredients of Astragalus mem-

branaceus in treating heart failure," *Zhongguo Zhong Xi Yi Jie He Za Zhi* 1995 Dec; 15(12): 707–09.

6. J. Ma, A. Peng, and S. Lin, "Mechanisms of the therapeutic effect of astragalus membranaceus on sodium and water retention in experimental heart failure," *Chin Med J* (Engl) 1998 Jan; 111(1): 17–23.

References for Bilberry

1. P. H. Canter, and E. Ernst, "Anthocyanosides of Vaccinium myrtillus (bilberry) for night vision—a systematic review of placebo-controlled trials," *Surv Ophthalmol* 2004 Jan–Feb; 49(1): 38–50.

2. G. E. Jayle, and L. Aubert, "Action of anthosyanin glycosides on the scotopic and mesoic vision of the normal subject," *Therapie* 1964 Jan–Feb; 19:171–85.

3. Y. Levy, and Y. Glovinsky, "The effect of anthocyanosides on night vision," *Eye* 1998; 12:967–69.

4. H. M. Mayser, and H. Wilhelm, "Effects of anthocyanosides on contrast vision," *Invest Ophthalmol Vis Sci* 2001; 42 (Suppl): 63.

5. E. Muth, J. Laurent, and P. Jasper, "The effect of bilberry nutritional supplementation on night visual acuity and contrast sensitivity," *Altern Med Rev* 2000; 5:164–73.

6. D. Zadok, Y. Levy, and Y. Glovinsky, "The effect of anthocyanosides in a multiple oral dose on night vision," *Eye* 1999; 13:734–36.

7. R. Alfieri, and P. Sole, "Influence des anthocyanosides administres par voie or-perlinguale sur l'adapto-electroretinogramme (AERG) en lumiere rouge chez l'homme," *Soc Biol Clermont-Ferrand* 1966; 160:1590–93.

8. L. Belleoud, D. Leluan, and Y. Boyer, "Etude des effets des glucosides d'anthocyane sur la vision nocturne du personnel navigant," *Rev Med Aeronaut Spat* 1967; 6:5–10.

9. G. E. Jayle, M. Aubry, H. Gavini, et al., "Etude concernant l'action sur la vision nocturne des anthocyanosides extrait du Vaccinium myrtillus," *Ann Ocul* 1965; 198:556–62.

10. A. Magnasco, and M. Zingirian, "Influence of anthocyanosides on the mesopic differential threshold of the retina," *Ann Ottalmol Clin Ocul* 1966; 92:188–93.

11. F. Ponte, and M. Lauricella, "Effect of Vaccinium myrtillus total extract on the recovery in the dark of the human electroretinogram," *Atti VII Simposio ISCERG* Istanbul (1969): 355–66.

12. D. Sala, P. L. Rossi, S. D. Rolando, et al., "Effetto degli antocianosidi sulle 'performances' visive alle basse luminanze," *Minerva Oftalmol* 1979; 21:283–85.

13. F. Sbrozzi, J. Landini, and M. Zago, "Night vision affected by antocyanosides. An electoretinographic test," *Minerva Oftalmol* 1983; 24:189–93.

14. G. E. Jayle, L. Aubert, op cit.

15. R. Alfieri, and P. Sole, "Influence of Anthocyanosides Administered Parenterally on the Adapto-Electroretinogram of the Rabbit," *C R Soc Biol* 1964; 158:2338–41.

16. G. Cavallacci, and C. Marconcini, "Appraisal of modification induced by anthocyanosides using ERG," *Minerva Oftalmol* 1979; 21:339.

17. F. Rouher, and P. Sole, "Can one improve the night vision of the automobile drivers?" *Ann Med Accid Traffic* (1965): 3–4.

18. H. Matsumoto, Y. Nakamura, S. Tachibanaki, S.

Kawamura, and M. Hirayama, "Stimulatory effect of cyanidin 3–glycosides on the regeneration of rhodopsin," *J Agric Food Chem* 2003 Jun 4; 51(12): 3560–63.

19. J. R. Sparrow, H. R. Vollmer-Snarr, J. Zhou, Y. P. Jang, S. Jockusch, Y. Itagaki, and K. Nakanishi, "A2E-epoxides damage DNA in retinal pigment epithelial cells. Vitamin E and other antioxidants inhibit A2E-epoxide formation," *J Biol Chem* 2003 May 16; 278(20): 18207–13. E-pub, 2003 Mar 19.

20. N. Katsube, K. Iwashita, T. Tsushida, K. Yamaki, and M. Kobori, "Induction of apoptosis in cancer cells by Bilberry (*Vaccinium myrtillus*) and the anthocyanins," *J Agric Food Chem* 2003 Jan 1; 51(1): 68–75.

21. D. Bagchi, C. K. Sen, M. Bagchi, and M. Atalay, "Anti-angiogenic, antioxidant, and anti-carcinogenic properties of a novel anthocyanin-rich berry extract formula," *Biochemistry* (Mosc) 2004 Jan; 69(1): 75–80.

References for Black Cohosh

1. E. J. Kennelly, S. Baggett, P. Nuntanakorn, A. L. Ososki, S. A. Mori, J. Duke, M. Coleton, and F. Kronenberg, "Analysis of thirteen populations of black cohosh for formononetin," *Phytomedicine* 2002 Jul; 9(5): 461–67.

2. J. E. Burdette, J. Liu, S. N. Chen, D. S. Fabricant, C. E. Piersen, E. L. Barker, J. M. Pezzuto, A. Mesecar, R. B. Van Breemen, N. R. Farnsworth, and J. L. Bolton, "Black cohosh acts as a mixed competitive ligand and partial agonist of the serotonin receptor," *J Agric Food Chem* 2003 Sep 10; 51(19): 5661–70.

3. G. B. Mahady, "Is black cohosh estrogenic?" *Nutr Rev* 2003 May; 61(5 Pt 1): 183–86.

4. K. Hostanska, T. Nisslein, J. Freudenstein, J. Reichling, and R. Saller, "Cimicifuga racemosa extract inhibits proliferation of estrogen receptor–positive and negative human breast carcinoma cell lines by induction of apoptosis," *Breast Cancer Res Treat* 2004 Mar; 84(2): 151–60.

5. K. Hostanska, T. Nisslein, J. Freudenstein, J. Reichling, and R. Saller, "Evaluation of cell death caused by triterpene glycosides and phenolic substances from Cimicifuga racemosa extract in human MCF-7 breast cancer cells," *Biol Pharm Bull* 2004 Dec; 27(12): 1970–75.

6. H. Jarry, P. Thelen, V. Christoffel, B. Spengler, and W. Wuttke, "Cimicifuga racemosa extract BNO 1055 inhibits proliferation of the human prostate cancer cell line LNCaP," *Phytomedicine* 2005 Mar; 12(3): 178–82.

7. B. Kligler, "Black cohosh," *Am Fam Physician* 2003; 68:114–16.

8. M. Thomsen, and M. Schmidt, "Hepatotoxicity from Cimicifuga racemosa? Recent Australian case report not sufficiently substantiated," *J Altern Complement Med* 2003 Jun; 9(3): 337–40.

9. B. Kligler, et al., op. cit.

10. J. S. Jacobson, A. B. Troxel, J. Evans, L. Klaus, L. Vahdat, D. Kinne, K. M. Lo, A. Moore, P. J. Rosenman, E. L. Kaufman, A. I. Neugut, and V. R. Grann, "Randomized trial of black cohosh for the treatment of hot flashes among women with a history of breast cancer," *J Clin Oncol* 2001 May 15; 19(10): 2739–45.

11. T. Nisslein, and J. Freudenstein, "Effects of an isopropanolic extract of Cimicifuga racemosa on urinary

crosslinks and other parameters of bone quality in an ovariectomized rat model of osteoporosis," *J Bone Miner Metab* 2003; 21(6):370–76.

12. W. Wuttke, D. Seidlova-Wuttke, and C. Gorkow, "The Cimicifuga preparation BNO 1055 vs. conjugated estrogens in a double-blind, placebo-controlled study: effects on menopause symptoms and bone markers," *Maturitas* 2003 Mar 14; 44 Suppl 1:S67–77.

References for Borage

1. Violet Schafer, *Herbcraft: A Compendium of Myths, Romance and Commonsense* (San Francisco: Yerba Buena Press, 1971).

2. E. A. Miles, T. Banerjee, and P. C. Calder, "The influence of different combinations of gamma-linolenic, stearidonic and eicosapentaenoic acids on the fatty acid composition of blood lipids and mononuclear cells in human volunteers," *Prostaglandins Leukot Essent Fatty Acids* 2004 Jun; 70(6): 529–38.

3. L. J. Leventhal, E. G. Boyce, and R. B. Zurier, "Treatment of rheumatoid arthritis with gammalinolenic acid," *Ann Intern Med* 1993 Nov 1; 119(9): 867–73.

4. R. B. Zurier, R. G. Rossetti, E. W. Jacobson, D. M. DeMarco, N. Y. Liu, J. E. Temming, B. M. White, and M. Laposata, "Gamma-Linolenic acid treatment of rheumatoid arthritis. A randomized, placebo-controlled trial," *Arthritis Rheum* 1996 Nov; 39(11): 1808–17.

5. B. M. Henz, S. Jablonska, P. C. van de Kerkhof, G. Stingl, M. Blaszczyk, P. G. Vandervalk, R. Veenhuizen, R. Muggli, and D. Raederstorff, "Double-blind, multicentre analysis of the efficacy of borage oil in patients with atopic eczema," *Br J Dermatol* 1999 Apr; 140(4): 685–88.

6. A. Takwale, E. Tan, S. Agarwal, G. Barclay, I. Ahmed, K. Hotchkiss, J. R. Thompson, T. Chapman, and J. Berth-Jones, "Efficacy and tolerability of borage oil in adults and children with atopic eczema: randomised, double-blind, placebo-controlled, parallel group trial," *BMJ* 2003 Dec 13; 327(7428): 1385.

7. C. J. van Gool, C. Thijs, C. J. Henquet, A. C. van Houwelingen, P. C. Dagnelie, J. Schrander, P. P. Menheere, and P. A. van den Brandt, "Gamma-linolenic acid supplementation for prophylaxis of atopic dermatitis—a randomized controlled trial in infants at high familial risk," *Am J Clin Nutr* 2003 Apr; 77(4): 943–51.

8. V. A. Ziboh, S. Naguwa, K. Vang, J. Wineinger, B. M. Morrissey, M. Watnik, and M. E. Gershwin, "Suppression of leukotriene B4 generation by ex-vivo neutrophils isolated from asthma patients on dietary supplementation with gammalinolenic acid-containing borage oil: possible implication in asthma," *Clin Dev Immunol* 2004 Mar; 11(1): 13–21.

9. J. E. Gadek, S. J. DeMichele, M. D. Karlstad, E. R. Pacht, M. Donahoe, T. E. Albertson, C. Van Hoozen, A. K. Wennberg, J. L. Nelson, and M. Noursalehi, "Effect of enteral feeding with eicosapentaenoic acid, gamma-linolenic acid, and antioxidants in patients with acute respiratory distress syndrome," Enteral Nutrition in ARDS Study Group, *Crit Care Med* 1999 Aug; 27(8): 1409–20.

10. M. S. Fewtrell, R. A. Abbott, K. Kennedy, A. Singhal, R. Morley, E. Caine, C. Jamieson, F. Cockburn, and A. Lucas, "Randomized, double-blind trial of long-chain

polyunsaturated fatty acid supplementation with fish oil and borage oil in preterm infants," *J Pediatr* 2004 Apr; 144(4): 471–79.

11. B. K. Saevik, K. Bergvall, B. R. Holm, L. E. Saijonmaa-Koulumies, A. Hedhammar, S. Larsen, and F. Kristensen, "A randomized, controlled study to evaluate the steroid sparing effect of essential fatty acid supplementation in the treatment of canine atopic dermatitis," *Vet Dermatol* 2004 Jun; 15(3): 137–45.

References for Cascara Sagrada

1. P. F. Giavina-Bianchi Jr, F. F. Castro, M. L. Machado, and A. J. Duarte, "Occupational respiratory allergic disease induced by Passiflora alata and Rhamnus purshiana," *Ann Allergy Asthma Immunol* 1997 Nov; 79(5): 449–54.

2. A. Pierce, *The American Pharmaceutical Association Practical Guide to Natural Medicines* (New York: Stonesong Press, 1999).

3. P. P. But, B. Tomlinson, and K. L. Lee, "Hepatitis related to the Chinese medicine Shouwu Pian, manufactured from Polygonum multiflorum," *Veterinary and Human Toxicology* 1996; 38(4): 280–82.

4. G. J. Park, S. P. Mann, and M. C. Ngu, "Acute hepatitis induced by Shouwu Pian, a herbal product derived from Polygonum multiflorum," *Journal of Gastroenterology and Hepatology* 2001; 16(1): 115–17.

5. A. Nair, D. Reddy, and D. H. Van Thiel, "Cascara sagrada induced intrahepatic cholestasis causing portal hypertension: case report and review of herbal hepatotoxicity," *American Journal of Gastroenterology* 2000; 95(12): 3634–37.

6. P. F. D'Arcy, "Adverse reactions and interactions with herbal medicines, Part 1," *Adverse Drug Reactions and Toxicology Reviews* 1991; 10(4): 189–208.

7. E. Mereto, M. Ghia, and G. Brambilla, "Evaluation of the potential carcinogenic activity of Senna and Cascara glycosides for the rat colon," *Cancer Lett* 1996 Mar 19; 101(1): 79–83.

8. N. Mascolo, E. Mereto, F. Borrelli, P. Orsi, D. Sini, A. A. Izzo, B. Massa, M. Boggio, and F. Capasso, "Does senna extract promote growth of aberrant crypt foci and malignant tumors in rat colon?" *Dig Dis Sci* 1999 Nov; 44(11): 2226–30.

9. C. P. Siegers, E. von Hertzberg-Lottin, M. Otte, and B. Schneider, "Anthranoid laxative abuse—a risk for colorectal cancer?" *Gut* 1993 Aug; 34(8): 1099–101.

References for Catnip

1. J. A. Duke, *CRC Handbook of Medicinal Herbs* (Boca Raton, FL: CRC Press, 1985).

2. K. C. Osterhoudt, S. K. Lee, J. M. Callahan, and F. M. Henretig, *Veterinary and Human Toxicology* 1997; 39:373–75.

3. C. Peterson, and J. Coates, *Pesticide Outlook* 2001; 12(4): 154–58.

4. A. Pierce, *The American Pharmaceutical Association Practical Guide to Natural Medicines* (New York: Stonesong Press, 1999).

References for Cat's Claw

1. M. Sandoval, R. M. Charbonnet, N. N. Okuhama, J. Roberts, Z. Krenova, A. M. Trentacosti, and J. M. Miller, "Cat's claw inhibits TNFalpha production and scavenges free radicals: role in cytoprotection," *Free*

Radic Biol Med 2000 Jul 1; 29(1): 71–78.

2. S. Lamm, Y. Sheng, and R. W. Pero, "Persistent response to pneumococcal vaccine in individuals supplemented with a novel water-soluble extract of Uncaria tomentosa, C-Med-100," *Phytomedicine* 2001 Jul; 8(4): 267–74.

3. Ibid.

4. J. Piscoya, Z. Rodriguez, S. A. Bustamante, N. N. Okuhama, M. J. Miller, and M. Sandoval, "Efficacy and safety of freeze-dried cat's claw in osteoarthritis of the knee: mechanisms of action of the species Uncaria guianensis," *Inflamm Res* 2001 Sep; 50(9): 442–48.

5. E. Mur, F. Hartig, G. Eibl, and M. Schirmer, "Randomized double-blind trial of an extract from the pentacyclic alkaloid-chemotype of uncaria tomentosa for the treatment of rheumatoid arthritis," *J Rheumatol* 2002 Apr; 29(4): 678–81.

6. C. Winkler, B. Wirleitner, K. Schroecksnadel, H. Schennach, E. Mur, and D. Fuchs, "In vitro effects of two extracts and two pure alkaloid preparations of Uncaria tomentosa on peripheral blood mononuclear cells," *Planta Med* 2004 Mar; 70(3): 205–10.

7. M. Sandoval, N. N. Okuhama, X. J. Zhang, L. A. Condezo, J. Lao, F. M. Angeles, R. A. Musah, P. Bobrowski, and M. J. Miller, "Anti-inflammatory and antioxidant activities of cat's claw (Uncaria tomentosa and Uncaria guianensis) are independent of their alkaloid content," *Phytomedicine* 2002 May; 9(4): 325–37.

References for Chamomile

1. D. Kavvadias, P. Sand, K. A. Youdim, M. Z. Qaiser, C. Rice-Evans, R. Baur, E. Sigel, W. D. Rausch, P. Riederer, and P. Schreier, "The flavone hispidulin, a benzodiazepine receptor ligand with positive allosteric properties, traverses the blood-brain barrier and exhibits anticonvulsive effects," *Br J Pharmacol* 2004 Jul; 142(5): 811–20.

2. A. Yamamoto, K. Nakamura, K. Furukawa, Y. Konishi, T. Ogino, K. Higashiura, H. Yago, K. Okamoto, and M. Otsuka, "A new nonpeptide tachykinin NK1 receptor antagonist isolated from the plants of Compositae," *Chem Pharm Bull* (Tokyo) 2002 Jan; 50(1): 47–52.

3. Y. C. Liang, Y. T. Huang, S. H. Tsai, S. Y. Lin-Shiau, C. F. Chen, and J. K. Lin, "Suppression of inducible cyclooxygenase and inducible nitric oxide synthase by apigenin and related flavonoids in mouse macrophages," *Carcinogenesis* 1999 Oct; 20(10): 1945–52.

4. P. Imming, S. Goeters, G. Pawlitzki, and B. Hempel, "Absolute stereochemistry of guaianolides, of matricin and its epimers, of yarrow proazulenes, and of chamazulene carboxylic acid," *Chirality* 2001 Jul; 13(7): 337–41.

5. P. Zanoli, R. Avallone, and M. Baraldi, "Behavioral characterisation of the flavonoids apigenin and chrysin," *Fitoterapia* 2000 Aug; 71 Suppl 1:S117–23.

6. H. Viola, C. Wasowski, M. Levi de Stein, C. Wolfman, R. Silveira, F. Dajas, J. H. Medina, and A. C. Paladini, "Apigenin, a component of Matricaria recutita flowers, is a central benzodiazepine receptors-ligand with anxiolytic effects," *Planta Med* 1995 Jun; 61(3): 213–16.

7. C. Wolfman, H. Viola, A. Paladini, F. Dajas, and J. H. Medina, "Possible anxiolytic effects of chrysin, a central benzodiazepine receptor ligand isolated from

Passiflora coerulea," *Pharmacol Biochem Behav* 1994 Jan; 47(1): 1–4.

8. J. H. Medina, A. C. Paladini, C. Wolfman, M. Levi de Stein, D. Calvo, L. E. Diaz, and C. Pena, "Chrysin (5,7–di-OH-flavone), a naturally-occurring ligand for benzodiazepine receptors, with anticonvulsant properties," *Biochem Pharmacol* 1990 Nov 15; 40(10): 2227–31.

9. J. B. Salgueiro, P. Ardenghi M. Dias, M. B. Ferreira, I. Izquierdo, and J. H. Medina, "Anxiolytic natural and synthetic flavonoid ligands of the central benzodiazepine receptor have no effect on memory tasks in rats," *Pharmacol Biochem Behav* 1997 Dec; 58(4): 887–91.

10. A. Gomaa, T. Hashem, A. Mohamed, and E. Ashry, "Matricaria chamomilla extract inhibits both development of morphine dependence and expression of abstinence syndrome in rats," *J Pharmacol Sci* 2003 May; 92(1): 50–55.

11. A. C. Paladini, M. Marder, H. Viola, C. Wolfman, C. Wasowski, and J. H. Medina, "Flavonoids and the central nervous system: from forgotten factors to potent anxiolytic compounds," *J Pharm Pharmacol* 1999 May; 51(5): 519–26.

12. H. J. Glowania, C. Raulin, and M. Swoboda, "Effect of chamomile on wound healing—a clinical double-blind study," *Z Hautkr* 1987 Sep 1; 62(17): 1262, 1267–71.

13. P. Aertgeerts, M. Albring, F. Klaschka, T. Nasemann, R. Patzelt-Wenczler, K. Rauhut, and B. Weigl, "Comparative testing of Kamillosan cream and steroidal (0.25% hydrocortisone, 0.75% fluocortin butyl ester) and non-steroidal (5% bufexamac) dermatologic agents in maintenance therapy of eczematous diseases," *Z Hautkr* 1985 Feb 1; 60(3): 270–77.

14. R. Patzelt-Wenczler, and E. Ponce-Poschl, "Proof of efficacy of Kamillosan(R) cream in atopic eczema," *Eur J Med Res* 2000 Apr 19; 5(4): 171–75.

15. O. Kyokong, S. Charuluxananan, V. Muangmingsuk, O. Rodanant, K. Subornsug, and W. Punyasang, "Efficacy of chamomile-extract spray for prevention of postoperative sore throat," *J Med Assoc Thai* 2002 Jun; 85 Suppl 1:S180–85.

16. P. Fidler, C. L. Loprinzi, J. R. O'Fallon, J. M. Leitch, J. K. Lee, D. L. Hayes, P. Novotny, D. Clemens-Schutjer, J. Bartel, and J. C. Michalak, "Prospective evaluation of a chamomile mouthwash for prevention of 5-FU-induced oral mucositis," *Cancer* 1996 Feb 1; 77(3): 522–25.

17. W. Carl, and L. S. Emrich, "Management of oral mucositis during local radiation and systemic chemotherapy: a study of 98 patients," *J Prosthet Dent* 1991 Sep; 66(3): 361–69.

18. S. de la Motte, S. Bose-O'Reilly, M. Heinisch, and F. Harrison, "Double-blind comparison of an apple pectin-chamomile extract preparation with placebo in children with diarrhea," *Arzneimittelforschung* 1997 Nov; 47(11): 1247–49.

19. D. F. Birt, D. Mitchell, B. Gold, P. Pour, and H. C. Pinch, "Inhibition of ultraviolet light–induced skin carcinogenesis in SKH-1 mice by apigenin, a plant flavonoid. *Anticancer Res* 1997 Jan–Feb; 17(1A): 85–91.

20. H. Wei, L. Tye, E. Bresnick, and D. F. Birt, "Inhibitory effect of apigenin, a plant flavonoid, on epidermal ornithine decarboxylase and skin tumor promotion in mice," *Cancer Res* 1990 Feb 1; 50(3): 499–502.

21. D. M. Lepley, and J. C. Pelling, "Induction of p21/WAF1 and G1 cell-cycle arrest by the chemopreventive agent apigenin," *Mol Carcinog* 1997 Jun; 19(2): 74–82.

22. D. M. Lepley, B. Li, D. F. Birt, and J. C. Pelling, "The chemopreventive flavonoid apigenin induces G2/M arrest in keratinocytes," *Carcinogenesis* 1996 Nov; 17(11): 2367–75.

23. P. W. Zheng, L. C. Chiang, and C. C. Lin, "Apigenin-induced apoptosis through p53-dependent pathway in human cervical carcinoma cells," *Life Sci* 2005 Feb 4; 76(12): 1367–79. E-pub, 2004 Dec 10.

24. L. Liu, J. Fang, Q. Zhou, X. Hu, X. Shi, and B. H. Jiang, "Apigenin inhibits VEGF expression and angiogenesis in human lung cancer cells: implication of chemoprevention of lung cancer," *Mol Pharmacol.* E-pub, 2005 Jun 9.

25. J. Fang, C. Xia, Z. Cao, J. Z. Zheng, E. Reed, B. H. Jiang, "Apigenin inhibits VEGF and HIF-1 expression via PI3K/AKT/p70S6K1 and HDM2/p53 pathways," *FASEB J* 2005 Mar; 19(3): 342–53.

References for Chaste Tree

1. T. K. Schulz, R. Hänsel, and V. E. Tyler, *Rational Phytotherapy: A Physician's Guide to Herbal Medicine* (Berlin: Springer-Verlag, 1997).

2. J. Liu, J. E. Burdette, Y. Sun, S. Deng, S. M. Schlecht, W. Zheng, D. Nikolic, G. Mahady, R. B. van Breemen, H. H. Fong, J. M. Pezzuto, J. L. Bolton, and N. R. Farnsworth, "Isolation of linoleic acid as an estrogenic compound from the fruits of Vitex agnus-castus L. (chaste-berry)," *Phytomedicine* 2004 Jan; 11(1): 18–23.

3. H. Jarry, B. Spengler, A. Porzel, J. Schmidt, W. Wuttke, and V. Christoffel, "Evidence for estrogen receptor beta-selective activity of Vitex agnus-castus and isolated flavones," *Planta Med* 2003 Oct; 69(10): 945–47.

4. A. Milewicz, E. Gejdel, H. Sworen, K. Sienkiewicz, J. Jedrzejak, T. Teucher, and H. Schmitz, "Vitex agnus castus extract in the treatment of luteal phase defects due to latent hyperprolactinemia. Results of a randomized, placebo-controlled, double-blind study," *Arzneimittelforschung* 1993 Jul; 43(7): 752–56.

5. L. M. Westphal, M. L. Polan, A. S. Trant, and S. B. Mooney, "A nutritional supplement for improving fertility in women: a pilot study," *J Reprod Med* 2004 Apr; 49(4): 289–93.

6. M. Atmaca, S. Kumru, and E. Tezcan, "Fluoxetine versus Vitex agnus castus extract in the treatment of premenstrual dysphoric disorder," *Hum Psychopharmacol* 2003 Apr; 18(3): 191–95.

7. R. Schellenberg, "Treatment for the premenstrual syndrome with agnus castus fruit extract: prospective, randomised, placebo-controlled study," *BMJ* 2001 Jan 20; 322(7279): 134–37.

8. D. Berger, W. Schaffner, E. Schrader, B. Meier, and A. Brattstrom, "Efficacy of Vitex agnus castus L. extract Ze 440 in patients with pre-menstrual syndrome (PMS)," *Arch Gynecol Obstet* 2000 Nov; 264(3): 150–53.

9. E. G. Loch, H. Selle, and N. Boblitz, "Treatment of premenstrual syndrome with a phytopharmaceutical formulation containing Vitex agnus castus," *J Womens Health Gend Based Med* 2000 Apr; 9(3): 315–20.

10. M. Halaska, P. Beles, C. Gorkow, and C. Sieder,

"Treatment of cyclical mastalgia with a solution containing a Vitex agnus castus extract: results of a placebo-controlled, double-blind study," *Breast* 1999 Aug; 8(4): 175–81.

11. P. G. Merz, C. Gorkow, A. Schrodter, S. Rietbrock, C. Sieder, D. Loew, J. S. Dericks-Tan, and H. D. Taubert, "The effects of a special Agnus castus extract (BP1095E1) on prolactin secretion in healthy male subjects," *Exp Clin Endocrinol Diabetes* 1996; 104(6): 447–53.

12. J. S. Dericks-Tan, P. Schwinn, and C. Hildt, "Dose-dependent stimulation of melatonin secretion after administration of Agnus castus," *Exp Clin Endocrinol Diabetes* 2003 Feb; 111(1): 44–46.

References for Cinnamon

1. K. J. Jarvill-Taylor, R. A. Anderson, and D. J. Graves, "A hydroxychalcone derived from cinnamon functions as a mimetic for insulin in 3T3–L1 adipocytes," *J Am Coll Nutr* 2001 Aug; 20(4): 327–36.

2. A. Khan, M. Safdar, M. M. Ali Khan, K. N. Khattak, and R. A. Anderson, "Cinnamon improves glucose and lipids of people with type 2 diabetes," *Diabetes Care* 2003 Dec; 26(12): 3215–18.

3. Y. Nir, I. Potasman, E. Stermer, M. Tabak, and I. Neeman, "Controlled trial of the effect of cinnamon extract on Helicobacter pylori," *Helicobacter* 2000 Jun; 5(2): 94–97.

References for Cranberry

1. E. L. Weiss, R. Lev-Dor, N. Sharon, and I. Ofek, "Inhibitory effect of a high-molecular-weight constituent of cranberry on adhesion of oral bacteria," *Crit Rev Food Sci Nutr* 2002; 42(3 Suppl): 285–92.

2. T. Kessler, B. Jansen, and A. Hesse, "Effect of black-currant-, cranberry- and plum-juice consumption on risk factors associated with kidney stone formation," *Eur J Clin Nutr* 2002 Oct; 56(10): 1020–23.

3. R. J. Jepson, L. Mihaljevic, and J. Craig, "Cranberries for preventing urinary tract infections," *Cochrane Database Syst Rev* 2004(2): CD001321.

4. T. Kontiokari, et al., "Randomised trial of cranberry-lingon-berry juice and Lactobacillus GG drink for the prevention of urinary tract infections in women," *BMJ* June 30, 2001; 322:1571–73.

5. M. K. Terris, M. M. Issa, and J. R. Tacker, "Dietary supplementation with cranberry concentrate tablets may increase the risk of nephrolithiasis," *Urology* 2001 Jan; 57(1): 26–29.

6. Kessler, Jansen, and Hesse, op cit.

7. T. McHarg, A. Rodgers, and K. Charlton, "Influence of cranberry juice on the urinary risk factors for calcium oxalate kidney stone formation," *BJU Int* 2003 Nov; 92(7): 765–68.

References for Dandelion

1. T. K. Schulz, R. Hänsel, and V. E. Tyler, *Rational Phytotherapy: A Physician's Guide to Herbal Medicine* (Berlin: Springer-Verlag, 1997).

2. H. Y. Youn, H. S. Kang, D. H. Bhang, M. K. Kim, C. Y. Hwang, and H. R. Han, "Allergens causing atopic diseases in canine," *J Vet Sci* 2002 Dec; 3(4): 335–41.

3. M. Malawska, and B. Wilkomirski, "Accumulation rate of polychlorinated biphenyls (PCBs) in dandelion (*Taraxacum officinale*) in the conditions of soil contam-

ination with oil derivatives," *Rocz Panstw Zakl Hig* 2001; 52(4): 295–311.

4. J. Pichtel, K. Kuroiwa, and H. T. Sawyer, "Distribution of Pb, Cd and Ba in soils and plants of two contaminated sites," *Environ Pollut* 2000 Oct; 110(1): 171–78.

5. E. Gaitan, R. C. Cooksey, J. Legan, and R. H. Lindsay, "Antithyroid effects in vivo and in vitro of vitexin: a C-glucosylflavone in millet," *J Clin Endocrinol Metab* 1995 Apr; 80(4): 1144–47.

6. K. Bohm, "Choleretic action of various plant drugs," *Arzneimittelforschung* 1959 Jun; 9(6): 376–78.

7. R. Gebhardt, "Anticholestatic activity of flavonoids from artichoke (*Cynara scolymus L.*) and of their metabolites," *Med Sci Monit* 2001 May; 7 Suppl 1:316–20.

8. I. Hook, A. McGee, and M. Henman, "Evaluation of Dandelion for diuretic activity and variation in potassium content," *Int J Pharmacog* 31 (1993): 29–34.

References for Echinacea

1. J. A. Taylor, W. Weber, L. Standish, H. Quinn, J. Goesling, M. McGann, and C. Calabrese, "Efficacy and safety of echinacea in treating upper respiratory tract infections in children: a randomized controlled trial," *JAMA* 2003 Dec 3; 290(21): 2824–30.

2. R. J. Mullins, and R. Heddle, "Adverse reactions associated with echinacea: the Australian experience," *Ann Allergy Asthma Immunol* 2002 Jan; 88(1): 42–51.

3. R. J. Mullins, "Echinacea-associated anaphylaxis," *Med J Aust* 1998 Feb 16; 168(4): 170–71.

4. S. R. Hosein, "Are echinacea and HIV not a good mix?" *Treatment Update* 1999 Feb; 11(1): 3.

5. D. Melchart, E. Walther, K. Linde, R. Brandmaier, and C. Lersch, "Echinacea root extracts for the prevention of upper respiratory tract infections: a double-blind, placebo-controlled randomized trial," *Arch Fam Med* 1998 Nov–Dec; 7(6): 541–45.

6. W. Grimm, and H. H. Muller, "A randomized controlled trial of the effect of fluid extract of Echinacea purpurea on the incidence and severity of colds and respiratory infections," *Am J Med* 1999 Feb; 106(2): 138–43.

7. R. B. Turner, D. K. Riker, and J. D. Gangemi, "Ineffectiveness of echinacea for prevention of experimental rhinovirus colds," *Antimicrob Agents Chemother* 2000 Jun; 44(6): 1708–09.

8. E. Schwarz, J. Metzler, J. P. Diedrich, J. Freudenstein, C. Bode, and J. C. Bode, "Oral administration of freshly expressed juice of Echinacea purpurea herbs fail to stimulate the nonspecific immune response in healthy young men: results of a double-blind, placebo-controlled crossover study," *J Immunother* 2002 Sep–Oct; 25(5): 413–20.

9. B. P. Barrett, R. L. Brown, K. Locken, R. Maberry, J. A. Bobula, and D. D'Alessio, "Treatment of the common cold with unrefined echinacea. A randomized, double-blind, placebo-controlled trial," *Ann Intern Med* 2002 Dec 17; 137(12): 939–46.

10. J. A. Taylor, et al., op. cit.

11. S. J. Sperber, L. P. Shah, R. D. Gilbert, T. W. Ritchey, and A. S. Monto, "Echinacea purpurea for prevention of experimental rhinovirus colds," *Clin Infect Dis* 2004 May 15; 38(10): 1367–71. E-pub, 2004 Apr 26.

12. S. H. Yale, and K. Liu, "Echinacea purpurea therapy for

the treatment of the common cold: a randomized, double-blind, placebo-controlled clinical trial," *Arch Intern Med* 2004 Jun 14; 164(11): 1237–41.

13. R. B. Turner, R. Bauer, K. Woelkart, T. C. Hulsey, and J. D. Gangemi, "An evaluation of Echinacea angustifolia in experimental rhinovirus infections," *N Engl J Med* 2005 Jul 28; 353(4): 341–48.

14. B. Schulten, M. Bulitta, B. Ballering-Bruhl, U. Koster, and M. Schafer, "Efficacy of Echinacea purpurea in patients with a common cold. A placebo-controlled, randomised, double-blind clinical trial," *Arzneimittelforschung* 2001; 51(7): 563–68

15. V. Goel, R. Lovlin, R. Barton, M. R. Lyon, R. Bauer, T. D. Lee, and T. K. Basu, "Efficacy of a standardized echinacea preparation (Echinilin) for the treatment of the common cold: a randomized, double-blind, placebo-controlled trial," *J Clin Pharm Ther* 2004 Feb; 29(1): 75–83.

16. B. Vonau, S. Chard, S. Mandalia, D. Wilkinson, and S. E. Barton, "Does the extract of the plant Echinacea purpurea influence the clinical course of recurrent genital herpes?" *Int J STD AIDS* 2001 Mar; 12(3): 154–58

17. E. Speroni, P. Govoni, S. Guizzardi, C. Renzulli, and M. C. Guerra, "Anti-inflammatory and cicatrizing activity of Echinacea pallida Nutt. root extract," *J Ethnopharmacol* 2002 Feb; 79(2): 265–72.

References for Eleuthero

1. E. J. Park, J. X. Nan, Y. Z. Zhao, S. H. Lee, Y. H. Kim, J. B. Nam, J. J. Lee, and D. H. Sohn, "Water-soluble polysaccharide from Eleutherococcus senticosus stems attenuates fulminant hepatic failure induced by D-galactosamine and lipopolysaccharide in mice," *Basic Clin Pharmacol Toxicol* 2004 Jun; 94(6): 298–304.

2. J. M. Yi, S. H. Hong, J. H. Kim, H. K. Kim, H. J. Song, and H. M. Kim, "Effect of Acanthopanax senticosus stem on mast cell-dependent anaphylaxis," *J Ethnopharmacol* 2002 Mar; 79(3): 347–52.

3. M. Miyazawa, and M. Hisama, "Antimutagenic activity of phenylpropanoids from clove (*Syzygium aromaticum*)," *J Agric Food Chem* 2003 Oct 22; 51(22): 6413–22.

4. B. Glatthaar-Saalmuller, F. Sacher, and A. Esperester, "Antiviral activity of an extract derived from roots of Eleutherococcus senticosus," *Antiviral Res* 2001 Jun; 50(3): 223–28.

5. P. T. Pearce, I. Zois, K. N. Wynne, and J. W. Funder, "Panax ginseng and Eleuthrococcus senticosus extracts—in vitro studies on binding to steroid receptors," *Endocrinol Jpn* 1982 Oct; 29(5): 567–73.

6. D. T. Zava, C. M. Dollbaum, and M. Blen, "Estrogen and progestin bioactivity of foods, herbs, and spices," *Proc Soc Exp. Biol Med* 1998 Mar; 217(3): 369–78.

7. B. T. Gaffney, H. M. Hugel, and P. A. Rich, "The effects of Eleutherococcus senticosus and Panax ginseng on steroidal hormone indices of stress and lymphocyte subset numbers in endurance athletes," *Life Sci* 2001 Dec 14; 70(4): 431–42.

8. B. T. Gaffney, H. M. Hugel, and P. A. Rich, "Panax ginseng and Eleutheroccus senticosus may exaggerate an already existing biphasic response to stress via inhibition of enzymes which limit the binding of stress hormones to their receptors," *Med Hypotheses* 2001 May; 56(5): 567–72.

9. J. Jellin, P. J. Gregory, F. Batz, K. Hitchens, et al.,

Pharmacist's Letter/Prescriber's Letter, Natural Medicines Comprehensive Database, 6th ed. (Stockton, CA: Therapeutic Research Faculty, 2004).

10. L. F. Eschbach, M. J. Webster, J. C. Boyd, P. D. McArthur, and T. K. Evetovich, "The effect of siberian ginseng (*Eleutherococcus senticosus*) on substrate utilization and performance," *Int J Sport Nutr Exerc Metab* 2000 Dec; 10(4): 444–51.

11. E. A. Dowling, D. R. Redondo, J. D. Branch, S. Jones, G. McNabb, and M. H. Williams, "Effect of Eleutherococcus senticosus on submaximal and maximal exercise performance," *Med Sci Sports Exerc* 1996 Apr; 28(4): 482–89.

12. A. F. Cicero, G. Derosa, R. Brillante, R. Bernardi, S. Nascetti, and A. Gaddi, "Effects of Siberian ginseng (*Eleutherococcus senticosus maxim.*) on elderly quality of life: a randomized clinical trial," *Arch Gerontol Geriatr Suppl* 2004; (9): 69–73.

13. B. T. Gaffney, H. M. Hugel, and P. A. Rich, "The effects of Eleutherococcus senticosus and Panax ginseng on steroidal hormone indices of stress and lymphocyte subset numbers in endurance athletes," *Life Sci* 2001 Dec 14; 70(4): 431–42.

14. B. Bohn, C. T. Nebe, and C. Birr, "Flow-cytometric studies with eleutherococcus senticosus extract as an immunomodulatory agent," *Arzneimittelforschung* 1987 Oct; 37(10): 1193–96.

15. A. J. Hartz, S. Bentler, R. Noyes, J. Hoehns, C. Logemann, S. Sinift, Y. Butani, W. Wang, K. Brake, M. Ernst, and H. Kautzman, "Randomized controlled trial of Siberian ginseng for chronic fatigue," *Psychol Med* 2004 Jan; 34(1): 51–61.

16. J. L. Donovan, C. L. DeVane, K. D. Chavin, R. M. Taylor, J. S. Markowitz, "Siberian ginseng (*Eleutheroccus senticosus*) effects on CYP2D6 and CYP3A4 activity in normal volunteers," *Drug Metab Dispos* 2003 May; 31(5): 519–22.

References for Evening Primrose

1. D. F. Horrobin, K. M. Ells, N. Morse-Fisher, and M. S. Manku, "The effects of evening primrose oil, safflower oil and paraffin on plasma fatty acid levels in humans: choice of an appropriate placebo for clinical studies on primrose oil," *Prostaglandins Leukot Essent Fatty Acids* 1991 Apr; 42(4): 245–49.

2. M. Schalin-Karrila, L. Mattila, C. T. Jansen, and P. Uotila, "Evening primrose oil in the treatment of atopic eczema: effect on clinical status, plasma phospholipid fatty acids and circulating blood prostaglandins," *Br J Dermatol* 1987 Jul; 117(1): 11–19.

3. J. Jantti, T. Nikkari, T. Solakivi, H. Vapaatalo, and H. Isomaki, "Evening primrose oil in rheumatoid arthritis: changes in serum lipids and fatty acids," *Ann Rheum Dis* 1989 Feb; 48(2): 124–27.

4. M. Schalin-Karrila, et al., op cit.

5. P. F. Morse, D. F. Horrobin, M. S. Manku, J. C. Stewart, R. Allen, S. Littlewood, S. Wright, J. Burton, D. J. Gould, P. J. Holt, et al., "Meta-analysis of placebo-controlled studies of the efficacy of Epogam in the treatment of atopic eczema. Relationship between plasma essential fatty acid changes and clinical response," *Br J Dermatol* 1989 Jul; 121(1): 75–90.

6. C. A. Hederos, and A. Berg, "Epogam evening primrose oil treatment in atopic dermatitis and asthma,"

Arch Dis Child 1996 Dec; 75(6): 494–97.

7. K. Yoshimoto-Furuie, K. Yoshimoto, T. Tanaka, S. Saima, Y. Kikuchi, J. Shay, D. R. Horrobin, and H. Echizen, "Effects of oral supplementation with evening primrose oil for six weeks on plasma essential fatty acids and uremic skin symptoms in hemodialysis patients," *Nephron* 1999 Feb; 81(2): 151–59.

8. D. K. Whitaker, J. Cilliers, and C. de Beer, "Evening primrose oil (Epogam) in the treatment of chronic hand dermatitis: disappointing therapeutic results," *Dermatology* 1996; 193(2): 115–20.

9. S. Oliwiecki, J. Armstrong, J. L. Burton, and J. Bradfield, "The effect of essential fatty acids on epidermal atrophy due to topical steroids," *Clin Exp Dermatol* 1993 Jul; 18(4): 326–28.

10. S. Qureshi, and N. Sultan, "Topical nonsteroidal anti-inflammatory drugs versus oil of evening primrose in the treatment of mastalgia," *Surgeon* 2005 Feb; 3(1): 7–10.

11. J. Blommers, E. S. de Lange-De Klerk, D. J. Kuik, P. D. Bezemer, and S. Meijer, "Evening primrose oil and fish oil for severe chronic astalgia: a randomized, double-blind, controlled trial," *Am J Obstet Gynecol* 2002 Nov; 187(5): 1389–94.

12. R. E. Mansel, B. J. Harrison, J. Melhuish, W. Sheridan, J. K. Pye, G. Pritchard, P. R. Maddox, D. J. Webster, and L. E. Hughes, "A randomized trial of dietary intervention with essential fatty acids in patients with categorized cysts," *Ann NY Acad Sci* 1990; 586:288–94.

13. S. K. Khoo, C. Munro, and D. Battistutta, "Evening primrose oil and treatment of premenstrual syndrome," *Med J Aust* 1990 Aug 20; 153(4): 189–92.

14. J. Moodley, and R. J. Norman, "Attempts at dietary alteration of prostaglandin pathways in the management of pre-eclampsia," *Prostaglandins Leukot Essent Fatty Acids* 1989 Sep; 37(3): 145–47.

15. A. D'Almeida, J. P. Carter, A. Anatol, and C. Prost, "Effects of a combination of evening primrose oil (gamma linolenic acid) and fish oil (eicosapentaenoic + docahexaenoic acid) versus magnesium, and versus placebo in preventing pre-eclampsia," *Women Health* 1992; 19(2–3): 117–31.

16. R. Chenoy, S. Hussain, Y. Tayob, P. M. O'Brien, M. Y. Moss, and P. F. Morse, "Effect of oral gamolenic acid from evening primrose oil on menopausal flushing," *BMJ* 1994 Feb 19; 308(6927): 501–03.

17. E. J. Bassey, J. J. Littlewood, M. C. Rothwell, and D. W. Pye, "Lack of effect of supplementation with essential fatty acids on bone mineral density in healthy pre- and postmenopausal women: two randomized controlled trials of Efacal v. calcium alone," *Br J Nutr* 2000 Jun; 83(6): 629–35.

18. C. Haslett, J. G. Douglas, S. R. Chalmers, A. Weighhill, and J. F. Munro, "A double-blind evaluation of evening primrose oil as an antiobesity agent," *Int J Obes* 1983; 7(6): 549–53.

19. J. Jantti, et al., op. cit.

20. J. J. Belch, D. Ansell, R. Madhok, A. O'Dowd, and R. D. Sturrock, "Effects of altering dietary essential fatty acids on requirements for non-steroidal anti-inflammatory drugs in patients with rheumatoid arthritis: a double-blind, placebo-controlled study," *Ann Rheum Dis* 1988 Feb; 47(2): 96–104.

21. M. Brzeski, R. Madhok, and H. A. Capell, "Evening primrose oil in patients with rheumatoid arthritis and side-effects of non-steroidal anti-inflammatory drugs," *Br J Rheumatol* 1991 Oct; 30(5): 370–72.

22. P. Oxholm, R. Manthorpe, J. U. Prause, and D. Horrobin, "Patients with primary Sjögren's syndrome treated for two months with evening primrose oil," *Scand J Rheumatol* 1986; 15(2): 103–08.

23. E. Theander, D. F. Horrobin, L. T. Jacobsson, and R. Manthorpe, "Gammalinolenic acid treatment of fatigue associated with primary Sjögren's syndrome," *Scand J Rheumatol* 2002; 31(2): 72–79.

24. A. P. Jenkins, A. T. Green, and R. P. Thompson, "Essential fatty acid supplementation in chronic hepatitis B," *Aliment Pharmacol Ther* 1996 Aug; 10(4): 665–68.

25. C. F. van der Merwe, J. Booyens, H. F. Joubert, and C. A. van der Merwe, "The effect of gamma-linolenic acid, an in vitro cytostatic substance contained in evening primrose oil, on primary liver cancer. A double-blind, placebo-controlled trial," *Prostaglandins Leukot Essent Fatty Acids* 1990 Jul; 40(3): 199–202.

26. M. G. Aman, E. A. Mitchell, and S. H. Turbott, "The effects of essential fatty acid supplementation by Efamol in hyperactive children," *J Abnorm Child Psychol* 1987 Mar; 15(1): 75–90.

27. L. E. Arnold, S. M. Pinkham, and N. Votolato, "Does zinc moderate essential fatty acid and amphetamine treatment of attention-deficit/hyperactivity disorder?" *J Child Adolesc Psychopharmacol* 2000 Summer; 10(2): 111–17.

28. J. J. Belch, B. Shaw, A. O'Dowd, A. Saniabadi, P. Leiberman, R. D. Sturrock, and C. D. Forbes, "Evening primrose oil (Efamol) in the treatment of Raynaud's phenomenon: a double-blind study," *Thromb Haemost* 1985 Aug 30; 54(2): 490–94.

29. S. M. Greenfield, A. T. Green, J. P. Teare, A. P. Jenkins, N. A. Punchard, C. C. Ainley, and R. P. Thompson, "A randomized controlled study of evening primrose oil and fish oil in ulcerative colitis," *Aliment Pharmacol Ther* 1993 Apr; 7(2): 159–66.

References for Feverfew

1. R. J. Marles, J. Kaminski, J. T. Arnason, L. Pazos-Sanou, S. Heptinstall, N. H. Fischer, C. W. Crompton, D. G. Kindack, and D. V. Awang, "A bioassay for inhibition of serotonin release from bovine platelets," *J Nat Prod* 1992 Aug; 55(8): 1044–56.

2. J. J. Murphy, S. Heptinstall, J. R. Mitchell, "Randomised double-blind, placebo-controlled trial of feverfew in migraine prevention," *Lancet* 1988 Jul 23; 2(8604): 189–92.

3. E. S. Johnson, N. P. Kadam, D. M. Hylands, and P. J. Hylands, "Efficacy of feverfew as prophylactic treatment of migraine," *Br Med J (Clin Res Ed)* 1985 Aug 31; 291(6495): 569–73.

4. V. Pfaffenrath, H. C. Diener, M. Fischer, M. Friede, and H. H. Henneicke-von Zepelin, "The efficacy and safety of Tanacetum parthenium (feverfew) in migraine prophylaxis—a double-blind, multicentre, randomized placebo-controlled dose-response study," *Cephalalgia* 2002 Sep; 22(7): 523–32.

5. M. Pattrick, S. Heptinstall, and M. Doherty, "Feverfew in rheumatoid arthritis: a double-blind, placebo-controlled study," *Ann Rheum Dis* 1989 Jul; 48(7): 547–49.

References for Flax

1. W. Demark-Wahnefried, C. N. Robertson, P. J. Walther, T. J. Polascik, D. F. Paulson, and R. T. Vollmer, "Pilot study to explore effects of low-fat, flaxseed-supplemented diet on proliferation of benign prostatic epithelium and prostate-specific antigen," *Urology* 2004 May; 63(5): 900–04.

2. W. Demark-Wahnefried, D. T. Price, T. J. Polascik, C. N. Robertson, E. E. Anderson, D. F. Paulson, P. J. Walther, M. Gannon, and R. T. Vollmer, "Pilot study of dietary fat restriction and flaxseed supplementation in men with prostate cancer before surgery: exploring the effects on hormonal levels, prostate-specific antigen, and histopathologic features," *Urology* 2001 Jul; 58(1): 47–52.

3. E. J. Frische, A. M. Hutchins, M. C. Martini, W. Thomas, and J. L. Slavin, "Effect of flaxseed and wheat bran on serum hormones and lignan excretion in premenopausal women," *J Am Coll Nutr* 2003 Dec; 22(6): 550–54.

4. S. Tarpila, A. Aro, I. Salminen, A. Tarpila, P. Kleemola, J. Akkila, and H. Adlercreutz, "The effect of flaxseed supplementation in processed foods on serum fatty acids and enterolactone," *Eur J Clin Nutr* 2002 Feb; 56(2): 157–65.

5. A. M. Hutchins, M. C. Martini, B. A. Olson, W. Thomas, and J. L. Slavin, "Flaxseed consumption influences endogenous hormone concentrations in postmenopausal women," *Nutr Cancer* 2001; 39(1): 58–65.

6. P. D. Nesbitt, Y. Lam, and L. U. Thompson, "Human metabolism of mammalian lignan precursors in raw and processed flaxseed," *Am J Clin Nutr* 1999 Mar; 69(3): 549–55.

7. E. J. Frische, A. M. Hutchins, M. C. Martini, W. Thomas, and J. L. Slavin, "Effect of flaxseed and wheat bran on serum hormones and lignan excretion in premenopausal women," *J Am Coll Nutr* 2003 Dec; 22(6): 550–54.

8. C. J. Haggans, E. J. Travelli, W. Thomas, M. C. Martini, and J. L. Slavin, "The effect of flaxseed and wheat bran consumption on urinary estrogen metabolites in premenopausal women," *Cancer Epidemiol Biomarkers Prev* 2000 Jul; 9(7): 719–25.

9. C. J. Haggans, A. M. Hutchins, B. A. Olson, W. Thomas, M. C. Martini, and J. L. Slavin, "Effect of flaxseed consumption on urinary estrogen metabolites in postmenopausal women," *Nutr Cancer* 1999; 33(2): 188–95.

10. J. D. Brooks, W. E. Ward, J. E. Lewis, J. Hilditch, L. Nickell, E. Wong, and L. U. Thompson, "Supplementation with flaxseed alters estrogen metabolism in postmenopausal women to a greater extent than does supplementation with an equal amount of soy," *Am J Clin Nutr* 2004 Feb; 79(2): 318–25.

11. S. Dodin, A. Lemay, H. Jacques, F. Legare, J. C. Forest, and B. Masse, "The effects of flaxseed dietary supplement on lipid profile, bone mineral density, and symptoms in menopausal women: a randomized, double-blind, wheat germ placebo-controlled clinical trial," *J Clin Endocrinol Metab* 2005 Mar; 90(3): 1390–97. E-pub, 2004 Dec 21.

12. J. D. Brooks, et al., op.cit.

13. E. A. Lucas, R. D. Wild, L. J. Hammond, D. A. Khalil, S. Juma, B. P. Daggy, B. J. Stoecker, and B. H. Arjmandi, "Flaxseed improves lipid profile without altering biomarkers of bone metabolism in postmenopausal women," *J Clin Endocrinol Metab* 2002 Apr; 87(4): 1527–32.

14. A. M. Hutchins, et al., op. cit.

15. A. Lemay, S. Dodin, N. Kadri, H. Jacques, and J. C. Forest, "Flaxseed dietary supplement versus hormone replacement therapy in hypercholesterolemic menopausal women," *Obstet Gynecol* 2002 Sep; 100(3): 495–504.

16. W. R. Phipps, M. C. Martini, J. W. Lampe, J. L. Slavin, and M. S. Kurzer, "Effect of flax seed ingestion on the menstrual cycle," *J Clin Endocrinol Metab* 1993 Nov; 77(5): 1215–19.

17. L. K. Ferrier, L. J. Caston, S. Leeson, J. Squires B. J. Weaver, and B. J. Holub, "alpha-Linolenic acid- and docosahexaenoic acid-enriched eggs from hens fed flaxseed: influence on blood lipids and platelet phospholipid fatty acids in humans," *Am J Clin Nutr* 1995 Jul; 62(1): 81–86.

18. D. J. Jenkins, C. W. Kendall, E. Vidgen, S. Agarwal, A. V. Rao, R. S. Rosenberg, E. P. Diamandis, R. Novokmet, C. C. Mehling, T. Perera, L. C. Griffin, and S. C. Cunnane, "Health aspects of partially defatted flaxseed, including effects on serum lipids, oxidative measures and ex vivo androgen and progestin activity: a controlled crossover trial," *Am J Clin Nutr* 1999 Mar; 69(3): 395–402.

19. M. L. Bierenbaum, R. Reichstein, and T. R. Watkins, "Reducing atherogenic risk in hyperlipemic humans with flax seed supplementation: a preliminary report," *J Am Coll Nutr* 1993 Oct; 12(5): 501–04.

20. E. A. Lucas, et al., op. cit.

21. S. Dodin, et al. op. cit.

22. S. C. Cunnane, S. Ganguli, C. Menard, A. C. Liede, M. J. Hamadeh, Z. Y. Chen, T. M. Wolever, and D. J. Jenkins, "High alpha-linolenic acid flaxseed (Linum usitatissimum): some nutritional properties in humans," *Br J Nutr* 1993 Mar; 69(2): 443–53.

23. S. C. Cunnane, M. J. Hamadeh, A. C. Liede, L. U. Thompson, T. M. Wolever, and D. J. Jenkins, "Nutritional attributes of traditional flaxseed in healthy young adults," *Am J Clin Nutr* 1995 Jan; 61(1): 62–68.

24. W. F. Clark, C. Kortas, A. P. Heidenheim, I. Garland, E. Spanner, and A. Parbtani, "Flaxseed in lupus nephritis: a two-year nonplacebo-controlled crossover study," *J Am Coll Nutr* 2001 Apr; 20(2 Suppl): 143–48.

25. W. F. Clark, A. Parbtani, M. W. Huff, E. Spanner, H. de Salis, I. Chin-Yee, D. J. Philbrick, and B. J. Holub, "Flaxseed: a potential treatment for lupus nephritis," *Kidney Int* 1995 Aug; 48(2): 475–80.

26. M. A. Allman, M. M. Pena, and D. Pang, "Supplementation with flaxseed oil versus sunflowerseed oil in healthy young men consuming a low-fat diet: effects on platelet composition and function," *Eur J Clin Nutr* 1995 Mar; 49(3): 169–78.

27. E. Mantzioris, M. J. James, R. A. Gibson, and L. G. Cleland, "Differences exist in the relationships between dietary linoleic and alpha-linolenic acids and their respective long-chain metabolites," *Am J Clin Nutr* 1995 Feb; 61(2): 320–24.

28. C. A. Francois, S. L. Connor, L. C. Bolewicz, and W. E. Connor, "Supplementing lactating women with flaxseed oil does not increase docosahexaenoic acid in their milk," *Am J Clin Nutr* 2003 Jan; 77(1): 226–33.

29. F. A. Wallace, E. A. Miles, and P. C. Calder, "Comparison

of the effects of linseed oil and different doses of fish oil on mononuclear cell function in healthy human subjects," *Br J Nutr* 2003 May; 89(5): 679–89.

30. S. Kew, T. Banerjee, A. M. Minihane, Y. E. Finnegan, R. Muggli, R. Albers, C. M. Williams, and P. C. Calder, "Lack of effect of foods enriched with plant- or marine-derived n-3 fatty acids on human immune function," *Am J Clin Nutr* 2003 May; 77(5): 1287–95.

31. F. Thies, E. A. Miles, G. Nebe-von-Caron, J. R. Powell, T. L. Hurst, E. A. Newsholme, and P. C. Calder, "Influence of dietary supplementation with long-chain n-3 or n-6 polyunsaturated fatty acids on blood inflammatory cell populations and functions and on plasma soluble adhesion molecules in healthy adults," *Lipids* 2001 Nov; 36(11): 1183–93.

32. D. C. Nordstrom, V. E. Honkanen, Y. Nasu, E. Antila, C. Friman, and Y. T. Konttinen, "Alpha-linolenic acid in the treatment of rheumatoid arthritis. A double-blind, placebo-controlled and randomized study: flaxseed vs. safflower seed," *Rheumatol Int* 1995; 14(6): 231–34.

33. I. A. Brouwer, M. B. Katan, and P. L. Zock, "Dietary alpha-linolenic acid is associated with reduced risk of fatal coronary heart disease, but increased prostate cancer risk: a meta-analysis," *J Nutr* 2004 Apr; 134(4): 919–22.

34. N. M. Attar-Bashi, A. G. Frauman, and A. J. Sinclair, "Alpha-linolenic acid and the risk of prostate cancer. What is the evidence?" *J Urol* 2004 Apr; 171(4): 1402–07.

35. M. Saadatian-Elahi, T. Norat, J. Goudable, and E. Riboli, "Biomarkers of dietary fatty acid intake and the risk of breast cancer: a meta-analysis," *Int J Cancer* 2004 Sep 10; 111(4): 584–91.

References for Garlic

1. M. Ali, "Mechanism by which garlic (*Allium sativum*) inhibits cyclooxygenase activity. Effect of raw versus boiled garlic extract on the synthesis of prostanoids," *Prostaglandins Leukot Essent Fatty Acids* 1995 Dec; 53(6): 397–400.

2. S. K. Banerjee, and S. K. Maulik, "Effect of garlic on cardiovascular disorders: a review," *Nutr J* 2002 Nov 19; 1(1): 4.

3. D. D. Ku, T. T. Abdel-Razek, J. Dai, S. Kim-Park, M. B. Fallon, and G. A. Abrams, "Garlic and its active metabolite allicin produce endothelium- and nitric oxide-dependent relaxation in rat pulmonary arteries," *Clin Exp Pharmacol Physiol* 2002 Jan–Feb; 29(1–2): 84–91.

4. M. Z. Ashraf, M. E. Hussain, and M. Fahim, "Endothelium mediated vasorelaxant response of garlic in isolated rat aorta: role of nitric oxide," *J Ethnopharmacol* 2004 Jan; 90(1): 5–9.

5. L. Liu, and Y. Y. Yeh, "Water-soluble organosulfur compounds of garlic inhibit fatty acid and triglyceride syntheses in cultured rat hepatocytes," *Lipids* 2001 Apr; 36(4): 395–400.

6. M. S. Chi, E. T. Koh, T. J. Stewart, "Effects of garlic on lipid metabolism in rats fed cholesterol or lard," *J Nutr* 1982 Feb; 112(2): 241–48.

7. L. Liu, and Y. Y. Yeh, "S-alk(en)yl cysteines of garlic inhibit cholesterol synthesis by deactivating HMG-CoA reductase in cultured rat hepatocytes," *J Nutr* 2002 Jun; 132(6): 1129–34.

8. Y. Y. Yeh, and L. Liu, "Cholesterol-Lowering Effect of Garlic Extracts and Organosulfur Compounds: Human and Animal Studies," *J Nutr* 2001; 131:989S–993S.

9. L. D. Lawson, and Z. J. Wang, "Low allicin release from garlic supplements: a major problem due to the sensitivities of alliinase activity," *J Agric Food Chem* 2001 May; 49(5): 2592–99.

10. S. K. Banerjee, and S. K. Maulik, "Effect of garlic on cardiovascular disorders: a review," *Nutr J* 2002 Nov 19; 1(1): 4.

11. L. D. Lawson, Z. J. Wang, and D. Papadimitriou, "Allicin release under simulated gastrointestinal conditions from garlic powder tablets employed in clinical trials on serum cholesterol," *Planta Med* 2001 Feb; 67(1): 13–18.

12. C. Stevinson, M. H. Pittler, and E. Ernst, "Garlic for Treating Hypercholesterolemia: A Meta-Analysis of Randomized Clinical Trials," *Ann Intern Med* 2000 Sep 19; 133(6): 420–29.

13. A. T. Fleischauer, C. Poole, and L. Arab, "Garlic consumption and cancer prevention: meta-analyses of colorectal and stomach cancers," *American Journal of Clinical Nutrition* 72(4): 1047–52, October 2000.

14. R. G. Leuschner, and V. Ielsch, "Antimicrobial effects of garlic, clove and red hot chilli on Listeria monocytogenes in broth model systems and soft cheese," *Int J Food Sci Nutr* 2003 Mar; 54(2): 127–33.

15. B. B. Adler, and L. R. Beuchat, "Death of Salmonella, Escherichia coli O157:H7, and Listeria monocytogenes in garlic butter as affected by storage temperature," *J Food Prot* 2002 Dec; 65(12): 1976–80.

16. S. M. Tsao, and M. C. Yin, "In-vitro antimicrobial activity of four diallyl sulphides occurring naturally in garlic and Chinese leek oils," *J Med Microbiol* 2001 Jul; 50(7): 646–69.

17. N. D. Weber, D. O. Andersen, J. A. North, B. K. Murray, L. D. Lawson, and B. G. Hughes, "In vitro virucidal effects of Allium sativum (garlic) extract and compounds," *Planta Med* 1992 Oct; 58(5): 417–23.

18. E. H. O'Gara, D. J. Hill, and D. J. Maslin, "Activities of garlic oil, garlic powder, and their diallyl constituents against Helicobacter pylori," *Appl Environ Microbiol* 2000 May; 66(5): 2269–73.

19. C. A. McNulty, M. P. Wilson, W. Havinga, B. Johnston, E. A. O'Gara, and D. J. Maslin, "A pilot study to determine the effectiveness of garlic oil capsules in the treatment of dyspeptic patients with Helicobacter pylori," *Helicobacter* 2001 Sep; 6(3): 249–53.

20. D. Y. Graham, S. Y. Anderson, and T. Lang, "Garlic or jalapeno peppers for treatment of Helicobacter pylori infection," *Am J Gastroenterol* 1999 May; 94(5): 1200–02.

21. E. Ledezma, K. Marcano, A. Jorquera, L. De Sousa, M. Padilla, M. Pulgar, and R. Apitz-Castro, "Efficacy of ajoene in the treatment of tinea pedis: a double-blind and comparative study with terbinafine," *J Am Acad Dermatol* 2000 Nov; 43(5 Pt 1): 829–32.

22. E. Ledezma, J. C. Lopez, P. Marin, H. Romero, G. Ferrara, L. De Sousa, A. Jorquera, and R. Apitz Castro, "Ajoene in the topical short-term treatment of tinea cruris and tinea corporis in humans. Randomized comparative study with terbinafine," *Arzneimittelforschung* 1999 Jun; 49(6): 544–47.

23. F. C. Groppo, J. C. Ramacciato, R. P. Simoes, F. M. Florio, and A. Sartoratto, "Antimicrobial activity of garlic,

tea tree oil, and chlorhexidine against oral microorganisms," *Int Dent J* 2002 Dec; 52(6): 433–37.

24. P. Josling, "Preventing the common cold with a garlic supplement: a double-blind, placebo-controlled survey," *Adv Ther* 2001 Jul–Aug; 18(4): 189–93.

25. M. E. St. Louis, S. H. Peck, D. Bowering, G. B. Morgan, J. Blatherwick, S. Banerjee, G. D. Kettyls, W. A. Black, M. E. Milling, A. H. Hauschild, et al., "Botulism from chopped garlic: delayed recognition of a major outbreak," *Ann Intern Med* 1988 Mar; 108(3): 363–68.

26. D. L. Morse, L. K. Pickard, J. J. Guzewich, B. D. Devine, and M. Shayegani, "Garlic-in-oil associated botulism: episode leads to product modification," *Am J Public Health* 1990 Nov; 80(11): 1372–73.

27. N. Lohse, P. G. Kraghede, and K. Molbak, "Botulism in a 38-year-old man after ingestion of garlic in chilli oil," *Ugeskr Laeger* 2003 Jul 21; 165(30): 2962–63.

References for Ginger

1. V. N. Dedov, V. H. Tran, C. C. Duke, M. Connor, M. J. Christie, S. Mandadi, and B. D. Roufogalis, "Gingerols: a novel class of vanilloid receptor (VR1) agonists," *Br J Pharmacol* 2002 Nov; 137(6): 793–98.

2. F. Borrelli, R. Capasso, A. Pinto, and A. A. Izzo, "Inhibitory effect of ginger (*Zingiber officinale*) on rat ileal motility in vitro," *Life Sci* 2004 Apr 23; 74(23): 2889–96.

3. H. C. Lien, W. M. Sun, Y. H. Chen, H. Kim, W. Hasler, and C. Owyang, "Effects of ginger on motion sickness and gastric slow-wave dysrhythmias induced by circular vection," *Am J Physiol Gastrointest Liver Physiol* 2003 Mar; 284(3): G481–89.

4. S. Gonlachanvit, Y. H. Chen, W. L. Hasler, W. M. Sun, and C. Owyang, "Ginger reduces hyperglycemia-evoked gastric dysrhythmias in healthy humans: possible role of endogenous prostaglandins," *J Pharmacol Exp Ther* 2003.

5. Mowray D, Clayson D, "Motion Sickness, Ginger, and Psychophysics," *Lancet.* 1982 Mar 20; 1(8273): 655–57.

6. G. Portnoi, L. A. Chng, L. Karimi-Tabesh, G. Koren, M. P. Tan, and A. Einarson, "Prospective comparative study of the safety and effectiveness of ginger for the treatment of nausea and vomiting in pregnancy," *Am J Obstet Gynecol* 2003 Nov; 189(5): 1374–77.

7. K. E. Willetts, A. Ekangaki, and J. A. Eden, "Effect of a ginger extract on pregnancy-induced nausea: a randomised controlled trial," *Aust N Z J Obstet Gynaecol* 2003 Apr; 43(2): 139–44.

8. C. Smith, C. Crowther, K. Willson, N. Hotham, and V. McMillian, "A randomized controlled trial of ginger to treat nausea and vomiting in pregnancy," *Obstet Gynecol* 2004 Apr; 103(4): 639–45.

9. T. Vutyavanich, T. Kraisarin, and R. Ruangsri, "Ginger for nausea and vomiting in pregnancy: randomized, double-masked, placebo-controlled trial," *Obstet Gynecol* 2001 Apr; 97(4): 577–82.

10. W. Fischer-Rasmussen, S. K. Kjaer, C. Dahl, and U. Asping, "Ginger treatment of hyperemesis gravidarum," *Eur J Obstet Gynecol Reprod Biol* 1991 Jan 4; 38(1): 19–24.

11. A. Keating, and R. A. Chez, "Ginger syrup as an antiemetic in early pregnancy," *Altern Ther Health Med* 2002 Sep–Oct; 8(5): 89–91.

12. A. M. Morin, O. Betz, P. Kranke, G. Geldner, H. Wulf, and L. H. Eberhart, "Is ginger a relevant antiemetic for postoperative nausea and vomiting?" *Anasthesiol Intensivmed Notfallmed Schmerzther* 2004 May; 39(5): 281–85.

13. S. Holtmann, A. H. Clarke, H. Scherer, and M. Hohn, "The anti-motion sickness mechanism of ginger. A comparative study with placebo and dimenhydrinate," *Acta Otolaryngol* 1989 Sep–Oct; 108(3–4): 168–74.

14. S. Gonlachanvit, Y. H. Chen, W. L. Hasler, W. M. Sun, and C. Owyang, "Ginger reduces hyperglycemia-evoked gastric dysrhythmias in healthy humans: possible role of endogenous prostaglandins," *J Pharmacol Exp Ther* 2003 Dec; 307(3): 1098–103. E-pub, 2003 Oct 08.

15. H. C. Lien, W. M. Sun, Y. H. Chen, H. Kim, W. Hasler, and C. Owyang, "Effects of ginger on motion sickness and gastric slow-wave dysrhythmias induced by circular vection," *Am J Physiol Gastrointest Liver Physiol* 2003 Mar; 284(3): G481–89.

16. I. Wigler, I. Grotto, D. Caspi, and M. Yaron, "The effects of Zintona EC (a ginger extract) on symptomatic gonarthritis," *Osteoarthritis Cartilage* 2003 Nov; 11(11): 783–89.

17. R. D. Altman, and K. C. Marcussen, "Effects of a ginger extract on knee pain in patients with osteoarthritis," *Arthritis Rheum* 2001 Nov; 44(11): 2531–38.

18. S. K. Verma, and A. Bordia, "Ginger, fat and fibrinolysis," *Indian J Med Sci* 2001 Feb; 55(2): 83–86.

19. A. Bordia, S. K. Verma, and K. C. Srivastava, "Effect of ginger (*Zingiber officinale Rosc.*) and fenugreek (*Trigonella foenumgraecum L.*) on blood lipids, blood sugar and platelet aggregation in patients with coronary artery disease," *Prostaglandins Leukot Essent Fatty Acids* 1997 May; 56(5): 379–84.

References for Ginkgo

1. M. Lenoir, E. Pedruzzi, S. Rais, K. Drieu, and A. Perianin, "Sensitization of human neutrophil defense activities through activation of platelet-activating factor receptors by ginkgolide B, a bioactive component of the Ginkgo biloba extract EGB 761," *Biochem Pharmacol* 2002 Apr 1; 63(7): 1241–49.

2. Y. Kubota, N. Tanaka, K. Umegaki, H. Takenaka, H. Mizuno, K. Nakamura, K. Shinozuka, and M. Kunitomo, "Ginkgo biloba extract-induced relaxation of rat aorta is associated with increase in endothelial intracellular calcium level," *Life Sci* 2001 Oct 5; 69(20): 2327–36.

3. Z. Li, Y. Nakaya, Y. Niwa, and X. Chen, "K(Ca) channel-opening activity of Ginkgo Biloba extracts and ginsenosides in cultured endothelial cells," *Clin Exp Pharmacol Physiol* 2001 May-Jun; 28(5–6): 441–45.

4. J. Birks, E. V. Grimley, and M. Van Dongen, "Ginkgo biloba for cognitive impairment and dementia," *Cochrane Database Syst Rev* 2002; (4): CD003120.

5. M. C. van Dongen, E. van Rossum, A. G. Kessels, H. J. Sielhorst, and P. G. Knipschild, "The efficacy of ginkgo for elderly people with dementia and age-associated memory impairment: new results of a randomized clinical trial," *J Am Geriatr Soc* 2000; 48:1183–94.

6. A. Wettstein, "Cholinesterase inhibitors and Ginkgo extracts—are they comparable in the treatment of dementia? Comparison of published placebo-controlled efficacy studies of at least six months' duration," *Phytomedicine* 2000; 6:393–401.

7. B. S. Oken, D. M. Storzbach, and J. A. Kaye, "The efficacy of Ginkgo biloba on cognitive function in Alzheimer's disease," *Arch Neurol* 1998; 55:1409–15.

8. M. H. Pittler, and E. Ernst, "Ginkgo biloba extract for the treatment of intermittent claudication: a meta-analysis of randomized trials," *Am J Med* 2000; 108:276–81.

9. S. Drew, and E. Davies, "Effectiveness of Ginkgo biloba in treating tinnitus: double-blind, placebo-controlled trial," *BMJ* 2001; 332:73.

10. B. Meyer, "Multicenter randomized double-blind drug vs. placebo study of the treatment of tinnitus with Ginkgo biloba extract" [in French], *Presse Med* 1986; 15:1562–64.

11. E. Ernst, and C. Stevinson, "Ginkgo biloba for tinnitus: a review," *Clin Otolaryngol* 1999; 24:164–67.

References for Ginseng

1. M. Blumenthal, "Farm Bill Bans Use of Name 'Ginseng' on Non-Panax Species: 'Siberian Ginseng' no longer allowed as commercial term," *HerbalGram* 2002; 56:54.

2. R. K. Siegel, "Ginseng abuse syndrome. Problems with the panacea," *JAMA* 1979, 241:1614–15.

3. Steven Foster, and Varro E. Tyler, *Tyler's Honest Herbal,* 4th ed. (New York: Haworth Herbal Press, 1999).

4. H. Sorensen, and J. Sonne, "A double-masked study of the effects of ginseng on cognitive functions," *Curr Ther Res Clin Exp* 1996; 57:959–68.

5. J. M. Ellis, and P. Reddy, "Effects of Panax ginseng on quality of life," *Ann Pharmacother* 2002; 36:375–79.

6. I. K. Wiklund, L. A. Mattsson, R. Lindgren, and C. Limoni, "Effects of a standardized ginseng extract on quality of life and physiological parameters in symptomatic postmenopausal women: a double-blind, placebo-controlled trial," Swedish Alternative Medicine Group, *Int J Clin Pharmacol Res* 1999; 19:89–99.

7. B. J. Cardinal, and H. J. Engels, "Ginseng does not enhance psychological well-being in healthy, young adults: results of a double-blind, placebo-controlled, randomized clinical trial," *J Am Diet Assoc* 2001; 101:655–60.

8. H. J. Engels, M. M. Fahlman, and J. C. Wirth, "Effects of ginseng on secretory IgA, performance, and recovery from interval exercise," *Med Sci Sports Exerc* 2003 Apr; 35(4): 690–96.

9. H. J. Engels, I. Kolokouri, T. J. Cieslak II, and J. C. Wirth, "Effects of ginseng supplementation on supramaximal exercise performance and short-term recovery," *J Strength Cond Res* 2001 Aug; 15(3): 290–95.

10. H. J. Engels, and J. C. Wirth, "No ergogenic effects of ginseng (Panax ginseng C.A. Meyer) during graded maximal aerobic exercise," *J Am Diet Assoc* 1997 Oct; 97(10): 1110–15.

11. H. J. Engels, J. M. Said, and J. C. Wirth, "Failure of chronic ginseng supplementation to affect work performance and energy metabolism in healthy adult females," *Nutr Res* 1996; 16:1295–1305.

12. H. Youl Kang, S. Hwan Kim, W. Jun Lee, and H. K. Byrne, "Effects of ginseng ingestion on growth hormone, testosterone, cortisol, and insulin-like growth factor 1 responses to acute resistance exercise," *J Strength Cond Res* 2002 May; 16(2): 179–83.

13. A. C. Morris, I. Jacobs, T. M. McLellan, A. Klugerman, L. C. Wang, and J. Zamecnik, "No ergogenic effect of ginseng ingestion," *Int J Sport Nutr* 1996 Sep; 6(3): 263–71.

14. J. D. Allen, J. McLung, A. G. Nelson, and M. Welsch, "Ginseng supplementation does not enhance healthy young adults' peak aerobic exercise performance," *J Am Coll Nutr* 1998; 17:462–66.

15. A. W. Ziemba, J. Chmura, H. Kaciuba-Uscilko, K. Nazar, P. Wisnik, and W. Gawronski, "Ginseng treatment improves psychomotor performance at rest and during graded exercise in young athletes," *Int J Sport Nutr* 1999 Dec; 9(4): 371–77.

16. B. T. Gaffney, H. M. Hugel, and P. A. Rich, "The effects of Eleutherococcus senticosus and Panax ginseng on steroidal hormone indices of stress and lymphocyte subset numbers in endurance athletes," *Life Sci* 2001 Dec 14; 70(4):431–42.

17. F. Scaglione, G. Cattaneo, M. Alessandria, and R. Cogo, "Efficacy and safety of the standardized Ginseng extract G115 for potentiating vaccination against the influenza syndrome and protection against the common cold [corrected]," *Drugs Exp Clin Res* 1996; 22:65–72.

18. F. Scaglione, F. Ferrara, S. Dugnani, M. Falchi, G. Santoro, and F. Fraschini, "Immunomodulatory effects of two extracts of Panax ginseng C. A. Meyer," *Drugs Exp Clin Res* 1990; 16(10): 537–42.

19. H. J. Engels, M. M. Fahlman, and J. C. Wirth, "Effects of ginseng on secretory IgA, performance, and recovery from interval exercise," *Med Sci Sports Exerc* 2003 Apr; 35(4): 690–96.

20. F. Scaglione, K. Weiser, and M. Alessandria, "Effects of the standardized ginseng extract G115 in patients with chronic bronchitis: a nonblinded, randomised, comparative pilot study," *Clin Drug Invest* 2001; 21:41–45.

21. T. K. Yun, S. Y. Choi, and H. Y. Yun, "Epidemiological study on cancer prevention by ginseng: are all kinds of cancers preventable by ginseng?" *J Korean Med Sci* 2001 Dec; 16 Suppl:S19–27.

22. F. Y. Xie, Z. F. Zeng, and H. Y. Huang, "Clinical observation on nasopharyngeal carcinoma treated with combined therapy of radiotherapy and ginseng polysaccharide injection," (Article in Chinese) *Zhongguo Zhong Xi Yi Jie He Za Zhi* 2001 May; 21(5): 332–34.

23. V. Vuksan, J. L. Sievenpiper, V. Y. Koo, T. Francis, U. Beljan-Zdravkovic, Z. Xu, and E. Vidgen, "American ginseng (Panax quinquefolius L) reduces postprandial glycemia in nondiabetic subjects and subjects with type 2 diabetes mellitus," *Arch Intern Med* 2000 Apr 10; 160(7): 1009–13.

24. V. Vuksan, M. P. Stavro, J. L. Sievenpiper, U. Beljan-Zdravkovic, L. A. Leiter, R. G. Josse, and Z. Xu, "Similar postprandial glycemic reductions with escalation of dose and administration time of American ginseng in type 2 diabetes," *Diabetes Care* 2000 Sep; 23(9): 1221–26.

25. J. L. Sievenpiper, J. T. Arnason, L. A. Leiter, and V. Vuksan, "Variable effects of American ginseng: a batch of American ginseng (Panax quinquefolius L.) with a depressed ginsenoside profile does not affect postprandial glycemia," *Eur J Clin Nutr* 2003 Feb; 57(2): 243–48.

26. J. L. Sievenpiper, J. T. Arnason, L. A. Leiter, et al., "Null and opposing effects of Asian ginseng (Panax ginseng C. A. Meyer) on acute glycemia," *J Am Coll Nutr* 2003; 22:524–32.

27. J. L. Sievenpiper, J. T. Arnason, L. A. Leiter, and V. Vuksan, "Decreasing, null and increasing effects of eight popular types of ginseng on acute postprandial glycemic indices in healthy humans: the role of ginsenosides," *J Am Coll Nutr* 2004 Jun; 23(3): 248–58.

28. H. J. Kim, D. S. Woo, G. Lee, and J. J. Kim, "The relaxation effects of ginseng saponin in rabbit corporal smooth muscle: is it a nitric oxide donor?" *Br J Urol* 1998 Nov; 82(5): 744–48.

29. G. S. Oh, H. O. Pae, B. M. Choi, E. A. Seo, D. H. Kim, M. K. Shin, J. D. Kim, J. B. Kim, and H. T. Chung, "20(S)-Protopanaxatriol, one of ginsenoside metabolites, inhibits inducible nitric oxide synthase and cyclooxygenase-2 expressions through inactivation of nuclear factor-kappaB in RAW 264.7 macrophages stimulated with lipopolysaccharide," *Cancer Lett,* 2004 Mar 8; 205(1): 23–29.

30. S. S. Choi, J. K. Lee, E. J. Han, K. J. Han, H. K. Lee, J. Lee, and H. W. Suh, "Effect of ginsenoside Rd on nitric oxide system induced by lipopolysaccharide plus TNF-alpha in C6 rat glioma cells," *Arch Pharm Res* 2003 May; 26(5): 375–82.

31. G. I. Scott, P. B. Colligan, B. H. Ren, and J. Ren, "Ginsenosides Rb1 and Re decrease cardiac contraction in adult rat ventricular myocytes: role of nitric oxide," *Br J Pharmacol* 2001 Nov; 134(6): 1159–65.

32. N. D. Kim, E. M. Kim, K. W. Kang, M. K. Cho, S. Y. Choi, and S. G. Kim, "Ginsenoside Rg3 inhibits phenylephrine-induced vascular contraction through induction of nitric oxide synthase," *Br J Pharmacol* 2003 Oct; 140(4): 661–70.

33. H. Yoshimura, N. Kimura, and K. Sugiura, "Preventive effects of various ginseng saponins on the development of copulatory disorder induced by prolonged individual housing in male mice," *Methods Find Exp Clin Pharmacol* 1998 Jan–Feb; 20(1): 59–64.

34. B. Hong, Y. H. Ji, J. H. Hong, K. Y. Nam, and T. Y. Ahn, "A double-blind crossover study evaluating the efficacy of korean red ginseng in patients with erectile dysfunction: a preliminary report," *J Urol* 2002 Nov; 168(5): 2070–73.

References for Gotu Kola

1. O. D. Laerum , O. H. Iversen, "Reticuloses and epidermal tumors in hairless mice after topical skin applications of cantharidin and asiaticoside," *Cancer Res.* 1972 Jul; 32(7):1463–9.

2. L. Incandela, G. Belcaro, M. T. De Sanctis, M. R. Cesarone, M. Griffin, E. Ippolito, M. Bucci, and M. Cacchio, "Total triterpenic fraction of Centella asiatica in the treatment of venous hypertension: a clinical, prospective, randomized trial using a combined microcirculatory model," *Angiology* 2001 Oct; 52 Suppl 2:S61–67.

3. M. T. De Sanctis, G. Belcaro, L. Incandela, M. R. Cesarone, M. Griffin, E. Ippolito, and M. Cacchio, "Treatment of edema and increased capillary filtration in venous hypertension with total triterpenic fraction of Centella asiatica: a clinical, prospective, randomized, dose-ranging trial," *Angiology* 2001 Oct; 52 Suppl 2:S55–59.

4. M. R. Cesarone, G. Belcaro, M. T. De Sanctis, L. Incandela, M. Cacchio, P. Bavera, E. Ippolito, M. Bucci, M. Griffin, G. Geroulakos, M. Dugall, S. Buccella, S. Kleyweght, and M. Cacchio, "Effects of the total triter-penic fraction of Centella asiatica in venous hypertensive microangiopathy: a prospective, placebo-controlled, randomized trial," *Angiology* 2001 Oct; 52 Suppl 2:S15–18.

5. M. R. Cesarone, G. Belcaro, A. Rulo, M. Griffin, A. Ricci, E. Ippolito, M. T. De Sanctis, L. Incandela, P. Bavera, M. Cacchio, and M. Bucci, "Microcirculatory effects of total triterpenic fraction of Centella asiatica in chronic venous hypertension: measurement by laser Doppler, TcPO2-CO2, and leg volumetry," *Angiology* 2001 Oct; 52 Suppl 2:S45–48.

6. J. P. Pointel, H. Boccalon, M. Cloarec, C. Ledevehat, and M. Joubert, "Titrated extract of Centella asiatica (TECA) in the treatment of venous insufficiency of the lower limbs," *Angiology* 1987 Jan; 38(1 Pt 1): 46–50.

7. M. R. Cesarone, G. Laurora, M. T. De Sanctis, L. Incandela, R. Grimaldi, C. Marelli, and G. Belcaro, "The microcirculatory activity of Centella asiatica in venous insufficiency. A double-blind study," *Minerva Cardioangiol* 1994 Jun; 42(6): 299–304.

8. G. V. Belcaro, A. Rulo, R. Grimaldi, "Capillary filtration and ankle edema in patients with venous hypertension treated with TTFCA," *Angiology* 1990 Jan; 41(1): 12–18.

9. G. P. Montecchio, A. Samaden, S. Carbone, M. Vigotti, S. Siragusa, and F. Piovella, "Centella Asiatica Triterpenic Fraction (CATTF) reduces the number of circulating endothelial cells in subjects with post phlebitic syndrome," *Haematologica* 1991 May–Jun; 76(3): 256–59.

10. M. R. Cesarone, L. Incandela, M. T. De Sanctis, G. Belcaro, P. Bavera, M. Bucci, and E. Ippolito, "Evaluation of treatment of diabetic microangiopathy with total triterpenic fraction of Centella asiatica: a clinical prospective randomized trial with a microcirculatory model," *Angiology* 2001 Oct; 52 Suppl 2:S49–54.

11. L. Incandela, G. Belcaro, M. R. Cesarone, M. T. De Sanctis, E. Nargi, P. Patricelli, and M. Bucci, "Treatment of diabetic microangiopathy and edema with total triterpenic fraction of Centella asiatica: a prospective, placebo-controlled randomized study," *Angiology* 2001 Oct; 52 Suppl 2:S27–31.

12. L. Incandela, G. Belcaro, A. N. Nicolaides, M. R. Cesarone, M. T. De Sanctis, M. Corsi, P. Bavera, E. Ippolito, M. Griffin, G. Geroulakos, M. Sabetai, G. Ramaswami, and M. Veller, "Modification of the echogenicity of femoral plaques after treatment with total triterpenic fraction of Centella asiatica: a prospective, randomized, placebo-controlled trial," *Angiology* 2001 Oct; 52 Suppl 2:S69–73.

13. M. R. Cesarone, G. Belcaro, A. N. Nicolaides, G. Geroulakos, M. Bucci, M. Dugall, M. T. De Sanctis, L. Incandela, M. Griffin, and M. Sabetai, "Increase in echogenicity of echolucent carotid plaques after treatment with total triterpenic fraction of Centella asiatica: a prospective, placebo-controlled, randomized trial," *Angiology* 2001 Oct; 52 Suppl 2:S19–25.

14. M. R. Cesarone, L. Incandela, M. T. De Sanctis, g. Belcaro, G. Geroulakos, M. Griffin, A. Lennox, A. D. Di Renzo, M. Cacchio, and M. Bucci, "Flight microangiopathy in medium- to long-distance flights: prevention of edema and microcirculation alterations with total triterpenic fraction of Centella asiatica," *Angiology* 2001 Oct; 52 Suppl 2:S33–37.

15. M. R. Arpaia, R. Ferrone, M. Amitrano, C. Nappo, G.

Leonardo, and R. del Guercio, "Effects of Centella asiatica extract on mucopolysaccharide metabolism in subjects with varicose veins," *Int J Clin Pharmacol Res* 1990; 10(4): 229–33.

16. C. L. Cheng, J. S. Guo, J. Luk, and M. W. Koo, "The healing effects of Centella extract and asiaticoside on acetic acid induced gastric ulcers in rats," *Life Sci* 2004 Mar 19; 74(18): 2237–49.

17. K. Sairam, C. V. Rao, and R. K. Goel, "Effect of Centella asiatica Linn on physical and chemical factors induced gastric ulceration and secretion in rats," *Indian J Exp Biol* 2001 Feb; 39(2): 137–42.

18. C. L. Cheng, and M. W. Koo, "Effects of Centella asiatica on ethanol induced gastric mucosal lesions in rats," *Life Sci* 2000 Oct 13; 67(21): 2647–53.

19. A. Shukla, A. M. Rasik, G. K. Jain, R. Shankar, D. K. Kulshrestha, and B. N. Dhawan, "In vitro and in vivo wound healing activity of asiaticoside isolated from Centella asiatica," *J Ethnopharmacol* 1999 Apr; 65(1): 1–11.

20. A. Shukla, A. M. Rasik, and B. N. Dhawan, "Asiaticoside-induced elevation of antioxidant levels in healing wounds," *Phytother Res* 1999 Feb; 13(1): 50–54.

21. M. H. Veerendra Kumar, and Y. K. Gupta, "Effect of different extracts of Centella asiatica on cognition and markers of oxidative stress in rats," *J Ethnopharmacol* 2002 Feb; 79(2): 253–60.

22. Y. K. Gupta, M. H. Veerendra Kumar, and A. K. Srivastava, "Effect of Centella asiatica on pentylenetetrazole-induced kindling, cognition and oxidative stress in rats," *Pharmacol Biochem Behav* 2003 Feb; 74(3): 579–85.

23. J. Bradwejn, Y. Zhou, D. Koszycki, and J. Shlik, "A double-blind, placebo-controlled study on the effects of Gotu Kola (Centella asiatica) on acoustic startle response in healthy subjects," *J Clin Psychopharmacol* 2000 Dec; 20(6): 680–84.

References for Grape

1. L. M. Szewczuk, and T. M. Penning, "Mechanism-based inactivation of COX-1 by red wine m-hydroquinones: a structure-activity relationship study," *J Nat Prod* 2004 Nov; 67(11): 1777–82.

2. J. G. Keevil, H. E. Osman, J. D. Reed, and J. D. Folts, "Grape juice, but not orange juice or grapefruit juice, inhibits human platelet aggregation," *J Nutr* 2000 Jan; 130(1): 53–56.

3. J. E. Freedman, C. Parker III, L. Li, J. A. Perlman, B. Frei, V. Ivanov, L. R. Deak, M. D. Iafrati, and J. D. Folts, "Select flavonoids and whole juice from purple grapes inhibit platelet function and enhance nitric oxide release," *Circulation* 2001 Jun 12; 103(23): 2792–98.

4. Y. K. Park, J. S. Kim, and M. H. Kang, "Concord grape juice supplementation reduces blood pressure in Korean hypertensive men: double-blind, placebo-controlled intervention trial," *Biofactors* 2004; 22(1–4): 145–47.

5. E. B. Rimm, A. Klatsky, D. Grobbee, and M. J. Stampfer, "Review of moderate alcohol consumption and reduced risk of coronary heart disease: is the effect due to beer, wine, or spirits," *BMJ* 1996; 312(7033): 731–36.

6. S. G. Wannamethee, and A. G. Shaper, "Type of alcoholic drink and risk of major coronary heart disease

events and all-cause mortality," *Am J Public Health* 1999; 89(5): 685–90.

7. D. Rein, T. G. Paglieroni, D. A. Pearson, T. Wun, H. H. Schmitz, R. Gosselin, and C. L. Keen, "Cocoa and wine polyphenols modulate platelet activation and function," *J Nutr* 2000 Aug; 130(8S Suppl): 2120S–6S.

8. D. I. Bernstein, C. K. Bernstein, C. Deng, K. J. Murphy, I. L. Bernstein, J. A. Bernstein, and R. Shukla, "Evaluation of the clinical efficacy and safety of grape-seed extract in the treatment of fall seasonal allergic rhinitis: a pilot study," *Ann Allergy Asthma Immunol* 2002 Mar; 88(3): 272–78.

9. S. L. Nuttall, M. J. Kendall, E. Bombardelli, and P. Morazzoni, "An evaluation of the antioxidant activity of a standardized grape seed extract, Leucoselect," *J Clin Pharm Ther* 1998 Oct; 23(5): 385–89.

10. N. Vogels, I. M. Nijs, and M. S. Westerterp-Plantenga, "The effect of grape-seed extract on 24 h energy intake in humans," *Eur J Clin Nutr* 2004 Apr; 58(4): 667–73.

11. J. Yamakoshi, A. Sano, S. Tokutake, M. Saito, M. Kikuchi, Y. Kubota, Y. Kawachi, and F. Otsuka, "Oral intake of proanthocyanidin-rich extract from grape seeds improves chloasma," *Phytother Res* 2004 Nov; 18(11): 895–99.

12. H. G. Preuss, D. Wallerstedt, N. Talpur, S. O. Tutuncuoglu, B. Echard, A. Myers, M. Bui, and D. Bagchi, "Effects of niacin-bound chromium and grape seed proanthocyanidin extract on the lipid profile of hypercholesterolemic subjects: a pilot study," *J Med* 2000; 31(5–6): 227–46.

13. G. B. Vigna, F. Costantini, G. Aldini, M. Carini, A. Catapano, F. Schena, A. Tangerini, R. Zanca, E. Bombardelli, P. Morazzoni, A. Mezzetti, R. Fellin, and R. Maffei Facino, "Effect of a standardized grape seed extract on low-density lipoprotein susceptibility to oxidation in heavy smokers," *Metabolism* 2003 Oct; 52(10): 1250–57.

14. J. F. Young, L. O. Dragsted, B. Daneshvar, S. T. Lauridsen, M. Hansen, and B. Sandstrom, "The effect of grape-skin extract on oxidative status," *Br J Nutr* 2000 Oct; 84(4): 505–13.

15. U. Kalus, J. Koscielny, A. Grigorov, E. Schaefer, H. Peil, and H. Kiesewetter, "Improvement of cutaneous microcirculation and oxygen supply in patients with chronic venous insufficiency by orally administered extract of red vine leaves AS 195: a randomised, double-blind, placebo-controlled, crossover study," *Drugs R D* 2004; 5(2): 63–71.

References for Guarana

1. J. S. Tolstrup, S. K Kjaer, C. Munk, L. B. Madsen, B. Ottesen, T. Bergholt, M. Gronbaek, "Does caffeine and alcohol intake before pregnancy predict the occurrence of spontaneous abortion?" *Hum Reprod* 2003 Dec; 18(12):2704–10.

2. J. C. Galduroz, and E. A. Carlini, "The effects of long-term administration of guarana on the cognition of normal, elderly volunteers," *Sao Paulo Med J* 1996 Jan–Feb; 114(1): 1073–78.

3. D. O. Kennedy, C. F. Haskell, K. A. Wesnes, and A. B. Scholey, "Improved cognitive performance in human volunteers following administration of guarana (*Paullinia cupana*) extract: comparison and interaction with Panax ginseng," *Pharmacol Biochem Behav* 2004

Nov; 79(3): 401–11.

4. T. Andersen, and J. Fogh, "Weight loss and delayed gastric emptying following a South American herbal preparation in overweight patients," *J Hum Nutr Diet* 2001 Jun; 14(3): 243–50.

5. A. R. Campos, A. I. Barros, F. A. Santos, and V. S. Rao, "Guarana (*Paullinia cupana Mart.*) offers protection against gastric lesions induced by ethanol and indomethacin in rats," *Phytother Res* 2003 Dec; 17(10): 1199–202.

6. C. N. Boozer, J. A. Nasser, S. B. Heymsfield, V. Wang, G. Chen, and J. L. Solomon, "An herbal supplement containing Ma Huang-Guarana for weight loss: a randomized, double-blind trial," *Int J Obes Relat Metab Disord* 2001 Mar; 25(3): 316–24.

7. T. Miura, M. Tatara, K. Nakamura, and I. Suzuki, "Effect of guarana on exercise in normal and epinephrine-induced glycogenolytic mice," *Biol Pharm Bull* 1998 Jun; 21(6): 646–48.

8. E. B. Espinola, R. F. Dias, R. Mattei, and E. A. Carlini, "Pharmacological activity of Guarana (*Paullinia cupana Mart.*) in laboratory animals," *J Ethnopharmacol* 1997 Feb; 55(3): 223–29.

9. S. P. Bydlowski, R. L. Yunker, and M. T. Subbiah, "A novel property of an aqueous guarana extract (*Paullinia cupana*): inhibition of platelet aggregation in vitro and in vivo," *Braz J Med Biol Res* 1988; 21(3): 535–38.

10. H. Fukumasu, T. C. Silva, J. L. Avanzo, C. E. Lima, I. I. Mackowiak, A. Atroch, H. D. Spinosa, F. S. Moreno, and M. L. Dagli, "Chemopreventive effects of Paullinia cupana Mart var. sorbilis, the guarana, on mouse hepatocarcinogenesis," *Cancer Lett* 2005 May 7.

11. A. R. Campos, et al., op. cit.

12. R. Mattei, R. F. Dias, E. B. Espinola, E. A. Carlini, and S. B. Barros, "Guarana (*Paullinia cupana*): toxic behavioral effects in laboratory animals and antioxidants activity in vitro," *J Ethnopharmacol* 1998 Mar; 60(2): 111–16.

References for Hawthorn

1. A. Muller, W. Linke, and W. Klaus, "Crataegus extract blocks potassium currents in guinea pig ventricular cardiac myocytes," *Planta Med* 1999 May; 65(4): 335–39.

2. S. Deprez, I. Mila, J-F Huneau, D. Tome, and A. Scalbert, "Transport of Proanthocyanidin Dimer, Trimer, and Polymer Across Monolayers of Human Intestinal Epithelial Caco-2 Cells," *Antioxidants and Redox Signaling* 2001 Dec; 3(6): 957–67(11).

3. M. H. Pittler, K. Schmidt, and E. Ernst, "Hawthorn extract for treating chronic heart failure: meta-analysis of randomized trials," *Am J Med* 2003 Jun 1; 114(8): 665–74.

References for Hoodia

1. O. L. Tulp, N. A. Harbi, and A. DerMarderosian, "Effect of Hoodia plant on weight loss in congenic obese LA/Ntul//-cp rats," *FASEB* 2002 March 20; 16(4): A648.

2. D. B. MacLean, and L. G. Luo, "Related Increased ATP content/production in the hypothalamus may be a signal for energy-sensing of satiety: studies of the anorectic mechanism of a plant steroidal glycoside," *Brain Res* 2004 Sep 10; 1020(1–2): 1–11.

References for Horse Chestnut

1. M. H. Pittler, and E. Ernst, "Horse chestnut seed extract for chronic venous insufficiency," *Cochrane Database Syst Rev* 2004; (2): CD003230.

2. C. Diehm, H. J. Trampisch, S. Lange, and C. Schmidt, "Comparison of leg compression stocking and oral horse-chestnut seed extract therapy in patients with chronic venous insufficiency," *Lancet* 1996 Feb 3; 347(8997): 292–94.

3. C. Diehm, and C. Schmidt, "Venostasin(r) retard gegen Plazebo und Kompression bei Patienten mit CVI II/IIIA. Final Study Report," *Klinge Pharma GmbH* (Munich) 2000 Nov 21.

4. U. Siebert, M. Brach, G. Sroczynski, and K. Berla, "Efficacy, routine effectiveness, and safety of horsechestnut seed extract in the treatment of chronic venous insufficiency. A meta-analysis of randomized controlled trials and large observational studies," *Int Angiol* 2002 Dec; 21(4): 305–15.

5. A. Ricci, I. Ruffini, M. R. Cesarone, U. Cornelli, M. Corsi, G. Belcaro, E. Ippolito, and M. Dugall, "Variations in plasma free radicals with topical aescin + essential phospholipids gel in venous hypertension: new clinical data," *Angiology* 2004 May–Jun; 55 Suppl 1:S11–14.

6. C. Bougelet, I. H. Roland, N. Ninane, T. Arnould, J. Remacle, and C. Michiels, "Effect of aescine on hypoxia-induced neutrophil adherence to umbilical vein endothelium," *Eur J Pharmacol* 1998 Mar 12; 345(1): 89–95.

7. X. M. Hu, Y. Zhang, and F. D. Zeng, "Effects of sodium beta-aescin on expression of adhesion molecules and migration of neutrophils after middle cerebral artery occlusion in rats," *Acta Pharmacol Sin* 2004 Jul; 25(7): 869–75.

8. F. Brunner, C. Hoffmann, and S. Schuller-Petrovic, "Responsiveness of human varicose saphenous veins to vasoactive agents," *Br J Clin Pharmacol* 2001 Mar; 51(3): 219–24.

9. F. Berti, C. Omini, and D. Longiave, "The mode of action of aescin and the release of prostaglandins," *Prostaglandins* 1977 Aug; 14(2): 241–49.

10. R. M. Facino, M. Carini, R. Stefani, et al., "Anti-elastase and anti-hyaluronidase activities of saponins and sapogenins from Hedera helix, Aesculus hippocastanum, and ruscusaculeatus: factors contributing to their efficacy in the treatment of venous insufficiency," *Arch Pharm* (Weinheim) 1995 Oct; 328(10): 720–24.

11. G. Hitzenberger, "The therapeutic effectiveness of chestnut extract," *Wien Med Wochenschr* 1989 Sep 15; 139(17): 385–89.

References for Kava Kava

1. K. Schirrmacher, D. Busselberg, J. M. Langosch, J. Walden, U. Winter, and D. Bingmann, "Effects of (+/-)-kavain on voltage-activated inward currents of dorsal root ganglion cells from neonatal rats," *Eur Neuropsychopharmacol* 1999 Jan; 9(1–2): 171–76.

2. J. Friese, and J. Gleitz, "Kavain, dihydrokavain, and dihydromethysticin non-competitively inhibit the specific binding of [3H]-batrachotoxinin-A 20-alphabenzoate to receptor site 2 of voltage-gated Na+ channels," *Planta Med* 1998 Jun; 64(5): 458–59.

3. H. B. Martin, M. McCallum, W. D. Stofer, and M. R. Eichinger, "Kavain attenuates vascular contractility

through inhibition of calcium channels," *Planta Med* 2002 Sep; 68(9): 784–89.

4. A. Jussofie, A. Schmiz, and C. Hiemke, "Kavapyrone-enriched extract from Piper methysticum as modulator of the GABA binding site in different regions of rat brain," *Psychopharmacology* (Berl) 1994 Dec; 116(4): 469–74.

5. L. P. Davies, C. A. Drew, P. Duffield, G. A. Johnston, and D. D. Jamieson, "Kava pyrones and resin: studies on GABAA, GABAB and benzodiazepine binding sites in rodent brain," *Pharmacol Toxicol* 1992 Aug; 71(2): 120–26.

6. G. Boonen and H. Haberlein, "Influence of genuine kavapyrone enantiomers on the GABA-A binding site," *Planta Med* 1998 Aug; 64(6): 504–06.

7. A. Jussofie, et al., op. cit.

8. J. Friese, A. Beile, A. Ameri, and T. Peters, "Anticonvulsive action of (+/-)-kavain estimated from its properties on stimulated synaptosomes and Na+ channel receptor sites," *Eur J Pharmacol* 1996 Nov 7; 315(1): 89–97.

9. S. S. Baum, R. Hill, and H. Rommelspacher, "Effect of kava extract and individual kavapyrones on neurotransmitter levels in the nucleus accumbens of rats," *Prog Neuropsychopharmacol Biol Psychiatry* 1998 Oct; 22(7): 1105–20.

10. J. Anke, and I. Ramzan, "Pharmacokinetic and pharmacodynamic drug interactions with Kava (*Piper methysticum Forst. f.*)" *J. Ethnopharmacol* 2004 Aug; 93(2–3): 153–60.

11. P. A. Whitton, A. Lau, A. Salisbury, J. Whitehouse, and C. S. Evans, "Kava lactones and the kava-kava controversy," *Phytochemistry* 2003 Oct; 64(3): 673–79.

12. S. A. Norton, and P. Ruze, "Kava dermopathy," *J Am Acad Dermatol* 1994 Jul; 31(1): 89–97.

13. S. Russmann, Y. Barguil, P. Cabalion, M. Kritsanida, D. Duhet, and B. H. Lauterburg, "Hepatic injury due to traditional aqueous extracts of kava root in New Caledonia," *Eur J Gastroenterol Hepatol* 2003 Sep; 15(9): 1033–36.

14. A. R. Clough, R. S. Bailie, and B. J. Currie, "Liver function test abnormalities in users of aqueous kava extracts," *Toxicol Clin Toxicol* 2003; 41(6): 821–29.

15. A. R. Clough, K. Rowley, and K. O'Dea, "Kava use, dyslipidaemia and biomarkers of dietary quality in Aboriginal people in Arnhem Land in the Northern Territory (NT), Australia," *Eur J Clin Nutr* 2004 Jul; 58(7): 1090–93.

16. P. V. Nerurkar, K. Dragull, and C. S. Tang, "In vitro toxicity of kava alkaloid, pipermethystine, in HepG2 cells compared to kavalactones," *Toxicol Sci* 2004 May; 79(1): 106–11.

17. Y. N. Singh, and A. K. Devkota, "Aqueous kava extracts do not affect liver function tests in rats," *Planta Med* 2003 Jun; 69(6): 496–99.

18. M. H. Pittler, and E. Ernst, "Kava extract for treating anxiety," *Cochrane Database Syst Rev* 2003; (1): CD003383.

19. F. P. Geier, and T. Konstantinowicz, "Kava treatment in patients with anxiety," *Phytother Res* 2004 Apr; 18(4): 297–300.

20. R. Thompson, W. Ruch, and R. U. Hasenohrl, "Enhanced cognitive performance and cheerful mood by standardized extracts of Piper methysticum (Kavakava)," *Hum Psychopharmacol* 2004 Jun; 19(4): 243–50.

21. D. L. Clouatre, "Kava kava: examining new reports of toxicity," *Toxicol Lett* 2004 Apr 15; 150(1): 85–96.

References for Lavender

1. M. Lis-Balchin, and S. Hart, "Studies on the mode of action of the essential oil of lavender (*Lavandula angustifolia P. Miller*)," *Phytother Res* 1999 Sep; 13(6): 540–42.

2. L. Re, S. Barocci, S. Sonnino, A. Mencarelli, C. Vivani, G. Paolucci, A. Scarpantonio, L. Rinaldi, and E. Mosca, "Linalool modifies the nicotinic receptor-ion channel kinetics at the mouse neuromuscular junction," *Pharmacol Res* 2000 Aug; 42(2): 177–82.

3. L. F. Silva Brum, T. Emanuelli, D. O. Souza, and E. Elisabetsky, "Effects of linalool on glutamate release and uptake in mouse cortical synaptosomes," *Neurochem Res* 2001 Mar; 26(3): 191–94.

4. A. Prashar, I. C. Locke, and C. S. Evans, "Cytotoxicity of lavender oil and its major components to human skin cells," *Cell Prolif* 2004 Jun; 37(3): 221–29.

5. H. K. Vaddi, P. C. Ho, and S. Y. Chan, "Terpenes in propylene glycol as skin-penetration enhancers: permeation and partition of haloperidol, Fourier transform infrared spectroscopy, and differential scanning calorimetry," *J Pharm Sci* 2002 Jul; 91(7): 1639–51.

6. E. Vernet-Maury, O. Alaoui-Ismaili, A. Dittmar, G. Delhomme, and J. Chanel, "Basic emotions induced by odorants: a new approach based on autonomic pattern results," *J Auton Nerv Syst* 1999 Feb 15; 75(2–3): 176–83.

7. M. A. Diego, N. A. Jones, T. Field, M. Hernandez-Reif, S. Schanberg, C. Kuhn, V. McAdam, R. Galamaga, and M. Galamaga, "Aromatherapy positively affects mood, EEG patterns of alertness and math computations," *Int J NeuroSci* 1998 Dec; 96(3–4): 217–24.

8. I. J. Romine, A. M. Bush, and C. R. Geist, "Lavender aromatherapy in recovery from exercise," *Percept Mot Skills* 1999 Jun; 88(3 Pt 1): 756–58.

9. C. Holmes, V. Hopkins, C. Hensford, V. MacLaughlin, D. Wilkinson, and H. Rosenvinge, "Lavender oil as a treatment for agitated behaviour in severe dementia: a placebo-controlled study," *Int J Geriatr Psychiatry* 2002 Apr; 17(4): 305–08.

10. S. G. Gray, and A. A. Clair, "Influence of aromatherapy on medication administration to residential-care residents with dementia and behavioral challenges," *Am J Alzheimers Dis Other Demen* 2002 May–Jun; 17(3): 169–74.

11. S. Akhondzadeh, L. Kashani, A. Fotouhi, S. Jarvandi, M. Mobaseri, M. Moin, M. Khani, A. H. Jamshidi, K. Baghalian, and M. Taghizadeh, "Comparison of Lavandula angustifolia Mill. tincture and imipramine in the treatment of mild to moderate depression: a double-blind, randomized trial," *Prog Neuropsychopharmacol Biol Psychiatry* 2003 Feb; 27(1): 123–27.

12. K. Soden, K. Vincent, S. Craske, C. Lucas, and S. Ashley, "A randomized controlled trial of aromatherapy massage in a hospice setting," *Palliat Med* 2004 Mar; 18(2): 87–92.

13. S. Cornwell, and A. Dale, "Lavender oil and perineal repair," *Mod Midwife* 1995 Mar; 5(3): 31–33.

References for Lemon Balm

1. G. Wake, J. Court, A. Pickering, R. Lewis, R. Wilkins, and E. Perry, "CNS acetylcholine receptor activity in

European medicinal plants traditionally used to improve failing memory," *J Ethnopharmacol* 2000 Feb; 69(2): 105–14.

2. H. Aoshima, and K. Hamamoto, "Potentiation of GABAA receptors expressed in Xenopus oocytes by perfume and phytoncid," *Biosci Biotechnol Biochem* 1999 Apr; 63(4): 743–48.

3. S. J. Hossain, H. Aoshima, H. Koda, and Y. Kiso, "Fragrances in oolong tea that enhance the response of GABAA receptors," *Biosci Biotechnol Biochem* 2004 Sep; 68(9): 1842–48.

4. H. Sadraei, A. Ghannadi, and K. Malekshahi, "Relaxant effect of essential oil of Melissa officinalis and citral on rat ileum contractions," *Fitoterapia* 2003 Jul; 74(5): 445–52.

5. D. O. Kennedy, W. Little, and A. B. Scholey, "Attenuation of laboratory-induced stress in humans after acute administration of Melissa officinalis (Lemon Balm)," *Psychosom Med* 2004 Jul–Aug; 66(4): 607–13.

6. D. O. Kennedy, G. Wake, S. Savelev, N. T. Tildesley, E. K. Perry, K. A. Wesnes, and A. B. Scholey, "Modulation of mood and cognitive performance following acute administration of single doses of Melissa officinalis (Lemon balm) with human CNS nicotinic and muscarinic receptor-binding properties," *Neuropsychopharmacology* 2003 Oct; 28(10): 1871–81.

7. D. O. Kennedy, A. B. Scholey, N. T. Tildesley, E. K. Perry, and K. A. Wesnes, "Modulation of mood and cognitive performance following acute administration of Melissa officinalis (lemon balm)," *Pharmacol Biochem Behav* 2002 Jul; 72(4): 953–64.

8. C. G. Ballard, J. T. O'Brien, K. Reichelt, and E. K. Perry, "Aromatherapy as a safe and effective treatment for the management of agitation in severe dementia: the results of a double-blind, placebo-controlled trial with Melissa," *J Clin Psychiatry* 2002 Jul; 63(7): 553–58.

9. S. Akhondzadeh, M. Noroozian, M. Mohammadi, S. Ohadinia, A. H. Jamshidi, and M. Khani, "Melissa officinalis extract in the treatment of patients with mild to moderate Alzheimer's disease: a double-blind, randomised, placebo-controlled trial," *J Neurol Neurosurg Psychiatry* 2003 Jul; 74(7): 863–66.

10. R. Koytchev, R. G. Alken, and S. Dundarov, "Balm mint extract (Lo-701) for topical treatment of recurring herpes labialis," *Phytomedicine* 1999 Oct; 6(4): 225–30.

References for Licorice

1. T. E. Strandberg, S. Andersson, A. L. Jarvenpaa, and P. M. McKeigue, "Preterm birth and licorice consumption during pregnancy," *Am J Epidemiol* 2002 Nov 1; 156(9): 803–05.

2. S. H. Lin, S. S. Yang, T. Chau, and M. L. Halperin, "An unusual cause of hypokalemic paralysis: chronic licorice ingestion," *Am J Med Sci* 2003 Mar; 325(3): 153–56.

3. L. Michaux, C. Lefebvre, and E. Coche, "Perverse effects of an apparently harmless habit," *Rev Med Interne* 1993 Feb; 14(2): 121–22.

4. A. Berlango Jimenez, L. Jimenez Murillo, F. J. Montero Perez, J. A. Munoz Avila, J. Torres Murillo, and J. M. Calderon de la Barca Gazquez, "Acute rhabdomyolysis and tetraparesis secondary to hypokalemia due to ingested licorice," *An Med Interna* 1995 Jan; 12(1): 33–35.

5. J. D. Blachley, and J. P. Knochel, "Tobacco chewer's hypokalemia: licorice revisited," *N Engl J Med* 1980 Apr 3; 302(14): 784–85.

6. A. R. Dehpour, M. E. Zolfaghari, T. Samadian, and Y. Vahedi, "The protective effect of liquorice components and their derivatives against gastric ulcer induced by aspirin in rats," *J Pharm Pharmacol* 1994 Feb; 46(2): 148–49.

7. G. Bianchi Porro, M. Petrillo, M. Lazzaroni, G. Mazzacca, F. Sabbatini, G. Piai, G. Dobrilla, G. De Pretis, and S. Daniotti, "Comparison of pirenzepine and carbenoxolone in the treatment of chronic gastric ulcer. A double-blind endoscopic trial," *Hepatogastroenterology* 1985 Dec; 32(6): 293–95.

8. K. D. Bardhan, D. C. Cumberland, R. A. Dixon, and C. D. Holdsworth, "Clinical trial of deglycyrrhizinised liquorice in gastric ulcer," *Gut* 1978 Sep; 19(9): 779–82.

9. U. Nussbaumer, M. Landolt, G. Rothlisberger, A. Akovbiantz, H. Keller, E. Weber, A. L. Blum, and P. Peter, "Postoperative stress hemorrhage: ineffective prevention with pepsin inhibitor and deglycyrrhizinized licorice extract. Prospective study," *Schweiz Med Wochenschr* 1977 Feb 26; 107(8): 276–79.

10. A. G. Morgan, W. A. McAdam, C. Pacsoo, and A. Darnborough, "Comparison between cimetidine and Caved-S in the treatment of gastric ulceration, and subsequent maintenance therapy," *Gut* 1982 Jun; 23(6): 545–51.

11. A. G. Turpie, J. Runcie, and T. J. Thomson, "Clinical trial of deglydyrrhizinized liquorice in gastric ulcer," *Gut* 1969 Apr; 10(4): 299–302.

12. D. Armanini, G. Bonanni, M. J. Mattarello, C. Fiore, P. Sartorato, and M. Palermo, "Licorice consumption and serum testosterone in healthy man," *Exp Clin Endocrinol Diabetes* 2003 Sep; 111(6): 341–43.

13. D. Armanini, M. J. Mattarello, C. Fiore, G. Bonanni, C. Scaroni, P. Sartorato, and M. Palermo, "Licorice reduces serum testosterone in healthy women," *Steroids* 2004 Oct–Nov; 69(11–12): 763–66.

14. D. Armanini, C. B. De Palo, M. J. Mattarello, P. Spinella, M. Zaccaria, A. Ermolao, M. Palermo, C. Fiore, P. Sartorato, F. Francini-Pesenti, and I. Karbowiak, "Effect of licorice on the reduction of body fat mass in healthy subjects," *J Endocrinol Invest* 2003 Jul; 26(7): 646–50.

15. J. Eisenburg, "Treatment of chronic hepatitis B. Part 2: Effect of glycyrrhizic acid on the course of illness," *Fortschr Med* 1992 Jul 30; 110(21): 395–98.

16. Y. Abe, T. Ueda, T. Kato, and Y. Kohli, "Effectiveness of interferon, glycyrrhizin combination therapy in patients with chronic hepatitis C," *Nippon Rinsho* 1994 Jul; 52(7): 1817–22.

17. M. Saeedi, K. Morteza-Semnani, and M. R. Ghoreishi, "The treatment of atopic dermatitis with licorice gel," *J Dermatolog Treat* 2003 Sep; 14(3): 153–57.

References for Milk Thistle

1. B. P. Jacobs, C. Dennehy, G. Ramirez, J. Sapp, and V. A. Lawrence, "Milk thistle for the treatment of liver disease: a systematic review and meta-analysis," *Am J Med* 2002 Oct 15; 113(6): 506–15. Review.

References for Nettle

1. M. Schottner, D. Gansser, and G. Spiteller, "Lignans from the roots of Urtica dioica and their metabolites

bind to human sex hormone binding globulin (SHBG)," *Planta Med* 1997 Dec; 63(6): 529–32.

2. A. Tahri, S. Yamani, A. Legssyer, M. Aziz, H. Mekhfi, M. Bnouham, and A. Ziyyat, "Acute diuretic, natriuretic and hypotensive effects of a continuous perfusion of aqueous extract of Urtica dioica in the rat," *J Ethnopharmacol* 2000 Nov; 73(1–2): 95–100.

3. A. Legssyer, A. Ziyyat, H. Mekhfi, M. Bnouham, A. Tahri, M. Serrhouchni, J. Hoerter, and R. Fischmeister, "Cardiovascular effects of Urtica dioica L. in isolated rat heart and aorta," *Phytother Res* 2002 Sep; 16(6): 503–07.

4. C. Randall, H. Randall, F. Dobbs, C. Hutton, and H. Sanders, "Randomized controlled trial of nettle sting for treatment of base-of-thumb pain," *J R Soc Med* 2000 Jun; 93(6): 305–09.

5. C. Randall, K. Meethan, H. Randall, and F. Dobbs, "Nettle sting of Urtica dioica for joint pain—an exploratory study of this complementary therapy," *Complement Ther Med* 1999 Sep; 7(3): 126–31.

6. A. Tahri, et al., op cit.

7. T. Schneider, and H. Rubben, "Stinging nettle root extract (*Bazoton-uno*) in long-term treatment of benign prostatic syndrome (BPS). Results of a randomized, double-blind, placebo-controlled multicenter study after 12 months," *Urologe A* 2004 Mar; 43(3): 302–06.

8. P. Mittman, "Randomized, double-blind study of freeze-dried Urtica dioica in the treatment of allergic rhinitis," *Planta Med* 1990 Feb; 56(1): 44–47.

9. S. K. Swanston-Flatt, C. Day, P. R. Flatt, B. J. Gould, and C. J. Bailey, "Glycaemic effects of traditional European plant treatments for diabetes. Studies in normal and streptozotocin diabetic mice," *Diabetes Res* 1989 Feb; 10(2): 69–73.

10. M. Bnouham, F. Z. Merhfour, A. Ziyyat, H. Mekhfi, M. Aziz, and A. Legssyer, "Antihyperglycemic activity of the aqueous extract of Urtica dioica," *Fitoterapia* 2003 Dec; 74(7–8): 677–81.

References for Parsley

1. U. Stein, H. Greyer, and H. Hentschel, "Nutmeg (myristicin) poisoning—report on a fatal case and a series of cases recorded by a poison information centre," *Forensic Sci Int* 2001 Apr 15; 118(1): 87–90.

2. H. Ahmad, M. T. Tijerina, and A. S. Tobola, "Preferential overexpression of a class MU glutathione S-transferase subunit in mouse liver by myristicin," *Biochem Biophys Res Commun* 1997 Jul 30; 236(3): 825–28.

3. G. Q. Zheng, P. M. Kenney, J. Zhang, and L. K. Lam, "Inhibition of benzo[a]pyrene-induced tumorigenesis by myristicin, a volatile aroma constituent of parsley leaf oil," *Carcinogenesis* 1992 Oct; 13(10): 1921–23.

4. C. Ciganda, and A. Laborde, "Herbal infusions used for induced abortion," *J Toxicol Clin Toxicol* 2003; 41(3): 235–39.

5. "Does the 'Internal Breath Freshener' Really Work?" *UC Berkeley Wellness Letter* 1997 Jan.

6. K. Lagey, L. Duinslaeger, and A. Vanderkelen, "Burns induced by plants," *Burns* 1995 Nov; 21(7): 542–43.

7. N. Gral, J. C. Beani, D. Bonnot, A. M. Mariotte, J. L. Reymond, and P. Amblard, "Plasma levels of psoralens after celery ingestion," *Ann Dermatol Venereol* 1993; 120(9): 599–603.

8. S. I. Kreydiyyeh, and J. Usta, "Diuretic effect and

mechanism of action of parsley," *J Ethnopharmacol* 2002 Mar; 79(3): 353–57.

9. S. I. Kreydiyyeh, J. Usta, I. Kaouk, and R. Al-Sadi, "The mechanism underlying the laxative properties of parsley extract," *Phytomedicine* 2001 Sep; 8(5): 382–88.

References for Peppermint

1. J. M. Hills, and P. I. Aaronson, "The mechanism of action of peppermint oil on gastrointestinal smooth muscle. An analysis using patch clamp electrophysiology and isolated tissue pharmacology in rabbit and guinea pig," *Gastroenterology* 1991 Jul; 101(1): 55–65.

2. L. T. Vo, D. Chan, and R. G. King, "Investigation of the effects of peppermint oil and valerian on rat liver and cultured human liver cells," *Clin Exp Pharmacol Physiol* 2003 Oct; 30(10): 799–804.

3. K. J. Goerg, and T. Spilker, "Effect of peppermint oil and caraway oil on gastrointestinal motility in healthy volunteers: a pharmacodynamic study using simultaneous determination of gastric and gall-bladder emptying and orocaecal transit time," *Aliment Pharmacol Ther* 2003 Feb; 17(3): 445–51.

4. G. Haeseler, D. Maue, J. Grosskreutz, J. Bufler, B. Nentwig, S. Piepenbrock, R. Dengler, and M. Leuwer, "Voltage-dependent block of neuronal and skeletal muscle sodium channels by thymol and menthol," *Eur J Anaesthesiol* 2002 Aug; 19(8): 571–79.

5. S. E. Jordt, D. D. McKemy, and D. Julius, "Lessons from peppers and peppermint: the molecular logic of thermosensation," *Curr Opin Neurobiol* 2003 Aug; 13(4): 487–92.

6. N. Hiki, H. Kurosaka, Y. Tatsutomi, S. Shimoyama, E. Tsuji, J. Kojima, N. Shimizu, H. Ono, T. Hirooka, C. Noguchi, K. Mafune, and M. Kaminishi, "Peppermint oil reduces gastric spasm during upper endoscopy: a randomized, double-blind, double-dummy controlled trial," *Gastrointest Endosc* 2003 Apr; 57(4): 475–82.

7. G. Micklefield, O. Jung, I. Greving, and B. May, "Effects of intraduodenal application of peppermint oil (WS(R) 1340) and caraway oil (WS(R) 1520) on gastroduodenal motility in healthy volunteers," *Phytother Res* 2003 Feb; 17(2): 135–40.

8. J. W. C. Gunn, "The Carminative Action of Volatile Oils," *J Pharmacol Exp Ther* 1920; 16:39–47.

9. T. Asao, H. Kuwano, M. Ide, I. Hirayama, J. I. Nakamura, K. I. Fujita, and R. Horiuti, "Spasmolytic effect of peppermint oil in barium during double-contrast barium enema compared with Buscopan," *Clin Radiol* 2003 Apr; 58(4): 301–05.

10. T. Asao, E. Mochiki, H. Suzuki, J. Nakamura, I. Hirayama, N. Morinaga, H. Shoji, Y. Shitara, and H. Kuwano, "An easy method for the intraluminal administration of peppermint oil before colonoscopy and its effectiveness in reducing colonic spasm," *Gastrointest Endosc* 2001 Feb; 53(2): 172–77.

11. M. J. Sparks, P. O'Sullivan, A. A. Herrington, and S. K. Morcos, "Does peppermint oil relieve spasm during barium enema?" *Br J Radiol* 1995 Aug; 68(812): 841–43.

12. M. Blumenthal, "FDA Declares 258 OTC Ingredients Ineffective: Many Herbs Included; Prunes are not an effective laxative, says FDA panel!" *HerbalGram* 1990 23:32–33, 49.

13. Steven Foster, and Varro E. Tyler, "Laws and Regulations,"

in *Tyler's Honest Herbal,* 4th ed. (New York: Haworth Herbal Press, 1999), 9–19.

14. M. H. Pittler, and E. Ernst, "Peppermint oil for irritable bowel syndrome: a critical review and meta-analysis," *Am J Gastroenterol* 1998 Jul; 93(7): 1131–35.

15. R. M. Kline, J. J. Kline, J. Di Palma, and G. J. Barbero, "Enteric-coated, pH-dependent peppermint oil capsules for the treatment of irritable bowel syndrome in children," *J Pediatr* 2001 Jan; 138(1): 125–28.

16. K. J. Goerg, and T. Spilker, "Effect of peppermint oil and caraway oil on gastrointestinal motility in healthy volunteers: a pharmacodynamic study using simultaneous determination of gastric and gall-bladder emptying and orocaecal transit time," *Aliment Pharmacol Ther* 2003 Feb; 17(3): 445–51.

17. H. Mascher, C. H. Kikuta, and H. Schiel, "Pharmacokinetics of carvone and menthol after administration of peppermint oil and caraway oil containing enteric formulation," *Wien Med Wochenschr* 2002; 152(15–16): 432–36.

18. K. Ushid, M. Maekawa, and T. Arakawa, "Influence of dietary supplementation of herb extracts on volatile sulfur production in pig large intestine," *J Nutr Sci Vitaminol* (Tokyo) 2002 Feb; 48(1): 18–23.

19. K. J. Goerg, and T. Spilker, "Effect of peppermint oil and caraway oil on gastrointestinal motility in healthy volunteers: a pharmacodynamic study using simultaneous determination of gastric and gall-bladder emptying and orocaecal transit time," *Aliment Pharmacol Ther* 2003 Feb; 17(3): 445–51.

20. T. E. Sullivan, J. S. Warm, B. K. Schefft, W. N. Dember, M. W. O'Dell, and S. J. Peterson, "Effects of olfactory stimulation on the vigilance performance of individuals with brain injury," *J Clin Exp Neuropsychol* 1998 Apr; 20(2): 227–36.

21. T. Satoh, and Y. Sugawara, "Effects on humans elicited by inhaling the fragrance of essential oils: sensory test, multi-channel thermometric study and forehead surface potential wave measurement on basil and peppermint," *Anal Sci* 2003 Jan; 19(1): 139–46.

22. A. Burrow, R. Eccles, A. S. Jones, "The effects of camphor, eucalyptus and menthol vapour on nasal resistance to airflow and nasal sensation," *Acta Otolaryngol* 1983 Jul–Aug; 96(1–2): 157–61.

23. R. Eccles, B. Lancashire, and N. S. Tolley, "The effect of aromatics on inspiratory and expiratory nasal resistance to airflow," *Clin Otolaryngol* 1987 Feb; 12(1): 11–14.

24. R. Eccles, "Menthol: effects on nasal sensation of airflow and the drive to breathe," *Curr Allergy Asthma Rep* 2003 May; 3(3): 210–14.

25. C. E. Wright, E. A. Laude, T. J. Grattan, and A. H. Morice, "Capsaicin and neurokinin A-induced bronchoconstriction in the anaesthetised guinea-pig: evidence for a direct action of menthol on isolated bronchial smooth muscle," *Br J Pharmacol* 1997 Aug; 121(8): 1645–50.

26. A. Schuhmacher, J. Reichling, and P. Schnitzler, "Virucidal effect of peppermint oil on the enveloped viruses herpes simplex virus type 1 and type 2 in vitro," *Phytomedicine* 2003; 10(6–7): 504–10.

27. R. S. Ramsewak, M. G. Nair, M. Stommel, and L. Selanders, "In vitro antagonistic activity of monoterpenes and their mixtures against 'toe nail fungus' pathogens," *Phytother Res* 2003 Apr; 17(4): 376–79.

28. H. Imai, K. Osawa, H. Yasuda, H. Hamashima, T. Arai, and M. Sasatsu, "Inhibition by the essential oils of peppermint and spearmint of the growth of pathogenic bacteria," *Microbios* 2001; 106 Suppl 1:31–39.

29. C. Foti, A. Conserva, A. Antelmi, L. Lospalluti, and G. Angelini, "Contact dermatitis from peppermint and menthol in a local action transcutaneous patch," *Contact Dermatitis* 2003 Dec; 49(6): 312–13.

References for Red Clover

1. N. Tsunoda, S. Pomeroy, and P. Nestel, "Absorption in humans of isoflavones from soy and red clover is similar," *J Nutr* 2002 Aug; 132(8): 2199–201.

2. J. B. Howes, K. Bray, L. Lorenz, P. Smerdely, and L. G. Howes, "The effects of dietary supplementation with isoflavones from red clover on cognitive function in postmenopausal women," *Climacteric* 2004 Mar; 7(1): 70–77.

3. J. A. Tice, B. Ettinger, K. Ensrud, R. Wallace, T. Blackwell, and S. R. Cummings, "Phytoestrogen supplements for the treatment of hot flashes: the Isoflavone Clover Extract (ICE) Study: a randomized controlled trial," *JAMA* 2003 Jul 9; 290(2): 207–14.

4. R. J. Baber, C. Templeman, T. Morton, G. E. Kelly, and L. West, "Randomized placebo-controlled trial of an isoflavone supplement and menopausal symptoms in women," *Climacteric* 1999 Jun; 2(2): 85–92.

5. D. C. Knight, J. B. Howes, and J. A. Eden, "The effect of Promensil, an isoflavone extract, on menopausal symptoms," *Climacteric* 1999 Jun; 2(2): 79–84.

6. J. A. Tice, et al., op. cit.

7. P. H. van de Weijer, and R. Barentsen, "Isoflavones from red clover (Promensil) significantly reduce menopausal hot flush symptoms compared with placebo," *Maturitas* 2002 Jul 25; 42(3): 187–93.

8. J. B. Howes, D. Sullivan, N. Lai, P. Nestel, S. Pomeroy, L. West, J. A. Eden, and L. G. Howes, "The effects of dietary supplementation with isoflavones from red clover on the lipoprotein profiles of post-menopausal women with mild to moderate hypercholesterolaemia," *Atherosclerosis* 2000 Sep; 152(1): 143–47.

9. S. J. Blakesmith, P. M. Lyons-Wall, C. George, G. E. Joannou, P. Petocz, and S. Samman, "Effects of supplementation with purified red clover (*Trifolium pratense*) isoflavones on plasma lipids and insulin resistance in healthy premenopausal women," *Br J Nutr* 2003 Apr; 89(4): 467–74.

10. C. Atkinson, W. Oosthuizen, S. Scollen, A. Loktionov, N. E. Day, and S. A. Bingham, "Modest protective effects of isoflavones from a red clover-derived dietary supplement on cardiovascular disease risk factors in perimenopausal women, and evidence of an interaction with ApoE genotype in 49–65 year-old women," *J Nutr* 2004 Jul; 134(7): 1759–64.

11. T. M. Schult, K. E. Ensrud, T. Blackwell, B. Ettinger, R. Wallace, and J. A. Tice, "Effect of isoflavones on lipids and bone turnover markers in menopausal women," *Maturitas* 2004 Jul 15; 48(3): 209–18.

12. J. B. Howes, D. Tran, D. Brillante, and L. G. Howes, "Effects of dietary supplementation with isoflavones from red clover on ambulatory blood pressure and endothelial function in postmenopausal type 2 diabetes," *Diabetes Obes Metab* 2003 Sep; 5(5): 325–32.

13. P. Nestel, M. Cehun, A. Chronopoulos, L. DaSilva, H.

Teede, and B. McGrath, "A biochanin-enriched isoflavone from red clover lowers LDL cholesterol in men," *Eur J Clin Nutr* 2004 Mar; 58(3): 403–08.

14. M. J. Campbell, J. V. Woodside, J. W. Honour, M. S. Morton, and A. J. Leathem, "Effect of red clover-derived isoflavone supplementation on insulin-like growth factor, lipid and antioxidant status in healthy female volunteers: a pilot study," *Eur J Clin Nutr* 2004 Jan; 58(1): 173–79.

15. P. B. Clifton-Bligh, R. J. Baber, G. R. Fulcher, M. L. Nery, and T. Moreton, "The effect of isoflavones extracted from red clover (Rimostil) on lipid and bone metabolism," *Menopause* 2001 Jul–Aug; 8(4): 259–65.

16. H. J. Teede, B. P. McGrath, L. DeSilva, M. Cehun, A. Fassoulakis, and P. J. Nestel, "Isoflavones reduce arterial stiffness: a placebo-controlled study in men and postmenopausal women," *Arterioscler Thromb Vasc Biol* 2003 Jun 1; 23(6): 1066–71. E-pub, 2003 Apr 24.

17. J. B. Howes, D. Tran, D. Brillante, and L. G. Howes, "Effects of dietary supplementation with isoflavones from red clover on ambulatory blood pressure and endothelial function in postmenopausal type 2 diabetes," *Diabetes Obes Metab* 2003 Sep; 5(5): 325–32.

18. Ibid.

19. S. J. Blakesmith, et al., op. cit.

20. C. Atkinson, J. E. Compston, N. E. Day, M. Dowsett, and S. A. Bingham, "The effects of phytoestrogen isoflavones on bone density in women: a double-blind, randomized, placebo-controlled trial," *Am J Clin Nutr* 2004 Feb; 79(2): 326–33.

21. P. B. Clifton-Bligh, et al., op. cit.

22. C. Atkinson, R. M. Warren, E. Sala, M. Dowsett, A. M. Dunning, C. S. Healey, S. Runswick, N. E. Day, and S. A. Bingham, "Red-clover-derived isoflavones and mammographic breast density: a double-blind, randomized, placebo-controlled trial," *Breast Cancer Res* 2004; 6(3): R170–79. E-pub, 2004 Feb 24.

23. G. E. Hale, C. L. Hughes, S. J. Robboy, S. K. Agarwal, and M. Bievre, "A double-blind randomized study on the effects of red clover isoflavones on the endometrium," *Menopause* 2001 Sep–Oct; 8(5): 338–46.

24. R. A. Jarred, M. Keikha, C. Dowling, S. J. McPherson, A. M. Clare, A. J. Husband, J. S. Pedersen, M. Frydenberg, and G. P. Risbridger, "Induction of apoptosis in low to moderate-grade human prostate carcinoma by red clover-derived dietary isoflavones," *Cancer Epidemiol Biomarkers Prev* 2002 Dec; 11(12): 1689–96.

References for Red Pepper

1. J. M. Jellin, P. J. Gregory, F. Batz, K. Hitchens, et al., *Pharmacist's Letter/Prescriber's Letter Natural Medicines Comprehensive Database,* 6th ed. (Stockton, CA: Therapeutic Research Faculty, 2004).

2. C. L. Deal, T. J. Schnitzer, E. Lipstein, J. R. Seibold, R. M. Stevens, M. D. Levy, D. Albert, and F. Renold, "Treatment of arthritis with topical capsaicin: a double-blind trial," *Clin Ther* 1991 May–Jun; 13(3): 383–95.

3. V. H. Morris, S. C. Cruwys, and B. L. Kidd, "Characterisation of capsaicin-induced mechanical hyperalgesia as a marker for altered nociceptive processing in patients with rheumatoid arthritis," *Pain* 1997 Jun; 71(2): 179–86.

4. C. P. Watson, K. L. Tyler, D. R. Bickers, L. E. Millikan,

S. Smith, and E. Coleman, "A randomized vehicle-controlled trial of topical capsaicin in the treatment of postherpetic neuralgia," *Clin Ther* 1993 May–Jun; 15(3): 510–26.

5. T. Forst, T. Pohlmann, T. Kunt, K. Goitom, G. Schulz, M. Lobig, M. Engelbach, J. Beyer, and A. Pfutzner, "The influence of local capsaicin treatment on small nerve fibre function and neurovascular control in symptomatic diabetic neuropathy," *Acta Diabetol* 2002 Apr; 39(1): 1–6.

6. W. Keitel, H. Frerick, U. Kuhn, U. Schmidt, M. Kuhlmann, and A. Bredehorst, "Capsicum pain plaster in chronic non-specific low back pain," *Arzneimittelforschung* 2001 Nov; 51(11): 896–903.

7. B. J. Mathias, T. R. Dillingham, D. N. Zeigler, A. S. Chang, and P. V. Belandres "Topical capsaicin for chronic neck pain. A pilot study," *Am J Phys Med Rehabil* 1995 Jan–Feb; 74(1): 39–44.

8. D. J. McCarty, M. Csuka, G. McCarthy, et al., "Treatment of pain due to fibromyalgia with topical capsaicin: A pilot study," *Semin Arth Rhem* 1994; 23:41–47.

9. M. Bortolotti, G. Coccia, G. Grossi, and M. Miglioli, "The treatment of functional dyspepsia with red pepper," *Aliment Pharmacol Ther* 2002 Jun; 16(6): 1075–82.

10. S. Rodriguez-Stanley, K. L. Collings, M. Robinson, W. Owen, and P. B. Miner Jr., "The effects of capsaicin on reflux, gastric emptying and dyspepsia," *Aliment Pharmacol Ther* 2000 Jan; 14(1): 129–34.

11. K. G. Yeoh, J. Y. Kang, I. Yap, R. Guan, C. C. Tan, A. Wee, and C. H. Teng, "Chili protects against aspirin-induced gastroduodenal mucosal injury in humans," *Dig Dis Sci* 1995 Mar; 40(3): 580–83.

12. D. Y. Graham, S. Y. Anderson, and T. Lang, "Garlic or jalapeno peppers for treatment of Helicobacter pylori infection," *Am J Gastroenterol* 1999 May; 94(5): 1200–02.

References for Sage

1. J. A. Robbers, and V. E. Tyler, *Tyler's Herbs of Choice: The Therapeutic Use of Phytomedicinals* (New York: Haworth Press, 1999).

2. P. J. Houghton, "Activity and Constituents of Sage Relevant to the Potential Treatment of Symptoms of Alzheimer's Disease," *HerbalGram* 61 (2004): 38–53.

3. M. L. Furey, P. Pietrini, G. E. Alexander, M. B. Schapiro, and B. Horwitz, "Cholinergic enhancement improves performance on working memory by modulating the functional activity in distinct brain regions: a positron emission tomography regional cerebral blood flow study in healthy humans," *Brain Res Bull* 2000 Feb; 51(3): 213–18.

4. M. L. Furey, P. Pietrini, and J. V. Haxby, "Cholinergic enhancement and increased selectivity of perceptual processing during working memory," *Science* 2000 Dec 22; 290(5500): 2315–19.

5. N. T. Tildesley, D. O. Kennedy, E. K. Perry, C. G. Ballard, S. Savelev, K. A. Wesnes, and A. B. Scholey, "Salvia lavandulaefolia (Spanish Sage) enhances memory in healthy young volunteers," *Pharmacol Biochem Behav* 2003 Jun; 75(3): 669–74.

6. K. M. Hold, N. S. Sirisoma, T. Ikeda, T. Narahashi, and J. E. Casida, "Alpha-thujone (the active component of absinthe): gamma-aminobutyric acid type A

receptor modulation and metabolic detoxification," *Proc Natl Acad Sci USA* 2000 Apr 11; 97(8): 3826–31.

7. J. Patocka, and P. Bohumil, "Pharmacology and Toxicology of Absinthe," *J. Applied Biomedicine* 2003; 1:199–205.

8. J. P. Meschler, and A. C. Howlett, "Thujone exhibits low affinity for cannabinoid receptors but fails to evoke cannabimimetic responses," *Pharmacol Biochem Behav* 1999 Mar; 62(3): 473–80.

9. J. Gruenwald, T. Brendler, and C. Jaenicke, eds. *PDR for Herbal Medicines* (Montvale, NJ: Thompson Medical Economics Company, 2000), 655–56.

10. S. Foster, and V. E. Tyler, *Tyler's Honest Herbal: A Sensible Guide to the Use of Herbs and Related Remedies,* 4th ed. (Binghamton, NY: Haworth Press, 1999), 327–29.

11 N. S. Perry, P. J. Houghton, J. Sampson, A. E. Theobald, S. Hart, M. Lis-Balchin, J. R. Hoult, P. Evans, P. Jenner, S. Milligan, E. K. Perry, "In-vitro activity of S. lavandulaefolia (Spanish sage) relevant to treatment of Alzheimer's disease," *J Pharm Pharmacol* 2001 Oct;53(10):1347–56.

12. A. Pierce, *The American Pharmaceutical Association Practical Guide to Natural Medicines* (New York: Stonesong Press, 1999), 563–65.

13. P. J. Houghton, et al., op. cit.

14. G. N. Farhat, N. I. Affara, and H. U. Gali-Muhtasib, "Seasonal changes in the composition of the essential oil extract of East Mediterranean sage (*Salvia libanotica*) and its toxicity in mice," *Toxicon* 2001 Oct; 39(10): 1601–05.

15. C. Chavkin, S. Sud, W. Jin, J. Stewart, J. K. Zjawiony, D. J. Siebert, B. A. Toth, S. J. Hufeisen, and B. L. Roth, "Salvinorin A, an active component of the hallucinogenic sage salvia divinorum is a highly efficacious kappa-opioid receptor agonist: structural and functional considerations," *J Pharmacol Exp Ther* 2004 Mar; 308(3): 1197–203.

16. S. Foster, et al., op. cit.

17. E. Holze, "Therapy of hyperhidrosis," *Hautarzt* 1984 Jan; 35(1): 7–15.

18. P. J. Houghton, et al., op. cit.

19. ibid.

20. S. Akhondzadeh, M. Noroozian, M. Mohammadi, S. Ohadinia, A. H. Jamshidi, and M. Khani, "Salvia officinalis extract in the treatment of patients with mild to moderate Alzheimer's disease: a double blind, randomized and placebo-controlled trial," *J Clin Pharm Ther* 2003 Feb; 28(1): 53–59.

21. N. S. Perry, C. Bollen, E. K. Perry, and C. Ballard, "Salvia for dementia therapy: review of pharmacological activity and pilot tolerability clinical trial," *Pharmacol Biochem Behav* 2003 Jun; 75(3): 651–59.

22. N. T. Tildesley, et al., op. cit.

References for Saw Palmetto

1. B. Hill, and N. Kyprianou, "Effect of permixon on human prostate cell growth: lack of apoptotic action," *Prostate* 2004 Sep 15; 61(1): 73–80.

2. J. P. Raynaud, H. Cousse, and P. M. Martin, "Inhibition of type 1 and type 2 5alpha-reductase activity by free fatty acids, active ingredients of Permixon," *J Steroid Biochem Mol Biol* 2002 Oct; 82(2–3): 233–39.

3. F. K. Habib, M. Ross, C. K. H. Ho, V. Lyons, and K. Chapman, "Serenoa repens (Permixon[R]) inhibits the 5alpha-reductase activity of human prostate cancer cell lines without interfering with PSA expression," *Int J Cancer.* E-pub, 2004 Nov 12.

4. M. Paubert-Braquet, J. M. Mencia Huerta, H. Cousse, and P. Braquet, "Effect of the lipidic lipidosterolic extract of Serenoa repens (Permixon) on the ionophore A23187-stimulated production of leukotriene B4 (LTB4) from human polymorphonuclear neutrophils," *Prostaglandins Leukot Essent Fatty Acids* 1997 Sep; 57(3): 299–304.

5. W. H. Goldmann, A. L. Sharma, S. J. Currier, P. D. Johnston, A. Rana, and C. P. Sharma, "Saw palmetto berry extract inhibits cell growth and Cox-2 expression in prostatic cancer cells," *Cell Biol Int* 2001; 25(11): 1117–24.

6. F. K. Habib, et al., op cit.

7. J. P. Raynaud, et al., op cit.

8. C. W. Bayne, M. Ross, F. Donnelly, and F. K. Habib, "The selectivity and specificity of the actions of the lipido-sterolic extract of Serenoa repens (Permixon) on the prostate," *J Urol* 2000 Sep; 164(3 Pt 1): 876–81.

9. F. Di Silverio, S. Monti, A. Sciarra, P. A. Varasano, C. Martini, S. Lanzara, G. D'Eramo, S. Di Nicola, and V. Toscano, "Effects of long-term treatment with Serenoa repens (Permixon) on the concentrations and regional distribution of androgens and epidermal growth factor in benign prostatic hyperplasia," *Prostate* 1998 Oct 1; 37(2): 77–83.

10. T. Wilt, A. Ishani, and R. MacDonald, "Serenoa repens for benign prostatic hyperplasia," *Cochrane Database Syst Rev* 2002; 3:CD001423.

11. T. J. Wilt, A. Ishani, G. Stark, R. MacDonald, J. Lau, and C. Mulrow, "Saw palmetto extracts for treatment of benign prostatic hyperplasia: a systematic review," *JAMA* 1998 Nov 11; 280(18): 1604–09.

12. M. Tarle, O. Kraus, D. Trnski, A. Reljic, B. Ruzic, J. Katusic, B. Spajic, and Z. Kusic, "Early diagnosis of prostate cancer in finasteride treated BPH patients," *Anticancer Res* 2003 Jan–Feb; 23(1B): 693–96.

13. J. C. Carraro, J. P. Raynaud, G. Koch, G. D. Chisholm, F. Di Silverio, P. Teillac, F. C. Da Silva, J. Cauquil, D. K. Chopin, F. C. Hamdy, M. Hanus, D. Hauri, A. Kalinteris, J. Marencak, A. Perier, and P. Perrin, "Comparison of phytotherapy (Permixon) with finasteride in the treatment of benign prostate hyperplasia: a randomized international study of 1,098 patients," *Prostate* 1996 Oct; 29(4): 231–40.

14. F. K. Habib, et al., op cit.

15. J. Morote, J. A. Lorente, C. X. Raventos, M. A. Lopez, G. Encabo, I. De Torres M. Lopez, and J. A. De Torres "Effect of finasteride on the percentage of free PSA: implications in the early diagnosis of prostatic cancer," *Actas Urol Esp* 1998 Nov-Dec; 22(10): 835–39.

16. J. K. Small, E. Bombardelli, and P. Morazzoni, "Serenoa repens (Bartram)," *Fitoterapia* 1997; 68:99–113.

17. A. A. Izzo, and E. Ernst, "Interactions between herbal medicines and prescribed drugs: a systematic review," *Drugs* 2001; 61(15): 2163–75.

18. J. S. Markowitz, J. L. Donovan, C. L. Devane, R. M. Taylor, Y. Ruan, J. S. Wang, and K. D. Chavin, "Multiple doses of saw palmetto (Serenoa repens) did not alter cytochrome P450 2D6 and 3A4 activity in normal volunteers," *Clin Pharmacol Ther* 2003 Dec; 74(6): 536–42.

19. S. A. Kaplan, M. A. Volpe, and A. E. Te, "A prospective, 1-year trial using saw palmetto versus finasteride in the treatment of category III prostatitis/chronic pelvic pain syndrome," *J Urol* 2004 Jan; 171(1): 284–88.

20. N. Prager, K. Bickett, N. French, and G. Marcovici, "A randomized, double-blind, placebo-controlled trial to determine the effectiveness of botanically derived inhibitors of 5-alpha-reductase in the treatment of androgenetic alopecia," *J Altern Complement Med* 2002 Apr; 8(2): 143–52.

References for Senna

1. H. A. Spiller, M. L. Winter, J. A. Weber, E. P. Krenzelok, D. L. Anderson, and M. L. Ryan, "Skin breakdown and blisters from senna-containing laxatives in young children," *Ann Pharmacother* 2003 May; 37(5): 636–39.

2. A. Valverde, J. M. Hay, A. Fingerhut, M. J. Boudet, R. Petroni, X. Pouliquen, S. Msika, and Y. Flamant, "Senna vs polyethylene glycol for mechanical preparation the evening before elective colonic or rectal resection: a multicenter controlled trial," *Arch Surg* 1999 May; 134(5): 514–19.

3. W. J. MacLennan, and A. F. W. M. Pooler, "A comparison of sodium picosulphate ("Laxoberal") with standardised senna ("Senokot") in geriatric patients," *Curr Med Res Opin* 1974–75; 2(10): 641–47.

4. P. P. But, B. Tomlinson, and K. L. Lee, "Hepatitis related to the Chinese medicine Shouwu Pian, manufactured from Polygonum multiflorum," *Veterinary and Human Toxicology* 1996; 38(4): 280–82.

5. G. J. Park, S. P. Mann, and M. C. Ngu, "Acute hepatitis induced by Shouwu Pian, a herbal product derived from Polygonum multiflorum," *Journal of Gastroenterology and Hepatology* 2001; 16(1): 115–17.

6. A. Nair, D. Reddy, and D. H. Van Thiel, "Cascara sagrada induced intrahepatic cholestasis causing portal hypertension: case report and review of herbal hepatotoxicity," *American Journal of Gastroenterology* 2000; 95(12): 3634–37.

7. P. F. D'Arcy, "Adverse reactions and interactions with herbal medicines, Part 1," *Adverse Drug Reactions and Toxicology Reviews* 1991; 10(4): 189–208.

8. N. Mascolo, E. Mereto, F. Borrelli, P. Orsi, D. Sini, A. A. Izzo, B. Massa, M. Boggio, and F. Capasso, "Does senna extract promote growth of aberrant crypt foci and malignant tumors in rat colon?" *Dig Dis Sci* 1999 Nov; 44(11): 2226–30.

9. National Toxicology Program, "NTP Toxicology and Carcinogenesis Studies of EMODIN (CAS NO. 518–82–1) Feed Studies in F344/N Rats and B6C3F1 Mice," *Natl Toxicol Program Tech Rep Ser* 2001 Jun; 493:1–278.

10. B. A. van Gorkom, A. Karrenbeld, T. van Der Sluis, J. Koudstaal, E. G. de Vries, and J. H. Kleibeuker, "Influence of a highly purified senna extract on colonic epithelium," *Digestion* 2000; 61(2): 113–20.

References for Soy

1. R. M. Weggemans, and E. A. Trautwein, "Relation between soy-associated isoflavones and LDL and HDL cholesterol concentrations in humans: a meta-analysis," *Eur J Clin Nutr* 2003 Aug; 57(8): 940–46.

2. X. G. Zhuo, M. K. Melby, and S. Watanabe, "Soy isoflavone intake lowers serum LDL cholesterol: a meta-analysis of 8 randomized controlled trials in humans," *J Nutr* 2004 Sep; 134(9): 2395–400.

3. J. W. Anderson, B. M. Johnstone, and M. E. Cook-Newell, "Meta-analysis of the effects of soy protein intake on serum lipids," *N Engl J Med* 1995 Aug 3; 333(5): 276–82.

4. S. Kreijkamp-Kaspers, L. Kok, D. E. Grobbee, E. H. de Haan, A. Aleman, J. W. Lampe, and Y. T. van der Schouw, "Effect of soy protein containing isoflavones on cognitive function, bone mineral density, and plasma lipids in postmenopausal women: a randomized controlled trial," *JAMA* 2004 Jul 7; 292(1): 65–74.

5. Z. K. Roughead, J. R. Hunt, L. K. Johnson, T. M. Badger, and G. I. Lykken, "Controlled substitution of soy protein for meat protein: effects on calcium retention, bone, and cardiovascular health indices in postmenopausal women," *J Clin Endocrinol Metab* 2005 Jan; 90(1): 181–89.   E-pub, 2004 Oct 13.

6. E. E. Krebs, K. E. Ensrud, R. MacDonald, and T. J. Wilt, "Phytoestrogens for treatment of menopausal symptoms: a systematic review," *Obstet Gynecol* 2004 Oct; 104(4): 824–36.

7. M. Penotti, E. Fabio, A. B. Modena, M. Rinaldi, U. Omodei, and P. Vigano, "Effect of soy-derived isoflavones on hot flushes, endometrial thickness, and the pulsatility index of the uterine and cerebral arteries," *Fertil Steril* 2003 May; 79(5): 1112–17.

8. S. Yamamoto, T. Sobue, M. Kobayashi, S. Sasaki, and S. Tsugane, "Soy, isoflavones, and breast cancer risk in Japan," *J Natl Cancer Inst* 2003 Dec 17; 95(24): 1881–82.

9. N. F. Boyd, J. Stone, K. N. Vogt, B. S. Connelly, L. J. Martin, and S. Minkin, "Dietary fat and breast cancer risk revisited: a meta-analysis of the published literature," *Br J Cancer* 2003 Nov 3; 89(9): 1672–85.

10. H. Akaza, N. Miyanaga, N. Takashima, S. Naito, Y. Hirao, T. Tsukamoto, T. Fujioka, M. Mori, W. J. Kim, J. M. Song, and A. J. Pantuck, "Comparisons of percent equol producers between prostate cancer patients and controls: case-controlled studies of isoflavones in Japanese, Korean and American residents," *Jpn J Clin Oncol* 2004 Feb; 34(2): 86–89.

11. A. H. Wu, D. Yang, and M. C. Pike, "A meta-analysis of soyfoods and risk of stomach cancer: the problem of potential confounders," *Cancer Epidemiol Biomarkers Prev,* 2000 Oct; 9(10): 1051–58.

12. H. M. Nan, J. W. Park, Y. J. Song, H. Y. Yun, J. S. Park, T. Hyun, S. J. Youn, Y. D. Kim, J. W. Kang, and H. Kim H, "Kimchi and soybean pastes are risk factors of gastric cancer," *World J Gastroenterol* 2005 Jun 7; 11(21): 3175–81.

13. D. Spector, M. Anthony, D. Alexander, and L. Arab, "Soy consumption and colorectal cancer," *Nutr Cancer* 2003; 47(1): 1–12.

14. B. Bruce, M. Messina, G. A. Spiller, "Isoflavone supplements do not affect thyroid function in iodine-replete postmenopausal women," *J Med Food* 2003 Winter; 6(4): 309–16.

15. B. L. Strom, R. Schinnar, E. E. Ziegler, K. T. Barnhart, M. D. Sammel, G. A. Macones, V. A. Stallings, J. M. Drulis, S. E. Nelson, and S. A. Hanson, "Exposure to soy-based formula in infancy and endocrinological and reproductive outcomes in young adulthood," *JAMA* 2001 Aug 15; 286(7): 807–14.

16. L. R. White, H. Petrovitch, G. W. Ross, K. Masaki, J. Hardman, J. Nelson, D. Davis, and W. Markesbery, "Brain aging and midlife tofu consumption," *J Am Coll Nutr* 2000 Apr; 19(2): 242–55.

References for St. John's Wort

1. S. Schulte-Lobbert, G. Holoubek, W. E. Muller, M. Schubert-Zsilavecz, and M. Wurglics, "Comparison of the synaptosomal uptake inhibition of serotonin by St John's wort products," *J Pharm Pharmacol* 2004 Jun; 56(6): 813–18.
2. J. F. Rodriguez-Landa, and C. M. Contreras, "A review of clinical and experimental observations about antidepressant actions and side effects produced by Hypericum perforatum extracts," *Phytomedicine* 2003 Nov; 10(8): 688–99.
3. L. Cervo, M. Rozio, C. B. Ekalle-Soppo, G. Guiso, P. Morazzoni, and S. Caccia, "Role of hyperforin in the antidepressant-like activity of Hypericum perforatum extracts," *Psychopharmacology* (Berl) 2002 Dec; 164(4): 423–28. E-pub, 2002 Sep 24.
4. V. Butterweck, M. Hegger, and H. Winterhoff, "Flavonoids of St. John's Wort reduce HPA axis function in the rat," *Planta Med* 2004 Oct; 70(10): 1008–11.
5. H. Murck, M. Uhr, K. Schaffler, and K. Seibel, "Effects of Hypericum extract (LI160) on the change of auditory evoked potentials by cortisol administration," *Neuropsychobiology* 2004; 50(2): 128–33.
6. C. Schroeder, J. Tank, D. S. Goldstein, M. Stoeter, S. Haertter, F. C. Luft, and J. Jordan, "Influence of St John's wort on catecholamine turnover and cardiovascular regulation in humans," *Clin Pharmacol Ther* 2004 Nov; 76(5): 480–89.
7. A. Denke, H. Schempp, D. Weiser, and E. F. Elstner, "Biochemical activities of extracts from Hypericum perforatum L. 5th communication: dopamine-beta-hydroxylase-product quantification by HPLC and inhibition by hypericins and flavonoids," *Arzneimittelforschung* 2000 May; 50(5): 415–19.
8. E. Kleber, T. Obry, S. Hippeli, W. Schneider, and E. F. Elstner, "Biochemical activities of extracts from Hypericum perforatum L. 1st Communication: inhibition of dopamine-beta-hydroxylase," *Arzneimittelforschung* 1999 Feb; 49(2): 106–09.
9. B. L. Fiebich, A. Hollig, and K. Lieb, "Inhibition of substance P-induced cytokine synthesis by St. John's wort extracts," *Pharmacopsychiatry* 2001 Jul; 34 Suppl 1:S26–28.
10. M. Gobbi, M. Moia, M. Funicello, A. Riva, P. Morazzoni, and T. Mennini, "In vitro effects of the dicyclohexylammonium salt of hyperforin on interleukin-6 release in different experimental models," *Planta Med* 2004 Jul; 70(7): 680–82.
11. G. Calapai, A. Crupi, F. Firenzuoli, G. Inferrera, G. Ciliberto, A. Parisi, G. De Sarro, and A. P. Caputi, "Interleukin-6 involvement in antidepressant action of Hypericum perforatum," *Pharmacopsychiatry* 2001 Jul; 34 Suppl 1:S8–10.
12. K. Hirano, Y. Kato, S. Uchida, Y. Sugimoto, J. Yamada, K. Umegaki, and S. Yamada, "Effects of oral administration of extracts of Hypericum perforatum (St John's wort) on brain serotonin transporter, serotonin uptake and behaviour in mice," *J Pharm Pharmacol* 2004 Dec; 56(12): 1589–95.
13. S. Kasper, and A. Dienel, "Cluster analysis of symptoms during antidepressant treatment with Hypericum extract in mildly to moderately depressed out-patients. A meta-analysis of data from three randomized, placebo-controlled trials," *Psychopharmacology* (Berl) 2002 Nov; 164(3): 301–08. E-pub, 2002 Sep 14.
14. G. Laakmann, G. Jahn, and C. Schule, "Hypericum perforatum extract in treatment of mild to moderate depression. Clinical and pharmacological aspects," *Nervenarzt* 2002 Jul; 73(7): 600–12.
15. E. Whiskey, U. Werneke, and D. Taylor, "A systematic review and meta-analysis of Hypericum perforatum in depression: a comprehensive clinical review," *Int Clin Psychopharmacol* 2001 Sep; 16(5): 239–52.
16. K. Linde, G. Ramirez, C. D. Mulrow, A. Pauls, W. Weidenhammer, and D. Melchart, "St John's wort for depression—an overview and meta-analysis of randomised clinical trials," *BMJ* 1996 Aug 3; 313(7052): 253–58.
17. U. Werneke, O. Horn, and D. M. Taylor, "How effective is St John's wort? The evidence revisited," *J Clin Psychiatry* 2004 May; 65(5): 611–17.
18. E. Whiskey, et al., op cit.
19. A. R. Bilia, S. Gallori, and F. F. Vincieri, "St. John's wort and depression: efficacy, safety and tolerability—an update," *Life Sci* 2002 May 17; 70(26): 3077–96.

References for Tea Tree Oil

1. "Feedback," issue 2492 of *New Scientist* magazine, 26 March 2005, p. 88.
2. I. B. Bassett, D. L. Pannowitz, and R. S. Barnetson, "A comparative study of tea-tree oil versus benzoylperoxide in the treatment of acne," *Med J Aust* 1990 Oct 15; 153(8): 455–58.
3. D. S. Buck, D. M. Nidorf, and J. G. Addino, "Comparison of two topical preparations for the treatment of onychomycosis: Melaleuca alternifolia (tea tree) oil and clotrimazole," *J Fam Pract* 1994 Jun; 38(6): 601–05.
4. M. M. Tong, P. M. Altman, and R. S. Barnetson, "Tea tree oil in the treatment of tinea pedis," *Australas J Dermatol* 1992; 33(3): 145–49.
5. A. C. Satchell, A. Saurajen, C. Bell, and R. S. Barnetson, "Treatment of interdigital tinea pedis with 25% and 50% tea tree oil solution: a randomized, placebo-controlled, blinded study," *Australas J Dermatol* 2002 Aug; 43(3): 175–78.
6. C. F. Carson, L. Ashton, L. Dry, D. W. Smith, and T. V. Riley, "Melaleuca alternifolia (tea tree) oil gel (6%) for the treatment of recurrent herpes labialis," *J Antimicrob Chemother* 2001 Sep; 48(3): 450–51.
7. D. M. Rubel, S. Freeman, and I. A. Southwell, "Tea tree oil allergy: what is the offending agent? Report of three cases of tea tree oil allergy and review of the literature," *Australas J Dermatol* 1998 Nov; 39(4): 244–47.

References for Tea

1. J. H. Hui, *Encyclopedia of Food Science and Technology* (New York: John Wiley, 1992).
2. S. Klaus, S. Pultz, C. Thone-Reineke, and S. Wolfram, "Epigallocatechin gallate attenuates diet-induced obesity in mice by decreasing energy absorption and increasing fat oxidation," *Int J Obes Relat Metab Disord*

2005 Jun; 29(6): 615–23.

3. G. W. Ross, R. D. Abbott, H. Petrovitch, D. M. Morens, A. Grandinetti, K. H. Tung, C. M. Tanner, K. H. Masaki, P. L. Blanchette, J. D. Curb, J. S. Popper, and L. R. White, "Association of coffee and caffeine intake with the risk of Parkinson disease," *JAMA* 2000 May 24–31; 283(20): 2674–79.

4. E. K. Tan, C. Tan, S. M. Fook-Chong, S. Y. Lum, A. Chai, H. Chung, H. Shen, Y. Zhao, M. L. Teoh, Y. Yih, R. Pavanni, V. R. Chandran, and M. C. Wong, "Dose-dependent protective effect of coffee, tea, and smoking in Parkinson's disease: a study in ethnic Chinese," *J Neurol Sci* 2003 Dec 15; 216(1): 163–67.

5. A. Ascherio, S. M. Zhang, M. A. Hernan, I. Kawachi, G. A. Colditz, F. E. Speizer, and W. C. Willett, "Prospective study of caffeine consumption and risk of Parkinson's disease in men and women," *Ann Neurol* 2001 Jul; 50(1): 56–63.

6. I. Hindmarch, P. T. Quinlan, K. L. Moore, and C. Parkin, "The effects of black tea and other beverages on aspects of cognition and psychomotor performance," *Psychopharmacology* (Berl) 1998 Oct; 139(3): 230–38.

7. P. J. Durlach, "The effects of a low dose of caffeine on cognitive performance," *Psychopharmacology* (Berl) 1998 Nov; 140(1): 116–19.

8. G. C. Curhan, W. C. Willett, F. E. Speizer, and M. J. Stampfer, "Beverage use and risk for kidney stones in women," *Ann Intern Med* 1998 Apr 1; 128(7): 534–40.

9. Z. Chen, M. B. Pettinger, C. Ritenbaugh, A. Z. LaCroix, J. Robbins, B. J. Caan, D. H. Barad, and I. A. Hakim, "Habitual tea consumption and risk of osteoporosis: a prospective study in the women's health initiative observational cohort," *Am J Epidemiol* 2003 Oct 15; 158(8): 772–81.

10. C. H. Wu, Y. C. Yang, W. J. Yao, F. H. Lu, J. S. Wu, and C. J. Chang, "Epidemiological evidence of increased bone mineral density in habitual tea drinkers," *Arch Intern Med* 2002 May 13; 162(9): 1001–06.

11. J. M. Geleijnse, L. J. Launer, A. Hofman, H. A. Pols, and J. C. Witteman, "Tea flavonoids may protect against atherosclerosis: the Rotterdam Study," *Arch Intern Med* 1999 Oct 11; 159(18): 2170–74.

12. J. M. Geleijnse, L. J. Launer, D. A. Van der Kuip, A. Hofman, and J. C. Witteman, "Inverse association of tea and flavonoid intakes with incident myocardial infarction: the Rotterdam Study," *Am J Clin Nutr* 2002 May; 75(5): 880–86.

13. D. J. Maron, G. P. Lu, N. S. Cai, Z. G. Wu, Y. H. Li, H. Chen, J. Q. Zhu, X. J. Jin, B. C. Wouters, and J. Zhao, "Cholesterol-lowering effect of a theaflavin-enriched green tea extract: a randomized controlled trial," *Arch Intern Med* 2003 Jun 23; 163(12): 1448–53.

14. K. Imai, and K. Nakachi, "Cross-sectional study of effects of drinking green tea on cardiovascular and liver diseases," *BMJ*, 1995 Mar 18; 310(6981): 693–96.

15. P. Chantre, and D. Lairon, "Recent findings of green tea extract AR25 (Exolise) and its activity for the treatment of obesity," *Phytomedicine* 2002 Jan; 9(1): 3–8.

16. E. M. Kovacs, M. P. Lejeune, I. Nijs, and M. S. Westerterp-Plantenga, "Effects of green tea on weight maintenance after body-weight loss," *Br J Nutr* 2004 Mar; 91(3): 431–37.

17. F. L. Chung, J. Schwartz, C. R. Herzog, and Y. M. Yang, "Tea and cancer prevention: studies in animals and humans," *J Nutr* 2003 Oct; 133(10): 3268S-3274S.

18. C. S. Yang, J. Y. Chung, G. Yang, S. K. Chabra, and M. J. Lee, "Tea and tea polyphenols in cancer prevention," *J Nutr* 2000 Feb; 130(2S Suppl): 472S-478S.

References for Turmeric

1. C. Sumbilla, D. Lewis, T. Hammerschmidt, and G. Inesi, "The slippage of the Ca2+ pump and its control by anions and curcumin in skeletal and cardiac sarcoplasmic reticulum," *J Biol Chem* 2002 Apr 19; 277(16): 13900–06. E-pub, 2002 Feb 13.

2. S. K. Biswas, D. McClure, L. A. Jimenez, I. L. Megson, and I. Rahman, "Curcumin induces glutathione biosynthesis and inhibits NF-kappa-B activation and interleukin-8 release in alveolar epithelial cells: mechanism of free radical scavenging activity," *Antioxid Redox Signal* 2005 Jan–Feb; 7(1–2): 32–41.

3. M. C. Heng, M. K. Song, J. Harker, and M. K. Heng, "Drug-induced suppression of phosphorylase kinase activity correlates with resolution of psoriasis as assessed by clinical, histological and immunohistochemical parameters," *Br J Dermatol* 2000 Nov; 143(5): 937–49.

4. M. E. Egan, M. Pearson, S. A. Weiner, V. Rajendran, D. Rubin, J. Glockner-Pagel, S. Canny, K. Du, G. L. Lukacs, and M. J. Caplan, "Curcumin, a major constituent of turmeric, corrects cystic fibrosis defects," *Science* 2004 Apr 23; 304(5670): 600–02.

5. Y. Song, N. D. Sonawane, D. Salinas, L. Qian, N. Pedemonte, L. J. Galietta, and A. S. Verkman, "Evidence against the rescue of defective DeltaF508-CFTR cellular processing by curcumin in cell culture and mouse models," *J Biol Chem* 2004 Sep 24; 279(39): 40629–33. E-pub, 2004 Jul 26.

6. J. Joshi, S. Ghaisas, A. Vaidya, R. Vaidya, D. V. Kamat, A. N. Bhagwat, and S. Bhide, "Early human safety study of turmeric oil (Curcuma longa oil) administered orally in healthy volunteers," *J Assoc Physicians India* 2003 Nov; 51:1055–60.

7. J. F. Innes, C. J. Fuller, E. R. Grover, A. L. Kelly, and J. F. Burn, "Randomised, double-blind, placebo-controlled parallel group study of P54FP for the treatment of dogs with osteoarthritis," *Vet Rec* 2003 Apr 12; 152(15): 457–60.

8. B. Lal, A. K. Kapoor, O. P. Asthana, P. K. Agrawal, R. Prasad, P. Kumar, and R. C. Srimal, "Efficacy of curcumin in the management of chronic anterior uveitis," *Phytother Res* 1999 Jun; 13(4): 318–22.

9. M. C. Heng, et al., op cit.

10. C. Prucksunand, B. Indrasukhsri, M. Leethochawalit, and K. Hungspreugs, "Phase II clinical trial on effect of the long turmeric (Curcuma longa Linn) on healing of peptic ulcer," *Southeast Asian J Trop Med Public Health* 2001 Mar; 32(1): 208–15.

11. C. Niederau, and E. Gopfert, "The effect of chelidonium- and turmeric root extract on upper abdominal pain due to functional disorders of the biliary system. Results from a placebo-controlled, double-blind study," *Med Klin* (Munich) 1999 Aug 15; 94(8): 425–30.

12. S. M. Plummer, K. A. Hill, M. F. Festing, W. P. Steward, A. J. Gescher, and R. A. Sharma, "Clinical development of leukocyte cyclooxygenase 2 activity as a

systemic biomarker for cancer chemopreventive agents," *Cancer Epidemiol Biomarkers Prev* 2001 Dec; 10(12): 1295–99.

13. R. A. Sharma, S. A. Euden, S. L. Platton, D. N. Cooke, A. Shafayat, H. R. Hewitt, T. H. Marczylo, B. Morgan, D. Hemingway, S. M. Plummer, M. Pirmohamed, A. J. Gescher, and W. P. Steward, "Phase I clinical trial of oral curcumin: biomarkers of systemic activity and compliance," *Clin Cancer Res* 2004 Oct 15; 10(20): 6847–54.

14. R. A. Sharma, H. R. McLelland, K. A. Hill, C. R. Ireson, S. A. Euden, M. M. Manson, M. Pirmohamed, L. J> Marnett, A. J. Gescher, and W. P. Steward, "Pharmacodynamic and pharmacokinetic study of oral Curcuma extract in patients with colorectal cancer," *Clin Cancer Res* 2001 Jul; 7(7): 1894–900.

References for Uva Ursi

1. M. P. Lostao, B. A. Hirayama, D. D. Loo, and E. M. Wright, "Phenylglucosides and the Na+/glucose cotransporter (SGLT1): analysis of interactions," *J Membr Biol* 1994 Nov; 142(2): 161–70.

2. S. Shiota, M. Shimizu, J. Sugiyama, Y. Morita, T. Mizushima, and T. Tsuchiya, "Mechanisms of action of corilagin and tellimagrandin I that remarkably potentiate the activity of beta-lactams against methicillin-resistant Staphylococcus aureus," *Microbiol Immunol* 2004; 48(1): 67–73.

3. L. Wang, and L. V. Del Priore, "Bull's-eye maculopathy secondary to herbal toxicity from uva ursi," *Am J Ophthalmol* 2004 Jun; 137(6): 1135–37.

4. D. Beaux, J. Fleurentin, and F. Mortier, "Effect of extracts of Orthosiphon stamineus Benth, Hieracium pilosella L., Sambucus nigra L. and Arctostaphylos uva-ursi (L.) Spreng. in rats," *Phytother Res* 1999 May; 13(3): 222–25.

5. G. Schindler, U. Patzak, B. Brinkhaus, A. von Niecieck, J. Wittig, N. Krahmer, I. Glockl, and M. Veit, "Urinary excretion and metabolism of arbutin after oral administration of Arctostaphylos uvae ursi extract as film-coated tablets and aqueous solution in healthy humans," *J Clin Pharmacol* 2002 Aug; 42(8): 920–27.

6. C. Siegers, C. Bodinet, S. S. Ali, and C. P. Siegers, "Bacterial deconjugation of arbutin by Escherichia coli," *Phytomedicine* 2003; 10 Suppl 4:58–60.

7. S. Choi, S. K. Lee, J. E. Kim, M. H. Chung, and Y. I. Park, "Aloesin inhibits hyperpigmentation induced by UV radiation," *Clin Exp Dermatol* 2002 Sep; 27(6): 513–15.

References for Valerian

1. M. S. Santos, F. Ferreira, C. Faro, E. Pires, A. P. Carvalho, A. P. Cunha, and T. Macedo, "The amount of GABA present in aqueous extracts of valerian is sufficient to account for [3H]GABA release in synaptosomes," *Planta Med* 1994 Oct; 60(5): 475–76.

2. E. Riedel, R. Hansel, and G. Ehrke, "Inhibition of gamma-aminobutyric acid catabolism by valerenic acid derivatives," *Planta Med* 1982 Dec; 46(4): 219–20.

3. B. Schumacher, S. Scholle, J. Holzl, N. Khudeir, S. Hess, and C. E. Muller, "Lignans isolated from valerian: identification and characterization of a new olivil derivative with partial agonistic activity at A(1) adenosine receptors," *J Nat Prod* 2002 Oct; 65(10): 1479–85.

4. R. Schellenberg, S. Sauer, E. A. Abourashed, U. Koetter, and A. Brattstrom, "The fixed combination of valerian and hops (Ze91019) acts via a central adenosine mechanism," *Planta Med* 2004 Jul; 70(7): 594–97.

5. Uwe Koetter, Ph.D., Glaxo Smith Kline, "From identification of compounds to clinical research: a comprehensive overview of recent research on valerian and hops," Arizona Center for Phytomedicine Research Seminar, 2002 October 14.

6. J. M. Jellin, P. Gregory, F. Batz, K. Hitchens, et al., eds. *Pharmacist's Letter/Prescriber's Letter. Natural Medicines Comprehensive Database,* 3rd ed. (Stockton, CA: Therapeutic Research Faculty, 2000).

7. L. B. Willey, S. P. Mady, D. J. Cobaugh, and P. M. Wax, "Valerian overdose: a case report," *Vet Hum Toxicol* 1995; 37: 364–65.

8. H. P. Garges, I. Varia, and P. M. Doraiswamy, "Cardiac complications and delirium associated with valerian root withdrawal," *JAMA* 1998; 280:1566–67.

9. A. Diaper, and I. Hindmarch, "A double-blind, placebo-controlled investigation of the effects of two doses of a valerian preparation on the sleep, cognitive and psychomotor function of sleep-disturbed older adults," *Phytother Res* 2004 Oct; 18(10): 831–36.

10. S. Gutierrez, M. K. Ang-Lee, D. J. Walker, and J. P. Zacny, "Assessing subjective and psychomotor effects of the herbal medication valerian in healthy volunteers," *Pharmacol Biochem Behav* 2004 May; 78(1): 57–64.

11. K. T. Hallam, J. S. Olver, C. McGrath, and T. R. Norman, "Comparative cognitive and psychomotor effects of single doses of Valeriana officianalis and triazolam in healthy volunteers," *Hum Psychopharmacol* 2003 Dec; 18(8): 619–25.

12. F. Donath, S. Quispe, K. Diefenbach, A. Maurer, I. Fietze, and I. Roots, "Critical evaluation of the effect of valerian extract on sleep structure and sleep quality," *Pharmacopsychiatry* 2000 Mar; 33(2): 47–53.

13. J. R. Glass, B. A. Sproule, N. Herrmann, D. Streiner, and U. E. Busto, "Acute pharmacological effects of temazepam, diphenhydramine, and valerian in healthy elderly subjects," *J Clin Psychopharmacol* 2003 Jun; 23(3): 260–68.

14. T. B. Klepser, and M. E. Klepser, "Unsafe and potentially safe herbal therapies," *Am J Health Syst Pharm* 1999 Jan 15; 56(2): 125–38.

15. D. R. Poyares, C. Guilleminault, M. M. Ohayon, and S. Tufik, "Can valerian improve the sleep of insomniacs after benzodiazepine withdrawal?" *Prog Neuropsychopharmacol Biol Psychiatry* 2002 Apr; 26(3): 539–45.

16. C. Stevinson, and E. Ernst, "Valerian for insomnia: a systematic review of randomized clinical trials," *Sleep Med* 2000 Apr 1; 1(2): 91–99.

References for Wild Yam

1. D. T. Zava, C. M. Dollbaum, and M. Blen, "Estrogen and Progestin Bioactivity of Foods, Herbs, and Spices," *Proceedings of the Society for Experimental Biology and Medicine* 1998 Mar; 217(3): 369–78.

2. R. S. Rosenberg Zand, D. J. Jenkins, and E. P. Diamandis, "Effects of natural products and nutraceuticals on steroid hormone-regulated gene expression," *Clin Chim Acta* 2001 Oct; 312(1–2): 213–19.

3. A. Pierce, *The American Pharmaceutical Association Practical Guide to Natural Medicines* (New York: Stonesong Press, 1999), 229–31.
4. M. Araghiniknam, S. Chung, T. Nelson-White, C. Eskelson, and R. R. Watson, "Antioxidant activity of dioscorea and dehydroepiandrosterone (DHEA) in older humans," *Life Sci* 1996; 59(11): PL147–57.
5. D. T. Zava, et al., op cit.
6. M. Araghiniknam, et al., op cit.
7. D. T. Zava, et al., op cit.
8. Ibid.
9. Ibid.
10. R. S. Rosenberg Zand, et al., op cit.

References for Wintergreen

1. P. Morra, W. R. Bartle, S. E. Walker, S. N. Lee, S. K. Bowles, and R. A. Reeves, "Serum Concentrations of Salicylic Acid Following Topically Applied Salicylate Derivatives," *Ann Pharmacother* 1996 Sep; 30(9): 935–40.
2. M. Battino, M. S. Ferreiro, D. Fattorini, and P. Bullon, "In Vitro Antioxidant Activities of Mouthrinses and their Components," *J. Clin. Periodontol* 2002 May; 29(5): 462–67.

References for Witch Hazel

1. S. Habtemariam, "Hamamelitannin from Hamamelis virginiana inhibits the tumour necrosis factor-alpha (TNF)-induced endothelial cell death in vitro," *Toxicon* 2002 Jan; 40(1): 83–88.
2. H. Masaki, T. Atsumi, and H. Sakurai, "Protective activity of hamamelitannin on cell damage induced by superoxide anion radicals in murine dermal fibroblasts," *Biol Pharm Bull* 1995 Jan; 18(1): 59–63.
3. C. Hartisch, H. Kolodziej, and F. von Bruchhausen, "Dual inhibitory activities of tannins from Hamamelis virginiana and related polyphenols on 5-lipoxygenase and lyso-PAF: acetyl-CoA acetyltransferase," *Planta Med* 1997 Apr; 63(2): 106–10.
4. H. C. Korting, M. Schafer-Korting, H. Hart, P. Laux, and M. Schmid, "Anti-inflammatory activity of hamamelis distillate applied topically to the skin. Influence of vehicle and dose," *Eur J Clin Pharmacol* 1993; 44(4): 315–18.
5. H. C. Korting, M. Schafer-Korting, W. Klovekorn, G. Klovekorn, C. Martin, and P. Laux, "Comparative efficacy of hamamelis distillate and hydrocortisone cream in atopic eczema," *Eur J Clin Pharmacol* 1995; 48(6): 461–65.
6. H. G. Knoch, W. Klug, and W. D. Hubner, "Ointment treatment of 1st degree hemorrhoids. Comparison of the effectiveness of a phytogenic preparation with two new ointments containing synthetic drugs," *Fortschr Med* 1992 Mar 20; 110(8): 135–38.
7. R. J. Royer, and C. L. Schmidt, "Evaluation of venotropic drugs by venous gas plethysmography. A study of procyanidolic oligomers," *Sem Hop* 1981 Dec 18–25; 57(47–48): 2009–13.

References for Yerba Maté

1. A. C. Leitao, R. S. Braga, "Mutagenic and genotoxic effects of maté (*Ilex paraguariensis*) in prokaryotic organisms," *Braz J Med Biol Res* 1994 Jul; 27(7): 1517–25.
2. D. E. Di Gregorio, H. Huck, R. Aristegui, G. De Lazzari, and A. Jech, "137Cs contamination in tea and yerba maté in South America," *J Environ Radioact* 2004; 76(3): 273–81.
3. D. Goldenberg, "Maté: a risk factor for oral and oropharyngeal cancer," *Oral Oncol* 2002 Oct; 38(7): 646–49.
4. A. Vassallo, P. Correa, E. De Stefani, M. Cendan, D. Zavala, V. Chen, J. Carzoglio, and H. Deneo-Pellegrini, "Esophageal cancer in Uruguay: a case-control study," *J Natl Cancer Inst* 1985 Dec; 75(6): 1005–09.
5. E. De Stefani, P. Correa, F. Oreggia, H. Deneo-Pellegrini, G. Fernandez, D. Zavala, J. Carzoglio, J. Leiva, E. Fontham, and S. Rivero, "Black tobacco, wine and maté in oropharyngeal cancer. A case-control study from Uruguay," *Rev Epidemiol Sante Publique* 1988; 36(6): 389–94.
6. E. De Stefani, L. Fierro, P. Correa, E. Fontham, A. Ronco, M. Larrinaga, J. Balbi, and M. Mendilaharsu, "Maté drinking and risk of lung cancer in males: a case-control study from Uruguay," *Cancer Epidemiol Biomarkers Prev* 1996 Jul; 5(7): 515–19.
7. E. De Stefani, L. Fierro, M. Mendilaharsu, A. Ronco, M. T. Larrinaga, J. C. Balbi, S. Alonso, and H. Deneo-Pellegrini, "Meat intake, 'maté' drinking and renal cell cancer in Uruguay: a case-control study," *Br J Cancer* 1998 Nov; 78(9): 1239–43.
8. E. De Stefani, P. Correa, L. Fierro, E. Fontham, V. Chen, and D. Zavala, "Black tobacco, maté, and bladder cancer. A case-control study from Uruguay," Department of Epidemiology, Instituto de Oncologia, Montevideo, Uruguay. *Cancer* 1991 Jan 15; 67(2): 536–40.
9. D. Goldenberg, A. Golz, and H. Z. Joachims, "The beverage maté: a risk factor for cancer of the head and neck," *Head Neck* 2003 Jul; 25(7): 595–601.
10. A. Martinet, K. Hostettmann, and Y. Schutz, "Thermogenic effects of commercially available plant preparations aimed at treating human obesity," *Phytomedicine* 1999 Oct; 6(4): 231–38.
11. T. Andersen, and J. Fogh, "Weight loss and delayed gastric emptying following a South American herbal preparation in overweight patients," *J Hum Nutr Diet* 2001 Jun; 14(3): 243–50.

References for Yohimbe

1. I. Saenz de Tejada, N. N. Kim, I. Goldstein, and A. M. Traish, "Regulation of pre-synaptic alpha adrenergic activity in the corpus cavernosum," *Int J Impot Res* 2000 Mar; 12 Suppl 1:S20–25.
2. B. B. Hoffman, "Catecholamines, sympathomimetic drugs, and adrenergic receptor antagonists," in J. G. Hardman, and L. E. Limbird, eds. *Goodman and Gilman's the Pharmacologic Basis of Therapeutics,* 10th ed. (New York: McGraw-Hill, 2001), 215–68.
3. P. Farley, "Terror Is the Best Remedy for Phobias," *New Scientist,* issue 2442, 10 April 2004, p. 16.
4. L. M. McKenry, and E. Salerno, eds. *Mosby's Pharmacology in Nursing,* 21st ed. St. Louis, MO: Mosby, 2003.
5. P. Kunelius, J. Hakkinen, and O. Lukkarinen, "Is high-dose yohimbine hydrochloride effective in the treatment of mixed-type impotence? A prospective, randomized, controlled double-blind crossover study," *Urology* 1997 Mar; 49(3): 441–44.
6. K. Reid, D. H. Surridge, A. Morales, M. Condra, C. Harris, J. Owen, and J. Fenemore, "Double-blind trial

of yohimbine in treatment of psychogenic impotence," *Lancet* 1987 Aug 22; 2(8556): 421–23.

7. H. J. Vogt, P. Brandl, G. Kockott, J. R. Schmitz, M. H. Wiegand, J. Schadrack, and M. Gierend, "Double-blind, placebo-controlled safety and efficacy trial with yohimbine hydrochloride in the treatment of nonorganic erectile dysfunction," *Int J Impot Res* 1997 Sep; 9(3): 155–61.

8. C. M. Meston, and M. Worcel, "The effects of yohimbine plus L-arginine glutamate on sexual arousal in postmenopausal women with sexual arousal disorder," *Arch Sex Behav* 2002 Aug; 31(4): 323–32.

9. T. Lebret, J. M. Herve, P. Gorny, M. Worcel, and H. Botto, "Efficacy and safety of a novel combination of L-arginine glutamate and yohimbine hydrochloride: a new oral therapy for erectile dysfunction," *Eur Urol* 2002 Jun; 41(6): 608–13.

10. J. E. Piletz, K. B. Segraves, Y. Z. Feng, E. Maguire, B. Dunger, and A. Halaris, "Plasma MHPG response to yohimbine treatment in women with hypoactive sexual desire," *J Sex Marital Ther* 1998 Jan-Mar; 24(1): 43–54.

11. F. M. Jacobsen, "Fluoxetine-induced sexual dysfunction and an open trial of yohimbine," *J Clin Psychiatry* 1992 Apr; 53(4): 119–22.

12. E. Hollander, and A. McCarley, "Yohimbine treatment of sexual side effects induced by serotonin reuptake blockers," *J Clin Psychiatry* 1992 Jun; 53(6): 207–09.

13. D. Michelson, K. Kociban, R. Tamura, and M. F. Morrison, "Mirtazapine, yohimbine or olanzapine augmentation therapy for serotonin reuptake-associated female sexual dysfunction: a randomized, placebo-controlled trial," *J Psychiatr Res* 2002 May–Jun; 36(3): 147–52.

ACKNOWLEDGMENTS

I OWE AN enormous debt of gratitude to all those who performed the real labor of researching and publishing their scientific discoveries on the therapeutic activities of plant molecules. You did the hard part—all I had to do was read your publications. Special thanks to author Harold McGee, the curious cook, for inspiring and encouraging my writing. For carefully placing me in the hands of Marlowe & Company, heartfelt thanks to Andrea Pedolsky. To the smart and capable Matthew Lore, who took on this project, and quickly steered my writing into a more comfortable style, I'll always be grateful, especially for his allowing this to expand into much larger book than was planned. Thanks to Jill Hughes, a copy editor who must have gone blind reading all the chemical names and removing all my excessive commas. Thanks to Pauline Neuwirth, for her lovely design, and Vince Kunkemueller for managing the production of this book. For getting the ball rolling, helping me organize and pair down to essentials, editors Peter Jacoby and Kylie Foxx deserve my thanks. To Renee Sedliar, who edited the bulk of this book, and did so with lightning speed, wisdom and grace, endless thanks. She's a delight to work with and every writer should be so lucky.

Thanks to my family for their continued love and for commenting on the many bits and pieces of drafts that I pelted you with over the years. Big hugs also to the sizeable, multitalented Erskine clan, who treat me like family. I especially owe my mom, Judy Wadyko, more than I can say, for nourishing my emotional and spiritual wellbeing, keeping alive my inner child, and for refraining from mailing me too many newspaper clippings on herbs when I was writing.

Thanks to the Department of Medicinal Chemistry at the University of Utah for unintentionally loaning me so much money, and to its faculty and staff, especially Dr. Art Broom and Dr. Chris Ireland. Thanks also for the longtime support from the faculty and staff of the Salt Lake Community College, especially Dr. Clifton Sanders and Dr. Peter Iles, for letting me neglect all those faculty meetings when I was writing. To Dr. Jeanette Roberts, now dean of pharmacy at the University of Madison, Wisconsin, thank you for teaching me so much in graduate school and for stimulating my interest in chemoprotection—the science of protecting yourself from chemicals by using other, different chemicals. I'm also always astonished by my students' overwhelming love and support, especially considering the exams I give them. My students have always provided the greatest stimulation for my scientific ideas.

Thanks to our good friends for sharing wine, food, and sustenance; Peter Hansen and Bea Lufkin of Salt Lake, for expanding us with exposures to low temperatures and independent films, and thanks for not including too many GHYITGA (Go Hang Yourself In The Garage Afterwards) and EDITE (Everyone Dies In The End) films. We promise not to show you too many RSFM (Ridiculous Science Fiction Movies). Thanks to Fred Henion, for his offerings of truffle oil, classroom antics, Wasatch mountain fungi, and pirate jokes. For the warm friendship of author JulieAnn Henneman and other members of SVUUS, bless you. Thanks to fellow cat saver and font of Buddhist advice, composer Vince Frates of Portland. For the generous support from retired attorney and continual mensch Michael Schwarz of New Paltz, Tim and I thank you from the bottoms of our hearts, and I apologize to everyone for never answering the phone.

Finally, this book would not be possible without my dear partner and illustrator, Tim Erskine, who long ago told me to quit whining about the absence of this sort of book, and to write it, instead. For his tender care over years while I daily assumed the posture of a disembodied brain with typing fingers that could not be disturbed, he is a saint. With his example of bravery in everyday life as a social activist, musician, programmer, engineer, and inventor with over 45 patents, his belief in me gave me the courage to write this book. And the answer is yes, Tim, I will marry you.